Sports Science and Medicine

Sports Science and Medicine

Editor: Ellis Baker

Callisto Reference
www.callistoreference.com

Callisto Reference,
118-35 Queens Blvd., Suite 400,
Forest Hills, NY 11375, USA

Visit us on the World Wide Web at:
www.callistoreference.com

ISBN: 978-1-63239-865-9 (Hardback)

Printed in China.

Cataloging-in-publication Data

Sports science and medicine / edited by Ellis Baker.
p. cm.
Includes bibliographical references and index.
ISBN 978-1-63239-865-9
1. Sports sciences. 2. Sports medicine. 3. Physical education and training. 4. Sports--Physiological aspects.
I. Baker, Ellis.
GV558 .S66 2017
613.71--dc23

Table of Contents

Preface

Sports science and sports medicine are two interrelated disciplines which are often studied together as they are complementary to each other. This book provides comprehensive insights into the field of sports science which is studied to investigate how a healthy body works during physical activity and exercise. On the other hand sports medicine focuses on the treatment as well as prevention of injuries and trauma related to sports. The text aims to bring about a confluence of the two fields so as to provide its reader a holistic understanding of the subject area. Coherent flow of topics, student-friendly language and extensive use of examples make this book an invaluable source of knowledge. It is a vital tool for all researching and studying sports science and sports medicine.

The world is advancing at a fast pace like never before. Therefore, the need is to keep up with the latest developments. This book was an idea that came to fruition when the specialists in the area realized the need to coordinate together and document essential themes in the subject. That's when I was requested to be the editor. Editing this book has been an honour as it brings together diverse authors researching on different streams of the field. The book collates essential materials contributed by veterans in the area which can be utilized by students and researchers alike.

Each chapter is a sole-standing publication that reflects each author´s interpretation. Thus, the book displays a multi-facetted picture of our current understanding of applications and diverse aspects of the field. I would like to thank the contributors of this book and my family for their endless support.

Editor

Comparison of Force Exertion Characteristics of Sustained Hand Grip and Toe Grip

Masakatsu Nakada[1,*], Shinichi Demura[2]

[1]National Defense Academy of Japan, 1-10-20 Hashirimizu, Yokosuka, Kanagawa, Japan
[2]Graduate School of Natural Science & Technology, Kanazawa University, Kakuma, Kanazawa, Ishikawa, Japan
*Corresponding author: nakada@nda.ac.jp

Abstract This study aimed to examine the differences in decreasing force during maximal sustained hand grip and toe grip exertions values. Fourteen males aged 18 to 22 years old performed hand and toe grip exertions for 6min. The sustained times of forces 40, 60, 70, and 80% of maximal strength (max), strength values at 90sec and 3min, and final strength value (% of max) were selected as evaluation parameters. The forces (% max) during both sustained grip exertions markedly decreased until about 60sec from their exertion onset, after which they slowly decreased, then decreased very little at 4-6min. Toe grip exertion values were significantly larger than hand grip exertion values until after 60sec from exertion onset (about 15% ～ 20% vs about 30% ～ 35%). Correlations among sustained time parameters (60%～80% max) were significant (r =0.657～0.960). The strength at 3 min in toe grip exertion significantly correlated to final strength, sustained time of forces 40% of max, and strength at 90sec. In summary, the forces during sustained hand grip and toe grip exertions show a similar decreasing tendency, but the latter's exertion values maintain a higher level than the former's after a marked decrease. The strength value at 3min for toe grip exertion may be useful as muscle endurance parameter.

Keywords: *hand, toe, grip, strength, muscle endurance*

1. Introduction

Movements using sustained hand grip are used frequently in daily life, i.e. holding onto an object or hanging onto a strap in a subway. Because a decrease in muscle endurance of the upper limbs interferes with daily life activities, adequate evaluation is necessary. Studies have been conducted evaluating muscle endurance based on the force decreasing phase of sustained grip exertion [1,2] and regarding the effects of different elbow positions on grip strength and grip endurance [3]. However, endurance of maximum toe grip has not been well studied.

Walking is the most basic activity in daily life. A decrease of muscle strength related to toe and proximal ankle joins is considered to largely affect the independent life of the elderly. In addition, a standing posture and walking have generally been continuously performed for a certain period, and strengths related to the above-stated joints are sustainably developed. It was reported that toe plantar flexion strength decreases with age [4]. Scott et al. [5] reported that the elderly have a slower walking speed and shorter step length as compared with young adults. Hence, evaluating adequately muscle endurance in addition to maximum strength of the toe is considered to be important.

The following aspects of sustained static maximal hand grip have been studied: the relationship of decreasing force and muscle oxygenation kinetics [6], the effect of measurement time on static muscle endurance [1], and the relationships among parameters of static muscle endurance [7]. In addition, Nakada and Demura [8] examined the change of exertion force during sustained toe grip exertion for 3 min. For an activity requiring the upper limbs, the dominant hand of the upper limb is usually used. But common movements, such as walking and running, require both lower limbs generally used simultaneously and continuously. Therefore, endurance characteristics of muscle groups related to gripping force may differ between the hands and toes. However, this difference has not been well studied.

According to Yamaji et al. [1], after sustained static hand gripping for 3 min, grip strength decreased until the final grip strength was about 20% of maximal grip strength. However, Nakada and Demura [8] reported that final strength after sustained toe gripping for 3 min was 39% of maximal toe grip strength. These reports indicate that the tendencies of grip force to decrease during maximal sustained hand and toe grip exertions are different. This study aimed to examine characteristics of grip force decreases during maximal sustained hand and toe grip exertions, and the relationships between muscle endurance parameters in both exertions.

2. Methods

2.1. Subjects

Fourteen males aged 18-22 years old were selected as subjects (height 170.7±5.0cm, weight 65.0±6.6kg). Thirteen of them belonged to athletic clubs. Informed consent was obtained after detailed explanation regarding experimental purpose and protocol.

2.2. Materials

Hand grip strength was measured using a handgrip sensor (EG-210, Sakai Medical. Co., Ltd., Tokyo, Japan), an indicator (EG-220, Sakai Medical. Co., Ltd., Tokyo, Japan), and the related software (EG-290, Sakai Medical. Co., Ltd., Tokyo, Japan). Exerted grip values were recorded at 20 Hz. Toe grip strength was measured using a toe finger dynamometer (T.K.K.3361, Takei Scientific Instruments Co., Ltd., Niigata, Japan). Exerted grip values were recorded at a 20 Hz sampling rate by an analog-to-digital interface (Power Lab/16sp, ADInstruments).

2.3. Experimental Procedure

2.3.1. Measurement Hand and Foot

Each subjects' dominant hand was determined as the hand mainly used in 4 activities (hammer, cutter knife, writing and throwing) based on Demura et al.'s report [9]. Among 14 subjects, 12 were judged to be right-handed. The dominant hand of all subjects was used for measuring hand grip. Each subjects' dominant leg was determined as the leg mainly used in 4 activities (hopping on one foot, stepping up on a chair, kicking a ball and stamping on an object) based on Demura et al.'s report [10]. Among 14 subjects, 13 were judged to be right-footed. The dominant foot was used to measure toe grip.

2.3.2. Measurement of Hand Grip Exertion Values

Maximal hand grip strength was measured while the subject was in a seated posture on a chair, before sustained hand grip exertion was measured. Subjects performed two maximal grip trials while keeping the arm supported by an armrest and the trunk at 90 degrees. The larger value was used as a representative value. For the sustained hand grip exertion measurement, subjects were instructed to exert maximal grip strength as fast as possible after a whistle signal, and to continue maximal exertion for 6 min in the same seated posture as above. To confirm reproducibility, all subjects performed the same test again on a different day.

2.3.3. Measurement of Toe Grip Exertion Values

Maximal toe grip strength was measured while the subject was in a seated posture on a chair with the knee joint angled at 90 degrees, before sustained toe grip exertion was measured. Subjects performed two maximal toe grip trials, and the larger value was used as a representative value. In the sustained toe grip exertion measurement, subjects were instructed to exert maximal toe grip as fast as possible after a whistle signal, and to continue maximal exertion for 6 min in the same seated posture as above. To examine reproducibility, all subjects performed the same test again on a different day. Of the 14 subjects, seven were measured in the order of the two hand grip exertion tests followed by the two toe grip exertion tests. The remaining seven were measured in reverse order.

2.4. Parameters

Parameters on sustained hand and toe grip exertions were selected by referencing previous studies [1,6]. The sustained times of 40, 60, 70, and 80% forces of maximal strength (max) were selected as the sustained time parameters. Grip strength at 90 sec, 3 min, and final strength (average at 1 sec before finishing) during the sustained grip test were selected as strength parameters. These strength parameters were expressed with percentage of maximal strength (% max).

2.5. Data Analysis

The cross-correlation coefficients were calculated to examine the reproducibility of the force during sustained hand and toe grip exertions. Changes of the forces (% max) in each elapsed time were examined by two-way repeated measure ANOVA (grip exertion style and elapsed time). Significant interaction or main effect was found, and multiple comparison was performed with Bonferroni post-test. The quadratic regression was calculated to examine changes of force values in each elapsed time. Pearson's correlation coefficient was calculated to examine the relationships among parameters in both grip exertions.

3. Results

Figure 1 shows the cross-correlation coefficients and the changes of force values during two maximal sustained hand grip and toe grip exertions. Both forces (% max) markedly decreased until about 60 sec after the onset of their grip exertions (hand grip: about 30% max, toe grip: about 45 % max), and then decreased more slowly. However, the force values decreased very little during the 4-6 min period (hand grip: about 25% max, toe grip: about 30% max). The cross-correlation coefficient was 0.995 (lag=0) in hand grip and 0.982 (lag=0) in toe grip. Hence, the reproducibility of each grip exertion was judged to be very high. The first trial data was used for the further analysis.

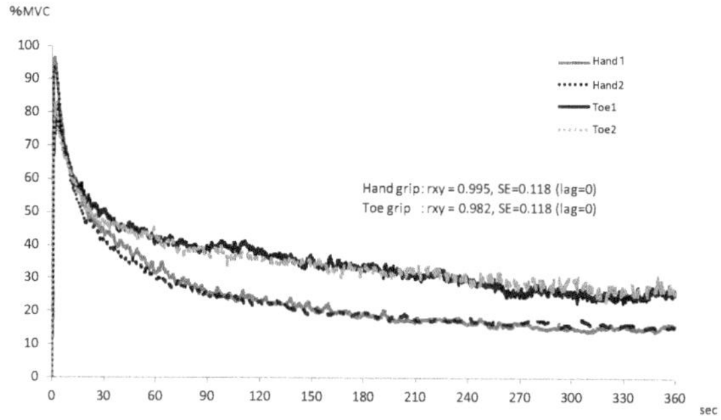

Figure 1. Cross-correlation coefficients and the changes of force values during two maximal sustained hand grip and toe grip exertions

Figure 2 shows the changes of the force values (% max) every 15sec (starting value at 1sec) in two maximal sustained hand and toe grip exertions, and the results of two-way repeated measure ANOVA (grip exertion style and elapsed time). A significant interaction was found. Results of multiple comparison showed that the forces were higher in the hand grip exertion than in the toe grip exertion at 1sec after the exertion onset, but higher in the latter exertion values from 60sec onward. In addition, results of multiple comparisons among mean force values at each elapsed time showed that no significant differences were found from 210sec in the hand grip exertion and from 240sec in the toe grip exertion. A significant quadratic regression between each elapsed time and the corresponding force was found, and the determination coefficient was about 79% in the hand grip exertion and about 90% in the toe grip exertion.

Table 1 shows the correlation coefficients among parameters of sustained hand and toe grip exertions. Correlations between each time parameter (40% ~ 80% max) were significant in the hand grip exertion. Their correlations in toe grip exertion were significant, but not between the 40% max sustained time and 70% max sustained time. In both grip exertions, there was no significant correlation between max strength and each parameter. In addition, no significant correlation between final strength and each sustained time parameter was found. In both grip exertions, no significant correlation between strength at 90 sec and final strength was found. However, significant correlation between strength at 3 min and final strength was found.

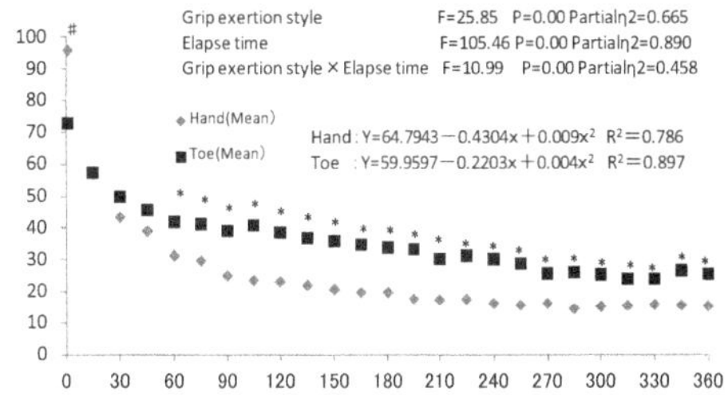

Note) *: p<0.05（Toe＞Hand）、#: p<0.05（Hand＞Toe）

Figure 2. Changes of the force values (% max) in two maximal sustained hand grip and toe grip exertions, and the result of two-way repeated measure ANOVA (grip exertion style and elapsed time)

Table 1. Correlation coefficients between parameters of sustained hand and toe grip exertions

			Mean	SD	1	2	3	4	5	6	7
Hand grip	1. Maximal strength	kg	46.4	5.7							
	2. 80% max sustained time	sec	5.2	3.8	0.156						
	3. 70% max sustained time	sec	9.2	6.7	0.139	0.896*					
	4. 60% max sustained time	sec	12.6	8.0	0.165	0.861*	0.960*				
	5. 40% max sustained time	sec	35.9	20.3	0.022	0.614*	0.764*	0.842*			
	6. Strength at 90 sec	%	24.9	7.1	-0.310	0.075	0.279	0.315	0.656*		
	7. Strength at 3 min	%	19.7	7.3	-0.181	-0.104	0.016	0.246	0.513	0.425	
	8. Final strength	%	15.3	5.1	-0.359	0.370	-0.336	-0.129	0.101	0.087	0.815*
Toe grip	1. Maximal strength	kg	15.6	2.5							
	2. 80% max sustained time	sec	2.2	2.0	-0.220						
	3. 70% max sustained time	sec	5.1	3.7	-0.008	0.769 *					
	4. 60% max sustained time	sec	11.5	11.2	-0.108	0.657 *	0.801*				
	5. 40% max sustained time	sec	58.3	57.9	-0.291	0.616 *	0.423	0.545 *			
	6. Strength at 90 sec	%	39.1	10.8	-0.254	0.372	0.290	0.411	0.827*		
	7. Strength at 3 min	%	33.8	11.1	-0.379	0.401	0.307*	0.368	0.561*	0.786*	
	8. Final strength	%	25.6	10.9	-0.382	-0.107	-0.129	-0.047	0.043	0.488	0.645*

Note)*: p<0.05

4. Discussion

The cross-correlation coefficients of two trials in each grip exertion were 0.995 in hand grip and 0.982 in toe grip. Nakada et al. [11] reported that the cross-correlation of grip force between trials on maximal repeated rhythmic grip exertion for 6 min was very high (r_{xy}=0.994). It is inferred that the reproducibility of the forces during both grip force exertions is very high.

Yamaji et al. [1] reported that the force exertion during sustained static maximal gripping decreased remarkably until about 30-60 sec after the onset of grip exertion, then decreased slowly, reaching 20% of maximal grip at about 3 min, 15% at about 4 min, and an almost steady state at 4-6 min. The decreasing force during the hand grip exertion in this study is similar to the results reported by Yamaji et al. [1]. In addition, Nakada and Demura [8] reported that the force during sustained toe grip exertion decreased markedly until about 30 sec after the start of exertion, then slowly decreased and reached about 40% of maximal toe grip strength at 3 min. The strength at 3 min in the present toe grip exertion was about 34% of max and was a little low as compared to the result of Nakada and Demura [8]. However, the decreasing tendency of forces was similar to that in the previous study [8].

The force was only higher in the hand grip exertion than in the toe grip exertion at 1 sec after beginning of the grip exertions. Time to max was 1.18±0.66 (Mean±SD) sec in the hand grip exertion and 2.02±1.00 (Mean±SD) sec in the toe grip exertion. In short, it is considered to be affected by the latter slowness. Miyata et al. [12] reported that the higher % FT fibers are, the faster its conduction velocity, and that the conduction velocity depends on the recruitment style of muscle fibers. It is inferred that muscle fiber composition related to hand and toe grip exertions as well as a difference in the recruitment style of muscle fibers affected the present results.

From 60 sec after the beginning of sustained grip exertions, the forces were higher in the toe grip exertion than in the hand grip exertion. Yamaji et al. [7] reported that, since oxygen saturation maintains low values by obstruction of the blood flow from the beginning of sustained static maximal hand gripping to 40-60 sec, the oxygenation supply of this time period will be decreased. In addition, Yamaji et al. [6] reported that from examination of muscle oxygenation kinetics during sustained static gripping, the regression coefficient in the Deoxy-Hb decreasing phase correlated significantly with decreasing force at 1-2 min. This parameter can evaluate the phase when resumption of the blood flow begins. However, this process of obstruction and resumption of blood flow may differ between the hand grip and the toe grip exertions. Ordway et al. [13] reported that the elbow flexors initially fatigued more rapidly, but reached a plateau at a relatively higher strength level than the knee extensors when comparing both via transformed scores to the same base. In addition, in the case of different muscle groups, fatigue tends to occur with a different rate even if comparing relative strengths [13]. It is now theorized that although the present results differed from those in previous studies, this depends on different characteristics of muscle groups in the upper and lower limbs. A difference of muscle group fibers recruited in each movement may affect strength levels at muscle fatigue.

There were no significant relationships between maximal strength and each sustained time parameter in both exertions. Each time parameter is thought to evaluate different abilities from max in both exertions. Yamaji et al. [1] reported that significant correlations (r=0.92-0.97) were found between parameters regarding time to 60, 70, and 80% of maximal grip during sustained static maximal gripping. In addition, Yamaji et al. [7] reported that persisting times of 80%, 70%, and 60% of max and the decrement size of exertion values for the first 1 min during sustained static maximal hand gripping for 12 min can evaluate a remarkable phase of strength decrease. On the other hand, Nakada and Demura [8] reported that significant correlations (r=0.786-0.958) were found between parameters at the sustained times of 60, 70, 80% forces of maximal toe grip strength during sustained toe grip exertion for 3 min. In the present results, significant correlations (r=0.614-0.960) were found between the times of 40-80% forces of maximal hand grip strength during sustained hand grip exertion. In addition, significant correlations (r=0.657-0.801) were found between the times of 60-80% max forces of maximal toe grip strength during sustained toe grip exertion. Strength at 3 min showed a significant correlation with final strength in both exertions (0.815 and 0.645), but significant correlation was only found between 40% max sustained time (0.561) and strength at 90 sec (0.786) in toe grip exertion. The force at 90 sec after start of exertion corresponds to the 20% max in hand grip exertion and the 40% max in toe grip exertion. From these results, the strength value at 3 min in toe grip exertion may be a useful parameter of toe grip endurance. On the other hand, it was reported that hand grip strength had significant correlation with isometric knee extensor strength [14]. However, a significant correlation between hand grip and toe grip strength was not found. In addition, no significant correlations among the same sustained time parameters in both exertions were found. The two grip exertions, even in the same limbs, are considered to evaluate different abilities.

5. Conclusions

This study examined characteristics of decreases in force exertion during maximal sustained hand and toe grip exertions, and the relationships between muscle endurance parameters in both exertions. The reproducibility of each grip exertion is high. Forces (% max) during both exertions markedly decreased until about 60 sec after the onset of their grip exertion (hand grip: about 30% max, toe grip: about 45% max.) The latter exertion values maintain a higher exertion level than the former after a marked decrease. Relationships between sustained time parameters (60-80% max) are high. Strength at 3min showed a relationship with final strength, 40% max sustained time, and strength at 90 sec in toe grip exertion. This parameter may be a useful parameter of toe grip endurance.

References

[1] Yamaji, S., Demura, S., Nagasawa, Y., Nakada, M. and Kitabayashi, T., "The effect of measurement time when evaluating static muscle endurance during sustained static maximal gripping." J Physiol Anthropol Appl Human Sci. 21. 151-158. 2002.

[2] Yamaji, S., Demura, S., Nagasawa, Y. and Nakada, M., "The influence of different target values and measurement times on the decreasing force curve during sustained static gripping work." J Physiol Anthropol. 25. 23-28. 2006.

[3] Shyam Kumar, A. J., Parmar, V., Ahmed, S., Kar, S. and Harper, W. M.,"A study of grip endurance and strengh in different elbow positions."J Orthop Traumatol. 9. 209-211. 2008.

[4] Menz, H. B., Zammit, G. V., Munteanu, S. E. and Scott, G., "Plantarflexion strength of the toes: age and gender differences and evaluation of a clinical screening test." Foot Ankle Int. 27. 1103-1108. 2006.

[5] Scott, G., Menz, H. B. and Newcombe, L., "Age-related differences in foot structure and function." Gait Posture. 26. 68-75. 2007.

[6] Yamaji, S., Demura, S., Nagasawa, Y. and Nakada, M., "Relationships between decreasing force and muscle oxygenation kinetics during sustained static gripping." J Physiol Anthropol Appl Human Sci. 23. 41-47. 2004.

[7] Yamaji, S., Demura, S., Nagasawa, Y., Nakada, M., Yoshimura, Y., Matsuzawa, Z. and Toyoshima, Y., "Examination of the parameters of static muscle endurance on sustained static maximal hand gripping." Japan J Phys Educ. 45. 695-706. 2000. [In Japanese with English Abstract].

[8] Nakada, M. and Demura, S., "The change of exertion force during sustained toe grip exertion and the relationships among toe muscle endurance parameters." J Educ Health Sci. 57. 253-257. 2012. [In Japanese with English Abstract].

[9] Demura, S., Sato, S. and Nagasawa, Y., "Re-examination of useful items for determining hand dominance." Gazz Med Ital – Arch Sci Med. 168. 169-177. 2009.

[10] Demura, S., Sato, S. and Sugiura, H., "Lower limb laterality characteristics based on the relationship between activities and individual laterality." Gazz Med Ital – Arch Sci Med. 169. 181-191. 2010.

[11] Nakada, M., Demura, S., Yamaji, S. and Nagasawa, Y., "Examination of the reproducibility of grip force and muscle oxygenation kinetics on maximal repeated rhythmic grip exertion." J Physiol Anthropol Appl Human Sci. 24. 1-6. 2005.

[12] Miyata, H., Sadoyama, T. and Katsuta, S., "Muscle fiber conduction velocity in human vastus lateralis during isometric contractions: relation to muscle fiber composition." J physical

Fitness Japan. 34. 231-238. 1985. [In Japanese with English Abstract].

[13] Ordway, G. A., Kearney, J. T. and Stull, G. A., "Rhythmic isometric fatigue patterns of the elbow flexors and knee extensors." Res Q. 48. 734-740. 1977.

[14] Samson, M. M., Meeuwsen, I. B., Crowe, A., Dessens, J. A., Duursma, S. A. and Verhaar, H. J., "Relationships between physical performance measures, age, height and body weight in healthy adults." Age Ageing. 29. 235-242. 2000.

2

Effects of Acute Consumption of L-Carnitine Tartrate (LCLT) Following an Exhaustive Aerobic Exercise on Serum Lipoproteins Levels in Iranian Elite Wrestlers

Mostafa Dehghani[1,*], Saeid Shakerian[2], Mohammad Kazem Gharib Nasseri[3], Massood Nikbakht[2], Sedigheh Heidari Nejad[4]

[1]Department of Physiology, Physical Education and Sports Science Faculty, Shahid Chamran University, Ahvaz, Iran
[2]Department of Physiology, Physical Education Faculty, Shahid Chamran University, Ahvaz, Iran
[3]Physiology Research Center, Jondishapoor Medical Sciences University, Ahvaz, Iran
[4]Department of Sports Management, Physical Education Faculty, Shahid Chamran University, Ahvaz, Iran
*Corresponding author: dehghani.m66@gmail.com

Abstract **Background and Objective**: In this study, the effect of LCLT supplementation was investigated on serum levels of high-density lipoprotein, low-density lipoprotein, and very low-density lipoprotein following an exhaustive aerobic exercise in elite wrestlers. **Materials and Methods**: Twenty healthy elite male wrestlers with a mean age of 22.05 ± 2.6 years, mean weight of 77.10 ± 11.65 kg, mean height of 1.79 ± 0.06 cm, and mean body mass index of 23.79 ± 2.45 kg/m^2 were participated in this single-blind clinical trial. The subjects were selectively divided into two groups of supplement and placebo. Ninety minutes before performing Conconi protocol, the supplement group received 3 g of LCLT dissolved in 200 ml water plus 6 drops of lemon juice and the placebo group received 200 ml water plus 6 drops of lemon juice. Blood samples were collected 90 min before exercise, immediately after exercise, and 30 min after exercise from brachial vein and their serum lipoprotein concentrations were measured. The obtained data were analyzed by SPSS-16. **Result**: The findings showed that acute consumption of 3 g LCLT tartrate in the experimental group, compared with the placebo group, had a significant positive correlation with increment of high-density lipoprotein and decrement of low-density lipoprotein following an exhaustive aerobic activity, while no significant change was observed in very low-density lipoprotein. **Conclusion:** The findings of the present investigation indicate that supplementation instant LCLT effect significant change was observed in HDL, LDL and VLDL and concentrations.

Keywords: *L-carnitine tartrate, high-density lipoprotein, low-density lipoprotein, very low-density lipoprotein, exhaustive aerobic activity*

1. Introduction

Nutrition is one of the most important topics of medical sciences and experts believe that observing nutrition principles may have a key role in health promotion and disease prevention in all periods of life [1]. Most athletes are familiar with dietary supplements which are used for improving athletic performance [2]; such as LCLT (3-hydroxy-4-N-trimethylammonio butanoate) with a molecular weight of 161 g/mol which was extracted from meat for the first time and is involved in the transport of fatty acids into mitochondria [3]. LCLT deficiency leads to impaired fats metabolism [4]. On the other hand, physical activity results in reduced LCLT in muscles [5]. Despite abundant reserves of triglycerides in the body, liver and muscle glycogen stores are limited, thus their depletion is expectable during exercise especially during prolonged endurance activities [6,7]. Several studies have been performed about the effects of LCLT on fatty acids consumption. In this context, some have indicated that supplementation with LCLT increases fat oxidation [8], decreases carbohydrate oxidation [9], improves exercise [10], and reduces the recovery time [11]; while, some studies have reported no effect on carbohydrate oxidation [12], no change in maximal oxygen consumption (VO_{2max}) [13], and no change in heart rate, oxygen consumption, and blood lactate concentration [14].

Research evidences show that the findings about acute effects of LCLT supplement on metabolic factors and athletic performance in athlete and non-athlete population are often disparate and inconsistent, such that some reports show the beneficial impacts of this supplementation on endurance performance and others not. Therefore, the aim of the present study was to evaluate the effects of acute consumption of 3 g LCLT on lipid metabolism in elite wrestlers performing exhaustive aerobic exercise, in order to provide new results along with other research findings.

2. Materials and Methods

The statistical population of this single-blind clinical trial consisted of elite wrestlers of Ahvaz. Following determination of sample size, 20 male wrestlers with full consent were selected as samples and signed the consent form. To measure their anthropometric variables, they were examined a few days before the test and the data on height, weight, and body mass index were determined. They were then specifically divided into two equal groups of supplement and placebo. The supplement group received 3 g of LCLT dissolved in 200 ml water plus 6 drops of lemon juice and the placebo group received 200 ml water plus 6 drops of lemon juice. The sample size was determined based on the findings of some studies on the effects of LCLT and sample size estimation for comparing the two groups, with a type I error at 5%. The confidence level for estimating sample size in this study was 95%. The subjects (Ahvaz elite wrestlers) hold national, Asian, and world championships, and they do not have any metabolic disease such as diabetes, asthma, or cardiovascular disease. Both experimental and control groups were prohibited to exercise 48 hours before the test. They were also asked to avoid consumption of coffee and dairy products at least a day before the test, to put themselves in normal conditions for the test, and to be fasting 12 to 14 hours before the test. LCLT tartrate (68.2% LCLT, 31.8% L-tartrate) was obtained as gift from the Shahr Darou Company.

Test performance: The supplement and placebo were consumed by the subjects 90 minutes before the exercise. Five milliliter blood sample was obtained from them at the test morning, after 15 min rest. To obtain serum, blood samples were centrifuged for 10 min at 2000 RPM. Serum high-density lipoprotein (HDL), low density lipoprotein (LDL), and very low-density lipoprotein (VLDL) were measured using standard kits (Bionic, Iran) with a sensitivity of 1 mg/dL (first stage). The exercise protocol; Conconi test (15), was performed 90 min after receiving the supplement and placebo as follows; after a warm-up, the participants start to run on a treadmill (Hp/cusmos-Germany) with an initial speed of 8 km/h which raised 0.5 km/h every 200 m and continued until the subject exhausted. Immediately after the test, the traveled distance was recorded and the second blood was sampled (second stage). The third blood sample was taken 30 min after the exercise (third stage) as mentioned earlier. Biochemical and physiological variables were compared in SPSS-16 using ANOVA inferential analysis (MANOVA). To evaluate normal distribution of original variables and to study homogeneity of variance, the parametric Kolmogorov-Smirnov test and the Leaven test were used, respectively. The significance level of mean difference was considered $p < 0.05$.

3. Results

A- The initial investigation showed that LCLT consumption had no side effects on the subjects, such as stomach ache or diarrhea which often occur following the consumption of some supplements. The participants were able to successfully complete the test protocol. Table 1 depicts the anthropometric characteristics of the two study groups in this exercise trial. As the results show, both groups were homogeneous in terms of anthropometric parameters and there are no significant differences in any of the characteristics.

Table 1. Anthropometric characteristics of subjects (mean ± SD)

Characteristics/Group	Experimental	Control
Age (years)	22.6 ± 1.42	21 ± 3.4
Height (m)	1.8 ± 1.06	1.79 ± 0.4
Weight (kg)	77.5 ± 10.62	76.7 ± 13.17
BMI (kg/m²)	23.87 ± 1.83	23.71 ± 3.06

B- Effect of LCLT on serum HDL

As in Figure 1, HDL levels shows no significant difference before and after exhaustive exercise in the experimental and control groups, while serum HDL was higher in the experimental group than the control group after resting ($p < 0.035$).

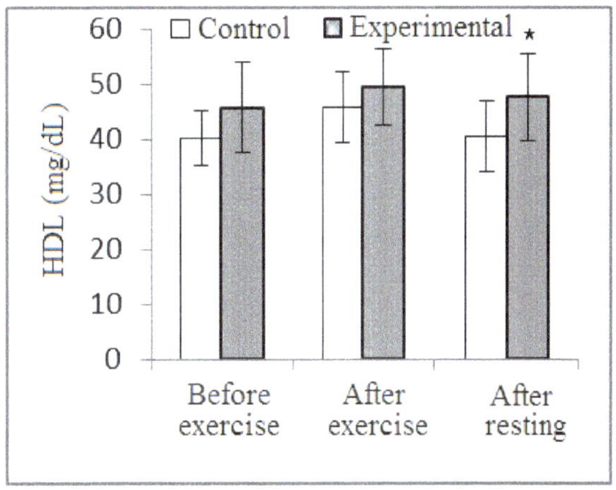

Figure 1. Effect of LCLT on serum HDL, 90 min before and immediately after exhaustive activity and 30 min after resting in control and experimental groups (10 persons per group). * Significant difference at $p < 0.05$

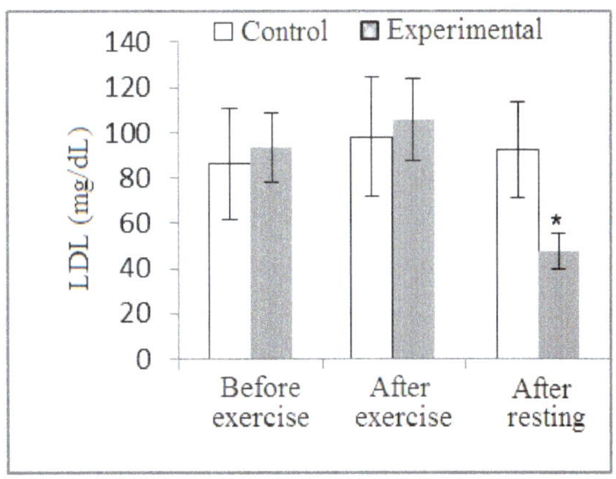

Figure 2. Effect of LCLT on serum LDL, 90 min before and immediately after exhaustive activity and 30 min after resting in control and experimental groups (10 persons per group). * Significant difference at $p < 0.05$

C- Effect of LCLT on serum LDL

As Figure 2 illustrates, the levels of LDL before and after exhaustive exercise have no significant difference in the experimental and control groups, while serum LDL is lower in the experimental group than the control group after resting ($p < 0.018$).

D- Effect of LCLT on serum VLDL

As in Figure 3, the level of VLDL before and after exhaustive exercise and resting has no significant difference in the experimental and control groups.

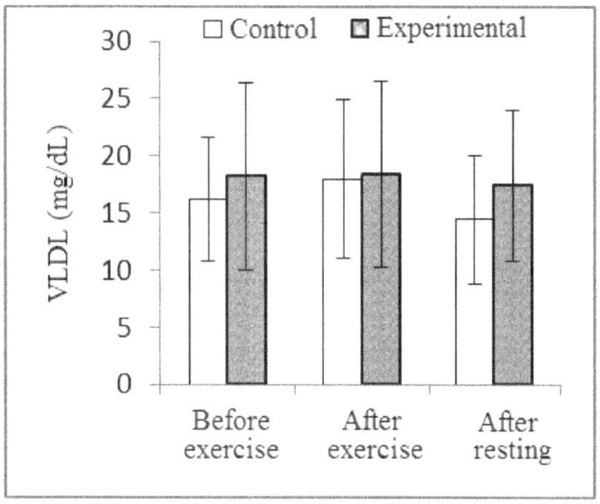

Figure 3. Effect of LCLT on serum VLDL, 90 min before and immediately after exhaustive activity and 30 min after resting in control and experimental groups (10 persons per group)

4. Discussion

To gain a competitive advantage and to achieve a higher level of health or physical performance, athletes experience various diet or artificial methods containing nutritional supplements or injectable medications [16]. Dietary supplements which improve athletic performance are familiar to most athletes [11]. The primary role of LCLT is focused on lipid metabolism however, scientific evidence confirms its role in carbohydrate metabolism as well and in fact, there is a strong correlation between muscle carnitine and Krebs cycle. Fat oxidation is triggered in rabbits following L-carnitine consumption [17]. Muscle carnitine concentration is directly proportional to muscle glycogen stores [18]. Studies show that L-carnitine improves fat metabolism and preserves glycogen [19]. Another study shows that L-carnitine increases fat oxidation and hence CO_2 elimination [20]. Other studies show ineffectiveness of L-carnitine on blood lipid levels [21]. What distinguishes the present research with these studies is the readiness of the subjects and the exercise type. Regarding the role of L-carnitine in transferring free fatty acids into mitochondria, particularly during sports, it is expected that its supplementation and thus its increase in plasma be associated with increased entry of free fatty acids into the cell's mitochondria; the main outcome of which is the preservation of liver and muscle glycogen to continue carbohydrate oxidation, particularly in the later stages of exercise and hence delayed exhaustion. These benefits have been confirmed by many scientific evidences.

5. Conclusion

Single-dose consumption of 3 g LCLT, 90 min before starting exercise can improve the performance through transporting of blood free fatty acids into mitochondria. The results of the present study showed that acute supplementation with LCLT tartrate increased HDL and decreased LDL, while not affected VLDL following an exhaustive aerobic activity. To improve fatty acid metabolism and their records, athletes of aerobic sports like wrestling (*e.g.* taekwondo and gymnastics) can be recommended to consume 3 g LCLT, 90 minutes before exercise. To analyze more confidently the results, it is suggests to measure glycogen concentration and LCLT in blood and muscle in future studies.

Acknowledgement

The authors of the paper would like to sincerely thank the Shahr Darou Company for providing L-carnitine.

References

[1] Shidfar, F. Mahan, L. Scout, S. Raymond, G. Background. Kraous food and the care process, 13th ed. Tehran: Khosravi; 2012; 254-5.

[2] Karlic H, Lohninger A, Laschan C .Downregulation of carnitine acyltransferases and organic cation transporter OCTN2 in mononuclear cells in healthy elderly and patients with myelodysplastic syndromes. *J Mol Med*; 2004; 81:435.

[3] Rebouche CJ, Chenard CA. Metabolic fate of dietary carnitine in human adults: identification and quantification of urinary and fecal metabolites. *J. Nutr* 1991; 121:539.

[4] Heinonen oj. Carnitine and physical exercise. Sport Med. 1996; 22 (2): 109-132.

[5] Zeyner A, Harmeyer J. Metablic functions of L-carnitine and its effects as feed additive in horses. Areview Arch Tiererahr. 1999 52; (2): 115-138.

[6] Robergs, R.A., Roberts S. Fundamental Principles of Exercise Physiology: For Fitness, Performance and Health. USA, McGraw Hill, 2000; pp 237-42.

[7] Maughan R, Gleeson M, Greenhaff P.L. Biochemistry of exercise & training. USA, Oxford Medical Publications, 1997; pp131-3.

[8] Ibrahim WH, Bailey N, Sunvold GD, Bruckner GG. Effects of carnitine and taurine on fatty acid metabolism and lipid accumulation in the liver of cats during weight gain and weight loss. Am J Vet Res 2003; 64(10):1265-77.

[9] Stephens FB, Constantin-Teodosiu D, Laithwaite D, Simpson EJ, Greenhaff PL. Anacute increase in skeletal muscle carnitine content alters fuel metabolism in resting human skeletal muscle. J Clin Endocrinol. Metab 2006; 91(12):5013-8.

[10] Guarnieri G, Biolo G, Vinci P, Massolino B, Barazzoni R. Advances in carnitine in chronic uremia. J Ren Nutr. 2007; 17(1):23-9.

[11] Karlic H, Lohninger A. Supplementation of L-carnitine in athletes: does it make sense? Nutrition 2004; 20(7):709-15.

[12] Abramowicz WN, Galloway SD. Effects of acute versus chronic L-carnitine L-tartrate supplementation on metabolic responses to steady state exercise in males and females. Int J Sport Nutr Exercise Metab 2005; 15(4):386-400.

[13] Ero ğ lu H, Senel O, Güzel NA. Effects of acute L-carnitine intake on metabolic and blood lactate levels of elite badminton players. Neuro Endocrinol Lett 2008; 29(2): 261-6.

[14] Stuessi C, Hofer P, Meier C, Boutellier U. L-carnitine and the recovery from exhaustive endurance exercise: a randomised, doubleblind, placebo-controlled trial. Eur J Appl Physiol 2005; 95(5-6): 431-5.

[15] Shuaa Kazmi, M. Kimiagar, M. RastManners R. Sarreshteh,m. Taleban, F. A. Acute supplementation of L - carnitine level, blood lactic acid and anaerobic threshold distance on the treadmill to Rsydnbh. Journal of Kurdistan University of Medical Sciences. Autumn 2006; 10: 43-52.

[16] Ghandchi, z. Mahan, L. Scout, S. Raymond, G . Nutrition in Exercise and Sport. Kraous food and the care process, 13th ed. Tehran: Khosravi; 2012: 13: 194-254.

[17] Bacurau R.F.P. Navarro, F. Bassit R.A. Does exercise training interfere with effects of L-carnitine supplementation? *Nutrition* 2003; 19 (4): 337-41.

[18] Horleys. L-carnitine. A division of naturalac nutrition. Level 2. [cited on 2003]. Available from: htpp://horlrys. com.

[19] Stephens, F.B. Constantin-Teodosiu D, Greenhaff PL. New insights concerning the role of carnitine in the regulation of fuel metabolism in skeletal muscle. J Physiol 2007; 581 (Pt 2): 431-44.

[20] Muller DM, Seim H, Kiess W, Loster H, Richter T. Effect of oral L-carnitine supplementation on in vivo long-chain fatty acid oxidation in healthy adult. Metabolism. 2002; 51(11): 1389-91.

[21] Colombani P, Wenk C, Kunz I. Effects of L-carnitine supplementation on physical performance and energy metabolism of endurance-trained athletes: a double-blind crossover field study. Eur J Appl Physiol Occup Physiol. 1996; 73: 434-439.

3

Effects of Daily Life Physical Activity on Obesity Indices, Cardiorespiratory Fitness and Association of the Latter Two with Academic Performance in Bengali Adolescents of India

Roan Mukherjee[1], Prakash C. Dhara[2,*]

[1]Department of Human Physiology, Hazaribag College of Dental Sciences and Hospital, Demotand, Hazaribag, Jharkhand, India
[2]Ergonomics and Sports Physiology Division, Department of Human Physiology with CommunityHealth, Vidyasagar University, Medinipore, West Bengal, India
*Corresponding author: prakashcdhara@gmail.com

Abstract This study examined the influence of daily life Physical Activity (PA) on obesity parameters (BMI: Body Mass Index, WHR: Waist Hip Ratio, Body fat percentage) and cardiorespiratory fitness or CRF (PFI: Physical Fitness Index). The influence of the later two on academic performance was also documented. The study was conducted on 720 healthy Bengali adolescents involving 240 subjects from each of the three age groups (Age group I: 13-14 yrs, Age group II:15-16 yrs, Age group III:17-18 yrs). Subjects of both the genders were chosen from urban and rural areas by random sampling method. Physical activity questionnaire for adolescents (PAQ-A) was used to classify adolescents into low, moderate and high PA levels. Obesity parameters and PFI was measured using standard techniques. Percentage (%) of the mean of the three years total marks of annual school examination was computed to get the academic score (%) of the participant. In most of the instances, obesity parameters were significantly ($p < 0.05$) varied among different PA levels. PFI also showed similar trend of results.It was seen that rural urban impact on obesity parameters may not always be necessarily present whereas in case of PFI it was consistently significant. Obesity parameters was found to have significant negative correlation ($p < 0.001$) with PA and academic performance. PFI possessed significant ($p < 0.001$) positive correlation with PA and academic performance.However, multiple regression analysis found that only body fat percentage independently and significantly predicted academic performance in both the genders. The present data highlighted the importance of practicing sufficient PA in daily life not only to keep check against increased body fat levels and prevent obesity but also to increase CRF. Additively, it indicated that higher levels of body fat and lower levels of CRF may possibly restrict performance in examination. PA induced lowering of body fat and improvements in CRF may be expected to bring about some positive changes in academic performance.

Keywords: *Bengali adolescents, physical activity, obesity parameters, cardiorespiratory fitness, academic performance*

1. Introduction

Several threats to health may be the consequence of being obese or overweight. These threats include, but are not limited to cardiovascular complications, hypertension, osteoporosis, diabetes, psychological disturbances like anxiety and depression.Obesity in an individual is characterised by the presence of excess amount of body fat [1]. Sophisticated methods like the use of dual-energy X-ray absorptiometry (DEXA), etc are available for direct measuring of body fat. Application of these methods are difficult in large scale studies [2]. However, there are indirect methods of determining body fat, which are based on the utilization of well known obesity parameters like BMI, WHR and Body fat % (estimated from skinfolds). These indirect methods are widely used in epidemiological studies and they well indicate whether the individual is carrying excessive body fat. Obesity may be noted not only in developed nations but also in developing nations [3]. In India, obesity had often found to coexist with undernourishment and it had been found to effect individuals of all age groups and socioeconomic status, particularly in an urban settlement [1]. Life style factors like over consumption of calories, due to dependency on non home based diet, with no control on ingrediants and amounts, absence of sufficient PA in daily life, prolonged engagement in sedentary screen based activities had been associated with obesity [3]. Moreover, easy ascess to motor driven vehicles [1] had allowed cutting down of walking/ cycling to school increasing the susceptibility of childrens and adolescents to obesity.

The negative relationship between PA and obesity parameters are well documented in other populations by several earlier studies [4-11] which depects the importance of PA in weight management. A study on the subjects of Kolkata, West Bengal documented similar findings [12]. Similarly, there are studies that noted positive relationship between PA and cardiorspiratory fitness / CRF (in terms of Physical fitness index/ PFI) [13,14]. Academic performance is known to reflect cognitive functions [15] and thus may act as a "proxy" for the same. Evidences had started to gather, which indicate that academic performance may posses negative relationship with obesity parameters [3,16,17,18] and a positive relationship with CRF [19,20]. In Bengali adolescent population of rural and urban areas, no empirical study has been conducted in context of these issues.

In view of these reports, this present study is intended to report the associations of daily life PA with obesity parameters and CRF as well as the association of the later two with academic performance in Bengali adolescents of both genders. The findings of the present study may support the implementation of adequate PA in daily life of adolescents to prevent obesity, improve CRF and academic performance.

2. Materials and Methods

A cross-sectional study was carried out among 720 (360: males and 360 females) Bengali (Indian) adolescents of age ranging from 13 to 18 years. The sample of adolescents were drawn by simple random sampling from West Bengal (Districts: Burdwan, Hooghly and Howrah), India. The samples of both the genders were selected from the following three age groups - group I: 13-14yrs, group II: 15-16 yrs, and group III: 17-18yrs. Each age group had 120 males and females respectively. Furthermore, samples for each of the three age groups were collected from rural and urban areas. Informed consent was obtained from the subjects to consider them as participants of the study. Permission from institutional human ethical committee were obtained for the study. Majority of the adolescents belonged to middle class strata of the society as per Kuppuswami scale [21].

The daily life PA of the sample was determined by PAQ-A [22] containing eight questions, which enquired about PA performed in a span of last 7 days. It may be mentioned that the validity of the instrument is good [23]. This present study was employed a modified version of this instrument, which was altered to add few common PA performed in Indian context. In addition, some uncommon physical activities, which were generally not performed by the Indian adolescents, were excluded. Final PA was computed according to the original version [22] and classification of adolescents into low, moderate and high PA level was done in the following way: Score $\leq$ 2: low PA, Score >2 and $\leq$ 3: moderate PA, Score > 3: high PA.

Body weight and height. Weight was determined using Human weighing machine. Height was measured using anthropometric rod.

Physical Fitness Index: PFI score was determined employing the procedure mentioned in the original Harvard Step test using the formula: PFI = (100 x test duration in seconds) / (2 x sum of heart beats in the recovery periods) [24].

2.1. Obesity Parameters/Indices

BMI was obtained by dividing weight in kilograms by height in squared meters. For the purpose of identification of overweight and obesity the cut off values of BMI set by the International Obesity Task Force (IOTF) were used [25] (Cole etal). Skin fold thickness were measured at the right tricep and calf using Holtain skin fold callipers.Computations of body fat % were done using tricep and calf skinfold equation [26] of Slaughter et al. The equations are as follows:

$$\text{Body fat\% for males} = 0.735(\text{triceps} + \text{calf skinfolds}) + 1.0$$

$$\text{Body fat\% for females} = 0.610(\text{triceps} + \text{calf skinfolds}) + 5.0$$

Waist circumference were measured just above the belly button. Geater trochanter were measured to get the hip circumference. Waist circumference was divided by hip circumference to get waist hip ratio (WHR).All the obesity parameters were measured in triplicate and their average were used in study.

2.2. "Proxy" Measure of Cognition

Academic performance may be altered by changes in cognition. In line to studies by other authors [27] and in continuation of the trend identified and utilised by our earlier study [15], academic performance was evaluated as an indicator of cognitive functions. The overall average marks scored in last three years annual school examination were obtained from files /report cards/ school data base.The mean of these three averages marks were computed. This was followed by calculation of the Percentage (%) of the obtained mean to derive academic score (%) of the subjects.

2.3. Statistical Evaluation

Means and standard deviation (SD) were computed for all the variables. Sex differences were tested using t- test. Two level nested ANOVA [28] showed whether or not all the obesity parameters and PFI significantly varied between low, moderate and high PA level. It also grossly indicated the presence or absence of subgroup variation i.e rural urban variation, nested within the PA levels. The variance between the PA levels in rural urban subgroups respectively were tested using one way ANOVA. Appropriate post hoc test were also employed following significant results of ANOVA. The exact location of rural urban difference within the subgroups were located employing t-tests. For finding the interrelationship between PA, PFI and obesity parameters Pearson's correlation coefficient were calculated to form a correlation matrix. Association of PFI and Obesity parameters with academic score were tested both by Pearson's correlation coefficient and multiple regression analysis.

3. Results

The means and standard deviation (SD) of the selected obesity parameters and PFI of the overall samples of male and females are presented according to different PA levels in Table 1. It showed that BMI of males and PFI of both the genders insignificantly varied among the different PA levels. The BMI of females, WHR and Body fat % of both the sexes was significanty different between the PA levels. In cases of significant variation of the study variables among different PA levels, the post hoc test conformed that the three PA levels (low, moderate and high) was significanty different from each other.

The results of the F statistics of the subgroup revealed that variation of BMI, WHR, Body fat % and PFI was present among the rural and urban subgroups, contained within the PA levels, excepting WHR and Body fat % of males (Table1).

The prevalence of overweight and obesity in the sample studied showed that in the overall sample of boys, 9.4% were overweight and 1.94 % were obese. On the contrary, in the overall sample of girls, 22.5% were overweight and 0.83 % were obese.

Table 1. Variation of selected Obesity parameters and PFI in different physical activity (PA) level male (M) and female (F)

Variables	Sex	Physical activity levels (Mean ± SD)			Two-level nested ANOVA		Post hoc Bonferroni-Multiple t- test
		Low(L)	Mod. (M)	High(H)	(F_G)	(F_{SG})	
BMI (kg/m²)	M	21.4 ± 3.32	18.2 ± 3.87	17.5 # ± 4.11	3.94 ns (17.9)	10.3***(11.1)	----------
	F	21.6 ± 288	18.4 ± 3.58	16.3 # ± 3.25	12.2* (31.9)	5.39***(4.7)	L≠M, L≠H, M≠H
WHR (cm)	M	1.06 # ± 0.27	0.95 # ± 0.17	0.85 # ± 0.11	20.4** (22.3)	1.79 ns(1.0)	L≠M, L≠H, M≠H
	F	0.96 # ± 0.21	0.83 # ± 0.15	0.75 # ± 0.07	11.5*(29.1)	5.00**(4.4)	L≠M, L≠H, M≠H
Body Fat(%)	M	20.8 # ± 5.09	16.7# ± 4.12	13.3 # ± 4.11	53.9**(41.7)	1.64 ns(0.61)	L≠M, L≠H, M≠H
	F	24.2 # ± 3.43	21.3 # ± 3.27	19.1 # ± 3.26	12.4*(33.6)	5.74 ***(4.9)	L≠M, L≠H, M≠H
PFI	M	52.7 # ± 9.14	57.1 # ± 8.63	60.4 # ± 9.63	2.16 ns(8.27)	10.9***(13.1)	----------
	F	46.1 # ± 7.59	52.1 # ± 6.43	55.2 # ± 8.98	4.08 ns(19.4)	10.9***(11.5)	----------

Males: low, n = 118, mod, n = 114, high, n = 128 ; Females: low, n= 109, mod, n =130, high, n =121

* ≤ 0.05; ** ≤ 0.01; *** ≤ 0.001, ns = not significant. (*Note: G = group and SG =subgroup)Figures in bracket under F statistics shows variance component percentage.*

Significantly different means, P ≤ 0.017 (0.05 /3) using post hoc Bonferroni corrected t-test following significant F_G in nested anova are shown in the table.

Means of Male Vs Female indicated with # in superscript in the same coloumne are significantly different by t -test (p ≤ 0.05).

The means and standard deviation of rural and urban adolescent males and females are presented according to different PA levels in Table 2. It was found that BMI, WHR, Body fat % and PFI significantly differed between the three PA levels.Post hoc test showed that in majority of the case the three PA levels differed from each other.

Table 2. Mean, SD, and ANOVA of selected obesity parameter and PFI of the subgroups (rural :R and urban: U) present within each PA group

Variables	Sex	Region	Physical activity levels (Mean ± SD)			One way ANOVA (F)	Post- hoc Scheffe 's test
			Low(L)	Mod. (M)	High(H)		
BMI(kg/m²)	M	R	20.5 # ± 3.31	17.4 # ± 4.19	16.0 # ± 1.69	28.7***(31.6)	L≠M, L≠H
		U	22.3 # ± 3.11	19.1 # ± 3.26	18.8 # ± 5.12	14.6***(18.60	L≠M, L≠H
	F	R	20.6 # ± 3.91	17.8 # ± 3.33	15.8 ± 2.99	28.4***(31.4)	L≠M,L≠H, M≠H
		U	22.7 # ± 3.58	19.0 # ± 3.74	16.8 ± 3.42	39.3***(39)	L≠M, L≠H, M≠H
WHR(cm)	M	R	1.04 ± 0.29	0.92 # ± 0.13	0.85 ± 0.06	16.1 ***(20.1)	L≠M, L≠H
		U	1.09 ± 0.26	0.98 # ± 0.21	0.86 ± 0.14	20.7 ***(24.8)	L≠M,L≠H, M≠H
	F	R	0.91 # ± 0.14	0.81 ± 0.12	0.74 ± 0.08	33.8 ***(35.4)	L≠M,L≠H, M≠H
		U	1.01 # ± 0.26	0.85 ± 0.17	0.76 ± 0.07	29.2***(32)	L≠M,L≠H, M≠H
BodyFat (%)	M	R	20.3 ± 3.56	16.1 ± 3.01	12.9 ± 3.42	70.8***(53.8)	L≠M,L≠H, M≠H
		U	21.3 ± 6.16	17.5 ± 5.10	13.6 ± 4.66	33.8***(35.5)	L≠M,L≠H, M≠H
	F	R	23.7 # ± 3.21	20.3 # ± 2.77	18.6 ± 2.66	44.9***(42.3)	L≠M,L≠H, M≠H
		U	24.8 # ± 3.59	22.2 # ± 3.46	19.5 ± 3.69	31.7 ***(34)	L≠M,L≠H, M≠H
PFI	M	R	54.5 # ± 9.38	59.3 # ± 7.40	64.0 # ± 7.89	19.6***(23.7)	L≠M,L≠H,M≠H
		U	51.1 # ± 8.80	54.3 # ± 9.44	57.1# ± 10.1	6.76***(8.8)	L≠H
	F	R	47.5 # ± 6.76	53.6 # ± 4.81	58.1# ± 4.92	41.1***(40)	L≠M,L≠H,M≠H
		U	44.4 # ± 7.01	50.2 # ± 6.57	52.6 # ± 10.9	14.7***(18.7)	L≠M,L≠H

Males R: low, n = 56, mod, n = 63, high, n = 61 ; Males U: low, n= 62, mod, n =51, high, n =67

Females R: low, n = 57, mod, n = 66, high, n = 57 ; Females U: low, n= 52, mod, n =64, high, n =64

* ≤ 0.05; ** ≤ 0.01; *** ≤ 0.001, ns = not significant

The variance component percentage are shown within parentheses under significant F statistics.

The PA groups having significantly different rural-urban subgroup are shown: Comparison (vertical coloumn wise) among same gender different region indicated by # in superscript are statistically different using t -test(p ≤ 0.05).

At different PA levels, BMI seemed to varry between rural urban adolescents, excepting in the case of high PA level females.Handful of instances of significant rural urban difference was present in case of WHR and Body fat % viz. WHR of moderate PA level males, and low PA level females, Body fat % of low and moderate PA level females. At all the PA levels, significant rural urban differences in PFI was present in both sexes.

Correlation Matrix: It is presented in Table 3. PA was found to possess significant negative correlation with all the obesity parameters in both the genders. It also showed that PA was positively and significantly correlated with PFI in both males and females. It was observed that PA possessed a higher degree of correlation coefficient with BMI of females and Body fat % of males than that of other cases. In general the degree of correlation was comparatively higher in females than that of males.

BMI had a significant positive correlation with WHR and Body fat % in males and females. WHR also possessed significant positive correlation with body fat % in both sexes. PFI was significantly and negatively correlated with obesity parameters in both male and females.

Table 3. Interrelationship between PA, obesity parameters and PFI

a. Correlation Matrix for males (n=360)					
Variables	PA	BMI	WHR	Body Fat %	PFI
PA	-				
BMI	-.34 ***	-			
WHR	-.39 ***	.20***	-		
Body fat %	-.52 ***	.25***	.12**	-	
PFI	.29 ***	-.19***	-.26***	-.23***	-
b. Correlation Matrix for females (n=360)					
Variables	PA	BMI	WHR	Body Fat %	PFI
PA	-				
BMI	-.52***	-			
WHR	-.50 ***	.37***	-		
Body fat %	-.53 ***	.59***	.33***	-	
PFI	.41***	-.33***	-.27***	-34***	-

* $\leq$ 0.05; ** $\leq$ 0.01; *** $\leq$ 0.001, ns = not significant

Academic Score of the subjects:

The mean academic score of males (M=43.7, SD=16.2) was found to be significantly ($p< 0.05$) lower than that of females (M=48.8, SD=14.6).

Association of Obesity parameters and Cardiorespiratory fitness (PFI) with academic score

A significant negative correlation between BMI and academic score in boys ($r = -.17$, $p < 0.001$), and girls ($r = -.29$, $p < 0.001$) was noted. It may be pointed out that the degree of correlation was higher in girls than that of boys. The academic score was also significantly and negatively correlated with WHR in boys ($r = -.20$, $p < 0.001$) and girls ($r= -.21$, $p < 0.001$). Similarly, significant negative correlation ($p<0.001$) was noted between Body fat % and academic score in both boys and girls. On the other hand there was a significant positive correlation ($p < 0.001$) between PFI and academic score in both the genders.

Table 4. Multiple regression analysis of Academic score with selected obesity parameters and Cardiorespiratory fitness (PFI)

	Male(n= 360)		Female(n= 360)	
R^2	12 %		13 %	
Variables	B (regression weights)	P	B (regression weights)	P
BMI (kg/m^2)	-0.30	> 0.05	-0.47	$\leq$ 0.05
WHR (cm)	-10.2	$\leq$ 0.01	-6.68	> 0.05
Body Fat (%)	-0.69	$\leq$ 0.001	-0.67	$\leq$ 0.01
PFI	0.13	> 0.05	0.14	> 0.05

After controlling for the other variables using multiple regression analysis, the following were found: In both the genders, the Body fat % had significant negative regression weights, indicating adolescents with lower body fat % were expected to have higher academic score, BMI possessed similar significant negative regression weights in females whereas WHR showed significant negative regression weights only in case of males. PFI was not significantly associated with academic score in males and females (Table 4).

4. Discussion

Earlier studies on adolescents and even adult populations reported decrement in BMI, WHR and fat % on being exposed to sufficient PA [4-11]. The findings of the present study confirmed the finding of these earlier studies in the present population (Bengali). It has been known that WHR gets lowered along with lowering of weight in individuals showing preponderance of adiposity in the abdomen [29,30,31]. The present study showed that PA may modify WHR in Bengali adolescents. This indicated that PA may mobilize fats from abdomen and thereby affect regional distribution of fats [32]. The findings of the present study on BMI, WHR and fat % implied that daily life PA may be helpful in weight management/ prevention of obesity. The effects of exercise /PA in regulating body weight are well accepted [33,34]. PA may be regarded to be one of the most important factors influencing obesity. Studies had noted that inactivity caused obesity although no accompanying more intake of energy through diet was present [35,36,37]. Thus every adolescent should adopt strategies to maintain sufficient PA in daily life in order to restrict obesity. Unlike the present study, reports of increase in weight, BMI, and other variables related to physical development following exercise or PA exists in the literature [38,39,40,41]. Thus it is evident that the effect of PA /exercise on body composition may differ among studies. These differences among studies may be attributed to be due to differences in methodology of estimation of body composition, duration and mode PA / exercise performed by the population [42]. Moreover, varried dietary practices by the population considered by these studies may also contributed to the differences among these studies. An earlier study [43] found that BMI of Bengali adolescents belonging to middle class strata of the society was much below than those belong to prosperous strata of the society. In light of this particular earlier finding, lower prevalence of obesity, found in the present study was not surprising.

The effects of PA leading to better PFI scores (cardiorespiratory fitness), as observed in the present study have been reported by many earlier studies [13,14]. Regular PA is known to improve PFI by improving recovery heart rate [44]. The efficient delivery and use of oxygen by the muscles and tissues (which in turn may lead to lower resting heart rate, higher stroke volume, higher arteriovenous O_2 difference and lower respiratory minute ventilation) [45] may be facilitated by exercise induced angiogenesis [46,47,48,49,50]. The improvement in PFI, on exposure to increasing levels of PA in the present study may be attributed to such physiological benefits of PA.

The higher BMI, WHR in boys and higher body fat % in girls in the present study is in line to a study on other population [51]. Earlier, Indian studies have also found BMI of male adolescents to be higher than females [52]. WHR is a measure of abdominal fat distribution [53]. Higher WHR in Bengali males in the present study suggest higher dominance of abdominal fats in males in comparison to Bengali females. This observation on WHR of Bengali males is supported by the fact that males show fat deposition especially in the truncal region. This includes subcutaneous and intra abdominal fat deposition [54]. Higher resting heart rate and more body fat in females may add to the differences in PFI values between male and females. Similar to our findings an earlier study on adult male and females using modified Harvard Step Test, found that the mean PFI score of females was lower than that of males [55]. This present study and even an earlier study [56] had shown that males with higher PFI showed lower amount of body fat. This indicated that body fat may influence PFI and since females show higher body fat than males, lower PFI values among females may be expected. Furthermore, earlier studies have noted that post exercise recovery heart rate of males drops back at a normal range earlier than females [57]. In addition females are known to be less physically active than males. Lower PFI in females in contrast to males in the present study may be due to above probable reasons.

Body fat levels may be influenced by dietary food habits. It may be that the dietary intakes of both rural and urban adolescents involved in the study were not much different from each other. This may had contributed to the inconsistency in rural urban differences, in context to obesity parameters. However, the PFI score was found to be consistently and significantly lower in urban individuals. This was in line to an earlier study [45]. This may be attributed to the comparatively lower daily physical activity level of urban boys and girls, in contrast to their rural counterpart.

In the present study, the observed positive relationship of BMI with other obesity parameters viz. WHR and body fat % was more pronounced in adolescent girls than that of the boys. These observations were in conformity with earlier studies on other population in which similar findings were obtained [58,59]. These findings of the present study implied that BMI to some extinct may be a better predictor of adiposity in girls than boys. Future studies need to conform this particular finding. The results of the present study also showed that higher PFI scores may be associated with lower values of obesity parameters. This implied that greater physiological fitness may lower the susceptibility of adolescents to develop obesity. Daily life PA is of much importance in achieving greater PFI as elucidated by the results of the present study. Increased adiposity may lower utilization of oxygen per unit of body mass. This may restrict proper functioning of heart especially during physical activities or exercises [60]. Thus on the basis of the present study it may be said that low PA level may result in higher mean values of BMI, WHR and body fat % which may be may be detrimental to cardiorespiratory fitness. Increased cardiorespiratory fitness (measured in terms of VO_2 Max) had been found to lower body fat % [60], BMI and WHR [61]. In light of these earlier studies and results of the present study it may be said that cardiorespiratory fitness whether measured in terms of either PFI or VO_2 Max may be expected to demonstrate a negative relationship with obesity parameters.

Academic scores of females in the present study was higher than that of males. This is in line to our previous study, performed with a different sample size of Bengali adolescents [15]. A number of studies [3,16,17,18] on other population reported that obese individuals were performing poorly in academics. This present study is possibly the first study on Bengali adolescents to report significant negative impact of BMI, WHR and Body fat % on academic performance in a sample of health, mostly non obese individuals. The findings were not surprising since individuals with more body fat may lack attentiveness and proper executive functions like flexibility in mental tasks [62]. However, some contradictory reports of no effect of excessive body fat on academic performance also exists in the literature [18,63]. In the present study, although initially it appeared from the correlation study that academic performance of girls may be little bit more adversely affected by increased obesity parameters, multiple regression analysis conformed the absence of any such trend. It showed no drastic differences in the effects of obesity parameters on academic performance between male and females. Consistent with a recent study [3] on Punjabi adolescents multiple regression analysis showed that BMI may have profound negative influence on academic performance of girls whereas it may not adversely affect academic performance in boys. An earlier study also found that BMI may not adversely influence cognition [64]. In elderly adults increased WHR had been found to be associated with impairment in cognitive ability [65,66]. The findings of the present study provided evidences that similar relationship between WHR and cognition may exists in adolescents. Furthermore, in the present study body fat % (rather than other obesity parameters) emerged as the most marked negative predictor of academic performance in both the genders. In the present study, multiple regression analysis showed lower explained variance in both boys and girls. This indicated that the various obesity parameters although not greatly but to a limited extinct may influence academic performance of Bengali adolescents.

Several explanations may be put forward to explain the negative relationship of obesity parameters with academic performance. Poor academic performance induced psychological disturbances may trigger excessive eating resulting in increased values of obesity parameters. Unfavourable attitude of teachers towards individuals with more body weight may lead to the assignment of lower marks/grades to them by teachers. Lack of discipline in personal life may prevent an individual from devoting time to both PA and academic tasks [67]. This in turn may increase their susceptibility to obesity and obtaining of poor grades in examinations. In individuals with higher BMI the amount of blood that is to be normally distributed to the brain gets distributed to other parts of the body. This compromised supply of blood to brain in individuals with higher BMI may lead to compromised academic performance or cognition. Lower self-esteem in overweight / obese individuals had also been linked to poor academic results [68].

Action of Leptin on brain affects synaptic plasticity and helps in removal of beta –amyloid which is thought to be beneficial for cognition. Raised leptin concentration in individuals with more body fat may hamper transportation of leptin across the blood brain barrier and may lead to the development of resistance to leptin. These events may result in the attenuation of the beneficial funcitions of leptin on brain. Thus persons with more body fat may show impaired cognition [69] and hence a negative influence of excessive body fat on academic performance will not be surprising and may be expected.

Greater cardiorespiratory fitness may promote executive control of working memory, attentive abilities, adjustment of cognitive skills, faster reaction time, activation of circuitry related to frontal and parietal regions of the brain, accuracies in response by individuals, memories related to arbitrary associations (relational memory), better hippocampal contribution to develop memories [70]. It may thus be expected that these physiological benefits in individuals who have good cardiorespiratory fitness, in conjunction with healthy body composition to some extinct may positively affect academic performance.

However, in the present study, positive relationship of lower magnitude was found to be present between cardiorespiratory fitness (PFI) and academic performance using correlation study. Moreover, multiple regression analysis found no independent associations between PFI and academic performance (a suppressor effect). Unlike some earlier studies on other population [19,20], the evidence obtained by the present study in support of the presence of positive impact of cardiorespiratory fitness on academics was fairly weak. Additively, literature had pointed out that depending on the technique or methodology of determination of cardiorespiratory fitness, the findings on the impact of the later on academic performance may vary [71]. Therefore further studies are needed to reach a definite conclusion regarding the association between CRF and academic performance in Bengali adolescents.

5. Conclusion

The findings documented herein found negative association of obesity parameters, viz., BMI, WHR and body fat % with PA. This provided evidences to support the fact that sufficient daily life PA may effectively prevent obesity. It may be said that obese adolescents may be able to lose weight owing to the implementation of adequate PA in their daily life. This present study confirmed that, increased cardiorespiratory fitness may be observed due to increment in PA. The results showed that increase in WHR and Body fat % may occur with increase in BMI, whereas decrease in BMI, WHR, Body fat % may take place due to increase in cardiorespiratory fitness. Poor performance in academics was linked to the presence of higher values of BMI, WHR and body fat %. Conversely, it was noted that greater cardiorespiratory fitness to a limited extent may be associated with better academic performance. Based on the findings of the present study, it may be said that sufficient PA in daily life may alter obesity parameters and cardiorespiratory fitness towards a healthy level which may positively influence academic performance by modulating cognition. The importance of daily life PA should not be restricted to only anti obesity campaign, instead its beneficial implications in relation to overall fitness and cognition should be promoted across all populations.

References

[1] Singh, R. "Childhood obesity: An epidemic in waiting?", *Int J Med. Public Health*, 3(1). 2-7. 2013.

[2] Vasudev, S., Mohan, A., Mohan, D., Farooq, S., Raj, D. and Mohan, V. "Validation of body fat measurement by skinfolds and two bioelectric impedance methods with DEXA–the Chennai Urban Rural Epidemiology Study [CURES-3]", *J Assoc Physicians India*, 52. 877-881. 2004.

[3] Rashmi and Jaswal, S. "Obesity and Academic Performance in Adolescents", *Int J Edu Sci*, 4(3). 275-278. 2012.

[4] Tudor-Locke, C.E and Myers, A.M. "Methodological considerations for researchers and practitioners using pedometers to measure physical (ambulatory) activity", *Res Q Exerc Sport*, 72. 1-12. 2001.

[5] Berkey, C.S., Rockett, H.R.H., Gillman, M.W. and Colditz, G.A. (2003). "One year changes in activity and in inactivity among 10- to 15-year-old boys and girls: relationship to change in body mass index", *Pediatrics*, 111.836-43. 2003.

[6] Mayo, M. J, Grantham, J.R, and Balasekaran,G. "Exercise-Induced Weight Loss Preferentially Reduces Abdominal Fat", *Med Sci Sports Exerc.* , 35(2). 207-13.2003.

[7] Kimm, S.Y.S., Glynn, N.W., Obarzanek, E., Kriska, A.M., Daniels, S.R., Barton, B.A., and Liu, K. "Relation between the changes in physical activity and body-mass index during adolescence: a multicentre longitudinal study" *Lancet*, 366. 301-07. 2005.

[8] Cuddihy T., Tomson, L.M., Jones, E.K. and Johnston, A.O. "E xploring the relationship between daily steps,body mass index and physical self-esteem in female Australian adolescents", *J Exerc Sci Fit*, 4 (1). 25-35. 2006.

[9] Mirhosseini, N.Z., Shahar, S., Yusoff, N.M., Mobarhan, M.G., Derakhshan, A.R. and Shakery, M.T. "Lower level of physical activity predisposes iranian adolescent girls to obesity and its metabolic consequences", *Pak. J Nutr*, 10(8). 728-734.2011.

[10] Shaikh, W.A., Patel, M.C. and Singh, S.K. "Association of physical activity and physical fitness with blood pressure profile in Gujarati Indian adolescents", *Indian J Physiol Pharmacol*, 55 (4). 322-328.2011.

[11] Mengistie, A.B., Reddy, R.C. and Babu, M.S. "The Effects of Combined Aerobic and Resistance Exercise Training on Obese Adults, Northwest Ethiopia", *Res. J Recent Sciences*, 2(1). 59-66. 2013.

[12] Mukhopadhyay, A., Bhadra, M. and Bose, K. "Physical exercise, body mass index, subcutaneous adiposity and body composition among Bengalee boys aged 10-17 years of Kolkata, India", *Anthropol Anz.*, 63(1). 93-101.2005.

[13] Bandyopadhyay, B. and Chattopadhyay, H. "Assessment of physical fitness of sedentary and physically active male college students by a modified Harvard step test", *Erogonomics*, 24(1). 15-20. 1981.

[14] Khodnapur, J. P., Dhanakshirur, G. B. and Aithala, M. "Role of Exercise and Nutrition on Cardiopulmonary Fitness", *Indian med Gaz*, 146(1). 6-9. 2012.

[15] Mukherjee, R. and Dhara, P.C. "Daily Physical Activity: The Link to Physical Fitness, Cognition and Academic Performance in Bengali (Indian) Adolescents of Rural and Urban Areas", *J. Biol. Chem. Research*, 30(2). 748-763. 2013.

[16] Sargent, J. D., and Blanchflower, D. G. "Obesity and stature in adolescence and earnings in young adulthood: Analysis of a British birth cohort", *Arch Pediatr Adolesc Med*, 148. 681-87. 1994.

[17] Crosnoe, R. and Muller. C. "Body mass index, academic achievement, and school context: Examining the educational experiences of adolescents at risk of obesity", J *Health Soc Behav*, 45. 393-407. 2004.

[18] Datar, A., Sturm, R. and Magnabosco, J. L. "Childhood overweight and academic performance: National study of kindergartners and first-graders". *Obesity Res, 12*(1). 58-68. 2004.

[19] Davis, C.L., Cooper, S. "Fitness, fatness, cognition, behavior, and academic achievement among overweight children: Do cross-

sectional associations correspond to exercise trial outcomes?", *Prev Med*, 52(suppl. 1). 65-69. 2011.

[20] Van Dusen, D.P., Kelder, S.H., Kohl, H.W., Ranjit, N.and Perry, C.L. "Associations of physical fitness and academic performance among school children", *J School Health*, 81(12). 733-740.2011.

[21] Kuppuswami, B. "*Manual of socio economic scale* ". Mansayan, Delhi, 1981.

[22] Kowalski, K.C., Crocker, P.R.E. and Kowalski, N.P. "Physical Activity Questionnaire for Adolescents", 1997. http://www.dapa-toolkit.mrc.ac.uk/documents/en/PAQ/PAQ_manual.pdf (Assessed October,2010).

[23] Kowalski, K.C., Crocker, P.R.E. and Faulkner, R.A. "Validation of the Physical Activity Questionnaire for Older Children", *Pediatric Exer Sci*, 9. 174-186. 1997.

[24] Brouha, L., Heath, C. W. and Graybiel, A. "A step test: A simple method of measuring physical fitness for hard muscular work in adult men", *Rev Cand Biol*,2. 86-91.1943.

[25] Cole, T.J., Bellizzi, M.C., Flegal, K.M.and Dietz, W.H. "Establishing a standard definition for child overweight and obesity worldwide: International survey", *BMJ*, 320. 1240-1243. 2000.

[26] Slaughter, M.H., Lohman, T.G., Boileau, R.A., Horewill, C.A., Stillman, R.J., VanLoan, M.D. and Bemben, D.A. "Skinfold equations for estimation of body fatness in children and youth", *Hum Biol*, 60. 709-723. 1988.

[27] Meo, S. A., Alkahlan, M. A., Al –Mubarak, M. A., Al-obayli, M. S., Melaibary, B. A., Bin Dous, A. N.and Alhassoun, A. I. "Impact of type 1 diabetes mellitus on academic performance", J. *Int. Med. Res.*, 41(3). 855-858. 2013.

[28] Sokal, R.R. and Rohlf, F.J. "*Biometry*", Freeman, New York. 2001.

[29] Casimirri, F., Pasquali, R., Cesari, M.P., Melchionda, N. and Barbara, L. "Interrelationships between body weight, body fat distributionand insulin in obese women before and after hypocaloricfeeding and weight loss", *Ann. Nutr. Metab.*, 33. 73-78. 1989.

[30] Wing, R.R., Jeffery, R.W., Burton, L.R., Thorson, C., Kuller, L.H.and Folsom, A. R. "Change in waist-hip ratio with weight loss and its association with change in cardiovascular risk factors", *Am J Clin Nutr.*, 55(6). 1086-92. 1992.

[31] Dennis, K.E. and Goldberg, A.P. " Differential effects of body fatness and body fat distribution on risk factors for cardiovascular disease in women: impact of weight loss," *Arterioscler. Thromb.*, 13:1487-1494, 1993.

[32] Mayo, M.J., Grantham, J.R. and Balasekaran, G. "Exercise-Induced Weight Loss Preferentially Reduces Abdominal Fat", *Med Sci Sports Exerc.*, 35(2). 207-13. 2003.

[33] Wing, R. R. And Hill, J. O. "Successful weight loss maintenance", *Annu. Rev. Nutr.* 21. 323-341. 2001.

[34] American College of Sports Medicine. "Appropriate intervention strategies for weight loss and prevention of weight regain for adults", *Med. Sci. Sports Exerc.*, 33. 2145-2156. 2001.

[35] Kimm, S.Y., Barton, B.A., Obarzanek, E., McMahon, R.P., Sabry, Z.I., Waclawiw, M.A., Schreiber, G.B., Morrison, J.A., Similo, S. and Daniels, S.R. "Racial divergence in adiposity during adolescence: the NHLBI Growth and Health Study", *Pediatrics*, 107. e34. 2001.

[36] Kimm, S.Y., Barton, B.A., Obarzanek, E., McMahon, R.P., Kronsberg, S.S., Waclawiw, M.A., Morrison, J.A., Schreiber, G.B., Sabry, Z.I. and Daniels, S.R. "Obesity development during adolescence in a biracial cohort: the NHLBI Growth and Health Study (NGHS),"*Pediatrics*, 110. e54. 2002.

[37] Kronsberg, S.S., Obarzanek, E., Affenito, S.G., Crawford, P.B., Sabry, Z.I., Schmidt, M., Striegel-Moore, R., Kimm, S.Y. and Barton, B.A. "Macronutrient intake of black and white adolescent girls over ten years: the NHLBI Growth and Health Study," *J Am Diet Assoc,* 103. 853-60. 2003.

[38] Park, T.S. "For the degree of contributions of socio-environmental factors and physical growth affecting physical development", *Korean J Growth Dev*, 1. 78-90. 1993.

[39] Lim, B.K.and Kim, H.G. "Assessment of health grade by physique and physical development index and healthy-life habits in elementary school students", *Korean J Growth Dev*, 12.17-28. 2004.

[40] Cho, K.O., Nam, S.N.and Kim, Y.S. "Assessments of nutrient intake and metabolic profiles in Korean adolescents according to exercise regularity using data from the 2008 Korean National Health and Nutrition Examination Survey", *Nutr Res Pract*,5(1). 66-72. 2011.

[41] Saha, S. "Somatic, body composition and anthropometric characteristics of college level men students", *Annals of Biol Res*, 4 (3). 95-100. 2013.

[42] Donnelly, J.E., Blair, S.N., Jakicic, J.M., Manore, M.M., Rankin, J.W., Smith, B.K. "American College of Sports Medicine Position Stand. Appropriate physical activity intervention strategies for weight loss and prevention of weight regain for adults," Med Sci Sports Exerc, 41. 459-471. 2009.

[43] Banerjee, I., Ghia, N., Bandopadhyay, S., Sayed, H.N. and Mukherjee, D. "Body mass index in Bengali adolescents", Indian Pediatr, 42. 262-267. 2005.

[44] Hattiwale, H.M.,.Maniyar, S.A.,.Das, K.K. and Dhundasi, S.A. "Role of BMI on PFI in two different age groups of healthy young males from north Karnataka", *Al Ameen J M ed Sci,*1(1). 50-54. 2008.

[45] Patil, R.B., Doddamani, B.R., Bhutkar, M. and Awanti, S.M. "A Comparative Study of Physical Fitness among Rural Farmers and Urban Sedentary Group of Gulbarga District", Al Ame en J Med Sci, 5 (1). 39-44. 2012.

[46] Ingjer, F. "Effects of endurance training on muscle fibre ATP-ase activity, capillary supply and mitochondrial content in man", *J Physiol*, 294. 419-32, 1979.

[47] Adolfsson, J., Ljungqvist, A., Tornling, G. and Unge, G. "Capillary increase in the skeletal muscle of trained young and adult rats", *J Physiol*, 310. 529-32, 1981.

[48] Holloszy, J.O. and Coyle, E.F. "Adaptations of skeletal muscle to endurance exercise and their metabolic consequences", *J Appl Physiol*, 56. 831-8, 1984.

[49] Wagner, P.D. "Skeletal muscle angiogenesis. A possible role for hypoxia", *Adv Exp Med Biol* 502. 21-38, 2001.

[50] Terjung, R.L., Zarzeczny, R.and Yang, H.T. "Muscle blood flow and mitochondrial function: Influence of aging", *Int J Sport Nutr Exerc Metab*, 12. 368-78, 2002.

[51] Hujova, Z. and Lesniakova, M. "Anthopometric risk factors of atherosclerosis:Differences between urban and rural East – Slovakian children and adolescent", *Bratisl Lek Listy*, 112(9). 491-496. 2011.

[52] Deshmukh, P.R., Gupta, S.S., Bharambe, M.S., Dongre, A.R., Maliye, C., Kaur, S. and Garg, B.(2006). "Nutritional status of adolescencts in rural wardah", *Indian J Pediatr*, 73(2). 139-141. 2006.

[53] Björntorp, P. "Abdominal fat distribution and the metabolic syndrome", *J Cardiovasc Pharmacol.*, 20 Suppl 8. S26-8. 1992.

[54] Rössner, S., Bo, W.J,.Hiltbrandt, E.,Hinson, W.,Karstaedt, N., Santago, P., Sobol, W.T. and Crouse, J.R. (1990). "Adipose tissue determinations in cadavers—a comparison between cross-sectional planimetry and computed tomography", *Int J Obes*, 14. 893-902. 1990.

[55] Das, S.K.,Mahapatre, S.,Bhattacharaya, G. and Mukherjee, D. "Determination of PFI with modified HST in young men and women",*Ind. J.Physiol and allied.Sci*, 47(2). 73-76. 1993.

[56] Häkkinen, A., Rinne, M., Vasankari, T., Santtila, M., Häkkinen, K. and Kyröläinen, H. "Association of physical fitness with health-related quality of life in Finnish young men", Health and Quality of Life Outcomes, 8. 15. 2010.

[57] Manssor, A.J., Al-janabi, H.O., Kamel, N.K.and Marbut, M.M. "A comparative study between male & female students attending submaximal exercise in regard to recovery heart rate & blood pressure", *Tikrit Med J*, 17(1): 156-160. 2011.

[58] Lean, M.E., Han, T.S. and Morrison, C.E. "Waist circumference as a measure for indicating need for weight management", *BMJ.*, 311(6998). 158-161. 1995.

[59] Ochiai, H., Shirasawa, T., Nishimura, R., Morimoto, A., Shimada, N., Ohtsu, T., Kujirai, E., Hoshino, H., Tajima, N. and Kokaze, A."Relationship of body mass index to percent body fat and waist circumference among schoolchildren in Japan--the influence of gender and obesity: a population-based cross-sectional study", *BMC Public Health.*, 10:493, 2010 [online] Available: http://www.biomedcentral.com/1471-2458/10/493. [Accessed October 10, 2013].

[60] Bandyopadhyay, A. "Cardiorespiratory fitness in obese girls", *Indian J Physiol Pharmacol*, 56(4). 393-395.2012.

[61] Chikuji, K., Motoyama, M., Ohto, H., Morita, T., Sunami, Y., Tanaka, M. and Shindo, M. "The effects of low intensity aerobic training on the physiological indexes and the quality of life in middle-aged white collar workers", *Sangyo Eiseigaku Zasshi.*, 41(3). 63-71. 1999.

[62] Lokken, K.L., Boeka, A.G., Austin, H.M., Gunstad, J.and Harmon, C.M. "Evidence of executive dysfunction in extremely obese adolescents: a pilot study", *Surg Obes Relat Dis*., 5:547-552. 2009.

[63] Mo-suwan, L., Lebel, L., Puetpaiboon, A. and Junjana, C. "School performance and weight status of children and young adolescents in a transitional society in Thailand" *Inter J Obes,* 23. 272-277. 1999.

[64] Gunstad, J., Spitznagel, M.B., Paul, R.H., Cohen, R.A., Kohn, M. et al. "Body mass index and neuropsychological function in healthy children and adolescents", *Appetite*, 50. 246-251.2008.

[65] Jagust,W., Harvey, D., Mungas, D. and Haan, M. " Central obesity and the aging brain", *Arch Neurol*., 62. 1545-1548.2005.

[66] Waldstein, S. R. And Katzel, L. I. "Interactive relations of central versus total obesity and blood pressure to cognitive function", *Int J Obes,* 30. 201-207. 2006.

[67] Sabia, J.J. "The effect of body weight on adolescent academic performance", *Southern Economic Journal,* 73(4). 871-900. 2007.

[68] Mohammad, A. "Relationship Between Self-esteem and Academic Achievement Amongst Pre-University Students", *J App Sci*, 10. 2474-2477. 2010.

[69] Zeki Al Hazzouri, A., Haan, M.N., Whitmer, R.A., Yaffe, K. and Neuhaus, J."Central Obesity, Leptin and Cognitive Decline: the Sacramento Area Latino Study on Aging", *Dement Geriatr Cogn Disord.,* 33(6). 400-9. 2012.

[70] Haapala, E.A. "Cardiorespiratory Fitness and Motor Skills in Relation to Cognition and Academic Performance in Children – A Review", *J Hum Kinet*., 36. 55-68. 2013.

[71] Dwyer, T., Sallis, J., Blizzard, L., Lazarus, R., and Dean, K.. "Relation of academic performance to physical activity and fitness in children", *Ped Exerc Sci*, 13(3). 225-237. 2001.

4

Evaluation of Joint Position Sense after ACL Reconstruction with Hamstring Tendon Auto Graft

Gholam A. Ghasemi[1,*], Vahid Zolaktaf[1], Khosravi Ibrahim[2], Minasian V[1]

[1]Department of Exercise science , University of Isfahan, Isfahan, Iran
[2]Department of Exercise Rehab, Faculty of Exercise Sciences, University of Isfahan, Isfahan, Iran
*Corresponding author: Gh. Ghasemi@yahoo.com

Abstract **Background:** Use of STG (Semitendinosus and gracilis) graft is one of the standard techniques for anterior cruciate ligament (ACL) reconstruction. The purpose of this study was the comparison of joint position sense (JPS) in involved and uninvolved knees of ACL reconstructed athletes and control group. **Methods:** Fifteen elite athletes (7 handballs, 8 soccer players) with a unilateral ACL rupture who had received a hamstring tendon auto grafts ACL reconstruction, matched by motor dominance and sport to fifteen healthy elite athletes, were subjects of our study. The injured group experienced an average of 19.9 months from surgery to participation in the research. The Biodex System III Isokinetic dynamometer and Active Angle Reproduction test with angle of 30° knee flexion were used for evaluation of knee JPS. **Results:** No significant difference was found between involved and uninvolved knees of ACL reconstructed group and between involved knee of ACL reconstructed and control group (p<0/05). **Conclusion:** The present study revealed that athletes with ACL reconstructed knee may have not experience JPS malfunction. This fact suggests that proprioceptive acuity has multimodal characteristics and is not always primarily dependent on the sensory information of ligament mechanoreceptors. There is the possibility of offsetting this deficit by regeneration of sensory neurons in the reconstructed ligament or by rehabilitation program.

Keywords: *joint position sense, anterior cruciate ligament reconstruction, hamstring (STG) tendon auto graft*

1. Introduction

ACL injury is more frequent in athletes, and usually causes long time absence from sports activities, and is associated with an increased risk of recurrent knee injury [1,2]. Estimated rates of reconstructions performed per year in the United States ranges from 60,000 to 175,000 [3,4]. Previous studies reported that in athletes the rate of return to sports was 70-80% [5,6]. However, there are some complications after ACL reconstruction. Contralateral ACL injury is one of the most serious complications after reconstruction [7].

Knee joint function is complex and does not depend on ligament stability alone, but also on the dynamic interaction between the central nervous system and the periarticular muscles. This is achieved by means of various mechanoreceptors and free nerve endings, which have been identified in the articular and periarticular knee joint structures [8]. They are found in particularly high numbers in the area close to the insertion of the ACL [9].

Proprioreceptors are the components of somatosensation that provides information about the orientation and motion of body segments and the state of the muscles. This information is conveyed largely through muscle spindles and Golgi tendon organs [10]. To investigate the role that Proprioreceptors plays in planning and controlling movements, proprioception has been removed through either surgery or by studying rare sensory neuropathy conditions, or has been distorted by the use of vibration [10]. Following the pioneering findings of Mott and Sherrington [10], many studies have examined the role of proprioception in movement control by examining movements in non-human primates who have undergone partial dorsal rhizotomy surgery, including the studies of Gilman et al. [11], Taub et al. [12], Polit and Bizzi [13] and Gauthier and Mussa Ivaldi [10], among others. It has been well established that animals proprioceptively differenced in this way show substantial impairments in accuracy and coordination during multijoint reaching and natural unrestricted movements [10].

Proprioception appears have critical role for controlling other aspects of limb mechanics, in addition to the effects of intersegmental dynamics. For example, Ghez et al. [14], showed that deafferented patients were unable to account for direction dependent variations in limb inertia during reaching movements, which resulted in substantial errors in movement distance and direction. Because direction dependent variations in limb inertia vary with limb configuration, this finding underscored the importance of proprioception in providing configuration information [14], showed that deafferented patients were unable to account for direction dependent variations in limb inertia during reaching movements, which resulted in substantial errors in movement distance and direction. Because direction dependent variations in limb inertia vary with limb configuration, this finding underscored the importance of proprioception in providing configuration information [14]. The critical role of proprioception in providing initial information of the postural state of the motor apparatus for movement planning is also supported by the study of Larish et al. [15]. This study also showed that when the limb was vibrated in the absence of visual feedback prior to the movement, final position was systematically altered [15]. Barrack et al.[16] reported decreased proprioception in knees with a ruptured ACL on the basis of an evaluation of the joint position sense. Ochi et al.[17] also studied joint position sense in knees with a ruptured ACL and demonstrated decreased joint position sense in patients with marked knee instability. However, there are also reports denying a relationship between ACL injury and changes in proprioception [5].

However, ACL injuries induces changes in the kinematics of the knee joint, instability, and proprioception impairment [18]. Injury to the ACL will result in a loss of both mechanical stability and proprioceptive feedback at the knee, directly affecting functional joint stability and can lead to further deterioration of the knee joint integrity [19]. Due to instability of the joint, repetitive injury and degenerative changes occur and the sports activity and even the daily life of the person are confused [20]. These cases determine the necessity for the ACL reconstruction surgery.

Therefore, it is becoming increasingly clear that knees with ruptured ACL gradually develop changes not only in performance but also in proprioception. However, as reported by Noyes et al. [21], we encounter individuals who readily perform high levels of athletic activities despite injury to the ACL [22].

Previous studies revealed that an integral element in achieving a favorable outcome following ACL reconstruction is participation in the postoperative rehabilitation [23]. The mechanical restraint and proprioceptive function of the ACL both help to provide functional joint stability of the knee during movement. Therefore, it is essential to monitor the restoration of proprioception after an ACL injury or ACL reconstruction/rehabilitation for safe and functional return to sport and should be considered in the evaluation of surgery results by orthopedic surgeons [24].

Although, different types of autograft and allograft have been used in ACL reconstruction for many years, recently the hamstring tendon has become the preferred autogenous graft [25,26]. In our comprehensive survey, we found that a few research has been done for the assessment of knee joint proprioceptive function after ACL reconstruction with STG graft. Hence, the aim of this research was to evaluate knee joint proprioception in elite athletes after ACL reconstruction with STG graft.

2. Materials and Methods

The participants were 30 male soccer and handball elite players who competing at premier leagues and Iranian national teams, and were classified as control (non-injured) and ACL-reconstructed (injured) groups. The participants in the control group consisted of 15 healthy elite athletes (8 soccer and 7 handball aged 23.06 ± 3.1 years, height 184.4 ± 7.8 cm, Weight of 85.2 ± 1.1 kg; mean ± s) with no previous history of lower-extremity orthopedic pathology. The participants in the ACL-reconstructed group consisted of 15 elite athletes (8 soccer and 7 handball mean aged 23.8 ± 3.5 years, Height 180.4 ± 7.6 cm, & Weight 76.4 ± 1.02 kg) who had undergone a unilateral ACL reconstruction with STG tendon graft. The injured group matched by motor dominance and sport with fifteen healthy elite athletes. The "accessible" sampling method was used for selecting the samples. The injured group experienced an average of 19.9 months (range 8 ± 60 months) from surgery to participation in the research. In this study we have some limitations to initiate the testing protocols, such as subjects and physicians permissions, and the number of subjects ready to take part in this study. All participants demonstrated a full, pain-free range of motion at the knee joint at the time of testing, and were excluded if they experienced any pain, effusion or edema during the test procedure.

Exclusion criteria included multiple surgical procedures in the involved knee, contralateral knee pathology, and age less than 18 years, limited ROM due to surgery, injury of the ankle and hip joint, time lapse of less than 6 months after ACL reconstruction, patellofemoral joint dysfunction and unstable co-existing cardiovascular, neurological, psychiatric or psychological conditions.

Biodex System 3 Isokinetic Dynamometer (Biodex Medical Inc., Shirley, NY, USA.) and active angle reproduction test were used to assess knee JPS. Visual cues were eliminated by a blindfold.

On the test day participants have to wear light clothes, and they completed a consent form. Personal information list completed with the investigator. Each subject was seated on the biodex isokinetic dynamometer with hip flexion of 100° and the axis of their knee joint aligned with the axis of the dynamometer arm. The ankle strap of the dynamometer arm was applied to the ankle 2 inches above the medial malleolus. The thigh strap also was applied. The dynamometer was calibrated by asking the participant to hold the knee at 0 degrees of extension, and the position checked using a hand held goniometer. The participant's knee was then returned to an angle of 90 degrees. Starting at 90° of knee flexion, the subject actively moved the limb to the target angle of 30° of flexion at an angular velocity approximating 5°·s. This angle is in the working range of the knee during daily weight-bearing activities. Subjects were instructed to voluntarily contract their muscles. The limb was maintained at the target angle for 10 seconds to enable the subject to remember the position. After the limb was passively returned to 90°, there was a 5-second pause, and the cycle was performed again. This time the subject activated a handheld stop button when he felt the target angle had been achieved. Once the button had been activated, patients were not permitted to correct the angle. The angle was identified from the onscreen goniometer. Three readings were taken, and the absolute difference between the perceived angle and the target angle was calculated for each reading. We used the average of these three scores as the error score for each subject.

SPSS software (ver. 16) was used for data analyzing. One-way ANOVA was used for comparing the average absolute error of the target angle for the operated knee, as regards with the healthy leg of the person himself and the matched knee of control group. Statistics significance were carried out at an alpha level of $P < 0.05$.

3. Results

Demographic data of the injured and healthy groups are shown in Table 1. The mean values and standard deviation of the reproduced angle absolute error for the injured and healthy group are shown in Table 2. Kolmogorov-Smirnov test ($P < 0.05$) was used to analyze the normality of the data and the Q-Q plots and box plots were also used for more assurance. ANOVA test showed that there is no significant difference between the average values of error score in ACL reconstructed knee as compare to contralateral knee and the knee of control group. ($F = 1.21$, $P = 0.3$).

Table 1. Demographics characteristics of Subjects (mean± standard deviation)

	Weight(kg)	Height(cm)	Age(y)
Injured group(n=15)	76.4 ± 1.02	180.43 ±7.63	23.86 ±3.58
Control group(n=15)	85.23 ± 1.17	184.47 ± 7.82	23.06 ± 3.10

Table 2. Absolute error of active angle reproduction test (Mean± standard deviation)

	Reconstructed knee	**Uninjured knee**	**Matched knee of Control group**
Absolute error	4.02 ± 1.55	3.12 ± 1.44	3.92 ± 2.11

4. Discussion

According to the results of this research, there was no significant difference between the JPS at the injured knee in comparison with contralateral knee and the knee of control group. As mentioned before the most important role of ligaments like ACL is providing the joint mechanical stability. Disruption of this support mechanism changes the joint kinematics and induces joint instability and osteoarthritic changes [27].

However, Kennedy et al. [28] reported that clinical symptoms characteristic of knees with ACL injury occur due to the disappearance of mechanoreceptor feedback in addition to altered kinematics. This report was followed by studies on proprioception of knees with a ruptured ACL [16,29,30]. Also some researcher like Barrack et al. [16] demonstrated a correlation between the magnitude of joint instability and the reduction of proprioception in knees with a ruptured ACL, and Ochi et al. [17] performed an electrophysiological study of knees with a ruptured ACL using somatosensory evoked potential (SEP) and concluded that SEP was low in patients with reduced joint position sense. Their findings also showed that sensory reinnervation occurred in the reconstructed human ACL and was closely related to the function of the knee [17]. Fremerey et al. [31] assessed knee proprioception using the angle reproduction test after reconstruction of the ACL. Six months after reconstruction, restoration of proprioception was seen near full extension and full flexion. In the intermediate motion range, no improvements could be demonstrated. Al-Othman [32] also demonstrated the complete recovery of proprioception following ACL. In a research by Hopper et al. [33] no significant difference observed in JPS between reconstructed and uninjured knees or between the flexion and extension tasks, that is compatible with the findings of our study.

Research by Risberg et al. [34] also indicates that there were no significant differences in proprioception between the ACL-reconstructed knee and the contra-lateral uninvolved knee 1 year or more after surgery. Bonfim et al. [20] did not find an improvement of proprioceptive function following ACL reconstruction in comparison with a control group. Other authors also report persistent impairment of proprioception [35,36]. Wilke and Froböse [37] found that the patient's position influenced the results of the joint position sense test. Proprioceptive information is different in the supine position as compared with standing and sitting positions because muscle recruitment is altered in the horizontal position.

Regarding the position of the knee, there are various results among different studies. The selected angle for the present research was chosen according to Grood and Noyes [38] investigation. The reason for this selection is that at 30° flexion of the knee, this joint is in a loose-packed position, where the ACL mechanical function is at its minimum. Hence, the neuromuscular mechanisms related to the joint stability of this ligament around this angle are most important. One research [33] also indicates that muscle-tendon receptors have greater role regarding joint receptors in providing JPS. Lephart et al. stated that the knee JPS could be improved by balance exercises [39]. In this study we examined subjects who were given rehabilitation by strength training, in the acute period after ACL injury and had no marked difficulty in daily activities including walking.

The existing differences between the studies could be related to the numbers of subjects involved, the surgery methods used in reconstruction of ACL, different angles in performing the test, rehabilitation programs, sport skills patterns and testing methods (active or passive, weight bearing or non-weight bearing). Therefore, regarding the unification between the two groups by consideration of sport activity levels, age and sex; it seems that lack of Proprioceptive information resulted from the reconstructed ligament to be offset by other proprioceptive sources. Also, there is the possibility for the joint mechanical receptors not to have a primary role in provision of JPS, or for the regeneration of sensory nerves in the reconstructed ligament to offset the loss of proprioception.

5. Conclusion

The following conclusions were reached from the results of our study, the results by this study showed that there is no significant difference in the knee JPS at the injured knee in comparison with contra-lateral knee and the knee of control group. It seems that the knee joint proprioception has a multimodal characteristic, not limiting to sensory information of the ligaments mechanoreceptors. There is also the possibility that the rehabilitation program or innervations of reconstructed ligament could offset this deficit.

References

[1] Roi GS NG, Tencone F. Time to return to professional soccer matches after ACL reconstruction. Sport Sci Health. 2006;1:142-5.

[2] Walden M HM, Ekstrand J. High risk of new knee injury in elite footballers with previous anterior cruciate ligament injury. Br J Sports Med. 2006;40:158-62.

[3] Frank CB JD. The science of reconstruction of the anterior cruciate ligament. J Bone Joint Surg Am. 1997;79:1556-76.

[4] Spindler KP WR. Clinical practice. Anterior cruciate ligament tear. N Engl J Med. 2008;359:2135-42.

[5] Katayama M HH, Kimura M, Kobayashi A, Hatayama K, Terauchi M, Takagishi K. Proprioception and performance after anterior cruciate ligament rupture. International Orthopaedics (SICOT). 2004;28:278-81.

[6] Nakase Junsuke TH, Kitaoka Katsuhiko,. Contralateral anterior cruciate ligament injury after anterior cruciate ligament reconstruction: a case controlled study. Sports Medicine, Arthroscopy, Rehabilitation, Therapy & Technology. 2012;4(46):1-4.

[7] Akoto Ralph HJ. Anterior cruciate ligament (ACL) reconstruction with quadriceps tendon autograft and press-fit fixation using an anteromedial portal technique. Musculoskeletal Disorders. 2012;13(161):1471-2474.

[8] Raunest J SM, Burgener E. Proprioceptive mechanisms in the cruciate ligaments: an electromyographic study on reflex activity in the thigh muscles. J Trauma. 1996;41:488-93.

[9] Adachi N OM, Uchio Y, Iwasa J, Ryoke K, Kuriwaka M. Mechanoreceptors in the anterior cruciate ligament contribute to the joint position sense. Acta Orthop Scand. 2002;73:330-4.

[10] Sarlegna FS, R. The Roles of Vision and Proprioception in the Planning of Reaching Movements. Adv Exp Med Biol. 2009;629:317-35.

[11] Gilman S CD, Hollenberg J. Kinematic effects of deafferentation and cerebellar ablation. Brain. 1976;99:99:311-30. [PubMed: 825186].

[12] Taub E GI, Taub P. Deafferentation in monkeys: pointing at a target without visual feedback. Exp Neurol. 1975 46( ):178-86. [PubMed: 1109336].

[13] Polit A BE. haracteristics of motor programs underlying arm movements in monkeys. J Neurophysiology. 1979;42:183-94. [PubMed: 107279].

[14] 14. Ghez C FM, Ghilardi MF, Gordon J, Bermejo R, Pullman S. Discrete and continuous planning of hand movements and isometric force trajectories. Exp Brain Res. 1997;115:217-33.

[15] Larish DD VC, Wallace SA. An empirical note on attaining a spatial target after distorting the initial conditions of movement via muscle vibration. J Mot Behav. 1984;16:76-83.

[16] Barrack RL SH, Buckley SL. Proprioception in the anterior cruciate deficient knee. Am J Sports Med. 1989;17:1-6.

[17] Ochi M IJ, Uchio Y, Adachi N, Sumen Y. The regeneration of sensory neurones in the reconstruction of the anterior cruciate ligament. J Bone Joint Surg [Br]. 1999;81:902-6.

[18] Angoules AG MA, Dimitriou R, Karzis K, Drakoulakis E, Michos J, Papagelopoulos PJ. Knee proprioception following ACL reconstruction: a prospective trial comparing hamstrings with bone-patellar tendon-bone autograft. knee. 2011;18:76-82.

[19] Lephart S SC, Fu F, Huxel K. Reestablishing neuromuscular control. Rehabilitation techniques for sports medicine and athletic training. 5 ed. new york: McGraw-Hill; 2011. 122-43 p.

[20] Bonfim TR JPCCBJ. Proprioception and behavior impairments in individuals with anterior cruciat ligament reconsruction knees. Archive of physical medicine rehabilitation. 2003;84:1217-23.

[21] Noyes FR BS, Mangine RE. Abnormal lower limb symmetry determined by function hop tests after anterior cruciate ligament rupture. Am J Sports Med. 1991;19:513-8.

[22] Fitzgerald GK AM, Snyder-Mackler. A decisionmaking scheme for returning patients to high-level activity with nonoperative treatment after anterior cruciate ligament rupture. Knee Surg Sports Traumatol Arthrosc. 2000;8:76-82.

[23] Shaw T WM, Chipchase LS. Do early quadriceps exercises affect the outcome of ACL reconstruction? A randomized controlled trial. Aust J Physiother. 2005;51:9-17.

[24] Cerulli G BD, Caraffa A, Ponteggia F (2001) Proprioceptive training and prevention of anterior cruciate ligament injuries in soccer. J Orthop Sports Phys Ther. 2001;31:655-61.

[25] Freedman K DAM, Nedeff D, Ari Kaz, Bach B. Arthroscopic anterior cruciate ligament reconstruction: a metaanalysis comparing patellar tendon and hamstring tendon autografts. Am J Sports Med. 2003;31:2-11.

[26] Valentin A EmB, Werner S. ACL reconstruction: patellar tendon versus hamstring grafts economical aspects. Knee Surg Sports Traumatol Arthrosc. 2006;4:536-41.

[27] Hawkins RJ MG, Merritt TR. Followup of the acute nonoperated isolated anterior cruciate ligament tear. Am J Sports Med. 1986;14:205-10.

[28] Kennedy JC AI, Hayes KC. Nerve supply of the human knee and its functional importance. Am J Sports Med. 1982;10:329-35.

[29] Corrigan JP CW, Brady MP. Proprioception in the cruciate deficient knee. J Bone Joint Surg [Br]. 1992;74:247-50.

[30] Friden T RD, Movin T, Wredmark T. Function after anterior cruciate ligament injuries. Influence of visual control and proprioception. Acta Orthop Scand. 1998;69:590-4.

[31] Fremerey RW LP, Zeichen J, Skutek M, Bosch U, Tscherne H. Proprioception after rehabilitation and reconstruction in knees with deficiency of the anterior cruciate ligament. A prospective longitudinal study. J Bone Joint Surg Br. 2000;82:801-6.

[32] AA A-O. Clinical measurement of proprioceptive function after anterior cruciate ligament reconstruction. Saudi Med J. 2004;25:195-7.

[33] Hopper Dm CM, Formby Pa, Goh Sc, Boyle Jj, Strauss Gr. Functional measurement of knee joint position sense after anterior cruciate ligament reconstruction. Arch Phys Med Rehabil. 2003;84(6):868-72.

[34] Risberg Ma BB, Peura Gd, Uh Bs. Proprioception after anterior cruciate ligament reconstruction with and without bracing. Knee Surg Sports Traumatol Arthrosc. 1999;7:303-9.

[35] Carter ND JT, Wilson D, Jones DW, Torode AS. Joint position sense and rehabilitation in the anterior cruciate ligament deficient knee. Br J Sports Med. 1997;31:209-12.

[36] MacDonald PB HD, Pacin O, Sutherland K. Proprioception in anterior cruciate ligament-deficient and reconstructed knees. Am J Sports Med. 1996;24:774-8.

[37] 37. Wilke C FI. Quantifizierung propriozeptiver Leistungen von Kniegelenken (Quantification of proprioceptive skills of the knee joint). Dtsch Z Sportmed. 2003;54:49-54.

[38] Grood ES NF. Diagnosis of knee ligaments injuries: Biomechanical precepts. In The Crucial Ligaments: Diagnosis and Treatment of Ligamentous Injuries About the Knee: New York: Churchill Livingstone; 1988. 245-60 p.

[39] Lephart Sm PD, Giraldo Jl, Fu FH. The role of proprioception in the management and rehabilitation of athletic injuries. Am J Sports Med. 1997;25(1):130-7.

5

A Pilot Study of the Physiological Demands of Futsal Referees Engaged in International Friendly Matches

D. Dixon*

Applied Sport and Exercise Sciences, School of Health Sport and Bioscience, University of East London. London, UK
*Corresponding author: d.dixon@uel.ac.uk

Abstract Futsal is a FIFA sanctioned form of 5-a-side football. It is controlled by two referees who run up and down the touchlines either side of the pitch ensuring the laws of the game are enforced. The match is played over two halves of 20 minutes, with the clock being stopped every time the ball goes out of play; so each half can last up to 40 minutes including stoppage time. To date there has been minimal research which has looked at the physiological demands of refereeing futsal. This pilot study was undertaken over consecutive days when two International futsal games took place involving four referees. Heart rate, core temperature, blood lactate and hydration status were monitored prior to the match, again at half time and at full time. The results showed that the referees operated at between 81 and 84% Heart Rate Maximum (HR_{max}). There was a marked difference between the first and second referee in both games and between the first and second halves. Core temperature increased during the game with the referees becoming progressively dehydrated towards the end of the game. Blood lactate was found on average to be higher at the end of the first half compared to the end of the second half (2.33 vs. 1.8 $mmol.l^{-1}$) and referees in the first game had readings higher than the second game (HT 2.8 vs. 1.9 $mmol.l^{-1}$; FT 2.4 vs. 1.2 $mmol.l^{-1}$). In conclusion, the major findings show that further investigation is needed into the physiological demands of Futsal Refereeing and that in future, activity profiling should also be considered.

Keywords: *heart rate, blood lactate, futsal, referee, indoor soccer, physiology*

1. Introduction

Futsal is the only 5-a-side form of football that is officially sanctioned by FIFA. It has been around since 1930, with the first world championships being played in 1971 under International Federation for Futebol de Sala, (FIFUSA) and finally coming under FIFA's umbrella, with the first World Cup being played in 1989 in Holland. The main differences between this version and 11-a-side soccer are that it is played indoors on a pitch that measures 40 x 20 metres and is played has an effective playing time of 20 minutes each way. The game itself is classed as an intermittent high-intensity sport with players changing directions / activity every 3.28 seconds [1] which is helped by the players being able to undergo unlimited substitutions without stopping play [2].

The Referee is responsible for enforcing the laws of the game in invasion type sports such as Futsal. However, unlike the 11 a side version of soccer, it employs two referees who operate up and down the touch lines. There is an increasing amount of research examining the physiological and psychological demands placed on the 11 a side soccer referee and assistant referees. Recently it has been reported that the demands of the futsal referee are similar to an FIFA Assistant Referee [4,13]. The research of [3,6,7] have been reported that assistant referees, undergo intense brief bouts of forward and sideways running. Although to date, there has little research that has examined the physiological demands of futsal referees. However, Rebelo et al [5] examined the physiological demands of experienced Futsal referees from the Portuguese first division. The referees were subject to lactate testing, heart rate (HR) measurement and motion analysis through video. The results showed that the referees covered an average of 5.89 Kilometres (Km), which is less than the 6.76 Km (S = 0.83; range = 5.20–8.21) [6] and 7.28 (s = 0.17) Km [6] reported to be covered by Assistant Referees during a game of 11-a-side soccer.

Rebelo et al [5] reported the average heart rate of the futsal referees during the match was 146 b.min-1, or 76% of their HRmax. This is higher than values measured by reference [6] for Danish assistant referees who recorded 137 b.min-1 (s = 3) or 73% of the HRmax and 124 b.min-1 (s = 15) for FIFA Assistant Referees found by Kustrup et al [6].

Reilly and Gregson [7] found that the assistant referees in professional games had blood lactate levels of 4.7 mmol.l-1 at half time and 4.8 mmol.l-1 at the end of their respective 11-a-side games, these lactate levels are in contrast to Kustrup et al [6] who reported values of 2.8 mmol.l-1 at the end of both halves. Similarly, Rebelo et al

[5] reported levels of 1.0, 2.0 and 1.5 mmol.l-1 1 in the Portuguese futsal referees when recorded before the match, at half time and at the end of the game respectively. These differences can be contributed to the futsal referees had sufficient breaks in play to allow sufficient recovery [5]. Therefore the suggestion would be that in these games there was limited use of the anaerobic glycolysis energy pathway and that the games in this particular research were not as intense as the games reported in previous player studies. Although another explanation may be that the lower values for heart rate and blood lactate were found in those officiating in their respective domestic leagues and as such the intensities found in International futsal may be similar to those found in the 11-a-side soccer games.

Humans attempt to maintain a constant core temperature (Tc) of 37°C [8] although core temperatures have been shown to be as high as 39.5°C in Swedish first division players at the end of their match [9]. This is thought to be a result of fluid loss as the lack of fluid will disrupt the cooling process. However, these games are usually played outdoors and futsal is played indoors during varying temperatures and as such core temperatures could be higher due to the lack of air velocity.

Therefore the purpose of this paper was to complete a preliminary investigation on whether the physiological demands of International futsal refereeing were more intense than refereeing futsal games in a professional domestic league. In addition the physiological demands will be compared to those undertaken by assistant referees in 11-a-side soccer.

2. Materials and Methods

Four high level futsal referees (3 FIFA and 1 National League) volunteered to participate in this study during two international friendly games. Prior to the data collection, the referees were informed about the procedures and the possible constraints before providing their informed consent.

Their mean height, body mass and age were 1.84m (s = 0.13), 82.15 Kg (s = 19.95) and 36 years (s = 9.02) respectively.

Heart rate was recorded continuously from each of the officials over the two matches every 5 seconds using Polar Team2 (version 1.4.5, Polar Electro Oy, Finland) from 1 hour before the game started and as such recorded heart rate values for the warm up, first half and the second half.

Core body temperature was measured via CorTemp monitoring System (CorTemp, HQInc, Palmetto, Florida) which consists of a ingestible thermometer which was consumed three hours before kick-off and the signal was then relayed to a hand held data recorder which was positioned against the lower back of the referee via a runners belt which was worn around the waist under the referees shirt. Data was recorded every 10 seconds starting about 1 hour before kick-off.

Blood lactate was collected from the referees via finger prick blood sample at rest and within 5 minutes of the end of the first and second halves in order to establish blood lactate concentration using a Lactate Pro (Arkray Global Business Inc, Japan).

Hydration status was monitored via the referees supplying a urine sample 1 hour before kick-off and then again at half time and full time. Urine samples were then marked and analysed with an Osmocheck (Vitech Scientific, West Sussex, England) which was calibrated with distilled water before and after each referees group of three samples.

The referees were instructed to continue with their normal pre-match routines and to drink fluid ad libitum before and during the matches.

For data analysis, periods of the match were divided into 10 minute segments as per the research of Rebelo et al. [5] Krustrup et al. [9], as the effective playing time is usually longer than the prescribed 20 minutes for each half. The last time period (30+ and 70+) in each half corresponds to the time that elapsed from 30 and 60 minutes respectively until the end of each half [5,9].

Statistical data is presented as mean and standard deviation.

3. Results

Heart rate and core temperature from a representative participant is shown in Figure 1. The mean heart rate was 136 beats.min-1 (s=23.34), 155 beats.min-1 (s=23.04) and 149 beats.min-1 (s=21.49) during the warm up, first half and second half respectively. This related to 74%, 84% and 81% of heart rate maximum (HRmax =184 beats.min-1 (s=9.02)). The mean heart rate was higher in the first half compared to the second and the overall values were higher for the first referee compared to the second referee.

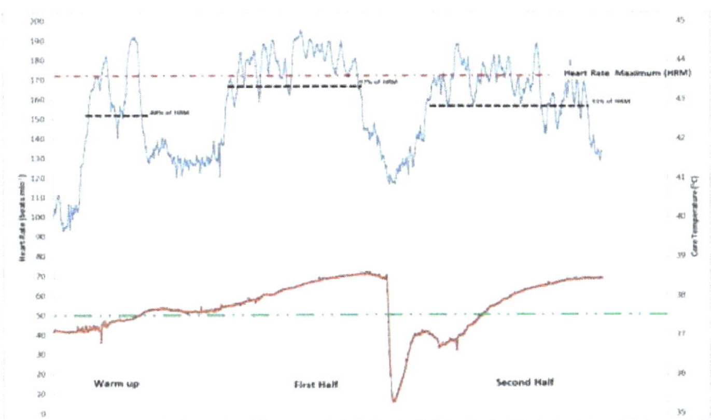

Figure 1. Heart Rate and Core Temperature Data

Also in Figure 1 is one of the referee's core temperature reading over the course of the match. The mean temperature over the course of the game was 38.58°C (s=0.6; range= 37.70 – 39.34). As can be seen from Figure 1 the core temperature of the referee gradually rose as each half went on, with the highest temperatures being recorded at the end of the match in each of the referees readings.

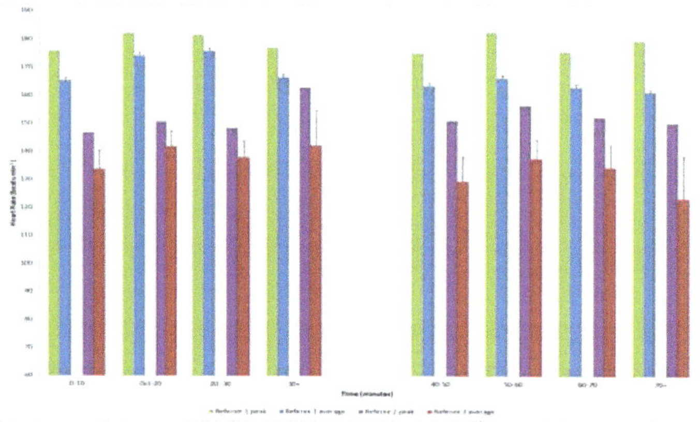

Figure 2. Peak and Average Heart rates of 1st and 2nd referees for each 10 minute spell of games

The above figure shows the peak and average heart rates from the 1st and 2nd Referees are shown over the two games. It can be seen that the 1st referees were operating at a high intensity than the 2nd referee in each of the 10 minutes. Although the 1st referees intensity seems to drop in the second half whereas the heart rate intensity seems to stay the same.

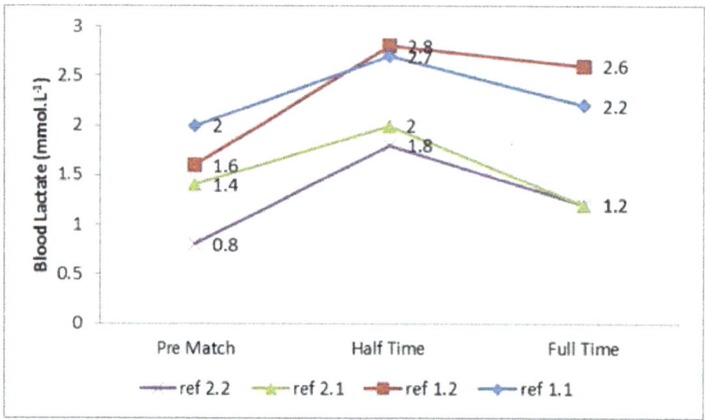

Figure 3. Blood Lactate readings of the Referees

As can be seen in Figure 3 above, blood lactate was 1.45 mmol.l-1 (s=0.50), 2.33 mmol.l-1 (s=0.5) and 1.8 mmol.l-1 (s=0.71) before, at half time and after the game respectively. Both the after match and half time values were higher than the resting values (pre match range = 0.8 – 2.0 mmol.l-1).

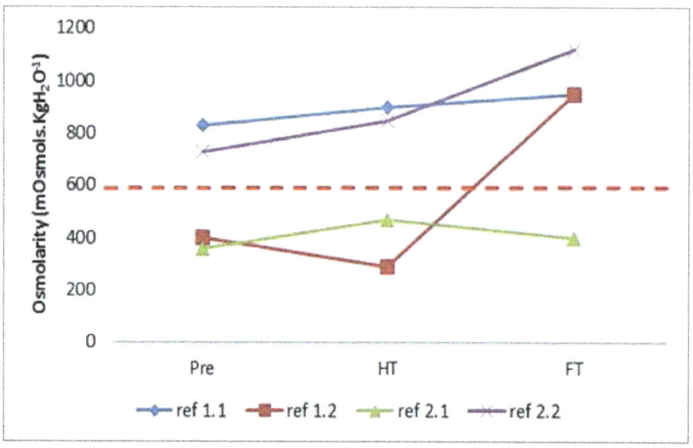

Figure 4. Osmolarity Readings of the Referees

Hydration status was found to be 580 mOsmols/kgH2O (range=360 – 830), 628 mOsmols/kgH2O (range=290-900) and 855 mOsmols/kgH2O (range= 400-1120), pre match, half time and full time respectively. Only one referee remained euhydrated throughout the match. Two referees were hypohydrated prior to the start of the match and as can be seen in Figure 4 three of the referees were hypohydrated at the end of the game which equated to 1.1 – 3.3 % loss in body weight over the course of the match.

4. Discussion

The results of this pilot study have revealed some interesting results which are worthy of further investigation.

The mean heart rate for the two international games were 155 beats.min-1 and 149 beats.min-1 during the first half and second half respectively which is higher than the mean in Portuguese domestic games. This may indicate a higher intensity of international futsal, however, similar to previous research the mean heart rate was higher in the first half compared to the second [5] and it tended to be lower at the end of the second half compared to the rest of the match for both referees.

In contrast to previous research a difference was found between the heart rate intensity of the first referee and the second referee for each of the ten minute period of the match (Figure 2), this warrants further investigation as to establish if this was unique to these games or is reflective of all futsal games.

Similar to Rebelo et al. [5] blood lactate levels taken for the referees before, half time and after the game were 1.45 mmol.l-1, 2..33 mmol.l-1 and 1.8 mmol.l-1 respectively, which suggests that the referees may not be reliant on anaerobic glycolysis metabolic system unlike their soccer colleagues in the 11-a-side version of the game where values of 5.1 mmol.l-1 and 4.8 mmol.l-1 have been reported in referees and in assistant referees respectively [5]. The heart rate data also supports the notion in that the first half elicited a greater heart rate response compared to the 2nd half. Blood lactate levels increased from resting levels and then showed a decline in the second half which is matched by the reduced HRmax of the referees in both halves and as such this may suggest higher workload in the first half compared to the second, which could be investigated further in future study's.

However, as illustrated by Figure 2 the referee's heart rate in the second game demonstrated a marked rate of decrease when compared to the referees in the first game. This may be as a result of the intensity of the game as these games were played on consecutive days and as such the players may have been experiencing some fatigue.

The hydration status of the referees showed that the referees actively dehydrated over the course of the game, although more may need to be done with the education of the referees as two were already dehydrated before the game started. Although on an individual basis the 1st referees dehydrated less than the 2nd Referees (1% vs. 3%). This may be important as a weight decrease of 2% has been shown to impair performance [10]. Further investigation is warranted as the highest core temperatures (>39°C) were recorded by the referees who showed the most dehydration. Reference [11] reports that performance may be adverse affected at body temperatures around 38.3 - 38.5°C which is above the average core temperature found in the referees in these games and lower than the peak temperature of the referees. Reference [11] also states that the performance would be exacerbated by progressive dehydration and that the performance included physical, cognitive and psychomotor aspects of skills. However, there is some debate as to whether dehydration has an impact performance. Although these arguments tend to revolve around wind speed, which is known to have has a cooling effect [12]. This would not be available in an indoor sport such as futsal. In addition to the authors knowledge there has been no investigation as to whether, hypohydration, core temperature and decision making are inter related in referees especially as normal cooling such as wind speed is not available.

Although this study offers a different examination of a futsal referees performance profile, it is not the full picture and as such future investigations should include video activity profiling. This would allow sport scientists to establish if there are different requirements between International and professional and non-professional domestic leagues and if there is a performance decline in movement and speed undertaking towards the end of the game [5,9].

5. Conclusions

To the authors knowledge only two studies have been completed examining futsal referees both of these examining referees operating in a professional league compared to over 10 years' worth of research into the referees operating in the 11 a side game.

This pilot study is based on 4 referees over two International matches and as such the results should be used with caution as the two previous studies have used 18 [5] and 16 [9] futsal referees respectively. Although having expressed this reservation there are a number of similarities with the previous studies. This study has also probably completed its role successfully in that more questions have been asked than have been answered and it would appear further investigation is required in this area, which should include time motion analysis of the activity profile of the futsal referees in domestic and international friendly matches which then allow better investigation to the workload of the futsal referee.

Acknowledgements

This study did not receive any funding. However we would like to thank the English Football Association and the effort from all the English Futsal referees involved in this study, without whose participation, this study would not have been possible.

Statement of Competing Interests

None.

List of Abbreviations

BASES	British Association of Sport and Exercise Scientists
beats.min-1	beats per minute
BMI	Body Mass Index

FIFA:	Fédération Internationale de Football Association
HRM	Heart Rate Maximum
HI	High Intensity
m	metres
mmol.l-1	millimoles per litre
mOsmols/kgH2O	milliosmols per kilogram of water
PARQ	Physical Activity Readiness Questionnaire
UEFA	Union of European Football Associations

References

[1] Do˘gramaci, SN, Watsford, ML, A comparison of two different methods for time-motion analysis in team sports. International Journal of Performance and Analysis in Sport, 6(1), pp73-83, 2006.

[2] Barbero, JC, Soto VM, Granda J, Match analysis and heart rate of futsal players during competition. Journal of Sports Sciences, 27, (1), pp1-11 2007.

[3] Krustrup, P, Mohr, M, and Bangsbo, J, Activity profile and physiological demands of top-class soccer assistant refereeing in relation to training status. *Journal of Sports Sciences*, 20, pp 861–871, 2002.

[4] UEFA *Futsal referees given fitness guidance* http://www.uefa.org/footballfirst/matchorganisation/refereeing/news/newsid=2024421.html, downloaded 13th November 2013.

[5] Rebelo, AN., Ascensão, AA., Magalhães, J. F., Bischoff, R., Bendiksen, M., & Krustrup, P. Elite futsal refereeing; activity profile and physiological demands, *The Journal of Strength and Conditioning Research*, 25(4), pp 980-987, 2011.

[6] Krustrup. P, Helsen, W, Randers, MB, Christensen, JF, MacDonald, C, Rebelo, AN, and Bangsbo, J, Activity profile and physical demands of football referees and assistant referees in international games, *Journal of Sports Sciences*, 27, (11), pp 1167-1176, 2009.

[7] Reilly T, and Gregson, W Special populations: the referee and assistant referee, *Journal of Sports Sciences*, 24, (7), 795-801, 2006.

[8] Draper, N, and Marshall, H, *Exercise physiology for health and sport performance*, Pearson education Limited, Harlow, England, 2013.

[9] Krustrup P., Randers, MB., Horton, J., Brito, J. and Rebelo, A. Ecological validity of the Yo-Yo SFIE2 test. *International Journal of Sports Medicine*, 33; pp432-438, 2012.

[10] MacLaren, D. Nutrition. In Reilly, T. and Williams, A.M. Science and Soccer 2nd Edition. Routledge, London, 2003.

[11] Reilly, T. *Environmental Stress*. In Reilly, T. and Williams, A.M. Science and Soccer 2nd Edition. Routledge, London, 2003.

[12] Noakes, T. *Waterlogged.* Champaign Il, Human Kinetics, 2012.

[13] UEFA. Referees urged to set standards http://www.uefa.org/footballfirst/matchorganisation/refereeing/news/newsid=1990079.html. Downloaded 3rd September 2013.

A Retrospective Study of the Yo-Yo IE2 Test: Can It be Used to Differentiate Between Different Levels of Futsal Referees?

D. Dixon*

Applied Sport and Exercise Sciences, School of Health Sport and Bioscience, University of East London. London, UK
*Corresponding author: d.dixon@uel.ac.uk

Abstract Recently FIFA have called on referees to be fitter and to look like athletes therefore the aim of this research was to retrospectively examine the results from the fitness test results undertaken by Futsal referees operating in and below the National Futsal League. Futsal is the FIFA sanctioned form of 5 a side football and is controlled by two referees who operate up and down the touchlines either side of the pitch. Research has shown that the referees operating at an average intensity of 76% heart rate maximum (HRmax)HRMAX and spent more time sprinting and working at high intensity compared to referees in the 11 a side game. Currently FIFA recommend a. and as such the current 1000 m run, but this is not thought to match the actual movements or intensity of futsal referees or matches. As such the Yo-Yo IE2 test was introduced this season as it has been found to correlate highly with high intensity running ($r=0.75$; $p<0.05$). Twenty-two National group and 36 Non-national group futsal referees underwent pre-season testing which in-cooperating the Yo-Yo Intermittent Endurance Level 2 Fitness Test, a 40 m sprint test and a 70 m agility run test. The result showed a trivial effect size difference for Yo-Yo IE2 test distance (0.21), a small effect size difference for 40 m speed test and a extremely large effect size difference for 70 m agility run. A moderate to large correlation was found between age and Yo-Yo IE2 distance ($r=-0.577$) and BMI and Yo-Yo IE2 distance ($r=-0.452$). Therefore the Yo-Yo IE2 can be used to differentiate between different levels of futsal referees and it may be possible to use the test to identify those referees who show the fitness attributes for further development.

Keywords: *fitness testing, Yo-Yo IE2, futsal, referee, indoor soccer, physiology*

1. Introduction

Futsal is the only 5-a-side form of football that is officially sanctioned by FIFA. The main differences between this type of football and its 11 a side version are that it is played indoors on a pitch that measures 40 x 20 metre and is played over a time of 20 min each way. However, in Futsal the clock is stopped every time the ball goes out of play so in reality each half usually lasts between 30 and 40 min. The game itself is classed as an intermittent high-intensity sport with players changing directions / activity about every 3.28 seconds [1] which is helped by the players being able to undergo unlimited substitutions without stopping play [2].

The Referee is responsible for enforcing the laws of the game in invasion type sports such as Futsal. However, unlike the 11 a side version, it is refereed by two referees who operate up and down the touch lines. Although there is an increasing amount of research examining the physiological and psychological demands of the 11 a side referee and assistant referees, which have shown that Assistant referees, undergo intense brief bouts of forward and sideways running [3]. However, there have been very few papers which examine the physiological demands of futsal referees. Research by [4] examined the physiological demands of Futsal referees using the Portuguese first division referees. It was found that the average heart rate of the futsal referees during matches was 146 beats.min-1 which equated to 76% of their HRmax. Research by [4] showed that Futsal referees undergo different movement patterns compared to their 11 a-side counterparts and for the majority of the game, futsal referees spend more time completing high intensity (HI) and maximal sprints, although these bouts of HI and maximal sprints are for a shorter periods of time.

1.1. Referee Futsal Fitness Test

Currently the futsal referees have a battery of test which include an endurance run (1000 m in 4 min), a sprint test (2x 40 metre sprint in less than 10 seconds) and an agility test (to be completed in less than 20 seconds and consisting of running, sprinting, sideways running and backwards running over a 30 metre course) [5]. All of these are usually conducted on a track in the weather conditions of the particular fitness test date, which in the English climate can be very variable and not conducive to the climate in which they would normally operate. Therefore it would be more appropriate if a test could be conducted indoors, the match environment, and in particular could differentiate between the different levels of referees.

1.2. Yo-Yo IE2 Fitness Test

The Yo-Yo IE2 fitness test is a test which can be used indoors over a 20 metre track. Research by [6] reports that the Yo - Yo test is highly correlated with high intensity running (HIR) ($r=0.75$; $p<0.05$). To the authors knowledge there has been only one study which has examined the use of the Yo Yo IE 2 test in which the data was compared to futsal referees [4]. In that paper the referees underwent the Yo Yo IE 2 where an average distance of 975 m was covered by the referees. A correlation was conducted between HIR and IE2 distance ($r=0.52$ $p<0.05$). A smaller significant correlation was found with total match distance covered $r=0.40$ $p<0.05$ and no correlation with match intensity (% of HR) $r=0.02$ $p>0.05$ [5] which according to [7] these would be classed as having a large correlation magnitude for HIR and IE2, a moderate magnitude for the match distance and IE2 and a trivial magnitude for IE2 and match intensity.

The test used needs to fit in with the ethos of FIFA to get the best referees, refereeing the best games, this test would seem to be able to differentiate between the referees from both groups as there was a significant difference in the total distance run between the two groups. This would be important for the development of referees on the national list and to allow the management of the game to know who would be in line for nomination to FIFA especially as this International organisation can work outside the European laws on age discrimination. As such they only allow referees to be nominated who are between 23 and 35 years [8].

Therefore the selected test needs to relate to the ability of the referee to officiate in matches which involve a large amount of time at high intensity running. It is also important that the test has some relationship with the actual movements in a futsal match and that the test being administered has been shown to deliver repeatable and consistent results.

2. Material and Methods

Fifty Eight referees (56 male and 2 female) undertook the Yo-Yo IE-2. However, the test was conducted on two different days to reflect the two different groups undertaking the test.

The first group was made up of thirty six referees (34 male and 2 female) undertaking the test in order to seek promotion into the National Group. These referees were made up of those who act as third official on the National League and either referee National League Division 2 or University Futsal matches.

The second test day was made up of twenty two referees (22 male) who were all referees within the current National group who referee on the National and Super Futsal League.

The Anthropometric data for the two groups reproduced in Table 1.

Prior to both tests an informed consent form, BASES health questionnaire and PARQ were completed by each referee, all referee who answered 'Yes' to any of the questions had to bring the information to my attention. Following the completion of the form, the referees were required to complete three tests, the Yo-Yo IE2 test, a 40 metre sprint test and a sixty metre agility test.

2.1. Yo-Yo Test IE2

This test consists of two cones placed 20 m apart with a further third cone positioned 2.5 m behind the start cone. The object of the test is to run between the two 20 metre cones reaching each end exactly at the time signal given by the test CD. After each 40 m the referee has a 5 second break in which to run slowly around the third cone and back to the start ready for the next signal. If the referee is too quick, they must wait at the marker until the next signal. If the referee is too slow a warning is given and on the second time the test is stopped [9].

On both occasions the referees were allowed to warm up for 10 min prior to the start of the Yo-Yo IE2 test.

During the second bank of testing test heart rate was recorded continuously for eight of the twenty-two referees taking part. The heart rates were sampled every 5 seconds using Polar Team2 (version 1.4.5, Polar Electro Oy, Finland) from about 20 min before the test started until the completion of all the tests.

Two other tests were also conducted on each day, a forty metre sprint test where the participant is required to run 40 m between two lines 10 m apart and a seventy metre agility test where the participant is required to 70 m running forwards, sideways and backwards [5]. Speed Light Timing gates placed 1 metre above ground were used to record the individual referee sprint and agility times (Brower Timing Systems, Utah, USA).

The data is presented as means and standard deviation. The correlations were established using the Pearsons product moment test and the magnitude were considered in accordance with Hopkins definitions [7].

3. Results

Anthropometric and fitness data are presented in Table 1. With regard to the referees' anthropometric data, the national group of referees were older and heavier than the non-national group of referees. For fitness test performance, national group of referees covered more distance on the Yo - Yo IE 2 test and recorded faster 40 m and 70 m sprint times.

Table 1. Anthropometric charteristic and test results of the groups (mean±SD)

	Nation Group Mean ± SD	Non-nation Group Mean ± SD	Effect size for the different (± 90% confidence interval)
Age (Yrs)	36.9 ± 9.9	32.0 ± 11.5	0.35(-0.10 to 0.79)**
Weight (Kg)	81.3 ± 10.3	79.8 ± 10.4	0.17(-0.28 to 0.61)*
Height (m)	178.3 ± 9.0	177.0 ± 8.1	0.19(-0.25 to 0.63)*
BMI (Kg/m^2)	25.6 ± 2.3	25.5± 3.3	0.00(-0.44 to 0.44)
YoYo (m)	1002 ± 325.1	927 ± 304	0.21(-0.24 to 0.65)*
40m test (s)	9.9 ± 0.5	10.2 ± 0.6	-0.48(-0.92 to -0.03)**
70m test (s)	18.7 ± 0.8	19.41 ± 1.9	10.51(8.71 to 12.02)***

The data in Figure 1 below is from the eight referees who wore the monitors and it would appear that all eight referees were close to their maximal values (172-204 beats.min-1) at the point of volition and as such the test has tested them fully and is a valid test for the referees. The average for the eight referees over the whole test was 164.76 beats.min-1 (s= 16.49) which equates to about 89% of heart rate maximum (HRmax) based on the average age of the eight referees was 35 years (range 17 – 49 years), although the HRmax range was 88-104%.

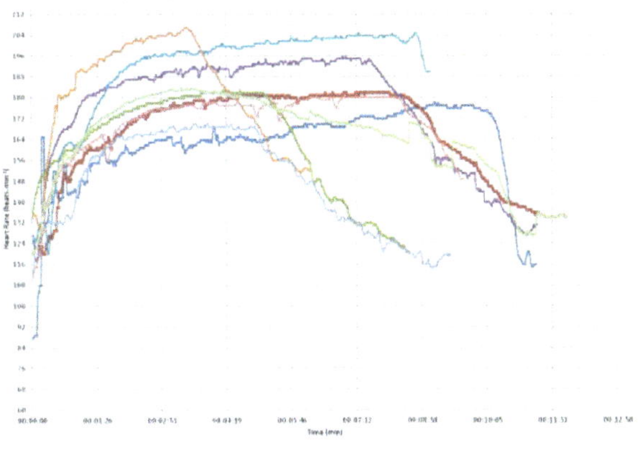

Figure 1. Heart Rate Data for National Group YO-YO IE2 Test

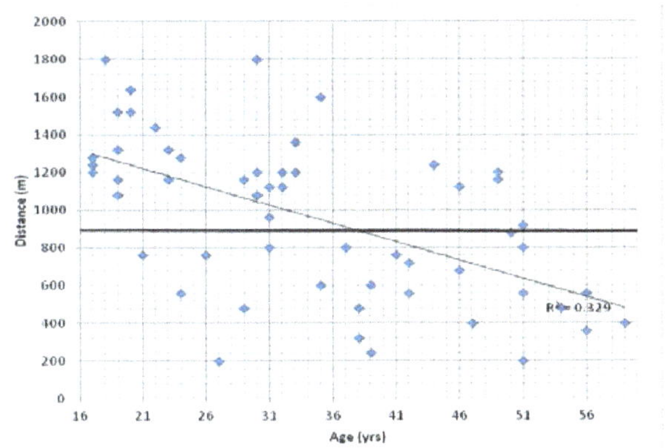

Figure 2. Comparison of referees Age vs. Distance travelled during YO – YO IE2 Test for both National and Non National Groups

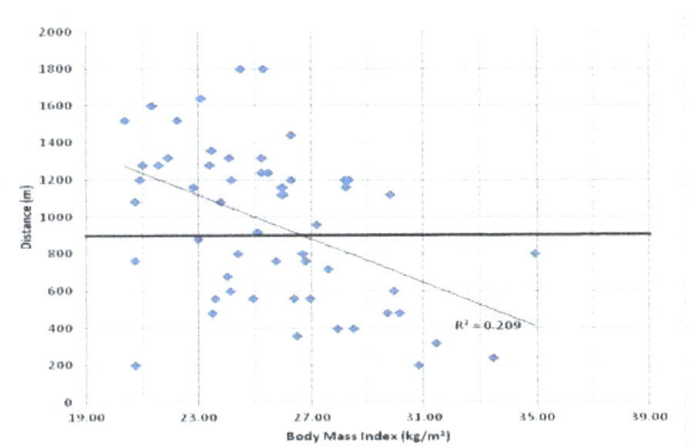

Figure 3. Comparison of referees BMI vs. Distance travelled during YO – YO IE2 Test for both National and Non National Groups

Analysis on the combined data of the two groups to see if there was a relationship between any of the variables and the distance covered in the Yo-Yo test. Moderate-large correlations were observed between referee age and Yo - Yo IE 2 distance (r = -0.577; 90% confidence interval –0.71 to -0.41) (Figure 2) and referee BMI and Yo - Yo IE 2 distance (r = -0.452; -0.61 to -0.2) (Figure 3).

4. Discussion

This initial study showed that the Yo-Yo IE2 can be used to differentiate between age and BMI. It can also be used as a form of talent identification for those referees who may be fit enough to work as potential FIFA referees and that the heart rates

In relation to talent identification of future FIFA referees, the Yo - Yo IE 2 test showed that there was a trivial for Yo - Yo IE2 distance (1002 vs. 927), a small effect for the 40 metre sprint test (9.9 vs. 10.2 seconds) and an extremely large effect for the 70 metre agility test (18.7 vs 19.4 seconds). As such the test would seem to be suitable to differentiate between the different levels of the referees with the national group running further and being faster in the 40 metre speed and 70 metre agility tests. Although in relation to the 40 metre and 70 metre tests the time taken to do each test was below that set by FIFA for their international referees (40 metre being 10 seconds and 70 metre being 20.5 seconds) [5] which then asks the question whether the time set for these tests sufficiently reflects the amount of training required and the speed of the game at the elite level. As such more research should be completed in this area.

Unlike other research in this area, there is no positional or intra and inter seasonal data. However, at the recent gathering of referees by FIFA an emphasis was placed on the fact that referees needed to become athletes and that fitness and body composition is becoming an important factor in their selection process [8,12]. The data from these tests indicates that there was a moderate to large correlation between the distance covered in the Yo –Yo IE2 test and the age of the participants and their BMI. As such the Yo – Yo IE2 could be used to identify the referees who may meet these new areas set by FIFA and UEFA [8,10]. However, BMI is not the best test of body composition in relation to physically active participants, and in such circumstance % body fat should be used. However, it was not possible to test everyone during this testing period, although a similar moderate correlation was found between % body fat and the distance completed in the Yo-Yo IE2 (r = -0.378; 90% confidence interval –0.65 to -0.02) [11] when a twenty two of the fifty eight referees were tested. As such further investigation could be made into whether percentage body fat is a sole factor or part of a number of factors which dictate the distance covered in the Yo-Yo IE2.

The heart rates sampled during the test show that the referee's heart rate increased as the test became harder and in such cases the heart rate is said to reflect the amount of oxygen taken up by the body [12] and at exhaustion the heart rate was on average 89% of HRmax. This is below those reported in other research [13], but the age range of the referee group is considerable wider than that found in player research. Although it may have been better if Blood Lactate samples had been taken to confirm that the aerobic system was sufficiently taxed and as such the anaerobic system has been stimulated [9].

The distance covered by the national group in the Yo-Yo IE2 test were slightly higher than the mean result found in the 18 elite Portuguese Futsal referees 1002m versus 975m, [4], but the non-national group mean was less than the elite referee group (927 vs. 975 m), although both groups were considerable less than the average distance said to be covered by elite soccer players (2600 m) [9]. However, the Yo - Yo IE 2 test has been shown to have a moderate to large correlation with the match distance covered both by elite soccer players (r2 = 0.55) [13] and elite referees (r2 = 0.4) [4]. As can be seen that there is a larger correlation with the players this may be due to the referees being reactive to the tactics employed by the players. However, as there has been only one study involving futsal referees in a professional league, more research should be conducted in a non-professional environment.

In the research by [4] a moderate to high correction was found between match distance and high Intensity running. However, there was no report as to whether there was any correction between the distance covered in the Yo-Yo IE 2 test and the distance covered moving side wards. This would be an important factor as this was the second highest movement pattern of the referee (911m) [4] and is reports as 1610m of the 5780m in another study of Portuguese referees [14], the latter being similar to that covered by FIFA Assistant referees [15]. However, in [14] there was no correlation found in the distance covered in the Yo-Yo SFIE2 (also called ARIET) and side wards movement, although this test may have more validity as it includes an element of side wards running as part of the test. Although it would appear that referees with poor physical fitness test results preforming the most side wards running [14]. However, as this is not an official futsal fitness test there is as the author understands it no minimum standard for the referees to pass which may be a factor in the results.

5. Conclusions

The results of this study have established that the Yo-Yo IE2 can be used to differentiate between different levels of futsal referees who operate in the National Futsal Division One and Two. The test can also be used to possible identify those referees who show the fitness attributes for further development based on the criteria of age and body composition as suggest by FIFA. Unfortunately it was not possible to capture any actual match activity profiles during this stage of testing and as such further research is needed to explore whether there is a correlation between the high intensity movements, side wards running and /or match distance covered by futsal referees in national league games and the distance covered in the Yo - Yo IE2 test compared to professional leagues [4].

More recently the Yo-Yo SFIE2 which is the same type of test as the Yo-Yo test with the addition of a side wards movement leg in between each run may be more akin to the movement of futsal referees. This new test has also shown a large correlation with match values [14] from professional futsal leagues. Therefore further research needs be conducted into the validity of the Yo-Yo IE2/ Yo-Yo SFIE2 and match values for match distance, HIR and sprinting by referees operating in non-professional futsal leagues.

Acknowledgement

This study did not receive any funding. However we would like to thank the English Football Association and the effort from all the English Futsal referees involved in this study, without whose participation, this study would not have been possible.

Statement of Competing Interests

None.

List of Abbreviations

ARIET	Assistant Referee Intermittent Endurance Test
BASES	British Association of Sport and Exercise Scientists
BMI	Body Mass Index
FIFA:	Fédération Internationale de Football Association
HRmax	Heart Rate Maximum
HI	High Intensity
m	metres
PARQ	Physical Activity Readiness Questionnaire
SFIE2	Sidewards-Forwards Intermittent Endurance Level 2
UEFA	Union of European Football Associations

References

[1] Dŏgramaci, SN, Watsford, ML, A comparison of two different methods for time-motion analysis in team sports. International Journal of Performance and Analysis in Sport, 6(1), pp73-83, 2006.

[2] Barbero, JC, Soto VM, Granda J, Match analysis and heart rate of futsal players during competition. Journal of Sports Sciences, 27, (1), pp1-11, 2007.

[3] Krustrup, P, Mohr, M, and Bangsbo, J, Activity profile and physiological demands of top-class soccer assistant refereeing in relation to training status. Journal of Sports Sciences, 20, pp 861-871, 2002.

[4] Rebelo, AN., Ascensão, AA., Magalhães, J. F., Bischoff, R., Bendiksen, M., & Krustrup, P. Elite futsal refereeing; activity profile and physiological demands, The Journal of Strength and Conditioning Research, 25(4), pp 980-987, 2011.

[5] FIFA Regulations on the Organisation of Refereeing in FIFA Member Associations. http://www.fifa.com/mm/document/tournament/competition/01/28/10/42/defs_regulationsorganisationrefereeinginfifama_inhalt.pdf. Downloaded on 15th November 2013.

[6] Weston, M., Castagna, C., Impellizzeri, F.M., Bizzini, M., Williams, A.M., and Gregson, W. Science and medicine applied to soccer refereeing: an update. Sports Medicine 42, pp 615-31, 2012.

[7] Batterham, AM. and Hopkins, WG. 'Making meaningful inferences about magnitudes', International Journal of Sports Physiology and Performance, 1 (1), pp.50-57, 2006.

[8] UEFA Futsal referees given fitness guidance http://www.uefa.org/footballfirst/matchorganisation/refereeing/news/newsid=2024421.html, downloaded 13th November 2013.

[9] Bangsbo, J. & Mohr, M. Fitness Testing in Football: fitness training in Soccer II. Bangsosport, 2011.

[10] UEFA. Referees urged to set standards http://www.uefa.org/footballfirst/matchorganisation/refereeing/news/newsid=1990079.html. Downloaded 3rd September 2013.

[11] Dixon D. (2013). Unpublished data from fitness testing of FA Futsal referees.

[12] Saltin B. Physiological effects of physical conditioning. Medicine and Science in Sport. 1(1). pp50-56, 1969.

[13] Bradley, P. S., Mohr, M., Bendiksen, M., Randers, M. B., Flindt, M., Barnes, C., Hood, P., Gomez, A., Andersen, JL., Di Mascio, M., Bangsbo, J. and & Krustrup, P. Sub-maximal and maximal Yo–Yo intermittent endurance test level 2: heart rate response, reproducibility and application to elite soccer. European journal of applied physiology, 111(6), pp969-978, 2011

[14] Krustrup P., Randers, MB., Horton, J., Brito, J. and Rebelo, A. Ecological validity of the Yo-Yo SFIE2 test. International Journal of Sports Medicine, 33; pp432-438, 2012.

[15] Castagna, C., Bendiksen, M., Impellizzeri, F. M. & Krustrup, P. Reliability, sensitivity and validity of the assistant referee intermittent endurance test (ARIET) – a modified Yo-Yo IE2 test for elite soccer assistant referees, Journal of Sports Sciences, 30(8), pp767-775, 2012.

7

Age-related Differences in Countermovement Vertical Jump in Soccer Players 8-31 Years Old: the Role of Fat-free Mass

Nikolaidis P.T.[1,2,*]

[1]Department of Physical and Cultural Education, Hellenic Army Academy, Athens, Greece
[2]Exercise Physiology Laboratory, Nikaia, Greece
*Corresponding author: pademil@hotmail.com

Abstract The aim of this study was to examine the effect of age on leg muscle power in male soccer players and to provide reference data. Male soccer players, all members of competitive soccer clubs and classified into six age groups (younger than 10 yr, U10, n = 17; U12, n = 27; U14, n = 70; U16, n = 92; U18, n = 33; older than 18 yr, Adults, n=36), participated in our study. They were examined for anthropometric characteristics, body composition, and performed the arm-swing countermovement vertical jump (CVJ) as a measure of leg muscle power. A one-way analysis of variance revealed significant differences between age groups with respect to CVJ ($F_{5,269} = 76.46$, $p < 0.001$, $\eta^2 = 0.59$). Our findings indicated that the older the age group, the higher the CVJ (e.g., 19.8±3.9 cm in U10, 30.0±5.9 cm in U14 and 41.8±6.0 cm in adult group). This result was in agreement with the significant and large correlation coefficient between age and CVJ ($r = 0.68$, $p < 0.001$). Although the cross-sectional design of our study did not allow inferring causal relationship between age and CVJ, it is reasonable to support that there are large gains in leg muscle power with development in soccer players. These gains are accompanied by large increase of FFM during the same period. The findings of this study could be useful for coaches and trainers in the context of talent identification and training optimization.

Keywords: *youth, lower limbs, muscle power, strength, football*

1. Introduction

In soccer, performance is influenced in great extent by leg muscle power [1]. In adolescence, this parameter of physical fitness is important in the context of talent identification and training monitoring. For instance, the measures of anaerobic power in young players aged 13-16 yr could partially determine if someone followed a career as an international, professional or amateur player in adulthood [2]. In spite of the popularity of soccer in adolescence, only a few studies have been carried out regarding physical traits and motor abilities of these athletes in a laboratory setting, especially with regard to leg muscle power.

We have recently investigated the development of anthropometric characteristics, body composition, physique [3], flexibility [4], isometric muscle strength [5], muscle endurance [6], force-velocity characteristics [7], performance in Wingate anaerobic test [8] and aerobic power in young soccer players [9]. The main findings of these studies revealed (a) significant differences between adolescent and adult players, (b) differences between the players in the lower spectrum and those in the higher spectrum of adolescence, and (c) better scores in soccer players than in general population.

Vertical jump has been used as a measure of leg muscle power in soccer [10,11,12,13] and to identify bilateral differences [14,15]. Moreover, recent research has supported an association between vertical jump and sport performance; vertical jump correlated with both 10 m and 30 m sprint time ($r = -0.72$ and $r = -0.60$, $p < 0.001$, respectively) [13]. In the case of adolescent players, there is limited information on their leg muscle power assessed by a vertical jump test. For instance, only one research has been ever carried out in a large sample of young players, aged 11-17 yr [16]. However, that study was not able to identify significant differences among age groups partially due to the number of participants (n = 184), and did not examine its findings with regard to children and adult values.

New normative data would be helpful to coaches and fitness trainers in order to select players and evaluate their training. Therefore, the aim of this study was to examine two relevant research hypotheses with regard to vertical jump; (a) adolescent had higher scores than children and lower scores than adult players, (b) players in the lower spectrum were outscored by those in the higher spectrum of adolescence.

2. Methods

Participants and procedures. In this investigation, a descriptive-correlation design was used to examine the effect of age on the arm-swing countermovement vertical jump (CVJ) across adolescence. Testing procedures were performed in the beginning of competition period of season 2011-12. Written informed consent was received from all players or parents after verbal explanation of the experimental design and potential risks of study. Although it is difficult to define adolescence in terms of chronological age, because of variation in time of its onset and termination, it has been suggested to range between 10 and 22 y in boys [17]. For the purpose of our study, we followed this definition. Male soccer players, all members of competitive soccer clubs and classified into six age groups (younger than 10 yr, U10, n = 17; U12, n = 27; U14, n = 70; U16, n = 92; U18, n = 33; older than 18 yr, Adults, n=36), participated in our study (Table 1). They visited our laboratory once; anthropometric and body composition data were obtained followed by the CVJ.

Protocols and equipment. Height and body mass were measured using a stadiometer (SECA, Leicester, UK) and an electronic scale (HD-351, Tanita, Illinois, USA), respectively. Percent of body fat was calculated from the sum of 10 skinfolds using a skinfold calliper (Harpenden, West Sussex, UK), based on the formula proposed by Parizkova [18]. The participants performed the countermovement jumps with arm-swing [19] twice with 1-min break between the two trials and the best score was retained for subsequent analysis. The height of each jump was estimated using the Opto-jump (Microgate Engineering, Bolzano, Italy) and was expressed as cm. Measurements were recorded to the nearest 0.1 cm. CVJ has been shown to be a reliable test [20,21].

Table 1. Anthropometric data and vertical jump scores of participants.

	Age groups						
	U10 (n=17)	U12 (n=27)	U14 (n=70)	U16 (n=92)	U18 (n=33)	Adults (n=36)	ANOVA
Age (yr)	9.1±0.6	10.9±0.7	13.1±0.5	15.0±0.6	17.0±0.5	21.7±3.4	$F_{5,269} = 342.30$, $p < 0.001$ $\eta^2 = 0.86$
Weight (kg)	33.6±7.3	42.5±9.0	50.8±9.5	62.6±8.4	66.6±5.9	74.1±8.4	$F_{5,269} = 94.70$, $p < 0.001$, $\eta^2 = 0.64$
Height (cm)	137±6	146±7	160±9	171±7	175±6	177±5	$F_{5,269} = 139.14$, $p < 0.001$, $\eta^2 = 0.72$
BMI (kg·m^{-2})	17.8±2.4	19.6±2.7	19.7±2.6	21.2±2.2	21.9±1.8	23.6±2.4	$F_{5,269} = 21.82$, $p < 0.001$, $\eta^2 = 0.29$
BF (%)	16.4±4.4	19.3±4.8	16.1±5.1	15.4±3.8	14.4±3.3	15.9±3.5	$F_{5,269} = 83.40$, $p < 0.001$, $\eta^2 = 0.08$
FM (kg)	5.7±2.8	8.6±3.8	8.5±4.0	9.8±3.3	9.7±2.8	12.0±3.8	$F_{5,269} = 9.15$, $p < 0.001$, $\eta^2 = 0.15$
FFM (kg)	27.8 (4.7)	33.9 (5.4)	42.4 (6.6)	52.8 (6.3)	56.9 (4.3)	62.1 (5.0)	$F_{5,269} = 154.08$ $p < 0.001$, $\eta^2 = 0.74$
CVJ (cm)	19.8±3.9	22.8±3.6	30.0±5.9	36.1±5.9	40.8±5.6	41.8±6.0	$F_{5,269} = 76.46$, $p < 0.001$, $\eta^2 = 0.59$

BMI = body mass index, BF = body fat, FM = fat mass, FFM = fat-free mass, CVJ = countermovement vertical jump.

Data and statistical analysis. Results were presented as mean±standard deviation. The effect of age on CVJ was examined by Pearson moment correlation coefficient (*r*). Magnitude of correlation coefficients were considered as trivial ($r \leq 0.1$), small ($0.1 \leq r < 0.3$) moderate ($0.3 \leq r < 0.5$), large ($0.5 \leq r < 0.7$), very large ($0.7 \leq r < 0.9$) and nearly perfect ($r \geq 0.9$) and perfect ($r = 1$). Differences between age-groups were assessed using one-way analysis of variance. Correction for multiple comparisons was undertaken using the Bonferroni method. To interpret effect sizes for statistical differences in the ANOVA we used eta square classified as small ($0.010 < \eta^2 \leq 0.059$), medium ($0.059 < \eta^2 \leq 0.138$) and large ($\eta^2 > 0.138$) [22]. Significance level was set at alpha = 0.05. Statistical analyses were performed using IBM SPSS v.20.0 statistical software (SPSS Inc., Chicago, IL, USA).

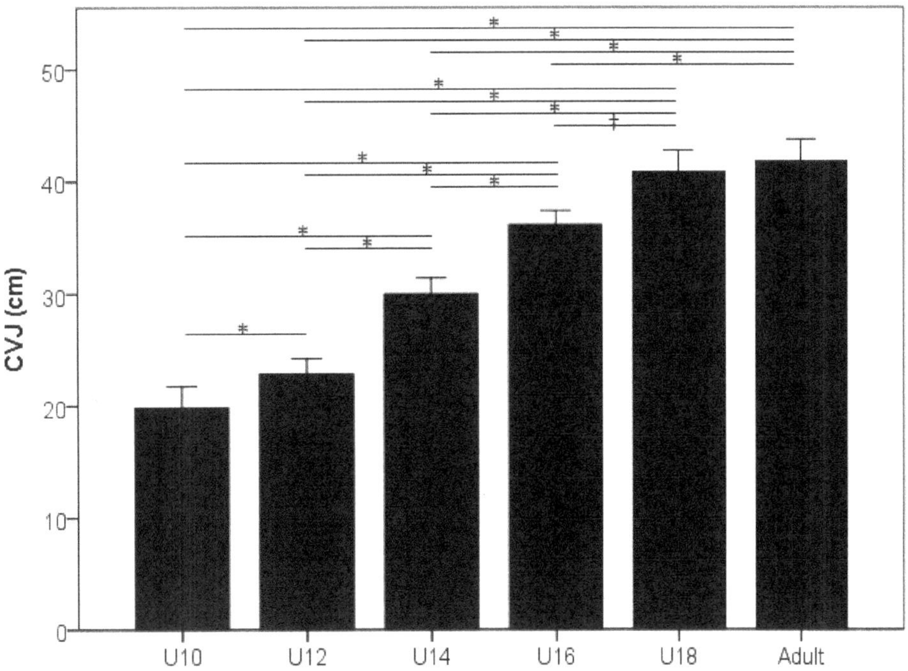

Figure 1. Differences in countermovement vertical jump (CVJ) between age groups. Error bars represent standard error. *p < 0.001, †p < 0.01

3. Results

The basic characteristics of participants can be seen in Table 1. Briefly, our sample was consisted by U10 (6%), U12 (10%), U14 (26%), U16 (34%), U18 (12%) and adult soccer players (13%). There were significant differences between age groups for age, weight, height, BMI, BF and CVJ. The older the age group, higher values were recorded. The relationship between age groups and age with CVJ can be found in Figure 1 and Figure 2. Taking into account the eta square as a measure of effect size, there was a large effect of age groups on CVJ. Accordingly, there was a large correlation between age and CVJ (r = 0.68, p < 0.001). We found also a large correlation of CVJ with weight and fat-free mass (Figure 3).

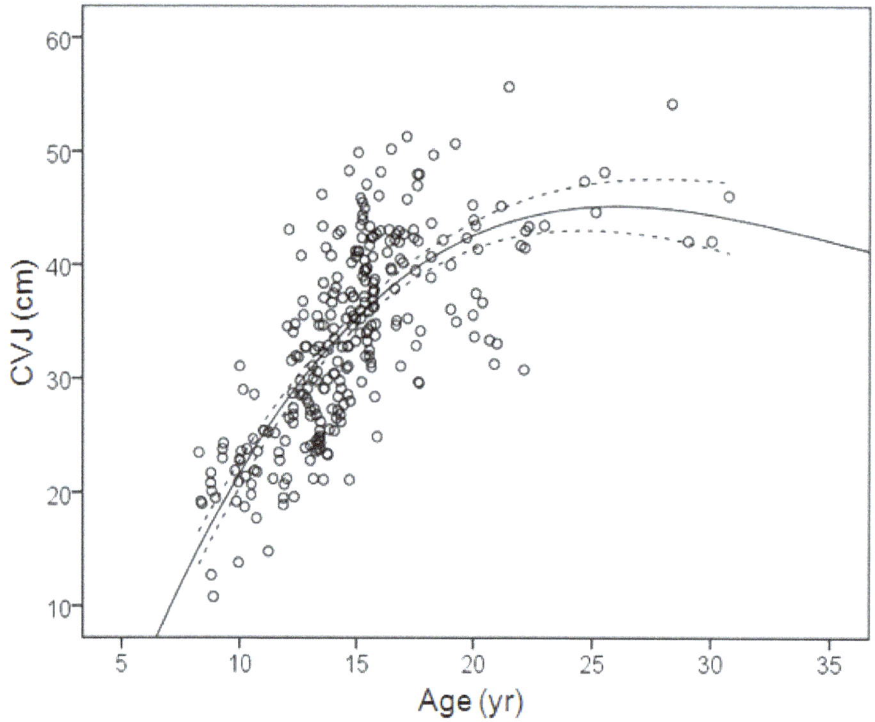

Figure 2. Relationship between age and countermovement vertical jump (CVJ) in participants. Dashed lines represent upper and lower 95% confidence intervals of the mean

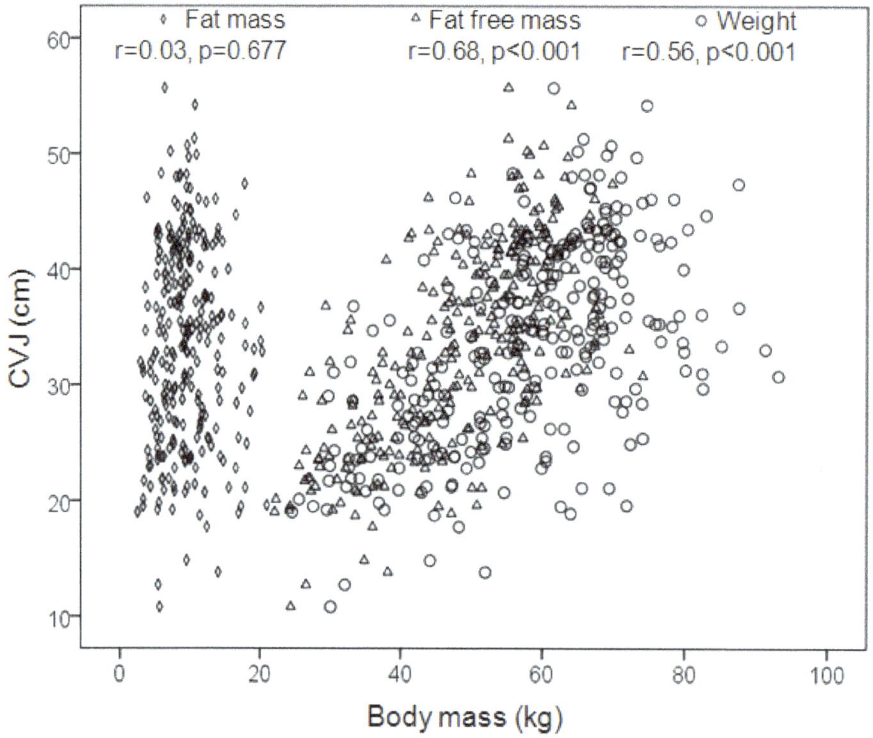

Figure 3. Relationship of countermovement vertical jump (CVJ) with fat mass, fat-free mass and total body weight

4. Discussion

The main finding of this study was that age is a very important factor on leg muscle power and this relationship seems to be attenuated after the age of 18 yr. There was no difference in CVJ between U18 and adult players. The smallest statistical difference was observed between U10 and U12, while the largest difference was between U12 and U14, followed by that between U14 and U16.

Compared with previous data on French soccer players [16], participants had lower score; 22.8 vs. 31.0 cm in U12, 30.0 vs. 34.3 cm in U14, 36.1 vs. 41.2 cm in U16 and 40.8 vs. 45.5 cm in U18. While there was a consistent difference between these two studies, both revealed important increase across this range of age (~79% vs. ~47%). The trend of CVJ increase during adolescence was similar with that reported in a recent study [23], which reported values of 24.2 cm, 27.7 cm, 32.6 cm, 36.7 cm and 36.7 cm in U11, U13, U15, U17 and U19 soccer players (~52%), respectively, as well as consistently higher values in trained than in untrained controls.

The similar values in CVJ between U18 and adults were in agreement with previous research [23,24]. For instance, the members of Italian national teams U17, U20 and U21 had similar CVJ (40.9 cm, 40.2 cm and 40.3 cm, respectively) [24]. Our interpretation for this finding is that muscle leg power does not discriminate between matured players independently from whether they are adults or in the highest spectrum of adolescence. Previous research which compared elite and non-elite players by playing position found higher CVJ in elite players only in the case of goalkeepers [25] showing that this fitness parameter does not discriminate players by performance level. The exception in the case of goalkeepers might be attributed to that they usually have higher vertical jump values when compared to outfielders [26].

From a physiological point of view, the large gains in CVJ were explained from the increase in FFM across adolescence. This finding confirmed previous research that suggested a large correlation between FFM and CVJ in 7-13 yr boys [27] and the directly proportional changes in FFM and CVJ in 11-16 yr boys [28]. Therefore, an increase of leg muscle power should be expected during growth independently from the stimulus of soccer training.

5. Conclusions

Although the cross-sectional design of our study did not allow inferring causal relationship between age and CVJ, it is reasonable to support that there are large gains in leg muscle power with development in soccer players. These gains are accompanied by large increase of FFM during the same period. The findings of this study could be useful for coaches and trainers in the context of talent identification and training optimization.

References

[1] Bangsbo J, Mohr M, Krustrup P. Physical and metabolic demands of training and match-play in the elite football player. J Sports Sci. 2006; 24(7): 665-74.

[2] Le Gall F, Carling C, Williams M, Reilly T. Anthropometric and fitness characteristics of international, professional and amateur male graduate soccer players from an elite youth academy. J Sci Med Sport. 2010; 13: 90-5.

[3] Nikolaidis P, Karydis NV. Physique and body composition in soccer players across adolescence. Asian J Sports Med. 2011; 2(2): 75-82.

[4] Nikolaidis PT. Age-related differences of hamstring flexibility in male soccer players. Baltic Journal of Physical Activity. 2012; 4(2): 110-5.

[5] Nikolaidis PT. Development of isometric muscular strength in adolescent soccer players. Facta Universitatis Series Physical Education and Sport. 2012; 10(3): 231-42.

[6] Nikolaidis P. Core stability of male and female football players. Biomed Hum Kinetics. 2010; 2: 30-3.

[7] Nikolaidis P. Age-related differences in force-velocity characteristics in youth soccer. Kinesiology. 2012; 44(2): 130-8.

[8] Nikolaidis P. Anaerobic power across adolescence in soccer players. Hum Movement. 2011; 12(4): 342-7.

[9] Nikolaidis P. Cardiorespiratory power across adolescence in male soccer players. Hum Physiol. 2011; 37(5): 636-41.

[10] Caldwell BP, Peters DM. Seasonal variation in physiological fitness of a semiprofessional soccer team. J Strength Cond Res. 2009; 23(5): 1370-7.

[11] Chlif M, Jullien H, Temfemo A, Mezouk A, Manouvrier C, Choquet D. Suivi physique et physiologique de footballeurs semi-professionnels: vers un entraînement individualisé par poste. Sci Sports. 2010; 25: 132-8.

[12] Lago-Penas C, Casais L, Dellal A, Rey E, Dominguez E. Anthropometric and physiological characteristics of young soccer players according to their playing positions: relevance for competition success. J Strength Cond Res. 2011;25(12):3358-67

[13] Wisloff U, Castagna C, Helgerud J, Jones R, Hoff J. Strong correlation of maximal squat strength with sprint performance and vertical jump height in elite soccer players. Br J Sports Med. 2004; 38(3): 285-8.

[14] Menzel HJ, Chagas MH, Szmuchrowski LA, Araujo SRS, De Andrade AGP, De Jesus-Moraleida FR. Analysis of lower limb asymmetries by isokinetic and vertical jump tests in soccer players. Journal of Strength and Conditioning Research. 2013 //; 27(5): 1370-7.

[15] Sannicandro I, Rosa RA, De Pascalis S, Piccinno A. The determination of functional asymmetries in the lower limbs of young soccer players using the countermovement jump. The lower limbs asymmetry of young soccer players. Science and Sports. 2012 //; 27(6): 375-7.

[16] Hertogh C, Micallef JP, Mercier J. Puissance anaérobie maximale chez l'adolescent (étude transversale). Sci Sports. 1992; 7(4): 207-13.

[17] Malina RM, Bouchard C, Bar-Or O. Growth, maturation and physical activity. Champaign: Human Kinetics; 2004.

[18] Parizkova J. Lean body mass and depot fat during autogenesis in humans. In: Parizkova J, Rogozkin V, editors. Nutrition, Physical Fitness and Health: International Series on Sport Sciences. Baltimore: University Park Press; 1978.

[19] Aragon-Vargas LF. Evaluation of four vertical jump tests: Methodology, reliability, validity, and accuracy. Meas Phys Educ Exerc Sci. 2000; 4: 215-28.

[20] Richter A, Räpple S, Kurz G, Schwameder H. Countermovement jump in performance diagnostics: Use of the correct jumping technique. Eur J Sport Sci. 2012; 12(3): 231-7.

[21] Markovic G, Dizdar D, Jukic I, Cardinale M. Reliability and factorial validity of squat and countermovement jump tests. J Strength Cond Res. 2004 Aug; 18(3): 551-5.

[22] Cohen J. Statistical power analysis for the behavioral sciences. 2nd ed. Hillsdale, NJ: Lawrence Erlbaum Associates; 1988.

[23] Keiner M, Sander A, Wirth K, Schmidtbleicher D. Is there a difference between active and less active children and adolescents in jump performance? Journal of Strength and Conditioning Research. 2013 //; 27(6): 1591-6.

[24] Castagna C, Castellini E. Vertical jump performance in Italian male and female national team soccer players. Journal of Strength and Conditioning Research. 2013 //; 27(4): 1156-61.

[25] Rebelo A, Brito J, Maia J, Coelho-E-Silva MJ, Figueiredo AJ, Bangsbo J, et al. Anthropometric characteristics, physical fitness and technical performance of under-19 soccer players by competitive level and field position. International Journal of Sports Medicine. 2013 //; 34(4): 312-7.

[26] Ziv G, Lidor R. Physical Characteristics, Physiological Attributes, and On-Field Performances of Soccer Goalkeepers. Int J Sports Physiol Perform. 2011; 6(4): 509-24.

[27] Aouichaoui C, Trabelsi Y, Bouhlel E, Tabka Z, Dogui M, Richalet JP, et al. The relative contributions of anthropometric variables to vertical jumping ability and leg power in Tunisian children. J Strength Cond Res. 2012 Mar; 26(3): 777-88.

[28] Temfemo A, Hugues J, Chardon K, Mandengue SH, Ahmaidi S. Relationship between vertical jumping performance and anthropometric characteristics during growth in boys and girls. European journal of pediatrics. 2009 Apr;168(4): 457-64.

8

Effect of Bharatnatyam Dancing on Body Composion of Bengalee Female Children

Shankarashis Mukherjee*, Neepa Banerjee, Surjani Chatterjee, Sandipan Chatterjee, Ayan Chatterjee, Tanaya Santra, Bijan Saha

Human Performance Analytics and Facilitation Unit, Department of Physiology, University of Calcutta, Kolkata, India
*Corresponding author: msasish@yahoo.co.in

Abstract Obesity, defined as abnormal or excessive fat accumulation that presents a risk to health, is on the rise including in the pediatric population in developed as well as less developed countries. As children are now fast adopting computer based activity both habitual and recreational with minimal level of physical effort, the prevalence of childhood obesity is a major concern. Indian dancing has been practised as a popular recreational activity for a long period of time. Bharatnatyam dancing is a traditional form of Indian classical dance which involves different body postures with continuous rhythmic body movements and therefore it may have some impact on body composition. A study has been undertaken in this backdrop, to assess the effect of Indian classical. Bharatanatyam dancing on body composition variables of girl children. Female individuals (12-18 year), receiving Bharatanatyam dancing training for at least a period of five years and practicing daily for an hour for 6 days in a week, constituted the Bharatanatyam dancing group (DG). Children of similar age and socioeconomic background with no regular physical activity including any form of dancing were randomly selected for constituting control group. It has been observed that training in Bharatnatyam dancing has significant ($P < 0.05$) favourable impact on the body composition parameters measured anthropometrically compared to the age and sex matched counterparts. It could therefore be concluded that Bharatnatyam dancing has specific beneficial impact on maintaining favourable body composition variables in children and thereby reducing the chance of obesity in adulthood.

Keywords: *childhood obesity, anthropometry, physical exercise, recreational activity, rhythmic movement*

1. Introduction

Overweight, defined as having excess body weight for a particular body height from fat, muscle, bone, water or a combination of these factors [1], have become a global problem in the last decade [2]. The scale of the obesity problem has a number of serious direct and indirect consequences for individuals and public health systems. The direct economic costs are medical costs for prevention, diagnosis, and treatment services for the obesity problem, while indirect costs relate to loss of income from decreased productivity, restricted activity, absenteeism, and bed days and lead to income loss by premature death. Together with rise in obesity in adults, the proportion of obesity in children have increased from 5% to 18% during 1980 to 2010 [3]. Children and adolescents who are obese are at greater risk for bone and joint problems, sleep apnoea, and social and psychological problems such as stigmatization and poor self-esteem ([4,5,6]). The greater concern is that the risks of overweight during childhood will persist into adolescence and adulthood [7]. The worldwide epidemic of excess weight is due to imbalance between physical activity and dietary energy intake, ective of the age of individuals. Sedentary lifestyle, unhealthy diet, and consequent overweight and obesity markedly increase the risk of cardiovascular diseases [8]. Physical activity plays an important role in the preventing one from becoming overweight and obese in childhood, reducing thereby the risk of suffering from obesity in adulthood [9]. Dance, a form of physical activity and a mode of exercise [10], performed by small groups of all ages [11], is a sequence of non verbal rhythmic body movements of creative nature and scope for expression. Bharatnatyam, an Indian classical dance, is a recreational activity since age old times.

It is a unique synchronization of music, rhythm and expression, where the dancer expresses the full gamut of human's experience through aesthetics. It includes some special movements like sitting, bending, standing, twisting etc and some complex movements like jumps and taut hand gestures. Some special types of exercise or initial basic steps, referred to as 'adavu', are required to be learnt before performing the dance. In this backdrop, a study was undertaken to see the effect of regular Bharatnatyam dancing on body composition in children.

2. Methodology

Initially institutions imparting training on Bharatnatyam dancing were approached and required permission was obtained. The names of initially interested volunteers were enlisted. The inclusion criteria was that the children (12-18 year) should have a minimum training of 5 years in Bharatnatyam and practice it regularly for at least an hour for 6 days in a week. Bharatnatyam dancing training for less than 5 years and being trained in other forms of exercise were considered as exclusion criteria for the study. Children of comparable age and socio-economic background, but not receiving training in any form of dance and also not exercising regularly constituted the Control Group (CG). Information about age (year), period for which individuals are receiving training in Bharatnatyam dancing, daily practicing time, nature and duration of daily activity, food habits, preliminary socio-economic condition and past incidence of major illness of self and parents were recorded in pre-designed schedule. Basic physical data like body height (cm) using Anthropometric rod with an accuracy of 0.1cm, body weight (kg) using a pre calibrated weighing scale with an accuracy of 0.1kg, with individuals in light clothing and without shoes, were measured and BMI was calculated. Waist circumference (WC), to the nearest of 0.5 cm, at the narrowest part of the iliac crest, and Hip circumference (HC), to the nearest of 0.5 cm, at the greatest circumference of the buttocks, with subjects in minimal inspiration were measured using a flexible measuring tape and waist hip ratio (WHR) was calculated. Body fat was estimated from skinfold measurement, using skin- fold calliper, obtained at three sites- tricep, subscapula and suprailiac. Obtained data were tabulated and used for further statistical analysis.

3. Results

The dancing group individuals and control group individuals do not differ significantly ($P > 0.05$) in respect of age.

In Figure 1a the mean Body Weight of individuals of DG (42.1kg) and CG (52.2 kg) are presented and there is significant difference ($P < 0.01$) between DG and CG individuals in respect of Body Weight. In Figure 1b the BMI (AM ± SD) of both DG (22.0) and CG (17.9) individuals are presented and there is significant difference ($P < 0.01$) between DG and CG individuals in respect of BMI. The Absolute Body Fat data of DG and CG individuals are presented in Figure 1c in AM ± SD form and significant difference ($P < 0.01$) between DG (9.2 kg) and CG (14.2kg) individuals in respect of Absolute Body Fat in kg is observed.

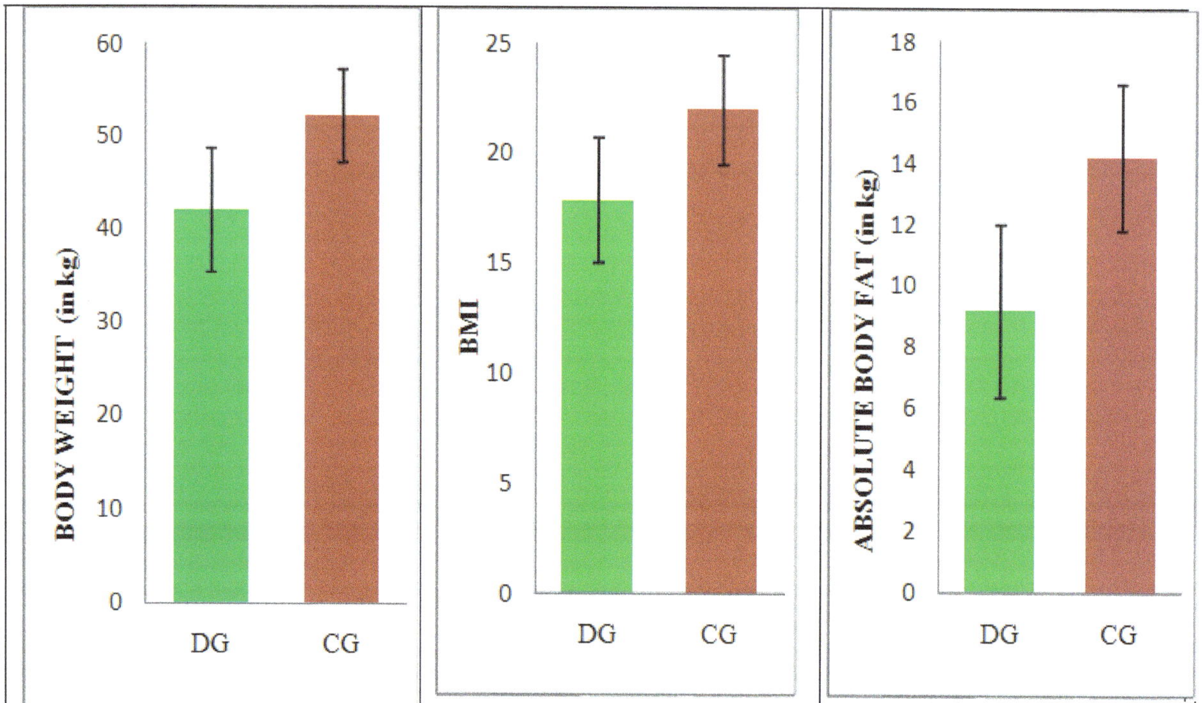

a) BODY WEIGHT**	b) BMI**	c) ABSOLUTE BODY FAT**

Figure 1. Comparison between DG and CG individuals in respect of BW, BMI and Absolute BF (**$P<0.01$)

The comparison between DG individuals and CG individuals is presented in respect of Waist Circumference (WC) in Figure 2a. It is observed that the WC is significantly ($P < 0.01$) lower in DG individuals (63.0cm) compared to their CG counterparts (70.5 cm).

In Figure 2b the Waist to Hip Ratio (WHR) status is presented for DG and CG individuals; the calculated values are respectively 0.76 and 0.78. It is observed that for the WHR, the DG individuals have significantly lower value ($P < 0.05$) compared to their CG counterparts.

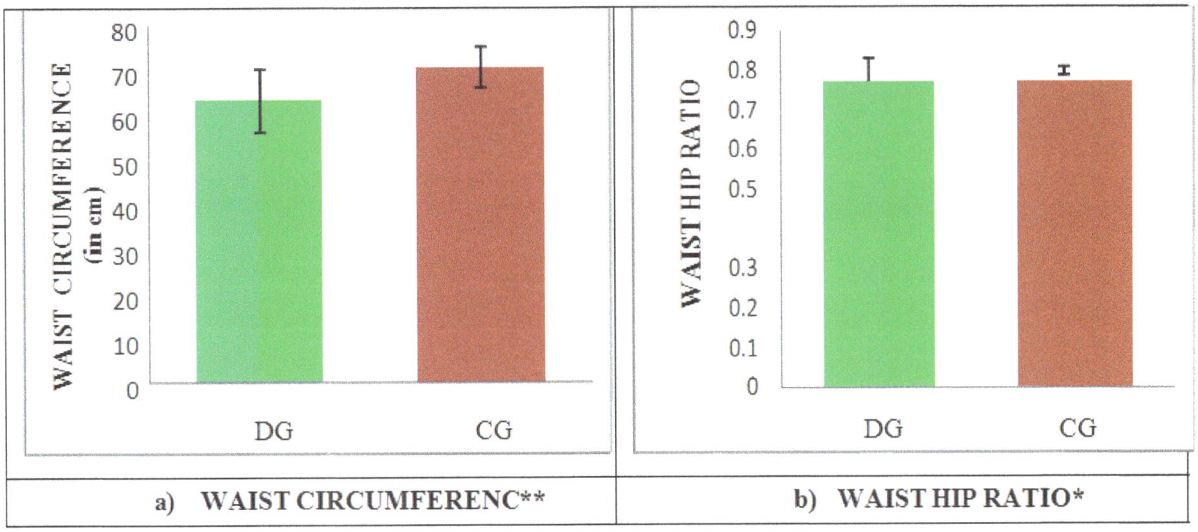

Figure 2. Comparison between DG and CG individuals in respect of WC and WHR (**P<0.01, *P< 0.05)

4. Discussions

The mean body height of the DG individuals was 153.5 cm and that of CG was 154.4 cm. As per WHO guideline on height for age for girls, the height for 14year and 15 year old girls are about 156cm and 160 cm respectively [12]. Body mass index (BMI, expressed in kg.m- 2), calculated as the ratio of subject's body weight (in kg) to the squared stature (m), and is now considered as one of the most commonly used indicator of obesity [13]. Children are defined as obese when BMI equals to or exceeds the age-gender-specific 95th percentile. Those with BMI equal to or exceeding the 85th but are below 95th percentiles are defined overweight and are at risk for obesity related co-morbidities [14]. In present study, the mean BMI of DG individuals is 17.9 which is significantly lower ($P < 0.01$), compared to their CG counterparts with mean BMI of 22.0; the trend of result of the present study are in agreement with the findings of Wyon [15]. The mean BMI of DG individuals is also found to be around the lower limit of the normal range of BMI values for girls aged between 5-19 years, in terms of WHO guideline; as per the latter, the BMI for 14 and 15 year old girls should be within 20 to 23.9. The favorable impact of Bharatnatyam dancing is again affirmed with assessment of the absolute body fat. The DG individuals have significantly lower ($P < 0.01$) absolute body fat, compared to their CG counterparts.

Waist Circumference (WC) and Waist Hip Ratio (WHR) are important indicators for defining central obesity and cardiovascular disease risk. The mean WC for DG children is 63.0 cm which is significantly lower ($P < 0.01$) compared to their CG counterparts having mean value of 70.5 cm. Present finding that DG individuals have lower value of WC is in agreement with the works of [16]; the mean WC of DG individuals are much lower than the cut off limit for Asians. A similar trend is observed for the WHR.

Earlier studies have found that dancing exercise plays an important role in the prevention of becoming overweight reducing the risk of obesity in adulthood [17]. Favorable impact of practicing Bharatnatyam dancing on body composition was observed previously in adult population [18], present study further affirmed that it has equally effective for female children.

5. Conclusion

On the basis of the study it could be concluded that Bharatnatyam dancing, if practiced regularly for at least an hour for 6 days in a week, has beneficial impact on maintaining favorable body composition variables, adjudged anthropometrically in children and thereby preventing the progression of onset of obesity and lower risk of suffering from specific diseases.

Acknowledgement

The authors are thankful to all the volunteers participating in the study for their cooperation and the concerned institutional authorities for their kind consent.

References

[1] Krebs NF, Hi mes JH, Jacobson D, Nicklas TA, Guilday P, Styne D, Assessment of child and adolescent overweight and obesity, *Pediatrics*, 120, 193-228, 2007.

[2] World Health Organisation, Obesity and Overweight, Global Strategy on Diet, *Physical Activity and Health*, 2006.

[3] Ogden CL, Carroll MD, Kit BK, Flegal KM. Prevalence of obesity and trends in body mass index among US children and adolescents, 1999-2010, *Journal of the American Medical Association,* 307(5), 483-490, 2012.

[4] Daniels SR, Arnett DK, Eckel RH, et al. Overweight in Children and Adolescents: Pathophysiology, Consequences, Prevention, and Treat ment. *Circulation,* 111, 1999-2002, 2005.

[5] Rockville, Office of the Surgeon General, *The Surgeon General's Vision for a Healthy and Fit Nation,* 2010.

[6] Dietz WH, Overweight in Childhood and Adolescence. *New England Journal of Medicine*, 350, 855-857. 2004.

[7] Kumari DJ, Krishna BS, Prevalence and Risk Factors for Adolescents (13-17 Years): Overweight and Obesity, *Current Science*, 100, February 2011.

[8] Lakka TA, Bouchard C, Physical Activity, Obesity and Cardiovascular Diseases, *Handb Exp pharmacol*, 170, 137-63, 2005.

[9] Hill AP, Andersen LB, Byrne NM, Physical Activity and Obesity in Children, *Br J Sports med,* 45(11):866-70, Sep 2011.

[10] Karageorghis CI, Terry PC, Today 5, *Sports Med*, 38-41, 2001.

[11] Mastura J, Fauzee MSO, Bahaman AS, Rashid S, Somchit MN, *Biol Sports*, 29, 63-69, 2012.

[12] Andreasi V, Michelin E, Rinaldi AEM, Burini RC, Physical fitness and Associations with Anthropometric Measurements in 7 to 15-year-Old School Children, *Jornal de Pediatria,* 86, 2010.

[13] Donohoue PA, Behrman RE, Kleigman RM, Jenson HB,Obesity. In, *Nelson Textbook of Pediatrics*, 17th ed, 173-7, 2004.

[14] Raj M, Kumar R, Obesity in children & adolescents, *Indian J Med Res,* 132, 598-607, Nove mber 2010.

[15] Wyon M, Allen N, Angioi M, Nevill A, Twitchett E, Anthropometric Factors Affecting Vertical Jump Height in Ballet Dancers, *Journal of Dance Medicine & Science,* 10, 106-110, 2006.

[16] Arslan F, The effects of an eight-week step-aerobic dance exercise programme on body composition parameters in middle- aged sedentary obese women, *International SportMed Journal*, 12, 160-168, 2011

[17] Kostić R, Đurašković R, Miletić D, Mikalački M, Body Composition of Women Under the Influence of the Aerobic Dance, *Physical Education and Sport,* 4, 59, 2006.

[18] S Mukherjee, N Banerjee, S Chatterjee, B Chakrabarti, Impact of Bharatnatyam Dancing Exercise in Reducing Central Obesity in Adult Bengalee Females, *Sci & Cult*, 79 (11-12), 503-506, 2013.

Is Futsal Kicking off in England? A Baseline Participation Study of Futsal

R. Moore*, J. Radford

Sport Industry Research Centre, Sheffield Hallam University, Sheffield, England
*Corresponding author: r.moore@shu.ac.uk

Abstract In England, there is a growing interest in futsal, driven by people who enjoy participating in the sport and others who see futsal as a development tool for those looking to succeed in football - dubbed the countries national sport. Nationally, the development of the sport has been overseen by futsal's governing body, The *Football Association* (FA), to improve the fortunes of the national futsal team and to provide a structure for the sport to grow at both grassroots and elite level. A lack of research into futsal exists, particularly around participation in the sport, and therefore there is insufficient knowledge to supply the elevated interest in the sport. The study establishes baseline measures to gain a greater understanding of futsal participation in England, to provide an indication of how many people participate in the sport; who participates, where, why and how? The study methodology was two-fold, firstly, analysis of primary and secondary data was undertaken to identify the number of teams and participants playing competitively between 7th January and 4th March 2013 - to provide a snapshot of futsal participation in England. The results, although indicative, show that during the course of this research there were 1975 teams playing organised competitive futsal and approximately 12,449 participants playing the sport during this period. Secondly, the research provides insight into participation trends of futsal from online survey responses of 108 futsal participants and 30 *County* FA coordinators, responsible for the development of the game nationwide. The evidence from respondents indicates that futsal is more popular than other variants of small sided football, with many respondents substituting or displacing their participation in other formats, to play futsal, while many also wish to increase their participation in the sport. Barriers to participation are also prevalent, particularly with regards to the availability and quality of facilities.

Keywords: *players, teams, facilities*

1. Introduction

1.1. Futsal

Futsal is *FIFA* and *UEFA's* recognised version of five-a-side football [1]. Consequently, because futsal is governed by football governing bodies it is structured similarly to football with worldwide competitions such as the *UEFA Futsal European Championships* and *FIFA World Cup* the pinnacles of the sport [2]. The English FA describe futsal as *'...an exciting, fast-paced small sided football game that is widely played across the world...'* [3]. Although futsal is an established worldwide sport in its own right, played both at amateur, semi-professional and professional level, its world wide appeal is supplemented by the fact that many elite football players endorse and speak of its importance to their own development [4].

1.2. English Futsal - Governance and Structure

Futsal is an emerging sport in England; played at grassroots and national level. The growth of futsal in England has been well documented, particularly as to many people it is a relatively new, fun, vibrant and fast paced sport in its own right, but partly because it is also employed as a tool, used by some football clubs, to develop young footballers. This vision is supported by *The FA* who state that the, '...game places a large emphasis on technical skill and ability in situations of high pressure, and is subsequently an excellent breeding ground for football competencies that can be translated into the 11-a-side format of the game' [3].

In relation to futsal as an independent sport, *The FA* has developed a *Small-Sided Football Strategy 2013-2017*, with one aspect to promote futsal participation in England and to develop the sport nationally, through the county FA structure [5]. This strategy incorporates elements of the *National Game Strategy* for football, targeting increased participation [5]. Part of this strategy is to maximise the potential of smaller sided formats which proposes fewer demands on time than traditional eleven-a-side football and aims to engage with footballers who no longer participate because of this time demand. The aims of the *Small Sided Football Strategy 2013-2017* are to increase participation nationally in the sport (youth participation, adult participation and elite development) and improve the fortunes of the English national team; to qualify for the showpiece global competitions; the *UEFA Futsal European Championship's* and the *FIFA World Cup.* Qualification for these events is of national importance, as, for example, The FIFA World Cup, attracts a 'global television audience', demonstrating the opportunity for international exposure, the potential inspirational effects for domestic participation growth and increased commercial revenues [6]. Furthermore, the FA has set an overall target of increasing the national number of small-sided teams to 30,000 by 2015 (28,370 in 2012), with futsal incorporated into this figure as part of the *National Game Strategy* [5].

In terms of elite participation, England players are selected from the *FA National Leagues*, the pinnacle of English competitive futsal [3]. Teams in these leagues are predominantly amateur and are grouped geographically according to their region (North, South and Midlands) and the season culminates in a national play off to decide the national champion [3].

At grassroots level, *The FA* also operates two participation initiatives. The *FA Futsal Fives* is designed to increase adult participation and is organised and facilitated by *County FA's* and through partnerships with commercial operators [3]. *FA Youth Futsal Festivals* are held nationally at under 12's, 14's, 16's in addition to the *FA National Under 19's Futsal Championships* which are held for both males and females [3]. Both schemes aim to grow and sustain grassroots participation and provide a pathway for players to progress into the FA National Leagues and potentially into the England national futsal team [3].

1.3. Futsal Participation

In addition to *FA* initiatives, the education sector provides further opportunities for competitive futsal to take place through organisations including *British Universities and Colleges Sport* (BUCS) and *British Colleges Sport* (BCS). Universities compete nationally, in leagues organised regionally, in conjunction with the academic year [7]. Furthermore, intramural futsal leagues in universities provide recreational playing opportunities for students [8]. *The FA* [3] has emphasised the significance of university futsal for increasing participation nationally.

Funded programmes which encompass futsal activity have enabled a wider audience to engage with the sport. For example, 39 professional English football clubs operate a futsal scholarship programme, which provide regular training in futsal linked to further education which enables young people to gain a recognised qualification [9]. Commercially, *@Futsal* arenas have revamped warehouses to create purpose-built, modernised centres to run futsal competitions around the UK [4]. At the time of this study @futsal operated five centres in total (Leeds, Stoke, Swindon, Sunderland, and Birmingham) but have since established a number of other facilities [4]. Other local providers also run commercial futsal leagues and run coaching clinics locally and in schools.

1.4. Academic Research into Futsal Participation

FIFA's Big Count participation study in 2006 reported that 265 million male and females are playing football worldwide [10]. The breakdown of the *Big Count* shows that there are just over 1 million male and females registered through their national governing bodies to play futsal [10]. Many people worldwide play futsal socially or in leagues not affiliated to governing bodies and therefore would not have been included in this calculation. It is expected that this figure will have increased significantly since this date. Furthermore, it is acknowledged in England that more people play futsal in Brazil than they do football, and that in Japan there are around 300,000 registered players, although no clear evidence is available in the English language.

The FA measures football participation against their own strategic aims, as a desire to increase participation collectively, thus boosting the chances of improving the national standard [11]. Therefore, measuring English futsal participation is fundamental to provide insight into strategizing an increase in futsal participation.

1.5. Barriers to Participation Growth

Although, there is a lack of research in relation to futsal, it is possible to identify barriers to participation in football which may also impact on futsal. For example, *The FA's National Facilities Strategy 2013-2015* surveyed football players, referees, coaches and administrators, finding that 84% of respondents identified 'poor facilities' as a barrier to participation [11]. Additionally, frequent responses pointed to concerns for the increased cost to use facilities and reduced maintenance of facilities [11]. As futsal is an indoor sport it could be argued that facility problems are more prevalent as they rely on the quality of indoor facilities - which football teams also use. Therefore it is of interest to identify any causality existing between facility conditions and barriers to participation particularly when assessing both supply and demand of futsal participation.

1.6. Justification for the Research

Academically, the body of evidence around participation in futsal is sparse. Little evidence exists in relation to futsal in England, and although it is anticipated the sport will continue to grow, it is important to understand more about futsal in terms of participation and the reasons why people play. This is particularly important, as The FA, the sport's governing body, aim to increase participation, while clubs at all levels seek to attract support to continue to develop. Little, if no research has been carried out to investigate futsal participants' perceptions of the game and how it is delivered in this country. Participation studies are notoriously difficult to conduct, but considering the constrained nature of futsal participation and the role of key organisations involved in its development it is possible to gain an indication of competitive participation in futsal.

2. Methodology

2.1. Secondary Analysis of Participation Data

To calculate a baseline figure for the number of clubs and participants involved in organised competitive futsal, it was crucial to identify organisations delivering competitive futsal opportunities. At the outset, support was gained from The FA, the largest provider of competitive futsal, to provide data pertaining to its various competitions. *The FA* provided data for the *FA Futsal Fives League, FA Youth Futsal Festival* (aged under 10 to under 16 competitions) and the *FA Under 18 Championship*, (currently the under 19 championship). This was significant, as although some of this data was available online, the majority was not, and therefore it was necessary that this support was provided.

The timeframe for collecting participation data was between the 7th January and the 4th March 2013. During this period, data was collected either online, via the telephone or provided through email. This period was chosen as the majority of leagues, identified prior to the study, were operating during this period. As a result, the decision was made to ensure that the data collated during this period would be representative of a single 'snapshot' in time. Furthermore, *BCS* futsal league was originally identified to form part of the study, but as the league was not running during this period, it was excluded from the study, so as to be consistent with the methodological approach.

The following considerations were made to identify participating futsal teams and leagues to participate in the study:

- Junior and Adult leagues providing competitive futsal opportunities.
- Male and female teams and participants.
- Availability of club and participant data.
- Leagues operating during the study period
- Only English teams were included

Once data was collected, the numbers of clubs in each league were calculated to provide a cumulative figure. Participant data was collected at source, if available. Missing participant data was either obtained by contacting appropriate personnel directly, or assumptions were made based on indicative figures, equivalent to five players per-team, which is conservative, but ensured that calculations were not overestimated. The following details how data was collected for each competition:

2.1.1. FA Youth Festival

The number of clubs participating in the *FA Youth Futsal Festival* was provided by *The FA*. Participant data was not included in the data provided and therefore an assumption was made for each team based on the minimum number of 5 players required to form a futsal team.

2.1.2. FA Futsal Fives

Team data was provided by *The FA* for all *County FA's* apart from Middlesex, and therefore this county were subsequently excluded from the study. Participant data was obtained for 7 *County FA's* from their official websites. An assumption was made for the remaining *County FA's*, based on a minimum of 5 players per team.

2.1.3. FA National Futsal League

The number of teams and participants data was obtained from *The FA Full time* website. Team lists were not provided for all teams and therefore squad lists were included, although it is possible, considering the study time period, that some participants did not play during this period.

2.1.4. @Futsal

The number of teams competing in *@futsal* leagues operating during the study period was obtained for 4 out of 5 centres. The data for the Stoke centre was not able to be identified and therefore this centre was excluded from the study. Participant data was obtained for two of the four centres from the *@futsal* website, while an assumption of 5 players per team was made based on the 2 centres where data was unable to be obtained.

2.1.5. British Universities Colleges Sport (BUCs)

Team data was captured from the *BUCs* website for all English teams competing in the futsal championships. Player data was obtained from thirty one universities who were contacted by either telephone or email. Participant data was not obtained from 11 universities, so an assumption was made based on 5 players per team.

2.1.6. FA National Under 18's Championships

Team data was provided by *The FA*. In the north, accurate player data was provided by 4 clubs who were contacted by email or telephone. Assumptions of 5 players per team were made for 6 teams. One team did not participate in the competition. In the midlands, 2 teams were contacted to obtain player data, and assumptions were made for 2 other teams. One team did not participate in the league. In the south, 12 teams were contacted to provide player data, 3 teams could not be contacted and therefore an assumption was made for these teams. One team did not compete in the competition.

2.1.7. Football League Trust Futsal League

The number of teams involved in this league were collected from the league website. No participant data was provided and therefore an assumption of 5 players per team was calculated.

2.2. Online Survey of Futsal Participants and County Football Association Staff

To capture views on futsal, participants and *County FA* staff were surveyed over a 3 week period in January. An online survey was designed to capture responses from each group. The survey was then distributed by *County FA's* and through social media. The purpose of the survey was to identify participation trends and individual perceptions of futsal. Surveys were electronic and were distributed via email and advertised through *FA Futsal Fives* and *FA National League* administrators and social network websites (Facebook and Twitter). In total, 148 survey responses were analysed; 108 from participants and 30 from *County FA's*.

3. Results

Table 1 displays the overall number of teams and participants playing competitive futsal during the 8 week snapshot.

Table 1. Number of futsal teams and participants

Provider	Total Teams	Total Participants	Average no. participants per team
FA Youth Futsal Festivals	1,100	5,500	5
@Futsal Centres	596	4,334	7.3
FA Futsal Fives	135	1,129	8.4
FA National Futsal Leagues	32	803	25.1
BUCS Futsal Championships	84	451	5.3
FA National Under 18's Championships	28	282	11.3
Football League Trust Futsal League	39	195	5
Total	**2,014**	**12,694**	**6.3**

Table 1 shows that 2,014 teams participated in futsal competition between the 7th January and 4th March 2013, providing opportunities for a total of 12,694 people playing futsal. The FA competitions provided opportunities for 64% (1295 teams) of teams and 61% (7714 players) of players. The highest number of teams and participants were competing at junior level in the *FA Youth Futsal Festival* (1,100), followed by participants in the *@futsal* centres (596 teams) which included both junior and adult teams. Commercial *@futsal* centres provided opportunities for 30% of clubs and 34% of participants demonstrating that it is a significant provider of participation alongside *The FA* competitions.

These figures demonstrate that futsal currently contributes 2,014 (7%) teams towards the FA's 2015 target for 30,000 small-sided teams. As the figure was previously 28,370 it can be assumed that other small-sided variations remain dominant. Although the figures presented are conservative, considering the limitations of the research, they do provide a baseline to measure future participation.

3.1. Participation trends

One hundred and eight futsal participants completed a survey regarding their involvement in the sport. The results show that 87% (94 participants) were male and 13% (14 participants) female and 76% (82 participants) were of 'White British' ethnic origin. The majority of respondents were aged between 21-25 (43%, 47 respondents), 26-35 (32%, 35 respondents) and 16-20 (19%, 21 respondents). The survey was targeted at adult participants and therefore this is reflected in the overall response.

The majority of respondents currently participate for between one (32%, 34 participants), two (24%, 26 participants) and three (33%, 35 participants) days per week, with 91% (97) of respondents training or playing in competitive matches for between one and six hours per week. Over half (53%) of participants had only been playing futsal for between one (36%, 39 participants) and two years (17%, 18 participants). This demonstrates, the emerging nature of futsal, with the majority of participants not experiencing the sport until recently.

It is interesting to note that 80% (75) of respondents participate more now in futsal than they have ever done, while 94% (101) of participants would like to participate in futsal more often. Evidently, these respondents have experienced the sport, and enjoy participating, which consequently has led them to participate more. It appears that there may also be latent demand, as participants want to participate more, but for some reason, do not. This is either because barriers exist to participation or because there is a lack of opportunities to play futsal. Furthermore, the view from *County FA's* is that futsal participation is increasing, according to 30 members of local county football associations who completed a survey for this study. Twenty-six (87%) members of *County FA's* stated that futsal participation is increasing, although 40% (12 *County FA's*) describe participation in their county as 'below average' demonstrating that they are aware that further development in the sport is required.

According to *County FA* staff, 73% (22 staff) felt that the most common reason for taking up futsal, was because it was relatively new in this country. Other reasons stated included 'skill development' (77%, 23 participants), and 'enjoyment' (77%, 23 participants). Key promoters of futsal include universities and colleges, as just under half (46%, 46) of participants first heard of futsal at college or university, while 14% (14 participants) of people heard of futsal through the *The FA*.

3.2. Participation Change

According to the results, the trend is that participants are playing more futsal and want to play more in the future. In relation to other formats of football, the literature shows that the 11 aside game is most popular, followed by other versions of 5 and 6 aside. The results demonstrate that displacement and substitution is occurring with regards to participation in other formats of football. For example, the results show that 98% (105) of respondents have already played 11-a-side football; 96% (103) 5-a-side football (not including futsal); 69% (74) 6-a-side and 75% (80) 7-a-side. As the majority of participants only took part in futsal 2 years ago, this suggests that the majority of futsal participants, were firstly engaged in another format of football, before participating in futsal. Evidently, 58% (63 respondents) still play 11 aside; 26% (28) 5-aside (26%, 28); 17% (18) 7-aside and 16% (18) 6-aside, which indicates that substitution is taking place, or participants are decreasing other football activity to find time to play futsal. Interestingly, 24% (26) only play futsal, with the largest drop in these respondents habits occurring when participants only play 5 aside (70%) rather than the 11 aside game (42%). This represents clear displacement, participants who completed the survey now favour futsal, ending their participation in other formats of football.

Furthermore, 94% (101) of people think that futsal is better than other versions of 5 aside, which is supported by 93% (28) of *County FA* staff while 76% (81 respondents) stated that futsal could become more popular than generic version of 5-aside, supported by 70% (21) of *County FA* staff. Participants stated that the structure of futsal, including the rules of play, speed, technical and tactical nature of the sport were all reasons why people were drawn to futsal.

3.3. Futsal Participation Sites

In terms of identifying where participation takes place, *BUCs* provided competition for 52 (55%) participants; *FA Futsal Fives* for 50 (53%) and *FA National Leagues* 41

(43%) participants. Competitive futsal players who completed the survey all played in multi-use facilities, which cater for a wide array of different sports. These include 'sports club or community association use facilities' (51%, 54 participants), 'pay and play facilities' (40%, 40), 'private use facilities' (38%, 40), and 'specialist *@futsal* facilities' (30%, 32 participants). Predominantly, the surfaces in the majority of facilities are marked out for other sports according to respondents with 91% (98 participants) of people playing on such surfaces. This is unsurprising given the competition for indoor space in sports that use similar facilities. Thirty nine percent (31) of respondents play futsal outside on facilities such as 'astroturf', 'tarmac' and 'grass'. Futsal is an indoor sport and therefore participation on such facilities could represent a barrier to future participation, if the reason for this usage is because of a lack of availability in indoor facilities or a lack of knowledge of how the sport should be played.

Futsal players also report a number of issues including availability (50%, 53 respondents), the condition of facilities and appearance of facilities (both 28%, 20 respondents). Twenty-one (70%, 21 staff) *County FA* staff stated that there are not enough suitable futsal facilities to maintain current demand in England for futsal to take place, while the 'cost of participating' (62%, 18 staff), and 'no opportunities to play train' (86%, 21 staff) were also cited as potential barriers.

3.4. Participation Impact on 11-aside Football

Interest in futsal as a sport, as the literature suggests, is often due to the potential development affect the sport may have on footballers. The majority of participants (96%, 102 respondents) and County FA staff (100%, 30) believe that futsal should be used as a development tool for football. County FA staff also think that using futsal as a development tool for football will help to increase participation in futsal, presumably because the link helps to promote the sport and allow more people to experience it. Seventy-six percent of County FA's believe that futsal can mirror the growth seen in other countries to eventually become a professional sport in this country.

4. Conclusion

The study provides a baseline calculation for futsal participation in England, to help contribute to the knowledge of the sports development in this country and to enable future studies to track the growth of the sport. Although there are certain limitations to the research, the study provides a comprehensive account for the number of teams and participants involved in futsal. The study also provides insight into the potential development of futsal providing evidence that participants are substituting and displacing participation in other formats of football, to take part in futsal. Furthermore, the study demonstrates that people are drawn to the sport, partly because it has a structure both nationally and internationally, but ostensibly because people enjoy the sport; the fast paced nature and technical and tactical aspects which differ from other formats. On the whole, survey respondents believe that futsal will continue to grow and will eventually become more popular than other small sided formats. There are though a number of barriers to participation which exist and could slow the development of the sport particularly regarding the availability and quality of facilities. Finally, the popularity of football means that their will continue to be a link between the two sports, which may help to increase participation, but could undermine the aspects of futsal which people enjoy, particularly if the sport is played in facilities traditionally used for football.

5. Limitations of the Study

There are certain limitations which affect the validity of the results in calculating a baseline number of futsal teams and participants involved in competitive futsal. The figures are indicative, predominantly because they do not include all competitive leagues and participants, due to the availability and accessibility of information. For example, it is anticipated that a number of private operators were not included in the study, partly because it was difficult to gain an overall picture of the number of futsal leagues, considering time, resource and the availability of information. Furthermore, university intra-mural leagues, who provide opportunities in futsal were excluded from the study as we could not confirm the number of teams participating nationwide during the study period.

The study was carried out during a limited period so as to decrease the possibility of double counting, when players play for more than one team or transfer to another team. However, there is still a possibility of this occurring particularly as some players may have played in national league competition, university competition and under 18 competition as well as *@futsal* sites. The study does not claim to provide data on all clubs and participants playing competitively in this country. It does however provide the most comprehensive account of the number of clubs and participants playing futsal in England during a 'snapshot' in time.

References

[1] FIFA (2013). *Futsal: Mission and Objectives.* (Online). Last accessed 19/3/13 at: http://www.fifa.com/aboutfifa/footballdevelopment/technicalsupport/futsal/mission.html

[2] UEFA STATUTES (2012). *Rules of Procedure of the UEFA Congress Regulations Governing the Implementation of the UEFA Statutes: 2012 Edition.* (Online). Last accessed 19/3/13 at: http://www.uefa.com/MultimediaFiles/Download/EuroExperience/uefaorg/WhatUEFAis/01/80/54/03/1805403_DOWNLOAD.pdf

[3] THE FOOTBALL ASSOCIATION (FA) (2013). *What is Futsal?* (Online). Last accessed 17/2/13 at: http://www.thefa.com/my-football/player/futsal/what-is-futsal.

[4] FUTSAL UK (2012). *10 Reasons to Play Futsal.* (Online). Last accessed 11/11/12 at: http://www.futsaluk.net/content/the-game.php.

[5] SMALL SIDED FOOTBALL STRATEGY (2012). *Good Practice Guide 2011-2012.* (Online). Last accessed 29/4/13 at: http://www.thefa.com/News/my-football/small-sided-football/ssf/2012/mar/~/media/A2E440D3BCE24BE8B63512B042D5BD48.ashx.

[6] FIFA (2012). *FIFA Futsal World Cup Thailand 2012.* (Online). Last accessed 11/11/12 at: http://www.fifa.com/futsalworldcup/matches/round=255907/match=300215828/index.html.

[7] BRITISH UNIVERSITIES & COLLEGES SPORT (BUCS) (2013). *Welcome to BUCS Futsal.* Last accessed 29/4/13 at: http://www.bucs.org.uk/sport.asp?section=14570&sectionTitle=Futsal.

[8] UNIVERSITY OF BATH (2011). *Futsal.* Last accessed 29/4/13 at: http://www.teambath.com/sport/football/futsal/.

[9] FOOTBALL LEAGUE TRUST (2012) *Futsal League Scholarship set for Kick-off.* (Online). Last accessed 29/4/13 at: http://www.football-league.co.uk/latestnews/20120828/futsal-league-scholarship-set-for-kick-off_2293301_2903020.

[10] FIFA (2007). *Big Count 2006: Statistical Summary Report*, FIFA Communications Division, 2007. [Online]. Available: http://www.fifa.com/mm/document/fifafacts/bcoffsurv/bigcount.summaryreport_7022.pdf. [Last accessed Jan. 27 2014].

[11] THE FOOTBALL ASSOCIATION (FA) (2011). *Strategic Plan 2011-2015.* Last accessed 30/3/13 at: http://www.thefa.com/~/media/files/pdf/about-the-fa/fa-strategic-plan-2011.ashx.

Heart Rate Variations in an Elite Futsal Player after Twelve Years of Maximum Performance

J. Álvarez-Medina[1,*], V. Murillo-Lorente[1], P. Manonelles-Marqueta[2], L. Giménez-Salillas[1]

[1]Faculty of Health Sciences, Department of Physical Medicine and Nursing, University of Zaragoza, Zaragoza, Spain
[2]Spanish Federation of Sports Medicine (FEMEDE), Pamplona, Spain
*Corresponding author: javialv@unizar.es

Abstract Compare cardiovascular responses and adaptations of a professional futsal player both at rest and in action over an uninterrupted twelve-year period. Cross-over case study. Data analysis was performed by descriptive analysis, which results are expressed as percentages (percentiles) and mean ± standard deviation (SD). The study was conducted between 1999 and 2012 sport seasons. Laboratory tests (Electrocardiogram and echocardiography, maximum stress test) and field test (competitive and training games).The VO2 max of our athlete decreased from 57.8 to 52.7 ml/kg/min however the anaerobic threshold significantly improved, as it increased from 80.4% to 92% of his heart rate maximum (HRmax). The athlete's HRmax changed from 194 bpm in 1999 to 176 bpm in 2012 and his mean heart rate (MHR) from 168.1 ± 13 bpm to 142 ± 13 bpm. In 1999 the athlete's performance was < 150 bpm 9.1% of time while in 2012 his heart rate (HR) was < 150 bpm 60.30% of time. In 1999, he had 150-170 bpm 32.9% of time, while in 2012 he was 39.7% of time with this HR. He changed from having a HR >170 bpm 57.8% of time in 1999 to not have this HR at any time in 2012. Comparative analysis indicated that intensity variability over a decade is < 10%, as it was 86.5% in 1999 and 80.6% in 2012. Conclusions: Age is the main factor causing heart rate variability in team sports players since maximum heart rate decreases with age. Using heart rate as an indicator of work intensity involves using relative values of percentage of work intensity with respect to their maximum heart rate.

Keywords: *team sports, adaptations, training, fitness, cardiovascular responses*

1. Introduction

Heart rate (HR) is widely accepted as an indicator of cardiovascular response [1,2,3] in many sports –including team sports– and is used for training load control [4-9]. The reason to using HR is that it can be easily measured, recorded, read and functionally applied. Moreover, it is a non-invasive parameter easily measurable by performance assessment teams.

HR variations have been reported in athletes performing the same work [10]. Such variations might be due to different causes, being the most relevant the age, competitive level and motivation of the athlete [11]. HR variations are greater in team sports as a result of individual playing style, playing positions, etc [12].

Researchers have found individual differences in the physiological profile of different sports modality players. However, scarce literature is available on the evolution of intrapersonal HR variations throughout a sports career.

In 1999 [13] we examined the physiological profiles of two futsal players: a young player performing at a very high HR, and an older player playing at a low HR. The profiles obtained led us wonder whether young players performing at so great absolute intensities maintain the same HR response over the years. To answer this question we conducted a ten-year follow-up study on a professional male futsal player. Accordingly, the aim of this study was to compare the cardiovascular responses and adaptations of a professional futsal player both at rest and in action over an uninterrupted ten-year period.

2. Material and Methods

This is a cross-over case study conducted between 1999 and 2012. Data analysis was performed by descriptive analysis, which results are expressed as percentages (percentiles) and mean ± standard deviation (SD).

The athlete provided informed consent to undergo all stress tests and was aware that he could quit the study at any moment.

As to the specific characteristics of the athlete, he did not have any relevant injury at any moment throughout the study period.

The first record was taken in 1999, when the athlete was 19 years of age, and the last was taken in the 2011-2012 season.

Futsal is an intermittent game based on brief intense actions interspersed by active and incomplete recovery periods including a sequence of highly demanding aerobic-anaerobic actions [13], where players frequently perform maximally [14].

This case study included the following studies:

Kinanthropometry: Height (cm) was measured by a 1-mm precision stadiometer "Seca". Weight was assessed by a 100g.-precision scale. Six skinfolds (mm) were measured with a "Holtain Crymich" 0.1 mm- scaliper.

Electrocardiograms and echocardiographies: We performed 12-lead electrocardiograms (Fukuda-Denshi FK-12) and echocardiographies (Ecocardiografo-Dopler "Hewlett Packard") with the subject at rest. These two tests were performed to find out whether professional training induces a different cardiovascular response at rest because of an adaptation of the heart. Electrocardiograms and echocardiographies were performed and read by the same observer.

Maximum stress tests were performed on a treadmill (Jaeger-LE5, Wuerburz, Germany): To determine the athlete's HR values and response to progressive-maximum stress we established work thresholds with a continuous progressive protocol set at a fixed 3% slope and 1 Km.h-1 load increases at 1-minute intervals. Pulmonary air flow and gas exchange were analyzed breath by breath (Medical Graphics CPX/MAX, St. Paul, Minnesota, USA).

We considered that maximum oxygen uptake (VO2 max) was reached:

When the oxygen uptake (VO2) although the training load was increased.

When the mean heart rate was > 90% of HR for age (220-age).

And when the gas exchange rate was > 1.15.

The ventilatory threshold was determined during stress tests by the V-Slope method [15].

Heart rate maximum (HRmax): Different studies indicate that HRmax is an individual parameter which is not sensitive to fitness status and is not affected or slightly affected by age, heredity etc. However, there are other factors such as fatigue, motivation or stress that may alter HRmax values [12]. At 32 years of age, the HRmax begins to decrease linearly. To determine the HRmax we used the maximum value obtained either in the laboratory test or during a game. The reason is that according to Barbero some players may have two or three more beats during a game than in lab tests [16,17].

Heart rate (HR) recorded in competitive and training games. We recorded the athlete's HR in eight matches – four throughout the 1999-2000 season and four throughout the 2011-2012 season. We considered that the sample size was appropriate as the results obtained were consistent with those obtained in previous studies [10,18]. Thus, previous studies have reported that HRmax values and mean HR (MHR) do not significantly vary from match to match, and each player has their own repeating performance pattern. Data were collected in the same conditions: type of work (futsal games); day time (in the afternoon); place and environmental conditions (indoor court); and constant hydration, since losing 1% of body weight negatively affects performance.

HR was measured using Polar heart rate monitors –the Accurex Plus model in 2000 and the 725X model in 2011– set to record HR at five-second intervals. The data collected in the field study were analyzed using the Polar Pro trainer interface.

It is noteworthy that two of the most relevant variables affecting HR –cognitive and emotional factors [19] – have changed over time.

3. Results

3.1. Laboratory Tests

In 1999: Age: 19 years old. Weight: 82.5 kg. Height: 181cm. ∑6skinfolds: 60.3 mm. Maximum oxygen uptake: 57.8 ml/kg/min. Loud reached in Maximum stress test 16 Km/h. Anaerobic Threshold: 156 bpm. HRmax: 194 bpm. Anaerobic Threshold % HRmax: 80.4%.

In 2012: Age: 32 years old. Weight: 84.1 kg. Height: 181.8 cm. ∑6skinfolds: 60.6 mm. Maximum oxygen uptake: 52.7 ml/kg/min. Loud reached in Maximum stress test 17 Km/h. Anaerobic Threshold: 162 bpm. HRmax: 176 bpm. Anaerobic Threshold % HRmax: 92.0%.

3.2. Competitive and Training Games

Cardiovascular response (Figure 1) and Work intensity by the percentage of maximum heart rate (Table 1):

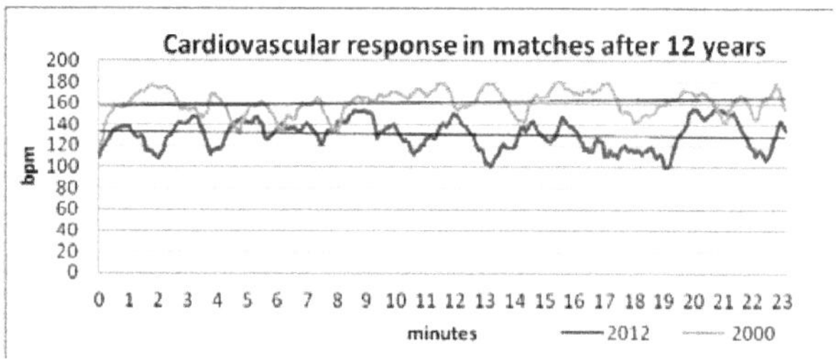

Figure 1. Cardiovascular response in matches after twelve years

Table 1. Cardiovascular response in matches

Season 1999-2000												
MHRa	%HRmaxb	>100	100-109	110-119	120-129	130-139	140-149	150-159	160-169	170-179	180-189	190-199
167±14	86.1	0.8	0	0.8	0.8	1.8	3.9	12	28.6	38	13	0.3
162±12	83.5	0.6	1	1.8	4	3.8	7	18.1	22.1	30.1	11.4	0
170±14	87.6	0.7	0.3	0.7	1.7	0.1	3.7	5	18.3	47.3	22.3	0
172±13	88.6	0	0.3	0.3	0.3	0.3	1.8	6.3	21.4	41.6	27.7	0
168±13	**86.5**	**0.5**	**0.4**	**0.9**	**1.7**	**1.5**	**4.1**	**10.3**	**22.6**	**39.2**	**18.6**	**0.1**
Season 2011-2012												
MHRa	%HRmaxb	>100	100-109	110-119	120-129	130-139	140-149	150-159	160-169	170-179	180-189	190-199
131±1	74.3	0.0	4.3	21.9	18.6	25.4	21.1	8.6	0.0	0.0	0.0	0.0
127±17	72.1	0.0	21.3	13.6	21.3	19.2	13.3	5.9	5.2	0.0	0.0	0.0
145±15	82.3	0.0	1.6	8.0	9.2	13.0	18.5	35.2	14.4	0.0	0.0	0.0
139±13	78.9	0.0	3.0	8.0	16.7	19.5	23.1	26.8	3.0	0.0	0.0	0.0
142±14	**80.6**	**0.0**	**2.3**	**8.0**	**12.9**	**16.2**	**20.8**	**31.0**	**8.7**	**0.0**	**0.0**	**0.0**

In 1999: HRmax was 194 bpm. In maches the work intensity by the percentage of HRmax was 86.5%. The player were <65% of their HRmax 2.8% of time; between 65-85% of their HRmax 31.6% of time, and >85% of their HRmax 65.5% of time.

In 2012: HRmax was 176 bpm. In maches the work intensity by the percentage of HRmax was 80.6%. The player were <65% of their HRmax 6.3% of time; between 65-85% of their HRmax 69.0% of time, and >85% of their HRmax 24.7% of time.

4. Discussion

4.1. Laboratory Tests

Anthropometric characteristics: Although the athlete changed from 82.5 to 84.1 kg of weight, his anthropometric characteristics did not change significantly over the 12-year study period. The reason is that in twelve years the athlete grew nearly one centimeter, and during the holidays the subject usually weighs one kilo more than during the pre-season ten years ago.

Electrocardiogram-echocardiography: In our study of the 1999 season [14] we found that over 80% of futsal players had sinus bradycardia. This is the case of our subject, who in 1999 presented a HR of 55 bpm at resting position and 45 bpm in 2012. The remaining parameters on the Electrocardiogram-echocardiography remained stable over the ten years and are similar to those found in similar sports players [20].

Maximum stress tests were performed at the beginning of the pre-season i.e when the player was not in his optimal fitness status. We found that, in spite of the years, the athlete maintained almost the same VO2 max, which was only slightly lower than ten years before. In addition, the athlete could endure greater training loads.

Maximal oxygen uptake (VO2 max): Firstly, we should take into account that VO2 max is not a limiting factor for maximal performance [21]. The reason is that the type of work performed in futsal is intermittent and correspond to short high-intensity training exercises that require high-intensity work. These methods involve a relatively low load to circulation and breathing by the introduction of brief sprinting-and-rest intervals appropriately separated (microbreaks). This physiological concept allows for older subjects or individuals with a lower VO2 max to perform intense work provided that work and recovery periods are appropriately regulated.

The VO2 max of our athlete decreased from 57.8 to 52.7 ml/kg/min, which is consistent with the findings of previous studies that suggest that the average rate of decline is 10% per decade after the age of 25. Increasing VO2 max is difficult. In fact, trained people only can increase their VO2 max by 10% approx [22]. The 52.7 ml/kg/min value obtained in this study in 2012 is lower than the value obtained in previous studies on futsal players (57.80±2.53 ml/kg/min) [21]. However, we think that such differences wouldn't exist if we had measured VO2 max during the in-season as in the referenced study. The values obtained in this study are consistent with those found in team sports players [21]. Thus, values < 50 ml/kg/min are considered deficient; between 50 and 55 ml/kg/min. are normal; 55-60 ml/kg/min. are good and > 60 ml/kg/min. are excellent VO2 max values.

HRmax: The athlete's HRmax decreased from 194 bpm in 1999 to 176 bpm in 2012, which accounts for a decline of 20 bpm approx. The age range of team sports players is wide as players can be 18-36 years of age. Consequently, their HRmax values also vary significantly, since age –and individual adaptation to stress– is directly related to HRmax. These two factors –age and individual adaptation– are the main cause of HR variations among team sports players undergoing the same stress.

Anaerobic threshold: Is the most reliable performance indicator and one of the primary goals of training. It can be increased by a maximum of 40% [23]. Training seasons are intended to make players progressively become more resistant to fatigue and increase their energy use, which can pass from 60% to 90% [24]. The anaerobic threshold of the player in our study significantly improved, as it increased from 80.4% to 92% of his HRmax, which accounts for a significant adaptation to high-intensity stress.

The VO2 max and anaerobic threshold values obtained in this study are consistent with those obtained by Parr et al. (1978) [25], who observed that although basket players do not present high oxygen uptake values, their anaerobic threshold is greater as compared to that of other sports players with a similar VO2 max.

4.2. Competitive and Training Games

Mean heart rate (MHR): Futsal is an indoor court sport with few players that is played in a small area with a limited number of changes. Consequently, all players perform considerable work and are in constant movement to search for spaces. When a player does not work with enough intensity, he is replaced with another player. As unlimited changes are allowed, futsal players present high MHR, as described in previous studies [13,16]. During a game, futsal players are 83% of time >85% of their HRmax, which is considered by Woolford and Argove [26] and the ACSM as a very vigorous intensity [17].

Accordingly, interpersonal HR variability is very important, and the dispersion of values around the mean HR value is very high. This was proven by Alvarez [10], who established a mean HR value of 165±10 bpm and a range of 141-181 bpm. Another study examining the HR of eight futsal players at the Division de Plata (second professional league) in five matches yielded a mean HR of 172.9±0.8 bpm [27].

The cardiovascular response of the athlete in our study changed over time. HR was always measured in the same conditions. The only factor that changed was the athlete's age and cognitive and emotional factors [19].

Age: The athlete's HRmax declined by 20 bpm approx. and his MHR changed from 168.1±13 bpm to 142±13 bpm. MHR should be associated with HRmax, which accounts for work intensity.

Cognitive and emotional factors: In 1999, the athlete was at the beginning of his professional career and wanted to earn a position in the team, so his performance was maximal in training sessions and competitive matches. After a decade, our athlete became a veteran player and had his place in the team, so he regulated his actions and avoided unnecessary stress, which reflects a better understanding of the game. In other words, he economized stress.

These data confirm that HR can be used as an indicator of stress provided that HRmax is related to relative intrapersonal intensity values rather than to absolute values.

HR distribution ranges (Figure 2): In 1999 the athlete's performance was < 150 bpm 9.1% of time while in 2012 his HR was < 150 bpm 60.30% of time. In 1999, he had 150-170 bpm 32.9% of time, while in 2012 he was 39.7% of time with this HR. He changed from having a HR >170 bpm 57.8% of time in 1999 to not have this HR at any time in 2012. These results are in agreement with those obtained by Barbero (2004) [16, 27], who found that players were <150 bpm 6.9% of time; 150-170 bpm 25.7% of time; and >170 bpm 67.4% of time during a match.

A possible explanation to this might be that the Barbero study was performed on players at the Division de Plata, where players are prevailingly young and have greater motivation and HRmax as compared to older players. This is confirmed by their HRmax, which were 192.1±0.8 bpm.

The decline in HR is not caused by a reduction in work intensity, but to the player's current inability to work at such a high HR due to a decline in his HRmax.

Work intensity by the percentage of HRmax: The results obtained in 1999 were similar to those reported by Barbero [16,27], who determined that futsal players are <65% of their HRmax 1.8% of time; between 65-85% of their HRmax 15% of time, and >85% of their HRmax 80.70% of time.

Comparative analysis indicated that intensity variability over a decade is < 10%, as it was 86.5% in 1999 and 80.6% in 2012.

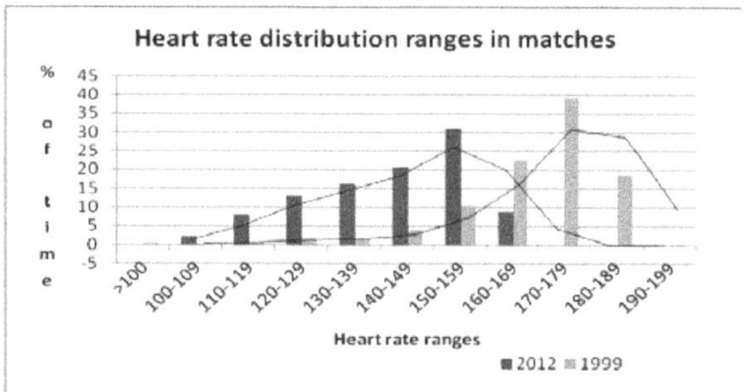

Figure 2. Heart rate distribution ranges in matches

We analyzed the interpercentile interval 65-85% – which is the interval used for the classification of training loads in team sports– and observed a significant increase in the 12-year study period. However, when we analyzed the 85% percentile we found a significant decrease [28]. The data obtained clearly show that the time spent at each intensity interval has changed over the years. Our athlete performed at < 65% of his HRmax 2.8% of time in 1999 and 6.3% in 2012. He played between 65-85% of his HRmax 31.6% of time in 1999 and 69% in 2012. He performed at > 85% of his HRmax 65.5% of time in 1999 and 24.7% in 2012. Over the years, the player reduced the time at >85% of his HRmax and increased the time spent at 65-85% of his HRmax.

Variability in work intensity can be explained by the adaptations induced by training, which are confirmed by an increased anaerobic threshold. An increased anaerobic threshold allows the player to do the same work at a lower intensity. In addition, his experience leads him economize stress.

5. Conclusions

- Age is the main factor causing heart rate variability in team sports players since maximum heart rate decreases with age.
- Older players know how to economize stress, since they have a better understanding of the game.
- Using heart rate as an indicator of work intensity involves:
  + Determining the cardiovascular profile of each player.
  + Determining their real maximum heart rate.
  + Using relative values of percentage of work intensity with respect to their maximum heart rate.

Practical Implications:

- The maximum heart rate of each player should be annually examined by stress tests.
- Training loads can be adapted by using the percentage of maximum heart rate of each player.
- Training loads can be controlled according to the cardiovascular response of each player.

Acknowledgement

This study was conducted thanks to the collaboration of the professional futsal team Sala 10-Zaragoza (Spain) and to the participation of its players, who so kindly accepted to participate in our intervention. No funding support was received for the purposes of this study.

Statement of Competing Interests

The authors transfer the ownership of copyright to the journal American Journal of Sports Science and Medicine. They state that the article is original, has not been submitted for publication in other journals and has not yet been published either wholly or in part. They state that they are responsible for the research that they have designed and carried out; that they have participated in drafting and revising the manuscript submitted, whose contents they approve.

In the case of studies carried out on human beings, the authors confirm that the study was approved by the ethics committee and that the patients gave their informed consent.

They also state that the research reported in the paper was undertaken in compliance with the Helsinki Declaration and the International Principles governing research on animals.

They agree to inform in the form below of any conflict of interest that might arise, particularly any financial agreements they may have with pharmaceutical or biomedical firms whose products are pertinent to the subject matter dealt with in the manuscript.

References

[1] Bangsbo, J., Mohr, M., Krustrup, P. "Physical and metabolic demands of training and match-play in the elite football player". J Sports Sci. 24 (7). 665-674. 2006.

[2] Buchheit, M., Lepretre, P.M., Behaegel, A.L., Millet, G.P., Cuvelier, G., Ahmaidi, S.L. "Cardiorespiratory responses during running and sport-specific exercises in hadball players". J Sci Med Sport. 12 (3). 399-405. 2009.

[3] Foster, C.D., Twist, C., Lamb, K.L., Nicholas, C.W. "Heart rate responses to small-sided games among elite junior rugby league players". J Strength Cond Res. 24 (4). 906-11. 2010.

[4] Alexiou, H., Coutts, A.J. "A comparison of methods used for quantifying internal training load in women soccer players". Int J Sports Psychiol Perform. 3 (3). 320-330. 2008.

[5] Borresen, J., Lambert, M.I. "Quantifying training load: A comparison of subjective and objective methods". Int. J Sports Psychiol Perform. 3 (1). 16-30. 2008.

[6] Coutts, A.J., Rampinini, E., Marcora, S.M., Castagna, C., Impellizzeri, F.M. "Heart rate and blood lactate correlates of perceived exertion during small-sided soccer games". J Sci Med Sport. 12 (1). 79-84. 2009.

[7] Álvarez, J., López, I., Echavarri, J.M., Quílez, J., Terreros, J.L., Manonelles, P. "Análisis científico de diferentes métodos de entrenamiento en el fútbol sala". Arch Med Deporte. 26. 93-103. 2009.

[8] Eston, R., Williams, J.G. "Reliability of rating of perceiver effort regulation of exercise intensity". Br J Sports Med. 22 (4). 153-155. 1998.

[9] Coutts, A.J., Rampinini, E., Marcora, S.M., Castagna, C., Impellizzeri, F.M. "Heart rate and blood lactate correlates of perceived exertion during small-sided soccer games". J Sci Med Sport. 12 (1). 79-84. 2009.

[10] Álvarez, J., Giménez, L., Corona, P., Manonelles, P. "Necesidades cardiovasculares y metabólicas del fútbol sala: análisis de la competición". Apunts. 67. 45-51. 2002.

[11] Jackson, A.S. "Estimación de la frecuencia cardiaca máxima de la edad. ¿Es una relación lineal?". Med Sci Sports Exerc. 39 (5). 822-829. 2007.

[12] Boudet, G., Garet, M., Bedu, M., Albuisson, E., Chamoux, A. "Median maximal heart rate calibration in different conditions: laboratory, field and competition". Int J Sports Med. 23 (4). 290-297. 2002.

[13] Álvarez, J., Corona, P., Giménez, L., Serrano, E., Manonelles, P. "Perfil cardiovascular en el fútbol-sala. Respuesta inmediata al esfuerzo". Arch Med Deporte. 83. 199-204. 2001.

[14] Álvarez, J., Corona, P., Giménez, L., Serrano, E., Manonelles, P. "Perfil cardiovascular en el fútbol-sala. Adaptaciones al esfuerzo". Arch Med Deporte. 82. 143-148. 2001.

[15] Beaver, W.L., Wassermann, K., Whipp, B.J. "A new method for detecting the anaerobic threshold by gas exchange". J Appl Physiol. 60. 2020-2027. 1986.

[16] Barbero-Alvarez, J.C., Soto, V.M., Barbero-Alvarez, V., Granda-Vera, J. "Match analysis and heart rate of futsal players during competition". J Sports Sci. 26 (1). 63-73. 2008.

[17] Castagna, C., D'Ottavio, S., Granda Vera, J., Barbero Alvarez, J.C. "Match demands of professional futsal: A case study". J Sci Med Sport. 12 (4). 490-494. 2009.

[18] Casamichana, D., Castellano, J., González, R. "Demanda fisiológica en juegos reducidos de fútbol con diferentes orientaciones del espacio". Int J Sports Sci. 2 (23). 141-154. 2011.

[19] O'Connor, P.J., Raglin, J.S., Morgan, W.P. "Psychometric correlates of perception during arm ergometry in males and females". Int J Sports Med. 17 (6). 462-466. 1996.

[20] Morganroth, J., Maron, B.J., Henry, W.L., Epstein, S.E. "Comparative left ventricular dimensions in trained athletes". Ann Intern Med. 82. 521-524. 1975.

[21] Álvarez, J., Giménez, L., Manonelles, P., Corona, P. "Importancia del VO2 máx. y de la capacidad de recuperación en los deportes de prestación mixta. Caso práctico: fútbol sala". Arch Med Deporte. 86. 577-583. 2001.

[22] Bouchard, C., Lortie, G. "Heredity and endurance performance". Sports Med. 1. 38-64. 1984.

[23] García, M., Leibar, X. Umbral Aeróbico y Umbral Anaeróbico. Entrenamiento de la resistencia de los corredores de medio fondo y fondo. Madrid, Gymnos, 1997.

[24] Lacour, J.R., Chatard, J.C. "Aspectos fisiológicos del fútbol". El entrenador Español de Fútbol. 5. 32-35. 1985.

[25] Parr, R.B., Wilmore, J.H., Bachman, D., Kerlan, R.K. "Professional basketball players. Atlethic profiles". Physician Sports Med. 6. 77-84. 1978.

[26] Wolford, S., Angove, M. "A comparison of training techniques and game intensities for national level netball players". Sports Coach. 14. 18-21. 1991.

[27] Barbero, J.C., Granda, J., Soto, V.M. "Análisis de la frecuencia cardiaca durante la competición en jugadores profesionales de fútbol sala". Apunts. 77. 71-78. 2004.

[28] Rubio, E., Rubio, A., Encarna, F. Estadística en ciencias sanitarias. Colección Monografías Didácticas nº 11. Universidad de Zaragoza. Capítulo 7, 2010.

Impact of a Strength Training Exercise Program on Body Composition and Cardiovascular Risk Factors in a Group of Obese Schoolchildren by Pubertal Stage

Fabian Vasquez*, Erik Diaz, Lydia Lera, Loretta Vasquez, Alyerina Anziani, Raquel Burrows

Institute of Nutrition and Food Technology (INTA), University of Chile
*Corresponding author: fvasquez@inta.cl

Abstract The purpose of this study was to evaluate the impact of a strength training exercise intervention on body composition and cardiovascular risk factors in obese children, by pubertal stage. The sample included 60 obese schoolchildren of both genders, aged 8 to 13 years, recruited from a school in the city of Santiago (Chile). The intervention included physical exercise (strength training 3 times per week), during 3 months. Multi-compartmental body composition was estimated using isotopic dilution, plethysmography, radiographic absorptiometry and 4C model as the gold standard. Presence of metabolic syndrome was diagnosed according to Cook criteria and cardiovascular risk factors were determined using anthropometric and biochemical indicators. We found differences in schoolchildren in pubertal stages III & IV. Compared to girls, boys showed significant reductions in body fat in kg and percentage (4-Component model) and isotopic dilution in kg ($p < 0,05$). Likewise, we observed an increase in the fat-free mass in kg, in the 4-Component Model ($p < 0,01$). In all groups, the prevalence of metabolic syndrome decreased from baseline to 3 months, but the reduction was significant only among boys of Tanner I & II ($p = 0.03$). Only this group showed a significant reduction in the prevalence of cardiovascular risk factors from baseline to 3 months ($p = 0.02$). This study provides evidence on the positive impact of a strength training physical exercise program on reductions of body fat, metabolic syndrome, and cardiovascular risk factors, supporting the use of exercise as a treatment for obesity and its comorbidities in schoolchildren.

Keywords: *obese schoolchildren, strength training exercise, metabolic syndrome, cardiovascular risk factors*

1. Introduction

Over the last decades, the prevalence of obesity has increased dramatically worldwide, reaching epidemic proportions and becoming a source of huge concern since the negative health consequences begin early in childhood. [1] In Chile, obesity in schoolchildren quadrupled from 1986 (4%) to 1998 (17%). In the 2000s, he prevalence of obesity among children entering the school system increased from 19,4% in 2006 to 22,1% in 2011. [2,3] To a great extent, the obesity epidemic is the result of changes in diet and activity patterns due to explosive economic growth, the so-called nutritional transition [4,5]

Consequences of childhood obesity include an increased risk of developing the Metabolic Syndrome (MS) (abdominal obesity, dyslipidemia, high blood pressure, and glucose intolerance), cardiovascular diseases, type 2 diabetes (DM2), non- alcoholic fatty liver disease, obstructive sleep apnea/hypoventilation, polycystic ovarian syndrome, infertility, asthma, orthopedic complications, psychiatric disease, and increased rates of cancer, among others [6,7].

The excessive accumulation of BF is deleterious to an individual's health, negatively affecting its physical and metabolic condition and contributing to insulin resistance and a chronic inflammatory state. Longitudinal studies show that MS in childhood quadruples the risk of DM2 and MS in adulthood. [8] These abnormalities may persist into adulthood without early interventions to prevent or treat obesity and restore cardiovascular and metabolic homeostasis. [9,10] The beneficial effect of physical exercise on the metabolism of lipids and carbohydrates, cardiovascular health, endothelium, and prevention and treatment of many metabolic, cardiovascular, and osteomuscular disorders associated with overweight has been well documented. [11] Dosed physical exercise (both aerobic and strength training) modify body composition, contributing to a conservation or increase in muscle mass and reductions of subcutaneous, visceral, and intramuscular fatty tissue. [12] Strength training physical exercise has been used to prevent and treat insulin resistance, as enhancement in muscular function improves glucose capture and transport as well as lipid oxidation [13,14,15,16].

Contractile activity initiates a series of molecular, physiological, and biochemical events in skeletal muscle cells, activating kinases and phosphates that produce multiple signal transduction events favoring metabolic homeostasis. [17,18] Furthermore, this type of exercise produces less cardiovascular overload, and the intermittent nature of strength training is familiar and compatible with the play and movement of schoolchildren. [19] The aim of this study was to evaluate the impact of a strength training exercise intervention on body composition and CVRF of obese children, by pubertal stage.

2. Materials and Methods

2.1. Subjects

The sample was made up of 60 obese (BMI $\geq 95^{th}$ percentile, according to CDC-NCHS charts) children of both sexes, aged 8 to 13, [20] recruited from an Elementary school in Macul, a district in Central East Santiago, Chile. The selection of establishment was by convenience, based on the school's proximity to the research center and professionals performing the intervention. Other inclusion criteria included full day attendance to the educational establishment, assent of the student to participate in the study, and consent form signed by the parent or legal guardian. Students were excluded if they had been diagnosed with a psychomotor disorder; used medications that alter body composition, physical activity, dietary intake, and/or biochemical parameters; or had physical abnormalities that would prevent them from participate in the exercise program. The study was approved by the institutional review board of the Institute of Nutrition and Food Technology (INTA), University of Chile, which meets national and international certification standards.

2.2. Description of Intervention

The exercise intervention took place within the educational establishment. Children were required to attend 45 minutes session, 3 times per week on non-consecutive days, for a period of 3 months (30 sessions in total). The intervention focused on localized strength training, using exercises that worked 6 muscle groups to fatigue: biceps (left and right), shoulders (left and right), pectorals (left and right), abdominals, calves (left and right), and thighs (left and right). The exercises used weighted arm bands for the arm exercises and body weight for the lower body exercises. The objective of the training was to rehabilitate muscle function, including both functional and working capacity, that had been lost due to physical inactivity. [21,22,23] The training circuit used the "1x2x3" method, which consists of 1 minute of exercise designed to fatigue the isolated muscle group, followed by 2 minutes of rest, repeated 3 times [23].

2.3. Biological Age

Pubertal development was classified using the Tanner scale according to female breast and male genital development [24].

Tanner stage was evaluated by visual inspection performed by a pediatric endocrinologist during the physical examination.

2.4. Anthropometry

Fasting weight and height were measured in early morning (7-8h). Children were just in underwear and stood on the scale, feet near the center, arms at their sides, and head neutral, so that the line from the corner of the eye to the origin of the ear was parallel with the floor. Weight was measured using an electronic precision scale (SECA® Model 767) with a sensitivity of 10 grams. Height was measured using a Holtain stadiometer (SECA) with a sensitivity of 0,1 cm. Both values were imported via Precision Hispana touch screen. Four skinfolds were measured (biceps, triceps, subscapular, and suprailiac) with a Lange caliper with millimetric precision (1 mm), using the technique described by Lohman et al., in triplicate. [25] All measurements (anthropometry, blood sampling) were performed in a single session.

2.5. Body Composition

2.5.1. Isotopic Dilution

Total body water was measured using deuterium dilution. The isotope was administered orally at a dose of 4 gr of deuterium oxide (99,8%), according to theparticipants' body weight. Body water values were derived from deuterium oxide concentrations, according to the Plateau method. Subjects fasted for a 3-hour equilibration period to minimize changes in total body water content. [26] A baseline saliva sample was taken (approximately 2 mL), and then the dose of deuterium was given, along with 20 ml of water. The post-dose saliva sample was taken after a 3-hour waiting period, during which the participants did not urinate or ingest other liquids or foods. The sample was frozen at a temperature of -20ºC. To analyze the deuterium content in the saliva, the sample was thawed and equilibrated with hydrogen gas, adding 5% platinum on alumina powder, for 3 days. The deuterium/hydrogen ratio in the resultant gas was analyzed using mass spectrometry (Hydra, Europa Scientific, Crewe, and Cheshire, UK).

2.5.2. Plethysmography

Body volume and density were measured using air-displacement plethysmography (BOD POD, mod 2000, Life Measurement, Inc, Concord, USA). Children were in underwear; only a swim cap covered their hair. Metalwork such as piercings and jewellry was removed. Children were weighed on a scale calibrated to a precision of 5g. This system first measures the pressure in the empty chamber and then measures the difference with the person inside using a 50-liter calibration cylinder, repeating the measurements 2-3 times. The total body volume calculated with this method is used as an input in the 4C equation.

2.5.3. Dual-energy X-ray Absorptiometry

Bone mineral density was estimated with dual-energy X-ray absorptiometry, using a latest-generation Ghc Lunar Prodigy DPX-NT (Lunar Radiology, WI, USA). This system evaluates the entire body in a five-minute cycle.

The children were positioned in supine on the exam bed, wearing underwear and covered with a sheet.

2.5.4. 2C Model

The 2C model divides the body into BF and FFM. Isotopic dilution, plethysmography, and DEXA were used to produce three estimates of body composition according to the 2C model.

2.5.5. 4C Model [27,28,29]

The 4C model divides the body into fat, water, protein, and minerals. Because the 4C model adjusts for mineral content, estimates of FFM hydration fraction and density are more precise as compared to the 3C model. The 4C model is considered the "gold standard" because it accounts for more of the sources of variability of its components. This equation has been validated previously in children of the same age group [30].

The 4C model uses the following equation:

$$\begin{aligned} \text{BF}\ (\text{Kg}) &= [(2.747*\text{BV}) - (0.710*\text{TBW})] \\ &\quad + [(1.460*\text{BMC}) - (2.050*\text{W})] \end{aligned}$$

Where BV is body volume in liters (plethysmography), TBW is total body water in liters (isotopic dilution), BMC is bone mineral content in kg (DEXA), and W is body weight in kg.

2.6. Cardiovascular Risk Factors

Waist circumference in centimeters was measured using a non-stretch metric tape (SECA®) with automatic locking, measured over the border of the iliac crest, passing over the umbilicus. The methodology was based on that described by NHANES III in American population. [31] Diastolic (DBP) and systolic (SBP) blood pressure were measured in mmHg, using a mercury sphygmomanometer with an *ad hoc* sleeve, according to the standard methodology. [32] Cholesterol profile (HDL-Chol and TG in mg/dl) was determined using the dry analytic methodology (Vitros, Johnson & Johnson, Clinical diagnostics Inc.).

Baseline insulin in uUI/dl was measured using RIA (RIA DCP Diagnostic Products Corporation LA USA), with intra-assay CV of 5,1% and inter-assay CV of 7,1% for 14,4 uUI/ml, and a sensitivity of 1,2 uUI/ml. Glycemia was measured in mg/dl, with a commercial kit using the GOD-PAP enzymatic colorimetric method (Química Clínica Aplicada S.A.). Baseline insulin sensitivity was calculated using the HOMA method (fasting insulin (uUI/dl) * Fasting glycemia (mmol/L) / 22,5). [33] The biochemical profiles required an 8 hour fast. For its determination it took venous blood samples of 10 ml. Samples were analyzed in a laboratory at the Institute of Nutrition and Food Technology (University of Chile).

2.7. Definition of MS

MS was diagnosed according to the Cook phenotype, including three or more of the following abnormalities [34]: waist circumference (WC) $\geq 90^{th}$ percentile, blood arterial pressure (BAP) $\geq 90^{th}$ percentile, triglycerides (TG) $\geq$ 110 mg/dl, HDL- Cholesterol (HDL-Chol) $\leq$ 40 mg/dl, and fasting hyperglycemia (GI) $\geq$ 100 mg/dl.

2.8. Statistical Analysis

Descriptive statistics including minimum, maximum, and frequency distribution were derived for all variables. The Shapiro Wilk goodness-of-fit test and homogeneity of variance test were performed for continuous variables. Normal variables were expressed as mean ± standard deviation. Where normality criteria were not satisfied, variables are expressed as median and interquartile range. Two-way ANOVA was performed for [(2) sex x (2) pubertal stage] to compare physical characteristics, body composition and CVRF between groups. The comparison of the change (before-after) in the anthropometric variables, body composition and CVRF between the two groups was performed using the Student's *t* tests or the Wilcoxon test for independent samples. The McNemar test was used for the dependent samples to measure the change (before-after). The Symmetry test was used to evaluate the change of prevalence CVRF from baseline to 3 months.

The significance level was set at $p < 0{,}05$. Data were analyzed using STATA 12.0 (StataCorp. 2011. Stata Statistical Software: Release 12. College Station, TX: StataCorp LP.).

3. Results

Table 1 shows the physical characteristics, body composition and CVRF of the sample, by gender and pubertal stage. There were significant differences by gender and pubertal stage, although there were no interaction effects between the two variables. Age, weight, height, total body water, and bone mineral density were significantly higher in males. Likewise, values of BF (kg) and FFM (kg) in the 4C model, isotopic dilution, DEXA, plethysmography and systolic blood pressure were significantly higher among males, whereas females of breast III & IV had higher values for HOMA-IR. Regarding pubertal stage, both males and females in more advanced stages showed significantly higher values of age, weight, height, total body water, and bone mineral density. They also had significantly higher values of BF (kg) and FFM (kg) in the 4C model, isotopic dilution, DEXA, plethysmography, systolic blood pressure and diastolic blood pressure.

Table 2 compares the groups in terms of change in physical characteristics, body composition and CVRF from baseline to 3 months. We found differences in schoolchildren in pubertal stages III & IV. Comparing males and females, the former showed significant reductions in BF in kg and percentage (4C Model) and isotopic dilution in kg. Similarly, in this groups we observed an increase in the FFM in kg, in the 4C Model.

In Table 3 and Table 4, only boys of Tanner I & II showed a significant reduction from baseline to 3 months in the prevalence of CVRF ($p = 0{,}02$). In addition, we highlight the following reductions from baseline to three month post intervention: one participant with two MS components decreased to zero component; three children with two risk factors decreased to one; and six participants with three risk factors decreased to zero component.

Figure 1 shows the change in the prevalence of MS from baseline to 3 months. A reduction in the prevalence of MS was observed in all groups, however, the variation was significant only among boys in Tanner stage I & II (p = 0,03).

Table 1. Physical characteristics, body composition and cardiovascular risk factors of the sample, by gender and pubertal stage

Variable	Boys		Girls	
	Genital I&II (n=19) Genital I (n=8) Genital II (n=11)	Genital III&IV (n=14) Genital III (n=8) Genital IV (n=6)	Breast I&II (n=5) Breast I (n=4) Breast II (n=1)	Breast III&IV (n=22) Breast III (n=15) BrIV (n=7)
Age (years)[1,2]	11,5 ± 1,1	13,6 ± 1,0	8,4 ± 0,8	11,5 ± 1,7
Weight (kg)[1,2]	60,9 ± 13,5	76,3 ± 11,7	38,5 ± 5,1	58,2 ± 14,3
Height (cm)[1,2]	149,4 ± 12,0	161,4 ± 4,8	131,1 ± 3,7	147,8 ± 8,0
Total body water (L)[1,2]	26,9 ± 5,5	35,6 ± 5,0	17,8 ± 2,1	25,6 ± 5,2
Bone mineral density (kg)[1,2]	1,8 ± 0,5	2,4 ± 0,3	1,2 ± 0,1	1,7 ± 0,4
4C Model				
BF (kg) [1,2]	25,3 ± 7,9	28,6 ± 9,3	14,4 ± 3,1	24,1 ± 8,5
BF (%)	41,2 ± 6,0	36,9 ± 7,9	37,2 ± 4,3	40,4 ± 6,2
FFM (kg)[1,2]	35,6 ± 7,7	47,7 ± 6,4	24,1 ± 2,6	34,1 ± 6,9
2C Model				
Isotopic dilution BF (kg)[1,2]	24,8 ± 7,8	28,4 ± 8,2	15,4 ± 2,9	24,4 ± 7,8
Isotopic dilution BF (%)	40,3 ± 5,7	36,8 ± 6,7	39,9 ± 3,6	41,3 ± 4,3
Isotopic dilution FFM (kg)[1,2]	36,1 ± 7,3	47,9 ± 6,8	23,1 ± 2,7	33,8 ± 7,1
DEXA BF (kg)[1,2]	25,6 ± 8,2	30,1 ± 8,8	14,8 ± 2,8	24,6 ± 8,0
DEXA BF (%)	41,5 ± 5,6	39,0 ± 7,0	38,3 ± 3,0	41,6 ± 4,7
DEXA FFM (kg)[1,2]	35,3 ± 6,7	46,2 ± 6,5	23,7 ± 2,6	33,6 ± 6,9
Plethysmography BF (kg)[1,2]	27,2 ± 8,3	30,6 ± 10,5	15,2 ± 3,6	25,5 ± 9,5
Plethysmography BF (%)	44,4 ± 6,7	39,2 ± 9,0	39,1 ± 6,1	42,6 ± 7,9
Plethysmography FFM (kg)[1,2]	33,7 ± 8,0	45,7 ± 5,9	23,3 ± 7,3	32,7 ± 7,0
Cardiovascular factors				
Waist circumference (cm)	91,8 ± 9,4	97,9 ± 9,3	77,3 ± 4,6	90,4 ± 11,3
Systolic blood pressure (mm Hg)[1,2]	106,3 ± 10,4	115,0 ± 11,5	92,5 ± 5,0	107,6 ± 11,9
Diastolic blood pressure (mm Hg)[2]	66,3 ± 7,2	69,6 ± 5,9	61,3 ± 2,5	66,9 ± 6,8
Glycemia (mg/dl)	93,4 ± 15,4	90,9 ± 8,9	88,4 ± 19,4	97,8 ± 17,1
HOMA-IR[1]	1,8 (1,2)	2,1 (1,2)	0,9 (1,6)	3,3 (2,5)
Total Cholesterol (mg/dl)	175,0 (38,0)	130,0 (20,0)	159,0 (67,5)	170,0 (57,0)
HDL-Cholesterol (mg/dl)	40,0 (14)	41,0 (16)	37,5 (12,5)	37,0 (8,0)
Triglycerides (mg/dl)	165,5 (69,0)	131,0 (75,0)	148,5 (192,0)	140,0 (74,0)

Data are presented as average ± standard deviation (SD) and mean (interquartile range)
[1]Significant difference by gender, p<0,05, [2]Significant different by pubertal stage, p<0,05.

Table 2. Change in physical characteristics, body composition and cardiovascular risk factors of the sample, by gender and pubertal stage

Variable		Girls	P value[1,2]	Boys	Girls	P value[1,2]
	Genital I &II (n=19) Genital I (n = 8) Genital II (n=11)	Breast I&II (n=5) Breast I (n=4) Breast II (n=1)		Genital III & IV (n=14) Genital III (n=8) Genital IV (n=6)	Breast III & IV (n = 22) Breast III (n = 15) BrIV (n = 7)	
Age (years)	0,3 ± 0,05	0,3 ± 0,05	0,28	0,3 ± 0,05	0,3 ± 0,04	0,74
Weight (kg)	1,9 ± 2,4	1,0 ± 1,6	0,50	0,8 ± 2,6	1,3 ± 3,5	0,68
Height (cm)	2,1 ± 1,1	2,0 ± 1,0	0,92	2,5 ± 1,2	1,9 ± 1,0	0,13
Total body water (L)	0,7 ± 0,9	0,5 ± 0,6	0,71	1,0 ± 1,1	0,5 ± 1,7	0,39
Bone mineral density (kg)	0,04 ± 0,07	0,05 ± 0,04	0,86	0,1 ± 0,1	0,09 ± 0,1	0,48
4C Model						
BF (kg)	0,8 ± 2,8	1,0 ± 1,2	0,87	-1,8 ± 2,8	0,2 ± 2,7	0,04
BF (%)	0,1 ± 3,9	1,6 ± 2,5	0,48	-2,8 ± 3,1	0,2 ± 3,9	0,03
FFM (kg)	0,9 ± 2,5	0,1 ± 1,4	0,47	2,6 ± 2,2	0,6 ± 2,8	0,03
2C Model						
Isotopic dilution BF (kg)	-9,4 ± 5,4	-7,1 ± 3,1	0,42	-20,4 ± 9,1	-9,0 ± 3,9	0,00
Isotopic dilution BF (%)	-0,2 ± 2,1	-0,6 ± 2,2	0,69	-1,2 ± 2,6	-0,5 ± 1,9	0,34
Isotopic dilution FFM (kg)	1,0 ± 1,5	0,8 ± 0,6	0,83	1,4 ± 1,4	0,7 ± 2,2	0,37
DEXA BF (kg)	0,4 ± 1,4	0,2 ± 1,5	0,75	-0,5 ± 2,8	0,3 ± 1,6	0,27
DEXA BF (%)	-0,6 ± 1,4	-0,5 ± 1,9	0,93	-1,1 ± 2,7	-0,2 ± 2,2	0,28
DEXA FFM (kg)	1,2 ± 1,5	0,8 ± 0,4	0,56	1,3 ± 1,6	0,5 ± 3,0	0,37
Plethysmography BF (kg)	0,9 ± 4,2	-0,06 ± 1,6	0,67	-1,5 ± 3,0	-0,2 ± 4,1	0,33
Plethysmography BF (%)	-0,1 ± 6,3	-1,3 ± 5,1	0,75	-2,3 ± 4,0	-0,3 ± 6,6	0,32
Plethysmography FFM (kg)	0,8 ± 3,6	1,0 ± 2,8	0,91	2,3 ± 2,9	1,0 ± 4,0	0,33
Cardiovascular factors						
Waist circumference (cm)	-0,4 ± 2,8	-1,3 ± 3,5	0,30	-0,9 ± 2,9	-0,8 ± 3,0	0,86
Systolic blood pressure (mm Hg)	-4,3 ± 7,4	0,0 ± 0,0	0,26	-4,2 ± 6,7	-3,3 ± 5,8	0,68
Diastolic blood pressure (mm Hg)	-1,3 ± 6,6	-1,3 ± 2,5	0,99	-2,7 ± 3,3	-2,6 ± 5,8	0,97
Glycemia (mg/dl)	-6,5 ± 14,6	2,1 ± 7,9	0,27	-6,5 ± 8,1	-12,5 ± 14,5	0,18
HOMA-IR	0,5 (1,0)	0,7 (1,4)	0,61	0,2 (1,8)	-0,3 (1,7)	0,35
Total Cholesterol (mg/dl)	2,5 (20,0)	-1,5 (22,5)	0,97	0,0 (16,0)	-4,0 (11,0)	0,05
HDL-Cholesterol (mg/dl)	1,0 (5,0)	3,5 (10,5)	0,46	2,0 (8,0)	1,0 (3,0)	0,96
Triglycerides (mg/dl)	-21,0 (69,0)	-57,5 (147,0)	0,93	-25,0 (40,0)	-17,0 (69,0)	0,51

Data are presented as average ± standard deviation (SD) and mean (interquartile range) [1]Student's *t* Test [2]Wilcoxon Rank sum Test

Table 3. Change in cardiovascular risk factors of boys at pubertal stages

Cardiovascular risk factors at baseline	Cardiovascular risk factors at 3-Month follow-up									
	Tanner 1[1,2]					Tanner 2[1]				
	0	1	2	3	4	0	1	2	3	4
0	0	0	0	0	0	1	0	0	0	0
1	0	0	1	1	0	1	2	0	0	0
2	1	3	0	0	0	0	2	1	0	0
3	0	1	6	2	0	0	0	1	3	1
4	0	0	0	3	1	0	0	0	1	1
Total	1	4	7	6	1	2	4	2	4	2

[1]Symmetry Test [2]p=0,02

Table 4. Change in cardiovascular risk factors of girls at pubertal stages

Cardiovascular risk factors at baseline	Cardiovascular risk factors at 3-Month follow-up										
	Tanner 1[1]					Tanner 2[1]					
	0	1	2	3	4	0	1	2	3	4	5
0	0	0	0	0	0	1	0	0	0	0	0
1	0	1	0	0	0	1	1	1	0	0	0
2	0	0	1	0	0	0	1	1	2	0	0
3	0	0	0	1	1	0	2	0	3	0	0
4	0	0	1	0	0	0	1	1	2	3	0
5	0	0	0	0	0	0	0	0	1	1	0
Total	0	1	2	1	1	2	5	3	8	4	0

[1]Symmetry Test

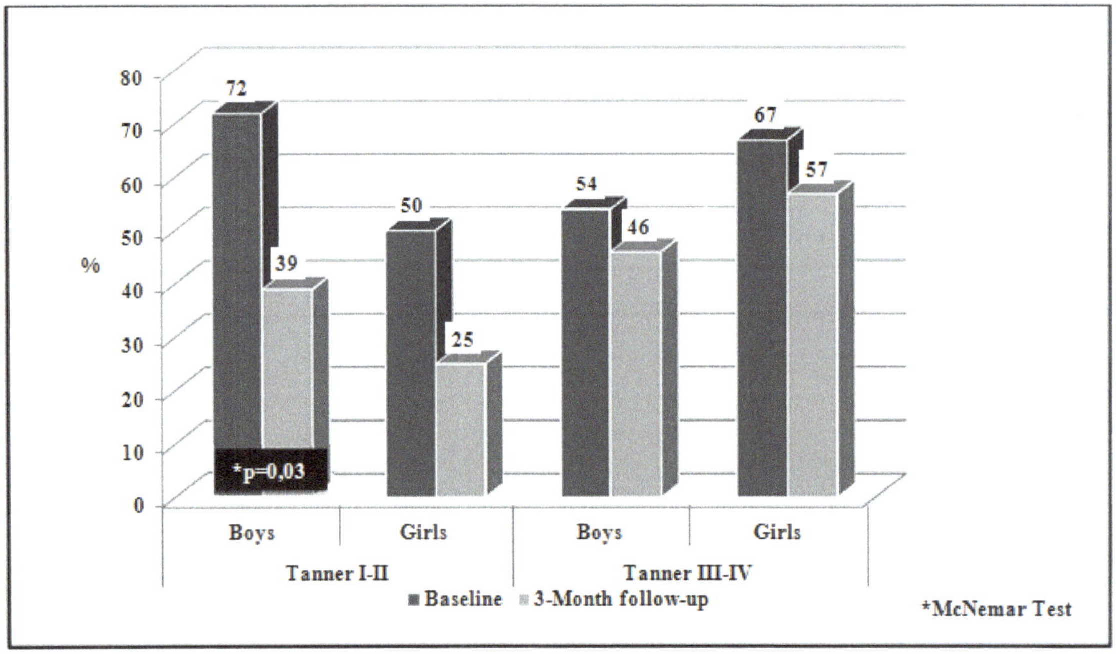

Figure 1. Change in prevalence of metabolic syndrome in boys and girls, from baseline to 3 months

4. Discussion

This study provides background on impact of exercise strength training interventions for obese schoolchildren carried out within the school system on body composition and CVRF, thus helping to increase the evidence available in both the country and the region. The 4C model quantifies BF and FFM more precisely than other methods because it directly measures mineral, water, and protein content rather than assuming a constant density of FFM. [35] In this research, it was chosen the 4C model as the reference standard to compare the sensitivity of other methods to estimate body composition (BF and FFM) in obese schoolchildren, by gender and pubertal stages. Concerning the impact on body composition (4 C model), the strength training intervention produced a significant reduction in BF (kg and %) and a significant increase in FFM (kg) in boys in Tanner stages III & IV, compared to girls girls. Instead, in the two-compartment model, a significant difference was also observed when comparing the reduction in BF (kg) in boys and girls, being higher in boys in Tanner III & IV. These findings are consistent with those provided by Ferguson et al. [36]. According to these authors, the effect of a 4 months of strength training exercise in obese children aged 7 to 11 years, reduced BF by 2,2% ($p < 0,001$). Similarly, a case-controlled intervention comprising strength training physical exercise intervention over ten weeks in overweight children aged 5 to 10 years result in a significant reduction in BF in the intervention group ($p < 0,01$) [37]. A similar outcome was observed after a four-month exercise program for obese children aged 7 to 11 years; reductions in percentage of BF were higher than 2% in the intervention group ($p < 0,01$). [38] McGuigan et al. [39] studied the effect of an eight-week strength training program in children with overweight or obesity, finding a reduction in BF of 2,6% ($p = 0,003$).

The research in children show that this type of exercise significantly lowers central and total adiposity, increases lean mass, and improves muscular strength. [40,41] However, an extensive review of the literature on the effect of physical exercise on obese children conclude that the magnitude of change in BF and FFM after exercise is associated with initial BF as well as the intensity and type of exercise [42,43,44]

In Chilean children and adolescents, the prevalence of MS is proportional to excess body weight (6.5% and 40.3% in overweight and severe obese children, respectively), whereas abdominal obesity increases the risk of MS by 17 times. [45] In Figure 1, both groups (girls and boys Tanner I-IV) showed lower rates of of MS, although the reduction was significant only among boys in Tanner I & II ($p = 0,03$). In the same groups we also observed a significant reduction in the number of risk factors after the intervention ($p = 0,02$) (Table 3), (Table 4). All groups achieved a reduction in abdominal obesity and hypertriglyceridemia, as well as a decrease in fasting hyperglycemia in boys in Tanner I-IV and girls in Tanner III & IV

Also, a decrease in total cholesterol in girls in Tanner I-IV along with an increase in HDL-Colesterol in boys and girls of Tanner I-IV were observed.

Similar results were reported in a research, in which a physical exercise intervention over a 6 weeks period led to a reduction in abdominal obesity ($p < 0,02$) and total cholesterol levels ($p < 0,05$). [6] Doyle et al. [37], whose intervention consisted of high- intensity physical exercise as well as nutritional and dietary education for children and their parents over 10 weeks, found a significant decrease in triglyceride levels in the intervention group as compared to the controls ($p = 0,0467$). Chang et al. [47] showed a decrease in the prevalence of fasting hyperglycemia, from 23,5% before intervention to 9% at 3 months and 0% at 9 months in the intervention group, vs. an increase from 23,1% at baseline to 29,4% at 12 months in the control group.

National and international studies concur that children's compliance rates with obesity treatment programs provided within the health care system are low. [48,49] The studies described above used conventional, individual treatment, in which the child is required to attend monthly or weekly sessions at a health care center. This design may partly explain the high attrition rate.

A strength of this study was that the program was provided in a group setting and targeted to obese schoolchildren. This design improved compliance and maintenance rates of the strength training exercise program over time.

A potential limitation is that the exposure-response relationship for the variable could not be analyzed due to the quasi- experimental design, resulting in a quality of evidence categorized as moderate rather than high as compared to randomized studies. [50] Thus, our results, although valid in our sample, cannot be generalized to the target population (obese school children aged 8 to 13). To achieve this type of findings, we recommend an effectiveness study.

5. Conclusions

This research measures the positive impact of a strength training physical exercise program on reductions of BF, MS, and CVRF. This program was provided in a group setting and designed especially for obese schoolchildren, which improved compliance and maintenance rates of the strength training exercise program. However, this kind of training in should be provided to all children within the school system, regardless of their nutritional status, to allow sustainability over time.

Acknowledgements

This research received financial support from the University of Chile Research Program, under grant Domeyko +++++, and the National Council for Research, Science and Technology (Chile), under grant FONDECYT Postdoctoral 3140344. We also thank the ongoing commitment of the participants, their families and schools..

Statement of Competing Interest

None of the authors had a conflict of interest.

List of abbreviation

Metabolic Syndrome: MS Cardiovascular
Risk Factors: CVRF Body Fat: BF
Fat-Free Mass: FFM
Dual-energy X-ray Absorptiometry: DEXA
4-Component Model: 4C Model
2-Component Model: 2C Model

References

[1] Global Health Observatory (GHO): Obesity 2008. World Health Organization 2013. [Online]. Available from: URL: http://www.who.int/gho/ncd/risk_factors/obesity_text/en/index.html. [Accessed Dec. 10, 2013].

[2] Muzzo S, Cordero J, Ramirez I, Burrows R. Trend in nutritional status and stature among school age children in Chile. *Nutrition.* 2004; 20 (10):867-973.

[3] National Council for School Assistance. Map Nutritional 2010. [Online]. Available from: URL: http://bpt.junaeb.cl:8080/MapaNutricionalGx/. [Accessed Jan. 23, 2014].

[4] Popkin BM, Gordon-Larsen P. The nutrition transition: worldwide obesity dynamics and their determinants. *Int J Obes Relat Metab Disord.* 2004; 28 Suppl 3:S2-S9.

[5] Popkin BM. An overview on the nutrition transition and its health implications: the Bellagio meeting. *Public Health Nutr.* 2002; 5 (1A):93-103.

[6] Bastien M, Poirier P, Lemieux I, Després JP. Overview of epidemiology and contribution of obesity to cardiovascular disease. *Prog Cardiovasc Dis.* 2014; 56 (4):369-381.

[7] Kelsey MM, Zaepfel A, Bjornstad P, Nadeau KJ. Age-Related Consequences of Childhood Obesity. *Gerontology*. 2014. [Epub ahead of print].

[8] Sun SS, Liang R, Huang TT, Daniels SR, Arslanian S, Liu K, Grave G, Siervogel R. Childhood obesity predicts adult metabolic syndrome: the Fels Longitudinal Study. *J Pediatr*. 2008; 152 (2):191-200.

[9] Hills AP, King NA, Armstrong TP. The contribution of physical activity and sedentary behaviors to the growth and development of children and adolescents: implications for overweight and obesity. *Sports Med*. 2007; 37 (6):533-545.

[10] Stein CJ, Colditz GA. The epidemic of obesity. *J Clin Endocrinol Metab*. 2004; 89 (6):2522-2525.

[11] Blair SN, Cheng Y, Holder JS. Is physical activity or physical fitness more important in defining health benefits?. *Med Sci Sports Exerc*. 2001; 33 Suppl 6:S379-S399.

[12] Saris WH. The role of exercise in the dietary treatment of obesity. *Int J Obes Relat Metab Disord*. 1993; 17 Suppl :S17-S21.

[13] Hawley JA. Exercise as a therapeutic intervention for the prevention and treatment of insulin resistance. *Diabetes Metab Res Rev*. 2004; 20 (5):383-393.

[14] Hawley JA, Lessard SJ. Exercise training-induced improvements in insulin action. *Acta Physiol (Oxf)*. 2008; 192 (1):127-135.

[15] Shaibi GQ, Cruz ML, Ball GD, Weigensberg MJ, Salem GJ, Crespo NC, Goran MI. Effects of resistance training on insulin sensitivity in overweight Latino adolescent males. *Med Sci Sports Exerc*. 2006; 38 (7):1208-1215.

[16] Watts K, Beye P, Siafarikas A, O'Driscoll G, Jones TW, Davis EA, Green DJ. Effects of exercise training on vascular function in obese children. *J Pediatr*. 2004; 144 (5):620-625.

[17] Diaz E, Saavedra C. Physical exercise and obesity, concepts and metabolic cellular level. In: Cruchet S, Rozowsky J. Editors. Obesity: A Comprehensive Approach. Santiago: Nestlé Chile SA, 2007, pp 51-63.

[18] Hood DA. Invited Review: contractile activity-induced mitochondrial biogenesis in skeletal muscle. *J Appl Physiol*. 2001; 90 (3):1137-1157.

[19] Faigenbaum AD. State of the art reviews: resistance training for children and adolescents: are there health outcomes?. *AJLM*. 2007; 1 (3):190-200.

[20] National Center for Health Statistical (NCHS) - Centers for Disease Control and Prevention (CDC). [Online]. Available from: URL:http://www.cdc.gov/GrowthCharts/. [Accessed Jan. 16, 2014].

[21] Chile. Ministry of Health. Program on Healthy Eating and Physical Activity for Chronic Disease Prevention in Women, Children, Adolescents and Adults 2008. [Online]. Available from: URL:http://webhosting.redsalud.gov.cl/minsal/archivos/alimentos ynutricion/estrategiaintervencion/orientacionespas af2008.doc. [Accessed Jan. 16, 2014].

[22] Diaz E, Saavedra C. Exercise and metabolic restoration. Nutrition, health and wellness. Magazine for health professionals (12), 26-40. 2008. Santiago: Nestlé Chile SA.

[23] Diaz E, Saavedra C, Meza J. Paper prepared for Ministry of Health. Contemporary Guide to exercise and health, 2007.

[24] Tanner JM. Fetus into man. Physical growth from conception to maturity. 2nd ed Harvard University Press, 1989.

[25] Lohman TG, Boileau RA, Slaughter RA. Body composition in children. In: Lohman TG. Editor. Human body composition. New York: Human Kinetics, 1984, pp 29-57.

[26] Schoeller DA. Hydrometry. In: Roche A, Heymsfield S, Lohman TG, editors. Human body composition. New York: Human Kinetics, 1996:25-43.

[27] Fuller NJ, Jebb SA, Laskey MA, Coward WA, Elia M. Four-component model for the assessment of body composition in humans: comparison with alternative methods, and evaluation of the density and hydration of fat-free mass. *Clin Sci (Lond)*. 1992; 82 (6):687-93.

[28] Bellisari A, Roche A. Anthropometry and Ultrasound. In: Heymsfield S, Lohman T, Wang Z, Going S. Editors. Human Body Composition. 2nd ed. United States: Human Kinetics, 2005, pp 109-128.

[29] Sopher A, Shen W, Pietrobelli A. Pediatric Body Composition Methods. In: Heymsfield S, Lohman T, Wang Z, Going S. Editors. Human Body Composition. 2nd ed. United States: Human Kinetics, 2005, pp 129-139.

[30] Wells J, Fuller N, Dewit O, Fewtrell M, Elia M, Cole T. Four-component model of body composition in children: density and hydration of fat-free mass and comparison with simpler models. *Am J Clin Nutr*. 1999; 69 (5):904-12.

[31] Fernandez J, Redden D, Pietrobelli A, Allison D. Waist circumference percentiles in nationally representative samples of African-American, European-American, and Mexican-American children and adolescents. *J Pediatric*. 2004; 145 (4):439-444.

[32] National high blood pressure education program working group on hypertension control in children and adolescents. Update on the 1987 task force report on high blood pressure in children and adolescents: a working group report from the national high blood pressure education program. *Pediatrics*. 1996; 98 (4 Pt 1):649-658.

[33] Matthews DR, Hosker JP, Rudenski AS, Naylor BA, Treacher DF, Turner RC. Homeostasis model assessment: insulin resistance and beta-cell function from fasting plasma glucose and insulin concentrations in man. Diabetologia 1985; 28 (7):412-419.

[34] Cook S, Weitzman M, Auinger P, Nguyen M, Dietz WH. Prevalence of a Metabolic Syndrome Phenotype in Adolescents: Findings From the Third National Health and Nutrition Examination Survey, 1988-1994. *Arch Pediatr Adolesc Med*. 2003; 157 (8):821-827.

[35] Wells JCK, Fuller NJ, Dewit O, Fewtrell MS, Elia M, Cole TJ. Four-component model of body composition in children: density and hydration of fat-free mass and comparison with simpler models. *Am J Clin Nutr*. 1999; 69 (5):904-912.

[36] Ferguson MA, Gutin B, Le NA, Karp W, Litaker M, Humphries M, Okuyama T, Riggs S, Owens S. Effects of exercise training and its cessation on components of the insulin resistance syndrome in obese children. *Int J Obes Relat Metab Disord*. 1999; 23 (8):889-895.

[37] Doyle-Baker PK, Venner AA, Lyon ME, Fung Tn. Impact of a combined diet and progressive exercise intervention for overweight and obese children: the B.E. H.I.P. study. *Appl Physiol Nutr Metab*. 2001; 36 (4):515-525.

[38] Owens S, Gutin B, Allison J, Riggs S, Ferguson M, Litaker M, Thompson W. Effect of physical training on total and visceral fat in obese children. *Med Sci Sports Exerc*. 1999; 31 (1):143-148.

[39] McGuigan MR, Tatasciore M, Newton RU, Pettigrew S. Eight weeks of resistance training can significantly alter body composition in children who are overweight or obese. *J Strength Cond Res*. 2009; 23 (1):80-85.

[40] Yoshioka M, Doucet E, St-Pierre S, Almeras N, Richard D, Labrie A, Despres JP, Bouchard C, Tremblay A. Impact of high-intensity exercise on energy expenditure, lipid oxidation and body fatness. *Int J Obes Relat Metab Disord*. 2001; 25 (3):332-339.

[41] Benson AC, Torode ME, Fiatarone Singh MA. The effect of high-intensity progressive resistance training on adiposity in children: a randomized controlled trial. *Int J Obes*. 2008; 32 (6):1016-1027.

[42] LeMura LM, Maziekas MT. Factors that alter body fat, body mass, and fat-free mass in pediatric obesity. *Med Sci Sports Exerc*. 2002; 34 (3):487-496.

[43] Nemet D, Barkan S, Epstein Y, Friedland O, Kowen G, Eliakim A. Short- and long-term beneficial effects of a combined dietary-behavioral-physical activity intervention for the treatment of childhood obesity. *Pediatrics*. 2005; 115 (4): e443-e4499.

[44] Sacher PM, Chadwick P, Wells JC, Williams JE, Cole TJ, Lawson MS. Assessing the acceptability and feasibility of the MEND Programme in a small group of obese 7-11-year-old children. *J Hum Nutr Diet*. 2005; 18 (1): 3-5.

[45] Burrows R, Leiva L, Weisstaub G. Metabolic syndrome in children and adolescents: association with insulin sensitivity and magnitude and distribution of obesity. *Rev Med Chil*. 2007; 135 (2):174-181.

[46] Woo KS, Chook P, Yu CW, Sung R, Qiao M, Leung S, Lam C, Metreweli C, Celermajer D. Effects of diet and exercise on obesity-related vascular dysfunction in children. *Circulation*. 2004; 109 (16):1981-1986.

[47] Chang C, Liu W, Zhao X, Li S, Yu C. Effect of supervised exercise intervention on metabolic risk factors and physical fitness in Chinese obese children in early puberty. *Obes Rev*. 2008; 9 Suppl 1:135-141.

[48] Barja S, Nuñez E, Velandia S, Urrejola P, Hodgson MI. Adherence and effectiveness in the medium term treatment of childhood obesity. *Rev Chil Pediatr*. 2005; 76 (2):151-158.

[49] Pinelli L, Elerdini N, Faith MS, Agnello D, Ambruzzi A, De Simone M, Leggeri G, Livieri C, Monetti N, Peverelli P, Salvatoni

A, Seminara S, Uasone R, Pietrobelli A. Childhood obesity: results of a multicenter study of obesity treatment in Italy. *J Pediatr Endocrinol Metab.* 1999;12 Suppl 3:795-799.

[50] Atkins D, Briss P, Eccles M, Flottorp S, Guyatt GH, Harbour RT, Hill S, Jaeschke R, Liberati A, Magrini N, Mason J, O'Connell D, Oxman AD, Phillips B, Schünemann H, Edejer TT, Vist GE, Williams JW Jr; GRADE Working Group. Systems for grading the quality of evidence and the strength of recommendations II: Pilot study of a new system. *BMC Health Serv Res.* 2005; 5 (1):25.

12

VO_2max Changes in English Futsal Players after a 6-Week Period of Specific Small-Sided Games Training

D. Berdejo-del-Fresno[1,*], R. Moore[2], M. W. Laupheimer[1,3]

[1]England Futsal National Squad, The Football Association and The International Futsal Academy (United Kingdom)
[2]Research Fellow, Sport Industry Research Centre, Sheffield Hallam University (United Kingdom)
[3]Senior Clinical Lecturer in Sports and Exercise Medicine, Queen Mary University of London (United Kingdom)
*Corresponding author: daniberdejo@gmail.com

Abstract Futsal is a high-intensity, intermittent sport where accelerations and short sprints are performed at maximal or sub-maximal intensity. These efforts are interspersed by brief recovery periods, during 2 halves of 20 minutes stopping clock. Aerobic endurance inevitably plays a key role in the players' performance. The aim of this study was to analyse the VO2 max progression and the agility (with and without ball) of English futsal players during a 6-week period of small-sided games practice. Two teams volunteered to participate in this study; an experimental group (EG), which performed a specialised small-sided training regime and a control group (CG) (normal training regime). VO2max was estimated from the results of the 20-metre Multi-Stage Fitness Test. The VO2max of the futsal players in the EG improved significantly (58.73±2.41 ml/kg/min vs. 60.11 ± 2.99 ml/kg/min, p=0.04). The same player's agility and agility with ball performance did not report any significant changes in either group. The results showed that periodisation, training sessions and methods based on small-sided games, which implied a change in the number of players, the size of the pitch and the task constraints, were adequate to increase aerobic endurance.

Keywords: *team sports, intermittent exercise, indoor soccer, aerobic endurance, physical condition*

1. Introduction

Futsal is a high-intensity, intermittent sport where accelerations and short sprints (usually with a duration of 1 to 4 seconds) are performed at maximal or sub-maximal intensity. These actions are interspersed by brief recovery periods (activities of low intensity or pauses). A match is organised in 2 halves of 20 minutes each with 10-15 minutes break between them. However, as the clock is stopped every time the ball goes out, a match can last from 75 to 80 minutes (Álvarez Medina et al., 2001a; Álvarez Medina et al., 2001b; Álvarez Medina et al., 2002; Barbero Álvarez et al., 2003; Barbero Álvarez et al., 2004a; Barbero Álvarez et al., 2004b). Consequently, it is deduced that, in order to improve their futsal performance, players should undertake specific futsal conditioning alongside resistance, sprint and agility training.

Although futsal is a relatively new sport, there are a large amount of articles analysing and studying the anthropometry of futsal players, the parameters of futsal, its physiological demands and the fitness level of the teams (Álvarez Medina et al., 2001a; Álvarez Medina et al., 2001b; Álvarez Medina et al., 2002; Barbero Álvarez et al., 2003; Barbero Álvarez et al., 2004a; Barbero Álvarez et al., 2004b; Castagna & Barbero Álvarez, 2010). However, there is no study that analyses the seasonal changes on fitness during a futsal season. This aspect is of great importance for the optimal construction of physical and sport-specific conditioning programmes to improve futsal performance. Since the main objective for a coach is to optimise athletic performance (Coutts and Aoki, 2009), the best performance improvements come from prescribing an optimal amount of physical training with proper recovery periods to allow for the greatest adaptation before competition (Gamble, 2006; Coutts & Aoki, 2009).

On the other hand, small-sided games are situations commonly used in the training of soccer, handball, basketball and futsal to develop technical and tactical skills (Jones and Drust, 2007), as well as to improve endurance (Hill-Haas et al., 2009b), and are used as part of generic training (Hill-Haas et al., 2009a). Impellizzeri et al. (2006) found that small-sided games were particularly advantageous in the case of young players, since the improvement of specific skills is closely related to the frecuency of practice. During this type of training, players experience similar situations to those they encounter in competitive matches (Owen et al., 2004), the only differences being the participation of fewer players, a reduced playing surface, the introduction of task constraints and the addition or modification of certain rules (Little, 2009).

However, no research has identified the impact of small-sided games and task constraints on fitness developments in futsal players in relation to seasonal changes. Only Duarte et al. (2009) have assessed the effects of exercise duration and number of players on heart rate responses and technical skills during small-sided futsal games.

Thus, the aim of this study was to analyse the fitness development of futsal players in a 6-week period, where small-sided games and modifications of the task constraints were applied. Particularly, the study analysed the development of VO2max calculated from the 20-metre Multi-Stage Fitness Test and the agility performance (with and without the ball) in the futsal players. The hypothesis was that an exhaustive periodisation using small sided games applied over a consecutive 6-week period would enhance the fitness level of the players and hence their aerobic performance more than standard training.

2. Method

Participants: Two teams volunteered to participate in this study after having signed the corresponding informed consent form. One team was the experimental group (EG) and the other was the control group (CG). The EG was made up by 12 elite level male futsal players with a football/futsal experience of 10.4 ± 1.2 years from a top-2 team that competes in the FA (The Football Association) Futsal National League. The CG was made up by 12 elite level male futsal players that compete in the FA (The Football Association) Futsal National League (football/futsal experience of 10.5 ± 1.6).

The task constraints used in the study were applied to the way in which players could score the goals. Five different ways where established following a progression: (a) real goals (3 x 2 m) and goalkeepers; (b) small goals (1 x 1 m) and no goalkeepers; (c) two small goals (1 x 1 m) per team and no goalkeepers; (d) big central line goal (10 m) and no goalkeepers; and (e) no goals and no goalkeepers, just possession game. These five different situations follow a progression from less to more intense (Casamichana and Castellano, 2009; (Casamichana and Castellano, 2010; Casamichana et al., 2011; Duarte et al., 2009; Duarte et al., 2010).

Procedures: The anthropometric and fitness tests were done in October at the end of the pre-season (week 10). The anthropometric values of the futsal players participating in this study are indicated in Table 1 and 2. The fitness tests were repeated in December after the 6-week specific small-sided games training period (week 17). All participants, coaches and managers were informed about the procedures and gave their written consent. The study was approved by the institutional Ethics Committe of the University of Castilla-La Mancha (Spain). All participants were familiar with all procedures used prior to the study.

Anthropometric Tests: Anthropometric measures were taken, following the Lohmann et al. (1988) instruction. Standing height was measured with a precision of 0.1 cm with a stadiometer (SECA Ltd. model 220., Hamburg, Germany). Body mass (kg) was recorded with a scale SECA (SECA Ltd., Hamburg, Germany) to the nearest 100 g., the subjects wearing light indoor clothing and no shoes. The Body Mass Index (BMI) was calculated using the Quetelet formula.

Table 1. The anthropometric values of the futsal players participating in this study (EG)

Experimental Group	n	Age (years)	Height (cm)	Weight (kg)	BMI (kg/m2)
All players	12	25.08 ± 2.57	177.25 ± 6.83	73.04 ± 7.58	23.23 ± 1.91
Max		30	185	90	26.58
Min		20	163	60	20.52
Range		10	22	30	6.06
Outfields	10	25.6 ± 2.22	175.11 ± 6.60	70.61 ± 5.48	23.05 ± 1.75
Max		30	185	78	25.99
Min		21	163	60	20.52
Range		9	22	18	5.47
Goalkeepers	2	22.50 ± 3.54	183.66 ± 0.58	80.33 ± 9.50	23.80 ± 2.69
Max		25	184	90	26.58
Min		20	183	71	21.2
Range		5	1	19	5.38

Table 2. The anthropometric values of the futsal players participating in this study (CG)

Control Group	n	Age (years)	Height (cm)	Weight (kg)	BMI (kg/m2)
All players	12	23.91 ± 2.97	179.05 ± 3.53	75.64 ± 4.58	23.59 ± 0.91
Max		29	185	90	26.29
Min		18	173	72	21.13
Range		11	12	18	5.16
Outfields	10	24.00 ± 3.39	177.11 ± 4.18	72.21 ± 4.28	23.02 ± 1.75
Max		29	185	80	25.70
Min		18	173	72	21.13
Range		11	12	8	4.57
Goalkeepers	2	23.66 ± 1.53	185.00 ± 0.00	87.50 ± 3.53	25.56 ± 1.02
Max		25	185	90	26.29
Min		22	185	85	24.84
Range		3	0	5	1.45

Fitness Tests: The fitness tests selection was based on validated batteries commonly used in sport in different cross-sectional and longitudinal studies. These tests are described in detail in an article by Ruiz et al., 2006. Each subject performed all tests on two separate non-consecutive days. On the first day, players performed the Speed of Movement-Agility (4x10-meter shuttle run) and the Speed of Movement-Agility with ball (4x10-meter shuttle run). On the second day, the 20-metre Multi-Stage Fitness Test was performed.

First day's Tests:

Speed of Movement-Agility (using the 4x10-meter shuttle run). The subjects had to run back and forth four times along a 10 m track at the highest speed possible. At the end of each track section, they had to step on the floor line. This allows measurement not only of speed of displacement but also of agility and change of direction (COD). Two non-consecutive repetitions were carried out and the best attempt was recorded.

Speed of Movement-Agility with ball (using the 4x10-meter shuttle run). In this test the subjects had to run back and forth four times along a 10 m track at the highest speed possible dribbling a ball. At the end of each track section they had to step on the floor line. This allows measurement not only of speed of displacement but also of agility and change of direction (COD) with ball. Two non-consecutive repetitions were carried out and the best attempt was recorded.

Second day's Test:

Cardiorespiratory fitness (20-metre Multi-Stage Fitness Test). In this test the initial speed is 8.5 km/h. which is then increased by 0.5 km/h per min (1 min equals one stage). The subjects ran in a straight line to pivot upon completing a shuttle, and to pace themselves in accordance to the audio signals given. The test is finished when the subject stops or fails to reach the end lines concurrent with the audio signals on two consecutive occasions. The equation of Léger and Gadoury (1989) was used to estimate the maximum oxygen uptake (VO2max):

$$\text{VO2max} = 20.6 + \text{Last stage completedx3}$$

Training Periodisation: The schedule of the performed season is shown in Figure 1.

		August		September				October					November				December			
Matches	Official							2		16				13	20	27	4			
	Friendly			4			25		9											
Tests											T1							T2		
Training Sessions												S1	S2	S3	S4	S5	S6			
Weeks		1	2	3	4	5	6	7	8	9	10	11	12	13	14	15	16	17	18	19
Beginning Monday		22	29	5	12	19	26	3	10	17	24	31	7	14	21	28	5	12	19	26
Training Schedule:		Pre-season						Competition I												Trans.

Figure 1. Schedule for the small-sided games periodization

The period lasted 6 weeks and began just after the pre-season. The players (both groups) trained twice a week, 1.5 hours on Tuesday and 2 hours on Thursday. The specific small-sided games were implemented on the Thursday sessions in the first 30 min on the EG. All the sessions consisted of 3 blocks of workout. Each block had a duration of 8 min, including the exercise time and the recovery time. The first week started with 4 min of workout and 4 min of rest; in every next week until the 4th week the workout time increased 1 min and the recovery time decreased 1 min (i.e. 7 min of work and just 1 min rest); then the workout time decreased 1 min every week and the rest time increased 1 min. A linear periodisation was being used. Linear training suggests the indefinite use of a constant training volume and loading scheme. Furthermore, five different situations were established following a progression from less to more intense (Casamichana and Castellano, 2009; Casamichana and Castellano, 2010; Casamichana et al., 2011; Duarte et al., 2009; Duarte et al., 2010). The progression was as follows: (a) real goals (3 x 2 m) and goalkeepers; (b) small goals (1 x 1 m) and no goalkeepers; (c) two small goals (1 x 1 m) per team and no goalkeepers; (d) big central line goal (10 m) and no goalkeepers; and (e) no goals and no goalkeepers, just possession game. This progression was applied following the linear periodisation as well. The sessions started with the habitual warm-up of the team, which consisted of patterned collective movements along the entire court without opposition during 10 minutes, followed by 5 minutes of static and dynamic stretching. All the specific small-sided games were played at 2-touch. The periodisation of the specific small-sided games applied to the EG was as follows:

Session 1: After the warm-up, the players performed 4v4 with goalkeepers and real goals (3 x 2 m) in half court (20 x 20 m) for 4 min, followed by an active break of 4 min during which the players carried out low intensity steady run. Then, the players played 3v3 without goalkeepers and small goals (1 x 1 m) in half court for 4 min, followed by 4 min of jogging. Finally, they performed 4v4 in half court without goalkeepers and two small goals (1 x 1 m) per team 6 m apart for 4 min, plus 4 min of slow jogging.

Session 2: After the warm-up, the players played 4v4 in half court without goalkeepers and two small goals (1 x 1 m) per team 6 m apart for 5 min, plus 3 min of slow jogging. Then, 3v3 without goalkeepers and big central line goals (10 m) in half court for 5 min, followed by 3 min of jogging. To score, players had to go through the goal dribbling the ball. The last drill was a possession game (without goals) of 4v4 in half court. To get a point, players had to perform ten consecutive passes. This task lasted 5 min followed by 3 min of slow steady run.

Session 3: After the warm-up, the players performed 3v3 with goalkeepers and real goals in half court for 6 min, followed by an active break of 2 min during which the players carried out low intensity steady run. Then, they played 2v2 without goalkeepers and small goals in a quarter of the court (10 x 20 m) for 6 min, followed by 2 min of jogging. Finally, the players performed 3v3 in half court without goalkeepers and two small goals per team 6 m apart for 6 min, plus 2 min of slow jogging.

Session 4: After the warm-up, the players played 3v3 in half court without goalkeepers and two small goals per team 6 m apart for 7 min, plus 1 min of slow jogging. Then, 2v2 without goalkeepers and big central line goals in a quarter of the court for 7 min, followed by 1 min of jogging. To score, players had to go through the goal dribbling the ball. The last drill was a possession game (without goals) of 3v3 in half court. To get a point, they had to perform ten consecutive passes. This task lasted 7 min followed by 1 min of slow steady run.

Session 5: After the patterned warm-up, the players performed 4v4 with goalkeepers and real goals in half court for 6 min, followed by an active break of 2 min when the players carried out low intensity steady run. Then, they played 3v3 without goalkeepers and small goals in half court for 6 min, followed by 2 min of jogging. Finally, they performed 4v4 in half court without goalkepeers and two small goals per team 6 m apart for 6 min, plus 2 min of slow jogging.

Session 6: In the last session, after the warm-up, they played 4v4 in half court without goalkepeers and two small goals per team 6 m apart for 5 min, plus 3 min of slow jogging. Then, 3v3 without goalkepeers and big central line goals in half court for 5 min, followed by 3 min of jogging. To score, players had to go through the goal dribbling the ball. The last drill was a possession game (without goals) of 4v4 in half court. To get a point, the players had to perform ten consecutive passes. This task lasted 5 min followed by 3 min of slow steady run.

The CG also followed the schedule indicated in Figure 1. The players performed the same number of weekly training sessions, and with the same duration. The only difference was the absence of the 30-minute intervention that was carried out on Thursday in the EG. Therefore, the head coach performed and led the whole of the sessions during the 6-week period following his own criteria. In those 30-minutes, the head coach performed warm-up exercises, technical drills (passing, shooting and dribling) possession games, tactical games and set pieces. The head coach in CG was said that the total training load of the sessions had to be similar to the total training load of the EG.

The training load of every session was controlled with heart rate monitors and rating of perceived exertion in both groups (EG and CG):

Heart Rate Control (HR): Heart rate was monitored for every player every 5 s in each training session using a heart rate monitor with individually coded transmitters via short-range radiotelemetry (Polar Team Sport System, Polar Electro, Finland). The variable used in this study was the mean heart rate for the whole practice. The data recorded during the briefing before the start of each training session were deleted. To reduce any heart rate recording errors during training, all players were regularly asked to check that their heart rate monitors were working and properly worn (at least every 10 min). In addition to this, one of the researchers was permanently looking at the portable PC screen, making sure that every player's heart rate monitor was transmitting the data. After every training session, the heart rate data were exported and analysed using the Excel software programme (Microsoft Corporation, U.S.).

Rating of Perceived Exertion (RPE): The RPE was measured using the 6-20 Borg scale (Borg, 1970). Each player's session-RPE was collected about 30 min after each training session to ensure that the perceived effort was referring to the whole session rather than the most recent exercise intensity. All players were taught and familiarized with this scale for rating perceived exertion during the 2 weeks prior to the start of the study. In the procedure, the player is shown the scale and asked "How was your workout?", and they must give a single number representing the training session.

Statistical Analyses: Descriptive statistics were performed for all the variables in order to check for the assumptions of normality. Mean ± standard deviation of the data was calculated. Normal distribution and homogeneity of the parameters were checked with Shapiro–Wilk and Levene's test. The statistical differences were assessed by using Student's t test. A P value of 0.05 or lower was considered as being statistically significant. An analysis was performed using SPSS version 16.0 (Chicago. IL. USA).

3. Results

All the variables were normally distributed. Levene's test showed no violation of homogeneity of variance. The EG characteristics were the following: they were aged 25.08 ± 2.57 with an age range of 10.00 years, had a Body Mass Index (BMI) of 23.23 ± 1.91, a weight of 73.04 ± 7.58 kg, and a height of 177.25 ± 6.83 cm (Table 1). The CG characteristics were as follows: they were aged 23.91 ± 2.97 with an age range of 11.00 years, had a Body Mass Index (BMI) of 23.59 ± 0.91, a weight of 75.64 ± 4.58 kg, and a height of 179.05 ± 3.53 cm (Table 2). Table 3 and 4 show all the fitness test results in the two respective moments (T1 and T2) (October and December) for the EG and the CG, respectively. EG and CG improved their performance in every test (agility, agility with the ball and 20-metre Multi-Stage Fitness Test), however only the 20-metre Multi-Stage Fitness Test and the VO2max (ml/kg/min) in the EG experienced a statiscally significant improvement. EG players increased their performance in the 20-metre Multi-Stage Fitness Test from 12.71 ± 0.80 stages in T1 to 13.17 ± 1.00 stages in T2. This improvement supposed a consequent increase in the VO2max (ml/kg/min), which enhanced from 58.73 ± 2.41 ml/kg/min in T1 to 60.11 ± 2.99 ml/kg/min in T2.

Table 3. Fitness test results of the elite male futsal players in the EG (n = 12) for Test 1 (October) and Test 2 (December)

EXPERIMENTAL GROUP FITNESS TESTS IN OCTOBER				
n = 12	Agility (s)	Agility ball (s)	Bleep test (stages)	VO2max (ml/kg/min)
Mean	9.49 ± 0.34	11.29 ± 0.49	12.71 ± 0.80	58.73 ± 2.41
Maximum	10.06	12.03	14.00	62.6
Minimum	9.03	10.41	11.50	55.1
Range	1.03	1.62	2.5	7.5
Outfields (n = 10)	9.39 ± 0.27	11.22 ± 0.51	12.70 ± 0.66	58.70 ± 1.99
Goalkeepers (n = 2)	9.98 ± 0.11	11.64 ± 0.11	12.75 ± 1.76	58.85 ± 5.03

EXPERIMENTAL GROUP FITNESS TESTS IN DECEMBER				
n = 12	Agility (s)	Agility ball (s)	Bleep test (stages)	VO2max (ml/kg/min)
Mean	9.38 ± 0.38	11.21 ± 0.38	13.17 ± 1.00	60.11 ± 2.99
Maximum	9.88	11.65	14.50	64.10
Minimum	8.88	10.38	12.00	56.60
Range	1.00	1.27	2.50	7.50
Outfields (n = 10)	9.32 ± 0.26	11.18 ± 0.41	13.21 ± 0.99	60.22 ± 2.98
Goalkeepers (n = 2)	9.71 ± 0.25	11.35 ± 0.01	13.00 ± 1.41	59.60 ± 4.24

Table 4. Fitness test results of the elite male futsal players in the CG (n = 12) for Test 1 (October) and Test 2 (December)

CONTROL GROUP FITNESS TESTS IN OCTOBER				
n = 12	Agility (s)	Agility ball (s)	Bleep test (stages)	VO2max (ml/kg/min)
Mean	9.50 ± 0.36	11.36 ± 0.56	12.61 ± 0.68	58.43 ± 2.41
Maximum	10.16	12.05	14.00	62.6
Minimum	9.15	10.40	10.50	52.1
Range	1.01	1.65	3.5	10.5
Outfields (n = 10)	9.40 ± 0.30	11.27 ± 0.59	12.70 ± 0.56	58.70 ± 1.79
Goalkeepers (n = 2)	10.01 ± 0.11	11.70 ± 0.11	12.00 ± 0.00	56.60 ± 0.00

CONTROL GROUP FITNESS TESTS IN DECEMBER				
n = 12	Agility (s)	Agility ball (s)	Bleep test (stages)	VO2max (ml/kg/min)
Mean	9.47 ± 0.30	11.29 ± 0.49	12.75 ± 1.00	58.85 ± 2.99
Maximum	9.98	11.83	14.00	62.60
Minimum	8.95	10.38	11.00	53.60
Range	1.03	1.45	3.00	9.00
Outfields (n = 10)	9.38 ± 0.16	11.23 ± 0.81	12.80 ± 0.79	59.00 ± 2.58
Goalkeepers (n = 2)	9.92 ± 0.25	11.62 ± 0.25	12.50 ± 0.00	58.10 ± 0.00

Table 5 shows the performance improvements (increase (Δ) and percentage increase (% Δ)) and P values between T1 (October) and T2 (December) in both groups (EG and CG). There were no significant differences between the groups (EG vs. CG) at the baseline (Test 1). Regarding the EG, agility improved by 1.15% from T1 to T2 (p = ns), agility with ball increased by 0.70% from T1 to T2 (p = ns), 20-metre Multi-Stage Fitness Test increased by 3.61% (p = 0.04), and VO2max increased by 2.34% (p = 0.04) from T1 to T2. In the CG, there were no significant improvements (i.e. agility improved by 0.31%, agility with ball increased its performance by 0.61%, 20-metre Multi-Stage Fitness Test increased by 1.15%, and VO2max improved by 0.71%) (Table 5).

The HR and RPE data obtained from both groups (EG and CG) during the 6-week in-season training phase did not show any statistical difference between both groups. In the EG group, the mean HR data ranged during the 12 sessions from 141.1 ± 9.2 to 138.9 ± 10.3 beats per minute (bmp) while the RPE was between 14.5 ± 2.1 to 14.1 ± 1.7. In the CG, the mean HR data were ranged between 143.1 ± 10.3 to 139.2 ± 9.3 bmp while the RPE was between 14.3 ± 1.1 to 14 ± 1.2. Therefore, it can be concluded that the trainind load applied to both groups was similar.

Table 5. Performance improvements and P value between Test 1 (October) and Test 2 (December) in both groups

Tests	EXPERIMENTAL GROUP			CONTROL GROUP		
	Test 1- Test 2			Test 1- Test 2		
	Δ	% Δ	p	Δ	% Δ	p
Agility (s)	0.11	1.15	ns	0.03	0.31	ns
Agility ball (s)	0.08	0.70	ns	0.07	0.61	ns
Bleep Test (Stages)	0.46	3.61	0.04	0.14	1.15	ns
VO2max (ml/kg/min)	1.38	2.34	0.04	0.42	0.71	ns

4. Discussion

The purpose of this study was to investigate the effects of a 6-week in-season small-sided game training phase on fitness parameters in elite male futsal players. The hypothesis was that small-sided futsal games applied over a consecutive 6-week period would increase the aerobic endurance of the futsal playersmore than standard training. The effects of the small-sided games periodisation allowed the EG futsal players to significantly increase their VO2max. However, the improvements achieved in both agility tests (with and without ball) were not significant. The CG futsal players did not obtain a significant increase in any of the tests. Thus, the results of this study confirm the above mentioned hypothesis.

Regarding the speed of the movement-agility test (with and without ball), Berdejo-del-Fresno (2012) used the same test (4x10 m shuttle run) to measure speed of movement and coordination in an integrated way (Ruiz et al., 2006) in another study that involved male futsal players. The speed of the movement-agility test constitutes a good way to measure the ability of futsal players to make changes in direction similar to those performed in a futsal game. Álvarez Medina et al. (2004) used the 5x10 m, 4x5 m and 2x5 m both with and without ball. However, it can be observed from the results that the modifications were not significant in any of the groups (EG and CG). Berdejo-del-Fresno (2012) found scores of 11.88, 11.86 and 10.80 seconds with the ball and 9.86, 10.02 and 9.21 seconds without the ball in three different moments in a season in futsal players from the same level. Maybe this is because the training protocol used (small-sided games) in this study is not the best way to improve this particular ability. Tessitore et al. (2011) proposed specific agility drills to increase its performance, thanks to which, after a 3-week pre-season programme with 20-minute specific agility drills, positive adaptations were obtained in 16 semi-professional male football players. Jones et al. (2009), in the same line as Graham-Smith and Pearson (2005), suggested that, to obtain basic improvements in COD and speed, athletes should seek to maximise their sprinting ability and enhance their eccentric knee flexor strength to allow effective neuromuscular control of the contact phase of the COD and speed task. Finally, Graham-Smith et al. (2009) added that the penultimate contact plays a significant role in deceleration when changing direction, i.e. greater braking forces in the penultimate contact are associated with faster agility times. Therefore, if futsal players wish to improve their agility capacity, they will need to work on their sprinting ability, eccentric knee flexor strength and body position before turning, as well as on the specific futsal agility drills.

Cardiorespiratory or aerobic endurance improved significantly throughout the 6-week period in the EG groups. VO2max increased in the EG probably due to the fact that the specific periodisation of small-sided futsal games had its effect, thanks to the high intensity bursts that game has itself. The final VO2max values in both groups were higher than those found by Álvarez-Medina et al. (2002) in professional Spanish players (57.80 ± 2.53 ml/kg/min) and non professional Spanish players (54.86 ± 3.21 ml/kg/min). The aerobic capacity in futsal is fundamental. A high level of this ability allows the player to be active during the whole game, especially in the last part of the match (Álvarez-Medina et al., 2002). Aerobic capacity also plays an important role in the process of regeneration. Thus, the team's performance might increase throughout the season if aerobic capacity improves (Álvarez Medina et al., 2001a; Álvarez Medina et al., 2001b; Álvarez Medina et al., 2002; Barbero Álvarez et al., 2003; Barbero Álvarez et al., 2004a; Barbero Álvarez et al., 2004b). It can be concluded that values lower than 50 ml/kg/min are deficient, values between 50-55 ml/kg/min are normal, values between 55-60 ml/kg/min are good, and values higher than 60 ml/kg/min are excellent (Álvarez Medina et al., 2002). Therefore, it can be concluded that the aerobic endurance of the players of this study was excellent for the EG (60.11 ± 2.99 ml/kg/min) and good for the CG (58.85 ± 2.99 ml/kg/min) at the end of the training phase. Both groups began with a good level (58.73 ± 2.41 ml/kg/min for the EG vs. 58.43 ± 2.41 ml/kg/min for the CG).

This study has shown that VO2max improved following a small-sided games periodisation that combines a change in the number of players involved in the exercises, together with the court size and the type of goals used (with or without goalkeeper, normal goals, small goals or line goals). Duarte et al. (2009) found that the decrease in the number of players resulted in intensity increases (heart rate) and more frequent individual tactical actions. Therefore, futsal coaches can increase the physiological demands of specific drills by reducing the number of players involved.. The results obtained in this study have shown that a 6-week period, where small-sided games and modifications of the task constraints were applied, the aerobic fitness level of futsal players can be enhanced.

5. Conclusion

The results obtained in the present study suggest that an adequate periodisation of small-sided games can be used to develop and increase the VO2max of futsal players. Having said this, in order to improve speed of movement-agility, both with and without ball, specific tasks and exercises should be performed as the small-sided game intervention used in the current study did not impact upon these parameters. These data indicate that futsal coaches may use small-sided games for training aerobic fitness and tactical-technical components concurrently by modifying the court dimension and the number of players involved in each task or exercise.

References

[1] Álvarez Medina, J., Serrano, E., Giménez, L., Manonelles, P. & Corona, P. (2001a) Perfil cardiovascular en el fútbol-sala: adaptaciones al esfuerzo. *Archivos de Medicina del Deporte* XVIII (82): 143-148.

[2] Álvarez Medina, J., Serrano, E., Giménez, L., Manonelles, P. & Corona, P. (2001b) Perfil cardiovascular en el fútbol-sala: respuesta inmediata al esfuerzo. *Archivos de Medicina del Deporte* XVIII (83):199-204.

[3] Álvarez Medina, J., Serrano, E., Giménez, L., Manonelles, P. & Corona, P. (2002) Necesidades cardiovasculares y metabólicas del fútbol sala: análisis de la competición. *Apunts: Educación física y deportes* 67: 45-53.

[4] Álvarez Medina, J., Manonelles, P., Giménez, L. & Corona, P. (2004) Entrenamiento, rendimiento y control de la vía anaeróbica aláctica y de la fuerza en el fútbol sala. *Archivos de Medicina del Deporte* XXI (102):307-314.

[5] Barbero Álvarez, J. C., Soto, V., & Granda, J. (2003) Temporary analysis during match play in futsal (indoor soccer) with photogrametric system. *Book of abstracts: Science and Football* 5, 266.

[6] Barbero Álvarez, J. C., Soto, V. & Granda, J. (2004a) Análisis de la frecuencia cardiaca durante la competición en jugadores profesionales de fútbol sala. *Apunts de educación física* 77:71-78.

[7] Barbero Álvarez, J. C., Soto, V. & Granda, J. (2004b) Effort profiling during indoor soccer competition. *Journal of Sports Sciences* 22:500-501.

[8] Berdejo-del-Fresno, D. (2012) Fitness seasonal changes in a first division English futsal team. *African Journal of Basic & Applied Sciences* 4(2): 49-54.

[9] Borg, G. (1970) Perceived exertion as an indicator of somatic stress. *Scandinavian Journal of Rehabilitation Medicine* 2, No. 2-3, 92-98.

[10] Casamichana, D. & Castellano, J. (2009) Análisis de los diferentes espacios individuales de interacción y los efectos en las conductas motrices de los jugadores: aplicaciones al entrenamiento en fútbol. *Motricidad. European Journal of Human Movement* 23:143-167.

[11] Casamichana, D. & Castellano, J. (2010) Time-motion, heart rate, perceptual and motor behaviour demands in small-sides soccer games: effects of pitch size. *Journal of Sports Sciences* 28(14):1615-1623.

[12] Casamichana, D., Castellano, J., González-Morán, A., García-Cueto, H. & García-López, J. (2011) Physiological demand in small-sided games on soccer with different orientation of space. *International Journal of Sport Science* 23(7):141-154.

[13] Castagna, C., & Barbero Álvarez, J. C. (2010) Physiological demands of an intermittent futsal-oriented high-intensity test. *Journal of Strength and Conditioning Research* 24(9):2322-2329.

[14] Coutts, A.J., & Aoki, M.S. (2009) Monitoring training in team sports. Olympic Laboratory: Technical Scientific Bulletin of the Brazilian Olympic Committee 9(2):1-3.

[15] Duarte, R., Batalha, N., Folgado, H. & Sampaio, J. (2009) Effects of exercise duration and Lumber of players in heart rate responses and technical skills during futsal small-sided games. *The Open Sports Sciences Journal* 2:37-41.

[16] Duarte, R., Araújo, D., Fernandes, O., Travassos, B., Folgado, H., Diniz, A. & Davids, K. (2010) Effects of different practice task constraints on fluctuations of player heart rate in small-sided football games. *The Open Sports Sciences Journal* 3:13-15.

[17] Gamble, P., (2006) Periodization of training for team sports athletes. *Strength and Conditioning Journal* 28(5):56-66.

[18] Graham-Smith, P. & Pearson, G. (2005) An investigation into the determinants of agility performance. *Proceeding of the 3rd International Biomechanics of the lower limb in health, disease and rehabilitation*; 2005 Sept 5-7; Manchester, United Kingdom.

[19] Graham-Smith, P., Atkinson, L., Barlow, R. & Jones, P. (2009) Braking characteristics and load distribution in 180 degree turns. (Abstract) In: *The Proceedings of the 5th annual UKSCA conference*, 6-7 June 2009, Wybosotn Lakes, Bedforshire, United Kingdom.

[20] Hill-Hass, S., Coutts, A., Rowsell, G. & Dawson, B. (2009a) Generic versus small-sided game training in soccer. *International Journal of Sports Medicine* 30:636-642.

[21] Hill-Hass, S., Dawson, B., Coutts, A., & Rowsell, G. (2009b) Physiological responses and time-motion characteristics of various small-sided soccer games in youth players. *Journal of Sports Science* 27:1-8.

[22] Impellizzeri, F.M., Marcora, S.M., Castagna, C., Reilly, T., Sassi, A., Iaia, F.M. & Rampini, E. (2006) Physiological and performance effects of generic versus specific aerobic training in soccer players. *International Journal od Sports Medicine* 27(6):483-492.

[23] Jones, P., Bampouras, T. & Marrin, K. (2009) An investigation into the physical determinants of change of direction speed. *The Journal of Sports Medicine and Physical Fitness* 49(1):97-104.

[24] Jones, S. & Drust, B. (2007) Physiological and technical demands of 4v4 and 8v8 games in elite youth soccer players. *Kinesiology* 39:150-156.

[25] Léger, L.A. &Gadoury, C. (1989) Validity of the 20 m shuttle run test with 1 min stages to predict VO_2max in adults. *Canadian Journal of Applied Sport Sciences* 14(1):21-26.

[26] Little, T. (2009) Optimizing the use of soccer drills for physiological development. Strength Conditioning Journal 31: 67-74.

[27] Lohmann, T.G., Roche, A.F. & Martorell, R. (1988) *Anthropometric standardization reference manual*. Champaign, IL: Ed. Human Kinetics.

[28] Owen, A., Twist, C. & Ford, F. (2004) Small-sided games: The physiological and technical effect of altering pitch size and player numbers. *Insight* 7: 50-53.

[29] Ruiz, J.R., Ortega, F.B., Gutierrez, A., Meusel, D., Sjöström, M. & Castillo, M.J. (2006) Health-related fitness assessment in childhood and adolescence: a European approach based on the AVENA, EYHS and HELENA studies. *Journal of Public Health* 14: 269-277.

[30] Tessitore, A., Perroni, F., Cortis, C., Meeusen, R., Lupo, C. & Capranica, L. (2011) Coordination of soccer players during preseason training. *Journal of Strength and Conditioning Research* 25(11): 3059-3069.

13

CESFM: A Proposal to FIFA for a new 'Continuous Evaluation Fuzzy Method' of Deciding the WINNER of a Football Match that Would Have Otherwise been Drawn or Tied after 90 Minutes of Play

Ranjit Biswas*

Department of Computer Science, Jamia Hamdard University, Hamdard Nagar, New Delhi, INDIA
*Corresponding author: ranjitbiswas@yahoo.com

Abstract In this research work the author consider only those cases of football matches for which the penalty shootout is a method for determining a winner, otherwise that would have been drawn or tied after 90 minutes of play. The existing method of penalty shootout is having a lot of criticisms due to its huge demerits. In this research work the author proposes an improved method to FIFA to select the winner by a continuous soft-computing evaluation method. The method is called by CESFM which is basically a fuzzy constructive method. But CESFM does not exclude five penalty kicks by each team as followed presently after 90 minutes of play. The result of five penalty kicks is one of the many components in the method of CESFM. This proposed fuzzy method can easily extract the real dominant team out of the two tied teams using a software called by CESFM-software with inputs from the Referee where some inputs are given by the Referee using his fuzzy pocket machines M. It is claimed that if FIFA implement this method of CESFM in World Cup Football, it will be a true justice to the football world, to the fans, to the players, to the teams (in particular to the looser team) and consequently it will give enormous justice to the 'football' if considered as a subject. CESFM is not to be applicable if the football game ends after 90 minutes with a result (not draw).

Keywords: *fuzzy set, FIFA, CESFM, positive parameters, negative parameters, CES-Score (CS), fuzzy pocket machine, CPS, CESFM-software*

1. Introduction

The penalty shootout is a method of determining a winner in Football matches that would have otherwise been drawn or tied after 90 minutes of play. A penalty shootout is normally used only in situations where a winner is needed and where other methods such as extra time and sudden death have failed to determine a winner. It avoids the delays involved in staging a replayed match in order to produce a result. The term *golden goal* was introduced by FIFA in 1993 along with the rule change because the alternative term, 'sudden death', was perceived to have negative connotations. Following a draw, two fifteen-minute periods of extra time are played. If any team scores a goal during extra time, that team becomes the winner and the game ends at once. The winning goal is known as the 'golden goal'. If there have been no goals scored after both periods of extra time, a penalty shootout decides the game.

The shoot-out is thus a test of individuals which may be considered inappropriate in a team sport; Football is a team sport and penalties is not a team, it is the individual. Inferior teams are tempted to play for a scoreless draw, calculating that a shoot-out offers their best hope of victory. The1990 FIFA World Cup was notable for many teams playing defensive football and using time wasting tactics, including a team of very high caliber, who scored only 5 goals but reached the final by winning two shootouts. Hence a common complaint about penalty shootouts is that they only determine the better team in the one, rather narrow, discipline of taking penalty shots, rather than fairly determining the better team in overall play. As a way to decide a football match, shoot-outs have been seen variously as a thrilling climax or as an unsatisfactory cop-out. The result is often seen as a lottery rather than a test of skill. Only a small subset of a footballer's skills is tested by a shoot-out. In this research article we propose a new soft-computing method for deciding the winner of a football match that would have otherwise been drawn or tied after 90 minutes of play.

This method is called by CESFM which stands for "Continuous Evaluation System for Football Matches". The proposed theory of CESFM uses fuzzy logic to compute the winner for such a draw or tied case.

2. About Fuzzy Set Theory

Since our proposed method of CESFM (Continuous Evaluation System for Football Matches) is based on fuzzy logic, we present here a preliminaries of fuzzy set theory [1,2,3,4,5] which will be used in this research article.

In the real world the human reasoning in most of the cases involves the use of variable whose values are fuzzy sets. Description of system behavior in the language of fuzzy rules lowers the need for precision in data gathering and data manipulation. Essentially, in a Fuzzy Set (FS) each element is associated with a point-value 'membership value' selected from the unit interval [0,1], which is also termed the 'degree of belongingness' or 'grade of membership' of the element in the fuzzy set.

If X be a universe of discourse, a fuzzy set A in X is a set of ordered pairs

$$A=\{(x,\mu_A(x)):x\in X\}$$

where $\mu_A: X \rightarrow [0,1]$ is a function called by "membership function" of the fuzzy set A. Thus, $0 \leq \mu_A(x) \leq 1 \ \forall \ x \in X$.

Here X is the universe of discourse, or universal set, which contains all the possible elements of concern in each particular context of applications. The membership function μ_A maps each element of X to a membership grade (or membership value) between 0 and 1.

Consider a decision parameter α[0,1]. An α-cut of a fuzzy set A is a crisp set Aα that contains all the elements of X that have membership value in A greater than or equal to α. i.e. $A_\alpha = \{x \mid A(x) \geq \alpha\}$.

A strong α-cut of a fuzzy set A is a crisp set $A_{\alpha+}$ that contains all the elements of X that have membership value in A strictly greater than α. i.e. $A_{\alpha+} = \{x \mid A(x) > \alpha\}$.

For details about the famous fuzzy set theory discovered by the great philosopher Prof. Zadeh [4], one could see any good book available in libraries/markets [1,2,3,4,5].

3. Theory of CESFM

Our proposed method of CESFM (Continuous Evaluation System for Football Matches) is applicable only to such cases of football matches that would have otherwise been drawn or tied after 90 minutes of play. This method is developed to replace the existing penalty shootout method. In the existing system, a penalty shootout is used to decide somehow a winner of a football match where the other methods such as extra time and sudden death have failed to determine a winner. The penalty shootout method has a lot of demerits, it does not give satisfaction to the looser. The spirit of the sport is not translated to the result, instead it becomes equivalent to a lottery game in many situations. The probability that the better team will win is not high, because it becomes like that 'the better goalkeeper will win, not necessarily the better team'. This is a genuine unsolved problem to the world football fans and teams and players, and thus to the football sport if considered as a subject of study and research.

In our work here we propose a new method CESFM based on continuous evaluation scores. The CESFM is a multi-criteria based decision making process. A team's performance, merits and demerits, can be evaluated on the basis of certain significant attributes.

3.1. Philosophy behind CESFM

For a draw/tied case, the main problem is : 'How to choose the better?'. It is fact that we must develop a new method such that the better team should win, not the weaker team by any chance.

The "Winner" must be

(i) the overall dominating team,

(ii) the overall better team by continuous performance shown by the team

who has contributed more substance of the subject 'football' in today's game by way of quality and performance.

The existing penalty shootout method of taking decision on the basis of the results of 5 penalty kicks to find the better or dominating team for declaring the 'Winner' is a weak method as it is a test for one player (Goalkeeper) only against one player of the opponent team (five players, one after another, of the opponent team for five penalty kicks). It does not give justice or satisfaction to the football world.

While a football match goes on, each team plays well revealing its merits in various criteria/attributes continuously at every second. It is very difficult to evaluate every second the merit-performance of both the teams. But each team also happens to commit mistakes during play, which are not happening continuously but in discrete moments of time. For example, a team commits one foul after 23 minutes, another foul after 12 minutes, then shown yellow card to one player of the team by the referee after 18 minutes, etc. These events if quantified by good mathematical techniques (using hybrid of soft-computing and hard-computing methods) can surely indicate the amount of discredits, amount of poor performance etc. of the concerned team. These events are well recorded in a database by the organizer for statistical analysis. In our proposed CESFM we input such discrete negative-events in a continuous manner during the 90 minutes of play, in addition to the positive events. Finally we compute the Continuous Evaluation System Score or CES-Scores or CS (in short) of both the teams comparing which we understand which team is the better performer today, i.e. which team is the dominant team. The team with higher CES-Score (CS) will be the winner. To compute the CS score of a team we compute CS values of few input parameters corresponding to the team.

3.2. Parameters in CESFM

FIFA World Cup is one of the most prestigious events happens on this earth! But for the draw cases under consideration here, what are the parameters on which one can decide the Winner? Can it be just one parameter (results of 5 penalty kicks at the penalty-shootout)?

Theory of CESM consider the following 16 parameters as its components for inputs to its software called by

CESFM-Software. The CESFM does not exclude penalty-shootout kicks (after 90 minutes of play) as one of its component inputs. But instead of existing practice of 5 kicks, theory of CESFM introduces 10 kicks with the following rule.

3.2.1. What is 'CESFM Penalty Shootout' (CPS)?

The 'CESFM Penalty Shootout' (CPS) consists of 10 penalty kicks by each team in the existing manner, with the condition that each player (except goalkeeper) of a team will kick once. None can kick twice. The CPS is one mandatory component in CESFM method in a football match. Replacement of Goalkeeper is allowed by a team as many times the team wants during CPS.

The philosophy behind this new norm of CPS is that it becomes a game of 11 players for each team upto certain extent. This philosophy is missing in the existing practice of penalty shootout in the FIFA rules.

3.2.2. What is 'Half-ground of the Opponent' for a Team?

We explain it by a figure. The Figure.1 shows that team X on the left hand side and team Y on the right hand side. For the team X, the Half-ground of the Opponent is shown by arrow mark. Similarly, for the team Y, the Half-ground of the Opponent is also shown by arrow mark. These two half-grounds are the partition of the complete ground into two equal halves by the middle half-line.

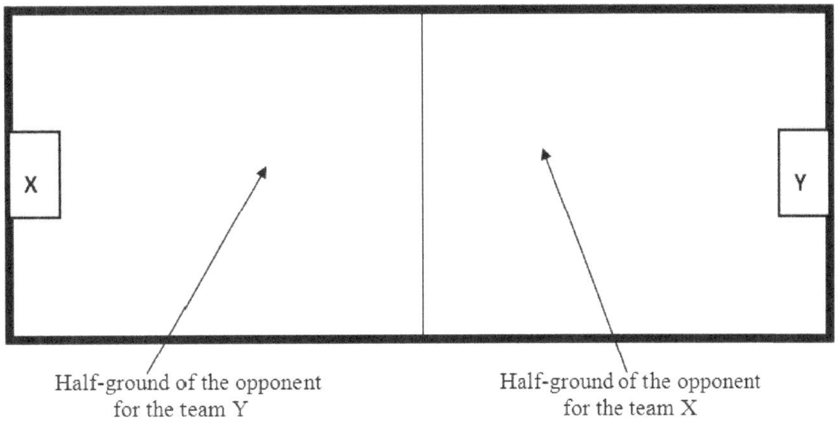

Figure 1. Half-ground of the Opponent for team X and team Y

3.2.3. Positive and Negative Parameters

There are 16 parameters in the theory of CESFM. Few of them are called negative parameters and rest of them are to be called positive parameters. There are seven negative parameters and nine positive parameters which are listed below (however, more number of decision contributing parameters, positive as well as negative, can be added in the theory of CESFM if decided).

Negative Parameters:

(i) F1 = Number of Simple Fouls committed (Not shown any card) during the 90 minutes of play.

(ii) F2 = Number of Yellow Cards shown by the Referee during the 90 minutes of play.

(iii) F3 = Number of Red Cards shown by the Referee during 90 minutes of play.

(iv) O = Number of Offsides committed during the 90 minutes of play

(v) H = Number of Handballs during the 90 minutes of play.

(vi) BPK = Number of Bad Penalty Kicks during CPS play. (by a 'bad penalty kick' of CPS we mean that the kicked ball goes outside the goalpost without touching the goalkeeper or barpost).

(vii) R = Number of Replacement of players made by the Coach (who are not injured) during 90 minutes of play.

Positive parameters:

(i) G = Number of Goals scored (during CPS only).

(ii) BPC = Percentage of Ball Possession at the complete ground during the 90 minutes of play.

(iii) BPH = Percentage of Ball possession at the half-ground of the opponent during 90 minutes of play.

(iv) SCB = Number of Shots which Collide at Barpost without scoring Goal during 90 minutes of play.

(v) CK = Number of Corner-kicks (CK) during 90 minutes play.

(vi) T = Number of Throws during 90 minutes of play.

(vii) 2G = Consecutive two goals scored (without any goal scored by the opponent in-between) during 90 minutes of play.

(viii) 3G = Consecutive three goals scored (without any goal scored by the opponent in-between) during 90 minutes of play.

(ix) nG = Consecutive four or more goals (n>3) scored (without any goal scored by the opponent in-between) during 90 minutes of play.

3.3. Categories of Fouls

Fouls in a football match are divided into three categories in our theory of CESFM :

(i) Category F1 : Simple Foul (not shown any card)

(ii) Category F2 : Shown Yellow Card Foul

(iii) Category F3 : Shown Red Card Foul

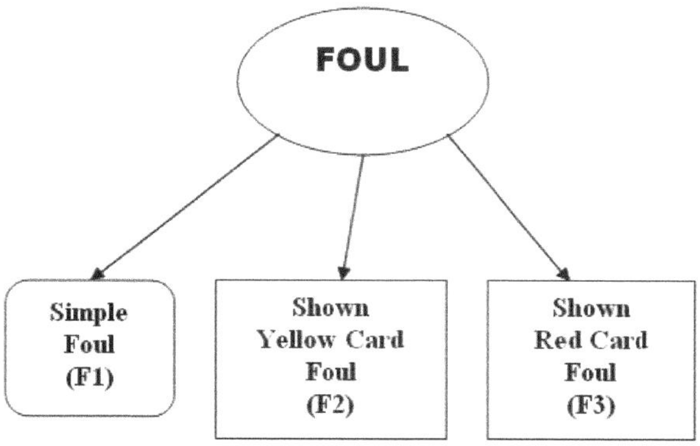

Figure 2. Three categories of Fouls in a football match

The simple fouls may have various amount of foul-gravity. Similarly the yellow-card fouls may have various foul-gravity, and also red-card fouls may have various amount of foul-gravity.

The foul gravity can be estimated by the Referee by his best possible intellectual judgment on the basis of finite number of significant criteria. For instance, FIFA could choose the following criteria to estimate the gravity of any foul (F1 or F2 or F3) :-

(i) 'bad intention mainly for making tactful physical collision',

(ii) 'unfair way of ball possession',

(iii) 'inappropriate body language',

(iv) 'argument with the opponent player(s)', and

(v) 'argument with the Referee'.

3.4. CS Value of a Foul (F1 or F2 or F3)

Fouls are negative parameters in the Theory of CESFM as mentioned in subsection-3.2. The CS value of a foul (F1 or F2 or F3) is a crisp value. But the referee awards a fuzzy value to it by his best possible intellectual judgment depending upon the gravity of the foul. This fuzzy value is then de-fuzzified by one of the three algorithms : Algo-1, Algo-2, Algo-3, to get the CS value of a foul.

For a foul (which could be F1 or F2 or F3), the universal set is the crisp set F given by F = $\{f_1, f_2, f_3, f_4, f_5\}$, where

f_1 = 'bad intention mainly for tactful physical collision',
f_2 = 'unfair way of ball possession',
f_3 = 'inappropriate body language',
f_4 = 'argument with the opponent player(s)', and
f_5 = 'argument with the Referee'.

Note: ***The elements f_i of the universal set F may be modified, number of elements may be increased/decreased and fixed by the FIFA experts. For the sake of hypothetical presentation here, we consider the five membered universal set for the Fouls.***

For every foul (F1 or F2 or F3) committed by a team, the Referee takes a fuzzy action against the team by awarding a fuzzy set A (of the universal set F) to the team. The fuzzy set A will be awarded to the team prior to the foul-kick to be kicked by the opponent team at the cost of hardly ten to twelve seconds.

3.4.1. Fuzzy Pocket Machine M for the Referee

There is a handy small fuzzy pocket machine M for the Referee using which the referee awards a fuzzy set A of F within a maximum of ten seconds. Once the Referee awards the fuzzy set, the data will be stored immediately in the concerned database in the FIFA-Server where there is a software called by "CESFM Software" which will be executed if and only if the situation after 90 minutes is a draw case, otherwise not.

The machine M will have three buttons in the name of F1, F2 and F3 respectively, twelve buttons in the name of : . (dot), 0, .1, .2, .3, .4, .5, .6, .7, .8, .9, and 1 respectively, and two more buttons in the name of 'ENTER' and 'EDIT'. In total there are 17 buttons in the fuzzy pocket machine M (as shown in Figure 3).

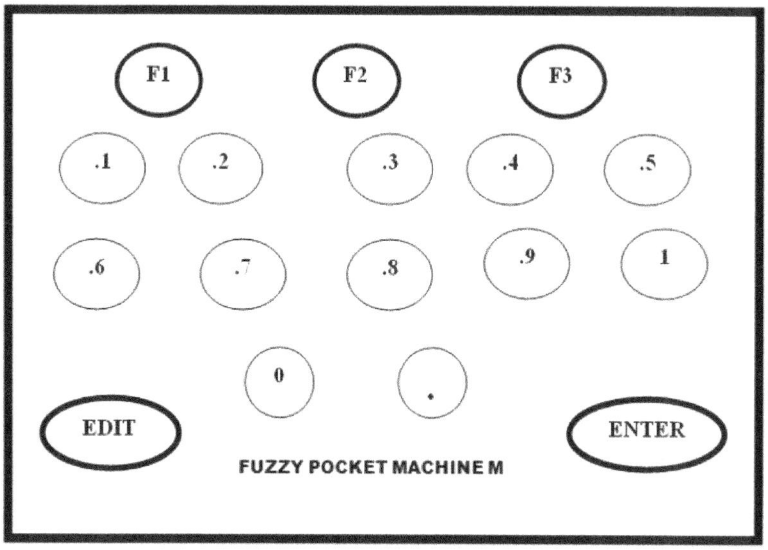

Figure 3. A Fuzzy Pocket Machine M for the Referee

For a committed Foul during play, depending upon the gravity of Foul, the Referee follows the following steps to award a fuzzy set A to the concerned team:

Step-1 : Referee press one of the buttons F1 or F2 or F3, and then the button 'ENTER'. (This signifies which of the three categories of fouls is awarded by the Referee).

Step-2 : Referee inputs one membership value from the closed interval [0,1] using one or more buttons : . (dot), 0, .1, .2, .3, .4, .5, .6, .7, .8, .9, and 1, and then the button 'ENTER'. (This is the membership value of the element f_1 for the fuzzy set A by best possible intellectual judgment of the Referee).

Step-3 : Referee inputs one membership value from the closed interval [0,1] using one or more buttons : . (dot), 0, .1, .2, .3, .4, .5, .6, .7, .8, .9, and 1, and then the button 'ENTER'. (This is the membership value of the element f_2 for the fuzzy set A by best possible intellectual judgment of the Referee).

Step-4 : Referee inputs one membership value from the closed interval [0,1] using one or more buttons : . (dot), 0, .1, .2, .3, .4, .5, .6, .7, .8, .9, and 1, and then the button 'ENTER'. (This is the membership value of the element f_3 for the fuzzy set A by best possible intellectual judgment of the Referee).

Step-5 : Referee inputs one membership value from the closed interval [0,1] using one or more buttons : . (dot), 0, .1, .2, .3, .4, .5, .6, .7, .8, .9, and 1, and then the button 'ENTER'. (This is the membership value of the element f_4 for the fuzzy set A by best possible intellectual judgment of the Referee).

Step-6 : Referee inputs one membership value from the closed interval [0,1] using one or more buttons : . (dot), 0, .1, .2, .3, .4, .5, .6, .7, .8, .9, and 1, and then the button 'ENTER'. (This is the membership value of the element f_5 for the fuzzy set A by best possible intellectual judgment of the Referee).

Referee can use the EDIT button to change his membership value. But after editing, he has to enter the modified data using ENTER button in order to save the modification in the memory of the FIFA-server. Using the fuzzy pocket machine M, the inputs of the Referee are transmitted to the server directly from the playground at real time.

3.4.2. Three Algorithms Algo-1, Algo-2 and Algo-3 for De-fuzzification

Corresponding to three categories of fouls, there are three cases which are explained below.

Case-1 : If the Foul is a Simple Foul

Consider a foul of category F1. The CS value of a foul F1 denoted by CS(F1) will be always one of the numbers 2, 3 and 4. Let A be the fuzzy set awarded by the Referee corresponding to this foul committed by a team. Then the following algorithm called by Algo-1 will be applicable on the basis of α-cut of the fuzzy set A.

Algo-1

If the .5-cut of A (i.e. the set $A_{.5}$) is a null set
then CS(F1) = 2. Stop. *else*
If the .8-cut of A (i.e. the set $A_{.8}$) is a null set
then CS(F1) = 3. Stop. *else*
CS(F1) = 4.

Case-2 : If the Foul is a Yellow Card Foul

Consider a foul of the category F2. The CS value of a foul F2 denoted by CS(F2) will be always one of the numbers 4, 5 and 6. Let A be the fuzzy set awarded by the Referee corresponding to this foul committed by a team. Then the following algorithm called by Algo-2 will be applicable on the basis of α-cut of the fuzzy set A.

Algo-2

If the .5-cut of A (i.e. the set $A_{.5}$) is a null set
then CS(F2) = 4. Stop. *else*
If the .8-cut of A (i.e. the set $A_{.8}$) is a null set
then CS(F2) = 5. Stop. *else*
CS(F2) = 6.

Case-3 : If the Foul is a Red Card Foul

Consider a foul of the category F3. The CS value of a foul F3 denoted by CS(F3) will be always one of the numbers 6, 7 and 8. Let A be the fuzzy set awarded by the Referee corresponding to this foul committed by a team. Then the following algorithm called by Algo-3 will be applicable on the basis of α-cut of the fuzzy set A.

Algo-3

If the .5-cut of A (i.e. the set $A_{.5}$) is a null set
then CS(F3) = 6. Stop. *else*
If the .8-cut of A (i.e. the set $A_{.8}$) is a null set
then CS(F3) = 7. Stop. *else*
CS(F3) = 8.

3.5. CS values of other Parameters of CESFM

Out of sixteen parameters in the theory of CESFM, there are seven number of negative parameters and nine number of positive parameters. The CS values of three negative parameters are discussed in the preceding subsection. In this subsection we discuss the CS values of other parameters.

3.5.1. CS Value of Negative Parameters

It is discussed in the preceding subsection that for a Simple Foul F1, the CS(F1)$\in\{2,3,4\}$. For a Yellow Card Foul F2, the CS(F2)$\in\{4,5,6\}$. For a Red Card Foul F3, the CS(F3)$\in\{6,7,8\}$.

For the other negative parameters, we propose the following CS values in the theory of CESFM.

(i) For each Offside, CS(O) = 1;
(ii) For each handball, CS(H) = 1;
(iii) For every Bad Penalty Kick, CS(BPK) = 1;
(iv) For Replacement of players (who are not injured during play), the CF value is given by the following norm :

$$CF(R) = \begin{cases} 1, & \text{if 1 or 2 players are Replaced during 90 minutes} \\ 2, & \text{if 3 or more players Replaced during 90 minutes.} \end{cases}$$

3.5.2. CS Value of Positive Parameters

For the positive parameters, we propose the following CS values in the theory of CESFM.

(i) For each Goal G scored during **CPS**, CS value CS(G) = 10.

(It is mentioned in subsection 3.2.1 that CPS is mandatory in CESFM method. The goals of the first 90 minutes of play are not to be considered in CESFM. They are ignored as the situation is a draw/tied case after 90 minutes of play).

(ii) If the Ball Possession of a team across the complete ground the during 90 minutes of play is = x%, then CS(BPC) = x/20.

(iii) If the Ball Possession of a team across the half-ground of the opponent during 90 minutes of play is = y%, then CS(BPH) = y/10.

(iv) For each Shot which Collides at Barpost without scoring Goal during 90 minutes of play, the CS value is CS(SCB) = 5. For each Shot which Collides at Barpost without scoring Goal during CPS play, the CS value is CS(SCB) = 1.

(However, if a Shot Collides at Barpost with a Goal during 90 minutes of play or during CPS, then there is no CS(SCB) value for this shot).

(v) For each corner kick during 90 minutes of play the CF value is given as below :-

CF(CK) = 1, if the corner-kick is a "Bad Corner Kick" (BCK) i.e. the ball of that corner-kick goes directly outside the play-ground without touching any player or inside-ground or barpost. Otherwise, for all other cases CF(CK) = 2. It is to be noted that in case the corner kick hits the barpost, the CS(SCB) value will also be considered as usual.

(vi) If a team gets a Throw, then for each such throw the CF value is given by CF(Throw) = 1

(vii) If a team scores two consecutive goals (without any goal scored by the opponent in-between) during 90 minutes of play, then for each such case the CF value is given by CF(2G) = 1.

This rule is not applicable during CPS play.

(viii) If a team scores three consecutive goals (without any goal scored by the opponent in-between) during 90 minutes of play, then for each such case the CF value is given by CF(3G) = 5 (in such case the CF value of 2G will not be considered).

This rule is not applicable during CPS play.

(viii) If a team scores n (n>3) consecutive goals (without any goal scored by the opponent in-between) during 90 minutes of play, then for each such case the CF value is given by CF(3G) = 10 (in such case the CF value of 2G or 3G will not be considered).

This rule is not applicable during CPS play.

3.6. CS Score of a Team

In a football match, suppose that two teams X and Y arrives at a Draw/Tied case after 90 minutes of play. Therefore this is a situation where the fuzzy method CESFM is applicable. To compute the CS Score of a Team X, the CESFM-software computes the following first of all :

(i) Total amount of CS values of all the negative parameters for the team X which is denoted by NCS(X).

(ii) Total amount of CS values of all the positive parameters for the team X which is denoted by PCS(X).

CS Score of the team X is then computed using the formula:

$$CS(X) = 1000 + PCS(X) - NCS(X).$$

Note: *In the above formula for CS(X), there is no significance of the amount 1000. It is added just to ensure that the value of CS(X) does not become a negative real number under any circumstances, for no other purpose. It is obvious that even if we do not added 1000 here, the final result of CESFM-software will not be changed.*

3.7. Who is the Winner by CESFM Method?

Suppose that after 90 minutes of play, situation is 'draw' case between the two teams X and Y. Then the CESFM-software will be executed in the FIFA-Server to compute the CS score of both the teams X and Y.

If CS(X) > CS(Y) then X is the Winner. Otherwise, if CS(X) < CS(Y) then Y is the Winner.

A very rare case is if CS(A) = CS(B). In that case the CPS (as introduced in subsection-3.2.1) will be repeated once more to run the CESFM-software. If the result yet comes 'draw' then CPS will be repeated once again and so on, untill the CESFM-software computes the Winner.

4. A Hypothetical Example

We explain here, with hypothetical data, an application of this fuzzy CESFM method in a football match between two teams X and Y which has become draw (2-2) after 90 minutes of play. Suppose that after CPS play, the following is the statistics for the two teams as recorded in the FIFA-server corresponding to the 16 parameters of CESFM, shown in Table 1:

Table 1. The statistics of 16 parameters for team X and Y

Serial No.	Parameters	Frequency (X) : Number of Occurrences for Team X	Frequency (Y) : Number of Occurrences for Team Y
1	F1	3	1
2	F2	2	1
3	F3	0	0
4	O	3	4
5	H	3	2
6	BPK	1	0
7	R	3	1
8	**G (CPS only)**	**4**	**3**
9	BPC	40%	60%
10	BPH	26%	50%
11	SCB	0	0
12	CK	3 (with one BCK)	5
13	T	6	9
14	2G	0	0
15	3G	0	0
16	nG(n>3)	0	0

Fouls committed by team X

In total there are five fouls committed by the team X, out of which there are three F1 fouls, two F2 fouls and nil number of F3 fouls.

The fuzzy sets corresponding to the three F1 fouls committed by the team X are given by the Referee via his fuzzy pocket machine M which are as below :

X(i) : the fuzzy set {(f_1, .85), (f_2, .8), (f_3, .95), (f_4, .85), (f_5, .9)}, and

X(ii) : the fuzzy set {(f_1, .95), (f_2, .85), (f_3, .9), (f_4, .95), (f_5, 1)}, and

X(iii) : the fuzzy set {(f_1, .85), (f_2, .6), (f_3, .95), (f_4, .85), (f_5, .8)}.

The fuzzy sets corresponding to the two F2 fouls committed by the team X are given by the Referee via his fuzzy pocket machine M which are as below :

X(iv) : the fuzzy set {(f_1, .95), (f_2, .9), (f_3, .95), (f_4, 1), (f_5, .95)}, and

X(v) : the fuzzy set {(f_1, .85), (f_2, .8), (f_3, .95), (f_4, .9), (f_5, 1)}.

While CESM-software executes its Algo-1 and Algo-2, it will get the following de-fuzzified CS values for the team X (see subsection 3.4):

$$CS(X(i)) = 4,\ CS(X(ii)) = 4, CS(X(iii)) = 4,$$

$$CS(X(iv)) = 6,\ CS(X(v)) = 6.$$

Fouls committed by team Y

In total there are two fouls committed by the team Y, out of which there is one F1 foul, one F2 foul and nil number of F3 fouls.

The fuzzy set corresponding to the one F1 fouls committed by the team Y is given by the Referee via his fuzzy pocket machine M which is as below :

Y(i) : the fuzzy set {(f_1, .2), (f_2, .1), (f_3, .15), (f_4, 0), (f_5,0)}.

The fuzzy set corresponding to the one F2 foul committed by the team Y is given by the Referee via his fuzzy pocket machine M which is as below :

Y(ii) :the fuzzy set {(f_1, .15), (f_2, .2), (f_3, .1), (f_4, 0), (f5,0)}.

While CESM-software executes its Algo-1 and Algo-2, it will get the following de-fuzzified CS values for the team Y (see subsection 3.4):

$$CS(Y(i)) = 2 \text{ and } CS(Y(ii)) = 2.$$

The CESFM-software will thus compute all the CS values (see subsection 3.4 and 3.5) which are shown in the Table 2.

Table 2. The CS values of 16 parameters for team X and Y

Serial No.	Parameters	Frequency (X)	CS Value (for X)	Frequency (Y)	CS Value (for Y)
1	F1	3	12	1	2
2	F2	2	12	1	4
3	F3	0	0	0	0
4	O	3	3	4	4
5	H	3	3	1	1
6	BPK	1	1	0	0
7	R	3	2	1	1
8	**G (CPS only)**	**4**	**40**	**3**	**30**
9	BPC	40%	2	60%	3
10	BPH	26%	2.6	50%	5
11	SCB	0	0	0	0
12	CK	3	5	5	10
13	T	6	6	9	9
14	2G	0	0	0	0
15	3G	0	0	0	0
16	nG (n>3)	0	0	0	0

The CESM-software then computes the following :

$$NCS(X) = 12+12+0+3+3+1+2\ = 33$$

$$\text{and } PCS(X) = 40+2+2.6+0+5+6+0+0 = 55.6.$$

$$NCS(Y) = 2+4+0+4+1+0+1 = 12$$

$$\text{and } PCS(Y) = 30+3+5+0+10+9+0+0 = 57.$$

Then, CS(X) = 1000 + PCS(X) – NCS(X) = 1022.6 and
CS(Y) = 1000 + PCS(Y) – NCS(Y) = 1045.

Final output of the CESM-software :

Since CS(Y) > CS(X), CESM outputs that Y is the Winner, X is the looser.

Declaration : The team Y is the Winner in today"s football match.

Comment:

In the above example, see that if the fuzzy CESFM method is not applied to this football match between two good teams X and Y then by the existing FIFA norms of Penalty-shootout method FIFA will declare the team X as the Winner(4-3) and the team Y as the looser. But any football-fan or expert will get psychologically shocked with this declaration witnessing the 90 minutes continuous play of both the team and also feeling about the real statistical data, visualized data.

It is not any fault of FIFA nor of any of the teams X and Y, nor of the Referee, nor of any football fans, nor of the venue, nor of the host country, nor of the weather-climate or any other reasons. Surely it is due to an obsolete method followed by FIFA on one of the most important issues of football game : "How to select the Winner if the result comes draw after 90 minutes of play?". It is due to non-availability of any new innovative modern mathematical (and philosophical) technique which can provide solution retaining the justice to the football, retaining the interest of the game, retaining the interest of the football fans and experts, retaining the interest of the football world as a whole. The author here claims that the soft computing method CESFM is a much improved method for this problem of football subject.

5. Conclusion

In this research work we propose a new theory called by Theory of CESFM to FIFA and Football-experts of the world with a claim that if FIFA incorporates this fuzzy method in the World Cup Football, there will be a huge improvement in the justice to the game 'football' if considered as a subject. The proposed method is a continuous evaluation method to compute the WINNER using a software known as CESFM-software to be executed at the FIFA server. The fuzzy pocket machine is a simple wireless machine M by which the inputs of the Referee transmitted to the server directly from the playground at real time. The hardware of this machine M can be manufactured by a good company dealing with electronics and communication engineering. The code of CESFM-software can be easily developed by a programmer. CESFM does not exclude the penalty-shootout results. Rather a modified and improved version of penalty-shootout is introduced called by CPS which is also a mandatory components in the CESFM method. The CPS is a much improved version in the sense of football-interest both meritoriously and philosophically than the existing penalty shootout method of FIFA presently being followed in World Cup Football matches. The proposed method CESFM can do huge justice to the football, can provide huge satisfaction to the football world, for the cases of football matches which have a draw situation after 90 minutes of play. A hypothetical example is presented to explain how the CESFM computes better results than the results applying the existing 'Penalty Shootout only' norms of FIFA. The CESFM is not to be applicable for a decided match in 90 minutes of play.

References

[1] Dubois,D. and Prade,H., Fuzzy Sets and Systems: Theory and Applications, Academic Press, New York, USA, 1980.

[2] Kaufmann, A., Introduction to theory of Fuzzy Subsets, Vol.I (Academic Press, New York, 1975).

[3] Klir, G. K. and Yuan,B., Fuzzy Sets and Fuzzy Logic, Theory and Applications, (Prentice Hall, New Jersey, 1995).

[4] Zadeh,L.A., Fuzzy sets, Information and Control, 8(1965) 338-353.

[5] Zimmermann, H.J., Fuzzy Set Theory and Its Applications, 2nd ed., Kluwer Academic Publishers, Boston/Dordrecht/London, 1991.

14

Effects of Wrist Taping Pressures on the Maximum Dorsal Flexion Angle

Kenji Takahashi[1,*], Shin-ichi Demura[2]

[1]Faculty of Community Health Care, Department of Judo Physical Therapy, Teikyo Heisei University, Uruidominami 4-1 Ichihara, chiba, Japan
[2]Graduate School of Natural Science & Technology, Kanazawa University, Kakuma, Kanazawa, Ishikawa, Japan
*Corresponding author: kenji.takahashi@thu.ac.jp

Abstract This study aimed to examine the effects of different taping pressures with or without external force on the maximum dorsal flexion angle (DFA). Twenty-two healthy male university students with >5 years of athletic experience participated. A qualified trainer wound a rigid tape thrice around subject's wrist joint. Taping pressure was measured using the pressure measuring system AMI3037-SB. Independent variables were five experimental conditions (5 hPa, 30 hPa, 60 hPa, and 90 hPa, and control) and two measurement conditions for the wrist joint DFA with non-external and external forces. In the former, the subject flexed the wrist joint himself (active DFA), while in the latter, a trainer helped in flexion (passive DFA). The dependent variable was the maximum DFA. Two-way repeated measures ANOVA (taping pressure × different DFA measurement) and multiple comparison tests showed that passive DFA was significantly larger than active DFA under all taping pressure conditions. Active DFA was smaller under 30-hPa condition than under the 5-hPa condition, and was smaller under 60-hPa conditions than under control and 5-hPa conditions, and was smaller under 90-hPa condition than under the other conditions. Passive DFA was smaller under 30- and 60-hPa conditions than under control and 5-hPa conditions, and was smaller under 90-hPa condition than under control, 5-, and 30-hPa conditions. In conclusion, the passive DFA is larger than the active DFA, regardless of taping pressure. Wrist taping with pressure over 30 hPa limits DFA, particularly at 90 hPa.

Keywords: *pressure measuring system, rigid tape, blood flow, competitive sports, wrist joint*

1. Introduction

Athletes such as sumo and other wrestlers, judo fighter, weightlifters, and gymnasts tape their wrists with the aim of preventing wrist disorders or injuries by limiting excessive motion of the wrist joints [1,2]. Many injuries occur to the wrist joints because of excessive dorsal flexion [3,4]. Therefore, taping, which limits dorsal flexion, may be effective in preventing disorders or injuries. There are various methods for taping the wrist joint. Constantinou and Brown [1] introduced the following two methods: taping around the wrist joint (Figure1-a. wrist taping) and X support taping using cross-bridge tape on the palmar surface (Figure 1-b. X taping).

Wrist taping has been primarily used to decrease load stress and prevent excessive dorsal flexion; however, the main purpose is the prevention of injuries [2]. Athletes have generally used this taping method because they can wind the tape themselves. This method slightly limits all movements of the wrist joint. However, the degree of limitation of the range of motion (ROM) has not been shown with an objective measurement value [1].

On the other hand, the X taping method is used instead of a brace after a wrist injury [1,2]. Yamamoto [5] reported that X taping limited an average 25° of the maximum dorsal flexion angle (DFA) in American football players. This taping method is considered to have a strong fixing force because it involves taping of the palmar surface. However, this method may have disadvantages. For example, the palmar response may become insensitive and slippery when the individual grips objects. Therefore, in competitive situations, wrist taping should be preferred over X taping. The fixing force of wrist taping is weaker than that of X taping. However, a fixing force similar to that used in X taping may be obtained by increasing taping pressure.

Constantinou and Brown [1] pointed out the need to control taping pressure when examining the effects of taping in a review of other studies. It is considered that differences in taping pressure affect various factors such as strength exertion and ROM. For example, strong pressure may decrease blood circulation and cause nerve compression [6], because a tape wound around the wrist joint can excessively limit ROM. Therefore, it is necessary to examine the effects of different taping pressures on ROM.

In clinical practice, passive ROM is generally used to evaluate ROM of patients after injuries or surgeries [7].

Active ROM is also measured together with passive ROM during ROM evaluation of patients with muscle paralysis. In competitive sports, although athletes bend the wrist joints voluntarily, there are cases in which dorsal flexion is forced when the athlete receives some external force. Therefore, it is necessary to examine the effects of the passive DFA and the active DFA. Passive ROM is generally greater than the active ROM in all joints [7].

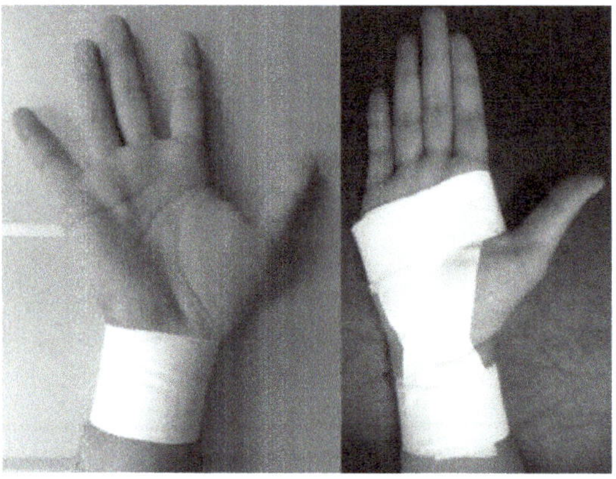

a: wrist taping b: X taping

Figure 1. Taping method of wrist joint

Therefore, we hypothesized that limitation effects on DFA become greater with increasing taping pressure because of the increased physical load on the wrist joint, and that the DFA is greater in the passive ROM measurement than in the active one, even if taping pressure is imposed on the wrist joint. This study aimed to examine the effects of different taping pressures on the passive and the active DFA.

From the present study, we may be able to judge the degree of taping pressure to decide a limited range of motion required when performing the wrist joint taping in the competitive situation.

2. Method

2.1. Subjects

Participants were 22 male university students (mean age, 19.4 ± 1.0 years) with >5 years of athletic experience and no history of wrist injuries such as sprain, fracture, or dislocation. Their sports were as follows: baseball (n = 8), soccer (n = 4), basketball (n = 4), track and field (n = 1), judo (n = 1), kendo (n = 1), karate (n = 1), rugby football (n = 1), and swimming (n = 1). Figure 1 shows the basic statistics [age, height, body weight, body mass index (BMI), wrist circumference, and competitive sports experience] of the subjects.

The aim and procedures of this study were explained in detail to all subjects prior to the experiment, and informed consent was obtained. This experimental protocol was approved by the Ethics Committee on Human Experimentation of the Faculty of Human Science, Kanazawa University (2012–18).

Table 1. The basic statistics for age, height, body weight, BMI and circumference of the dominant wrist joint of subjects (n=22)

	Mean	SD	MAX	MIN
Age (years)	19.4	1.0	22.0	18.0
Hight (cm)	171.3	6.6	185.3	158.7
Weight (kg)	65.2	10.1	88.1	50.0
BMI	22.2	2.9	28.4	18.3
Wrist circumference of dominant hand (cm)	15.8	0.6	17.2	14.9
Sports experience (years)	8.8	2.5	13.0	5.0

2.2. Tape and Taping Method

In this study, we used 50-mm rigid (non-elastic) tape manufactured by Johnson & Johnson (New Brunswick, NJ, USA). We adopted the wrist-taping method, in which one piece of rigid tape is wound thrice around the wrist joint, including the radius and ulnar styloid processes (Figure 1-a). An athletic trainer (Japan Sport Association) with >10 years of clinical experience performed the taping.

2.3. Pressure-Measuring Device

Taping pressure was measured using the pressure measuring system for stockings and bandages (AMI3037-SB, AMI-Techno. Tokyo, Japan.) (Figure 2). This system can measure pressure on the human body through clothing such as socks [8] and can detect the addition of constant pressure such as that from the use of an elastic bandage [9]. Therefore, this device is considered to be useful in measuring taping pressure. The measurement unit was hPa. A measurable range was 1–200 hPa, and the measurement error was ±3 hPa.

Taping was performed at the wrist joint of a participant's dominant hand. The dominant hand was judged according to Demura et al.'s handedness inquiry [10]. After a pressure sensor was placed on the palmaris longus muscle tendon 1.5 cm proximal to the palmar crease of the wrist, it was fixed with a cover tape (Figure 3 a, b, and c).

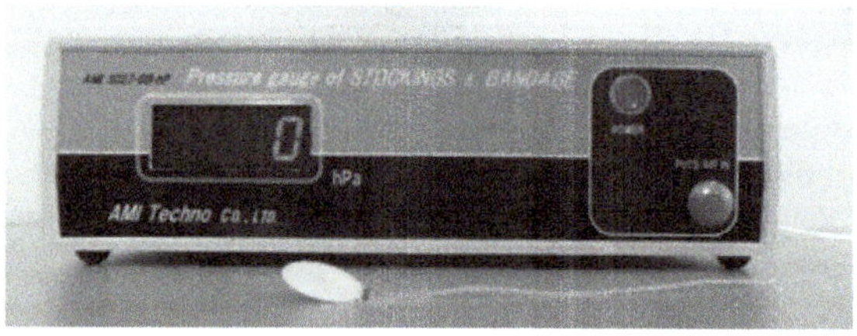

Figure 2. Pressure measuring system for stockings and bandages (AMI3037-SB)

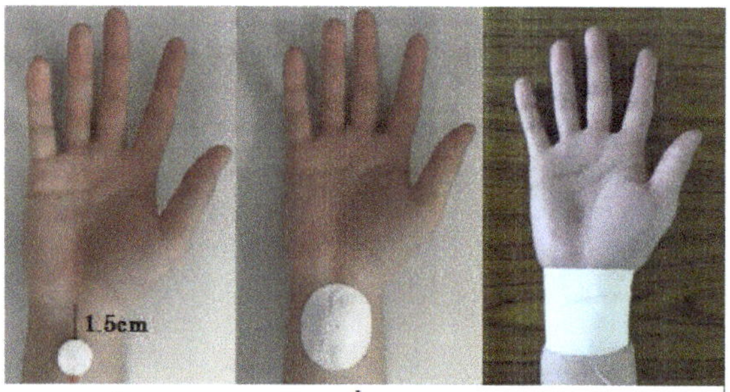

a b c

Figure 3. a: sensor only; **b**: sensor with cover tape; **c:** wrist joint taping with sensor & cover tape

2.4. Independent and Dependent Variables

The independent variables were five experimental conditions (pressure loads on the wrist joint), namely 4 pressure conditions of 5 hPa, 30 hPa, 60 hPa, and 90 hPa and a control condition (no tape) without tape attachment, and two measurement conditions of external force (passive DFA) applied by a trainer and no external force (active DFA). Under the 5-hPa condition, the tape was only wound around the wrist without any pressure. We assumed that these experimental conditions would reveal the effects of different taping pressures on DFA of the wrist joint. The 5-hPa condition was adjusted within an error range of ±1 hPa, whereas the other pressures were adjusted within a range of ±2 hPa. Dorsal flexion was measured under the following two conditions: under no external force, that is, when the subject flexed his own wrist joint maximally (active DFA), and under external force, when a qualified athletic trainer helped in flexion (passive DFA).

The dependent variable was the maximum DFA. The measurement unit was degree (°). A mean of three trials involving active and passive DFA measurements was used as an evaluation variable.

2.5. Experimental Procedure

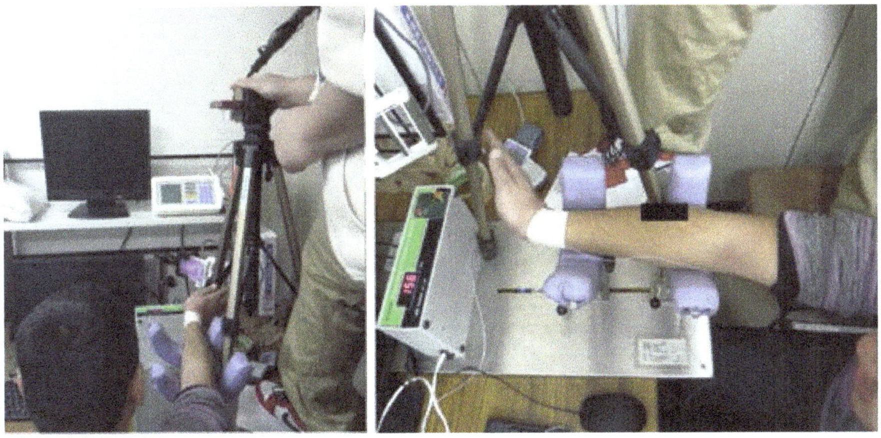

Figure 4. Measurement of (active) dorsal flexion angle using a digital camera with a leveler installed

Before the experiment, the subjects performed wrist warm-up exercises to prevent injury. Then, they assumed the following sitting posture: shoulder joint in 70–90° forward flexion, elbow joint in 15–30° flexion, forearm in the middle position between pronation and supination, and wrist joint in the neutral position. The metacarpophalangeal joint, the proximal interphalangeal joint, and the distal interphalangeal joint were kept in the extension state. Using a digital camera (DSC-W730/P, SONY, Tokyo, Japan) with a leveler installed, images of the measurements were acquired from directly above (Figure 4). Setting the stationary arm as the radius and the movable arm as the second metacarpal, we calculated DFA of the wrist joint using a posture evaluation program Ver. 1.0.1. (Takei, Tokyo, Japan) on the basis of the measurement images. Pressure experimental conditions were randomized for every subject, and active and passive DFAs were measured thrice in each condition without a rest time between trials. A rest time between conditions was >3 min. Passive and active DFA measurements were conducted alternately to eliminate any order effects. The tape was replaced in each pressure condition. The experiment was performed from 9:00 h to 13:00 h in a laboratory maintained at 26°C.

2.6. Statistical Analysis

Two-way repeated measures ANOVA (taping pressure × different DFA measurement) was used to reveal the mean differences among each condition using SPSS 18 (SPSS Inc., Chicago, IL). When significant effects were found, we performed a multiple comparison test using the Tukey's HSD method. The level of significance was set a priori to 0.05. The statistical power (1–β) of interaction and main effect obtained in ANOVA was calculated in *post-hoc* analysis using G*Power 3.1.7 software (http://www.psycho.uni-duesseldorf.de/abteilungen/aap/gpower3/) [12]. In addition, an effect size (ES) was calculated to examine the size of mean differences. ES was interpreted as follows: <0.2 as small, >0.5 as intermediate, and >0.8 as large.

3. Results

Table 2 shows the means and standard deviations of the active and passive DFAs under all experimental conditions. Results of the two-way repeated measures ANOVA (taping pressure × different DFA measurement) and the multiple comparison tests are also shown along with ES values. No significant difference was found in interaction (df = 4, F = 2.19, p = 0.08, partial $\eta 2 = 0.09$, $1 - \beta = 0.98$), and significance was found in both main factors of the measurement method (df = 1, F = 328.78 $p < 0.05$, partial $\eta 2 = 0.94$, $1 - \beta = 1$) and taping pressure (df = 4, F = 41.47, $p < 0.05$, partial $\eta 2 = 0.66$, $1 - \beta = 1$). Multiple comparison tests showed that the passive DFA was larger than the active DFA under all experimental conditions [ES (d) = 4.22-5.28]. Active DFA was smaller under the 30-hPa condition than under the 5-hPa condition [ES (d) = 0.58], and was smaller under the 60-hPa condition than under control and 5-hPa conditions [ES (d) = 0.50, 0.70], and was smaller under the 90-hPa condition than under other conditions [ES (d) = 0.51-1.14]. Passive DFA was smaller under 30- and 60-hPa conditions than under control and 5-hPa conditions [ES (d) = 0.73-1.58], and was smaller under the 90-hPa condition than under control, 5-hPa, and 30-hPa conditions [ES (d) = 0.66-1.93].

Table 2. Two-way repeated measures ANOVA (N=22)

		Dorsal flexion					Two-way ANOVA			Tukey's HSD	Effect size (d)
		Active DFA		Passive DFA							
		Mean	SD	Mean	SD		F-value	p-value	η2		
Taping pressure	Control	63.30	7.85	97.91	4.92	F1	328.78*			Active DFA: Con>60, 90 5>30, 60,>90.	 0.50, 0.96 0.51-1.14
	5hPa	64.79	7.51	96.03	5.58					Passive DFA:	
	30hPa	60.18	8.29	91.91	5.79					Con, 5>30, 60, 90 30<90	0.73-1.93 0.66
	60hPa	59.30	8.19	90.17	4.92	F2	41.47*	0.00	0.66	Con, 5, 30, 60, 90: Passive DFA>Active DFA	4.22-5.28
	90hPa	54.65	10.11	88.32	5.01	IN	2.19	0.08	0.09		

*: $p<0.05$
F1: Active DFA *Passive DFA F2: Taping pressure IN: interaction
Con: Control 5: 5hPa, 30: 30hPa, 60: 60hPa, 90: 90hPa

4. Discussion

Generally, ROM of the wrist joint becomes larger when an external force is added by the examiner than when individuals move the joint themselves. Norkin and White [7] reported that the margins protect the joint structure from external forces. Researchers have not considered the limiting effects of wrist-taping with taping pressure on ROM [1]. This study therefore clarifies that the passive DFA is larger than the active DFA, regardless of taping pressure magnitude. Therefore, DFA becomes larger under added external forces, even when the wrist is taped.

A taping pressure of >30 hPa limited both active and passive DFAs, whereas that of 5 hPa did not. In particular, the limiting effects were stronger under the 90-hPa condition than under the no-tape condition (ES = 0.96, 1.93). Therefore, regardless of external force, it can be said that the limiting effect of DFA cannot be expected by wrist-taping without pressure; it can be expected under the application of pressures >30 hPa, particularly 90 hPa.

The limiting effect probably occurred under the 30-hPa condition because the tape acts as a splint when a certain level of tension is applied. Conversely, no limiting effect was achieved under the 5-hPa condition, probably because the tension required for the tape to act as a splint was not achieved at a pressure of 5 hPa.

It is inferred that the strong limiting effect achieved under the 90-hPa condition is due to the splint effect and taping pressure applied to the joint structure. Shimawaki et al. [11] reported that veins were constricted on addition of a pressure of >60 mmHg (80 hPa) to the upper arm. Therefore, a pressure of up to 60 hPa was decreased by veins located just below the surface of the wrist joint; this pressure extends to the joint structure at 90 hPa. However, we believe that there was no difference in limiting effect between the 30- and 60-hPa conditions because only the splint effect was applied.

Under the 90-hPa (77.25 mmHg) condition in our study, we found a slight pressure change (1–3 hPa) in all subjects, as observed by the pulse and a change in complexion of the hand. We thought that taping pressure close to the diastolic blood pressure at the wrist joint may cause a slight pressure change. Shimawaki et al. [11] reported that blood volume in the finger increased gradually by increasing the pressure in increments, when applied with pressures of 20–80 mmHg over the upper arm. Moreover, a pressure close to the diastolic blood pressure causes constriction of veins and blood flow changes enough for individuals to feel their pulse. Therefore, in future, it will be necessary to examine blood flow change according to differences in taping pressure.

In this study, the procedure of attaching the tape, adjusting the pressure, and completing the measurements took approximately 4 min. In any case, we avoided prolonged taping of the wrist with a pressure of 90 hPa. We did not find a slight pressure change under the 60-hPa condition. However, in this condition, it may be possible to palpate the pulse because there is much individual variation in blood pressure. Regarding the problem of blood pressure and blood flow mentioned above, it would also be necessary to examine the 60-hPa condition in addition to the 90-hPa condition in relation to the duration of taping.

A change in the complexion of the hand was not found under the 30-hPa condition (approximately 4 min). The effect on the blood flow is small during wrist-taping with a pressure of 30 hPa. The limiting effect on dorsal flexion was not higher at the 60-hPa condition than at the 30-hPa condition. Therefore, if a taping pressure of 30 hPa can result in the same limiting effect as that with 60-hPa, we recommend that there is no requirement to increase the taping pressure to >30 hPa.

Constantinou and Brown [1] introduced some wrist joint taping methods such as wrist-taping and X support taping (X taping). Yamamoto et al. [5] reported considerable limitation effects by X taping. As mentioned above, wrist-taping with a pressure of >30 hPa also limited DFA. In the future, it will be necessary to compare the limiting effects of X taping and wrist-taping in the same subjects. In addition, it will be necessary to compare the limiting effects of both taping methods and examine the effects on other joint movements such as palmar, ulnar, and radial flexion under the same experimental conditions.

In competitive situations, high-pressure wrist-taping is considered effective to prevent disorders and injuries by limiting the maximum DFA. However, prolonged taping may inhibit blood flow and result in decreased performance. Therefore, it is necessary to adjust taping pressure according to the sport and duration of the competition.

As practical applications to competitive sports, wrist-taping with high pressure may not be adequately for athletes requiring consecutive strength exertion for a prolonged time, such as judo fighters, because they negatively affect their performance by the time to inhibition of blood flow becomes long. On the other hand, it will affect little performance of athletes such as weightlifters because the performance time is very short. In addition, when obtaining a limiting effect of dorsal flexion regardless of a difference of the athletic event, it may be necessary to use the taping pressure of >30 hPa.

There are some methods of wrist-taping other than that used in this study [2]. In addition, elastic tape has been also used in the athletic field. Therefore, it is considered that the effect of taping pressure differs on the basis of the type of tape and taping method, and one limitation of study is that the results of this study apply only to the taping method using in this study (i.e., rigid tape). Future studies must examine the effects of range of motion caused by different types of tapes and taping methods.

5. Conclution

This study examined the effects of different taping pressures on the maximum DFA using the wrist-taping method, in which one piece of rigid tape is wound thrice around the wrist joint. Regardless of the magnitude of taping pressure, the passive DFA is larger than the active DFA. In both active and passive DFA measurements, the limiting effects on DFA can be expected from a taping pressure of >30 hPa, particularly 90 hPa. However, a pressure of >90 hPa raises concerns about the negative effects of constricted blood flow. It is therefore necessary to adjust taping pressure according to the duration that the tape will be worn and the characteristics of the athlete and the sport.

References

[1] Constantinou, M., Brown, M., "Therapeutic taping for musculoskeletal conditions." Elsevier: Churchill Livingstone, 2010.

[2] Rose, M., "Pocketbook of Taping Techniques." Elsevier, Churchill Livingstone 2010.

[3] Linscheid, RL., Dobyns, JH., "Athletic injuries of the wrist." *Clin Orthop* 198:141-151, 1985.

[4] Thomas, S., "Wrist Injuries: Part I." *Dynamic Chiropractic* Feb 10, Vol. 15, Issue 04, 1997

[5] Yamamoto, I., Ichimiya, S., Kibamoto, K., Morita, H., Nakajima, T., Suzuki, A., "Athletic taping for preventing injury was performed for healthy athletes before exercise" [in Japanese]. *Bulletin of NSSU* 15 (2): 71-77, 1986.

[6] Hirata, K., Yoshida, M., "Effect of cuff compression intensity and cuff width on Skin blood flow measured by a laser-Doppler flowmeter" [in Japanese]. *J JRA for Textile End-Use* 36: 154-161, 1995.

[7] Norkin, CC., White, DJ., "Measurement of Joint Motion: Guide to Goniometry (4 edition)." F.A. Davis Company 2009.

[8] Ooizumi, Y., Matsuzawa, E., Iida, Kenichi., "Establishment of evaluation methods of clothing pressure of high supported clothes-The relation between clothing pressure of stretch clothes measured on a dummy and the human body" [in Japanese]. *Bulletin of TIRI* 2: 120-121, 2007.

[9] Hirai, M., "Clinical application of elastic stockings" [in Japanese]. *Jpn J Phle* 18 (5): 239-245, 2007.

[10] Demura, S., Sato, S., Nagasawa, Y., "Re-ex-amination of useful items for determining hand domi-nance" [in Japanese]. *Arch Sci Med (Torino)* 168: 169-177, 2009.

[11] Shimawaki, S., Sakai, N., Tamura, H., "Change in Blood Vessel Images in Human Finger Using Near-Infrared Radiation while Compressing the Upper Arm: Effect of the Compression Pressure and the Age of Subjects" [in Japanese]. *Transactions of the Jpn Society of Mechanical Engineers, Part C* 75 (756): 2280-2285, 2009.

[12] G*power 3.1.7 software. Heinrich Heine University Düsseldorf. (http://www.psycho.uni-duesseldorf.de/abteilungen/aap/gpower3/).

Measurement of Energy Expenditure among Free Living Active and Sedentary Women (18-23 Years): Results of Objective and Self-Reported Assessment

Mansi Chopra*, Anupa Siddhu

Department of Food and Nutrition, Lady Irwin College, Sikandra Road, New Delhi- 110001, University of Delhi, India
*Corresponding author: chopra.mansi2@gmail.com

Abstract **Background:** Heart rate monitoring has been advocated for assessing energy expenditure in field studies. The aim of the study is to determine and compare the energy requirements by heart rate method and factorial method and measure PWC_{170} for young active and sedentary women. **Methods:** A cross-sectional study on 30 collegiate women (18-23 years) was conducted. Young active (Group A) (n=15) and age matched sedentary women (Group S) (n=15) were selected based on an inclusion criterion. Using standard procedures, data was collected on general information, anthropometry, blood pressure, body composition, PWC_{170}, HR-VO_2 relationship, diet and physical activity to compute energy requirements. **Results:** Individual HR- VO_2 equations were developed. Mean TDEE by factorial method for Group A was 2256 ±246 kcal and for Group S was 1772 ± 163 kcal. Mean TDEE by heart rate method of Group A was 1952 ± 68 kcal and of Group S was 1579 ± 116 kcal. Mean PWC_{170} for Group A and Group S were 94.8 ± 6.9 and 93.5 ± 13.9 watts respectively. PAL for Group A was 32% higher than Group S. **Conclusion:** The heart rate technique is a useful tool for computing energy requirement of active groups because of its simplicity and potential use in free living conditions.

Keywords: *energy requirement, heart rate method, PWC_{170}, factorial method, total daily energy expenditure*

1. Introduction

The energy expenditure of individuals and groups are of vital interest to nutritionists for policy, therapeutic and research purposes. The body needs energy for maintaining body temperature and metabolic activity and for supporting physical work and growth. Energy balance is achieved when input (i.e. dietary energy intake) is equal to output (i.e. total energy expenditure), in adults. Human energy requirements are estimated from measures of energy expenditure plus the additional energy needs for growth, pregnancy and lactation [1]. Various methods, suitable for field studies, have been developed for computing energy expenditure. Evaluation of two of the methods, heart rate monitoring and activity diaries is addressed in this paper.

Heart rate monitoring is a method of estimating energy expenditure that is based on the strong positive correlation that exists between heart rate and oxygen consumption [2,3]. The development of small instruments which measure and store heart rate (HR) minute-by-minute for long periods of time has considerably improved the applicability of this technique to the measurement of total daily energy expenditure (TDEE). The relationship between HR and oxygen consumption (VO_2), is unique to each individual and is normally described as linear at energy expenditure above basal and below maximal output [4]. Individual calibration to obtain VO_2- HR relationship and is a cardinal feature of most studies using HR to obtain energy expenditure (EE) [2,5].

Physical activity is an integral part of everyday life. In general the capacity to transform chemical energy into mechanical work is the work capacity of the organism. Physical work capacity (PWC) is defined as the maximal amount of oxygen that a subject can consume during short term maximal exercise (1 or 2 min) [6]. The purpose of this study is to determine and compare the energy requirements by two methods namely heart rate and factorial method respectively, and measure PWC_{170} for young active and sedentary women in the age group of 18-23 years.

2. Subjects and Methods

Thirty healthy, collegiate women (18-23 years) participated in the study. Young active women in the college basketball team (n=15) and age matched sedentary women (n=15) were selected from Lady Irwin College, New Delhi. Active women were enrolled in the study based on an inclusion criteria of being unmarried, not suffering from any kind of respiratory illness and not having any history of diseases like diabetes, cardiovascular disease, asthma, hypertension, etc.; not consuming any hormones or drugs; being in their prefollicular/ preluteal phase of menstrual cycle and involved in active sport for one year, at least 1 hour/day, 5 times a week. Sedentary women were included based on a similar inclusion criterion except being actively involved in any sport for at least 1 hour/day, 5 times a week. The study had an institution ethical clearance. A formal informed consent was obtained from all subjects and they agreed to adhere to their regular food intake and activity patterns; and maintained their current training program throughout the course of the study.

2.1. Anthropometric Assessment

Body weight (to nearest 0.1 kg) was measured using a digital balance and height (to nearest 0.1 cm) was measured using anthropometric rod. Prior to the measurements the subjects were told to dress in light clothing and were instructed to stand barefoot and straight with the head in the Frankfurt plane. Body mass index was calculated as weight (kg) divided by height (m) squared. Mid- upper arm circumference was measured using a flexible non- stretchable tape made of fibre glass on the left hand at the midpoint of the upper arm, between the acromian process and tip of the olecranon, to the nearest 0.1 cm. Hip circumference was measured at the largest posterior extension of the buttocks and waist circumference was measured at the midpoint between subcostal and suprailiac landmarks. Waist circumference was measured using an inelastic tape, kept in contact with skin without pressing it [7]. Measurements were taken in duplicate.

Blood pressure was measured using sphygmomanometer. Two readings separated by 5 minutes were averaged to get a precise measurement. The TANITA Body Composition Analyzer (BC- 420 MA) was used to measure the body composition. Estimated values of Lean body mass (LBM), Body fat % (BF %) and Total body water (TBW) were obtained.

2.2. Cardio Respiratory Index- PWC_{170}

Cardio respiratory fitness or PWC_{170} (Physical Work Capacity) was assessed in Exercise Physiology Lab, Defence Institute of Physiology and Allied Sciences (DIPAS) using a modified physical working capacity test (PWC) on a Monark cycle ergometer that predicted the workload at an HR of 170 beats·min^{-1} (PWC_{170}). Participants were instructed to avoid vigorous exercise on the day of testing, and not to consume food, alcohol, caffeine or tobacco products two hours before testing. After briefing the subjects on the procedure of the test, each subject was given a warm up trial test at a lower load of 25 watts (W). Each test stage lasted for 2 minutes and the wattage was increased from 25W to 50 W to 75W to 100W to 125W depending on the subject's cardio respiratory fitness. Pedaling frequency throughout the test was to be kept at 60 rev·min^{-1}. At the end of each minute of the test, the heart rate was recorded, measured via Polar Sports tester heart rate monitor (RS 400) placed around the chest at the level of the xiphoid process of the sternum. The watch like receiver was worn on the wrist. The participant's heart rate at the end of the stage was used to determine the change in resistance for the next stage and resistance for each stage was recorded. Cycle ergometers were calibrated before each day's testing. The PWC_{170} was calculated by using the loads and the heart rates by the following Eq. (1) and Eq. (2) [8]:

When $Hf_2 > 170$, then,

$$PWC_{170} = L2 - L_2 - L_1 / Hf_2 - Hf_1\left(Hf_2 - 170\right) \quad (1)$$

When $Hf_2 < 170$, then,

$$PWC_{170} = L2 + L_2 - L_1 / Hf_2 - Hf_1\left(170 - Hf_2\right) \quad (2)$$

Where, PWC_{170} = Physical Work Capacity at Heart Rate 170, L_1 and L_2 are two different loads, and Hf_1 and Hf_2 are heart rates at L_1 and L_2.

2.3. Dietary Intake (24-hour Dietary Record)

To assess the intake pattern, the subjects maintained a 24-hour dietary record for one working day. A record sheet was given to the subjects. The energy intake was calculated by converting food items into raw ingredients and then calculating the calorific values from Nutritive Value of Indian Foods [9]. 'Diet soft' software version 1.1.7 was used to calculate the nutrient intake.

2.4. Heart Rate Method

The use of HR to estimate EE was based on the assumption of a close individual linear relationship between HR and VO_2 and thus also between HR and EE [2]. The heart rates were recorded using the Polar Sports tester heart rate monitor (RS 400). HR monitoring was done for one working day beginning at 7:00 am for active women and at 9:00 am for sedentary women; and ending at the same time next day. The heart rate recorder was disconnected when the subjects were bathing or sleeping during the day. The average length of HR monitoring was > 12 hours for each subject. The recorded data was transferred via the Infra-red device to Polar Pro Trainer 5 software for complete analysis. Aberrant readings, if observed, were replaced by the average of the previous and subsequent values.

2.5. Activity Record

Subjects completed 24 hour activity record for the same day of the HR monitoring to reflect the EE. The form included three columns; first column was time, second column was activity and the last column was remarks. A sample record of activities as a guideline was given to the study subjects prior to obtaining the information.

2.5.1. BMR Estimation

Basal metabolic rate of each subject was predicted by using equations based on body weight, age and sex [1]. The Eq. (3) used for females (18-30 years) was:

$$BMR 14.818 \times Body\ Weight\left(Kg\right) + 486.6. \quad (3)$$

The calculated BMR was used in computing day's requirement as described in FAO/WHO/UNU (2004). PAR and PAL was also computed for both the groups.

2.6. HR and VO_2 Measurement during Activities

HR and O_2 consumption (VO_2) were measured simultaneously. The subjects were briefed on the procedure of the test to obtain VO_2 and HR on a Monark ergometer (828 E) in Exercise Physiology lab, Defence Institute of Physiology and Allied Sciences (DIPAS). Daily records of ambient room temperature and relative humidity were recorded. The face mask was put on and held by stretchable rubber straps. The subjects were seated on the bicycle ergometer for 2 minutes and then the loads were increased till exhaustion. Two consecutive readings of VO_2 and HR were obtained with the subject sitting idle on the bicycle ergometer. The average of two readings was used as the RMR and it was expressed as shown by Eq. (4):

$$RMR\ (Kcal/\min) = 5 * VO_2\ (L/\min) \qquad (4)$$

A calorific equivalent of 5 kcal/l of oxygen [10] was used to convert the VO_2 values to EE. For HR above FHFLEX, corresponding EE was determined by using the regression equations applicable to individual subjects. Total Energy Expenditure (TEE) was computed using the Eq. (5):

$$TEE = (t1\ *\ BMR) + (t2 * RMR) + (t3 * dEE) \qquad (5)$$

Where, t1 = time spent at BMR, t2 = time spent at HR < FHFLEX and t3= time spent at different HR > FHFLEX.

2.7. Estimates of EE from HRM

Individual estimates of EE were made with HR monitoring technique. Individual regression equations were developed to predict EE in Kcal/min from HR. The regression was introduced as the relationship between HR and VO_2 over the range of heart rates. Regression equations were established from all sub maximal heart rates and VO_2 measurements. It is well documented that there is a different HR-VO_2 relationship at low and higher energy expenditure activities. Therefore, it was necessary to determine the point of inflection, which is referred to as FHFLEX. The heart rates above FHFLEX were used to calculate VO_2 from calibration curve/ regression equation and heart rates below the FHFLEX were calculated from different regression equations. Flex HR was calculated as the mean of the highest resting pulse and the lowest on exercise + ten [11]. The mean daily heart rate was applied to the single line regression equation to estimate the mean energy expenditure. The individual calibration data was used to predict minute-by-minute energy expenditure for each person.

2.8. Estimates of EE from Activity Record

EE was calculated from activity records using the energy cost of activities found in the literature. Typical training activities for active women playing basket ball included warming up, running, basketball practice, stretching exercises and residual time. For the sedentary women, the typical activities throughout the day were attending theory and practical classes and lunch time in between.

3. Statistical Analysis

The entire data was expressed in mean ± SD. Unpaired t test was used for comparison between active and sedentary women. Pearson's correlation was calculated for HR (≥ FHFLEX) and corresponding EE and individual linear regression equations were calculated to establish the relationship between HR and corresponding EE for active and sedentary subjects. Level of significance was kept at 0.05. Statistical analysis was done using SPSS (17.0) software.

4. Results

Several methods have been used to determine EE for computing energy requirements of groups of individuals. The findings of the study were based on thirty young collegiate women in the age range of 18-23 years. Mean age of young women belonging to the active and sedentary group was 20.0 years. Comparison of the anthropometric measurements between Group A and Group S are presented in Table 1.

Table 1. Anthropometric and body composition data of Group A and Group S (Group A, Active; Group S, Sedentary; BMI, body mass index; WC, waist circumference; HC, hip circumference; MUAC, mid-upper arm circumference; FFM, fat free mass; TBW, total body water; BMR, basal metabolic rate. Mean ± SD in rows; range in parentheses (all such values). 1 Equation used: BMR= 14.818 X Body Weight + 486.6 [1].)

Parameters	Group A (n = 15)	Group S (n = 15)
Height (cm)	156.96 ± 3.42 (153.4-163.0)	158.65 ± 4.93 (146-167.2)
Weight Kg)	52.25 ± 7.67 (40.0-65.0)	55.19 ± 6.5 (45-66.8)
BMI (Kg/m^2)	21.27 ± 3.02 (16.8-26.0)	22.08 ± 3.17 (18.3-29.1)
WC (cm)	71.6 ± 6.75 (58.4-83.8)	72.8 ± 8.14 (66.0-91.4)
HC(cm)	94.9 ± 7.5 (83.8-111.8)	96.4 ± 6.3 (86.4-107.9)
MUAC (cm)	24.4 ± 3.24 (20.3-30.0)	25.09 ± 2.57 (21.5-29)
Fat %	20.13 ± 7.26 (7.5-32.4)	22.07 ± 6.22 (11.4-30.2)
Fat mass (Kg)	11.7 ± 5.35 (3.9-22.9)	12.53 ± 4.77 (5.2-20.2)
FFM (Kg)	41.86 ± 2.89 (38-47.7)	42.56 ± 2.25 (39-46.6)
Muscle mass (Kg)	39.55 ± 2.93 (35.7-45.3)	40.47 ± 2.13 (37-44.2)
TBW (Kg)	29.03 ± 2.55 (25.6-34.0)	29.78 ± 1.82 (27.0-33.0)
TBW %	55.7 ± 4.69 (48.2-65.6)	54.35 ± 3.91 (47.6 - 60.0)
BMR(Kcal/d)[1]	1261 + 114 (1194-1505)	1304 ± 96 (1231-1453)

Mean systolic BP for Group A was 113.7 ± 4.73 mm Hg and for Group S was 118.3 ± 7.22 mm Hg. Mean diastolic BP for Group A was 73.5 ± 4.45 mm Hg and for Group S it was 75.06 ± 6.01 mm Hg. Mean systolic BP of Group S was 4% higher as compared to Group A and mean diastolic BP of Group S was 2% higher as compared to Group A. This difference was significant ($p < 0.05$) between Group A and Group S for systolic blood pressure.

Body composition was determined using TANITA Body Composition Analyzer (BC- 420 MA) for Group A and Group S. Comparison of body composition between Group A and Group S are given in Table 1. High correlations were observed between anthropometric and body composition variables for Group A and Group S (Table 2). BMI of Group S was higher as compared to the Group A by 3.8%. Mean PWC_{170} values for Group A and Group S were 94.8 ± 6.9 and 93.5 ± 13.9 watts respectively. PWC_{170} of Group A was just 5% higher than Group S.

Table 2. Correlation Analysis for Group A and Group S (Pearson correlation coefficient, p <0.01. Group A: Active; Group S: Sedentary; BMI-body mass index; FFM- fat free mass; TBW- total body water)

Group A	Weight (Kg)	Fat %	Fat mass (Kg)	FFM (Kg)	TBW (Kg)	TBW %	BMI (Kg/m^2)
Weight (kg)	1.00	0.98	0.92	0.91	0.97	-0.97	0.96
Fat %		1.00	0.9	0.84	0.92	-0.99	0.96
Fat mass (Kg)			1.00	0.94	0.91	-0.84	0.86
FFM (Kg)				1.00	0.97	-0.79	0.83
TBW (Kg)					1.00	-0.89	0.88
TBW %						1.00	-0.94
Group S	Weight (Kg)	Fat %	Fat mass (Kg)	FFM (Kg)	TBW (Kg)	TBW %	BMI (Kg/m^2)
Weight (kg)	1.00	0.92	0.97	0.84	0.87	-0.90	0.87
Fat %		1.00	0.99	0.58	0.63	-1.00	0.92
Fat mass (Kg)			1.00	0.94	0.91	-0.84	0.86
FFM (Kg)				1.00	1.00	-0.53	0.54
TBW (Kg)					1.00	-0.59	0.59
TBW %						1.00	-0.92

Table 3. TDEI and TDEE (HR and Factorial Method) of Group A and Group S ([1]Unpaired t test, p< 0.05. Group A: Active; Group S: Sedentary; HR- heart rate; TDEE- total daily energy expenditure; TDEI- total daily energy intake.)

Group A	TDEI[1] (Kcal/d)	TDEE[1](Kcal/d) HR Method	TDEE[1] (Kcal/d) Factorial Method	Group S	TDEI[1] (Kcal/d)	TDEE[1] (Kcal/d) HRMethod	TDEE[1] (Kcal/d) Factorial Method
A1	1620	2008	2526	S1	1687	1639	2014
A2	1720	2082	2528	S2	1424	1566	1671
A3	2243	2029	2133	S3	1507	1534	1794
A4	2040	2003	2295	S4	1549	1554	1952
A5	1467	1934	2330	S5	1478	1653	1526
A6	1912	1962	2149	S6	1555	1502	1979
A7	1665	1950	2591	S7	1441	1628	1826
A8	1697	1933	2377	S8	1542	1713	1590
A9	1783	1875	1975	S9	1313	1417	1707
A10	1655	1900	2395	S10	1975	1433	1737
A11	1930	1934	2043	S11	1462	1487	1701
A12	1884	1904	2603	S12	1634	1763	1963
A13	1883	1997	1979	S13	1556	1790	1921
A14	1564	1974	2075	S14	1444	1559	1553
A15	2085	1802	1846	S15	1339	1450	1647
MEAN	1810	1952	2256	MEAN	1527	1579	1772
SD	212	68	246	SD	159	116	163

4.1. Estimates of Total Daily Energy Intake (TDEI)

To compute TDEI, 24 hour dietary record was used for all the subjects. Intake was recorded for the same day as energy expenditure was measured. The energy intakes of active women were slightly higher than sedentary women (Table 3). Significant difference was obtained between Group A and Group S for TDEI ($p<0.05$).

4.2. Estimates of EE from Activity Record Method

The mean values of TDEE by the factorial method for Group A and Group S are presented in Table 3. Mean TDEE for Group A was 27% higher than the sedentary women. Significant difference was obtained between Group A and Group S for TDEE ($p<0.05$).

4.3. Estimates of EE from Heart Rate Method

Energy expenditures for a period of time were obtained by using the HRM. Estimates of TDEE were made for individual subjects by heart rate monitoring (Table 3). Mean TDEE of Group A was 1952 ± 68 Kcal and of Group S was 1579 ± 116 Kcal. Significant difference was obtained between Group A and Group S for TDEE ($p<0.05$).

It is well documented that there are different HR/EE relationships for low and high levels of activity. Therefore, FHFLEX was determined, above which HR/EE relationship can be applied and below which RMR was used. BMR value given by FAO/WHO/UNU report (2004) was used for duration of sleep [1]. FHFLEX i.e. the point of inflection was determined individually for all the subjects. Mean time spent in sleep by Group A and Group S subjects was 554 ± 50.8 minutes and 577 ± 72.9 minutes respectively. Mean time spent by Group A and Group S in activities >FHFLEX was 295 ± 75.3 and 175 ± 90.8 minutes respectively. Mean time spent in activities <FHFLEX by Group A and Group S subjects was 591 ± 104.8 and 688 ± 80.95 minutes respectively. No

significant difference between Group A and Group S for EE in sleep and below FHFLEX activities was obtained at $p<0.05$ level. However significant difference of EE in activities > FHFLEX was obtained at $p<0.05$. On an average the sample of active women spent 70 ± 9.4 minutes in sports and their mean EE was 164 ± 15.7 Kcal; 2.4 ± 0.3 Kcal/minute; or 3.23 ± 0.5 Kcal/ Kg BW.

HR method and factorial method separately gave a significant difference between Group A and Group S at $p<0.05$. Significant difference was also obtained between Group A and Group S with respect to the estimation of EE by the two methods. The factorial method gave nearly 16% higher values ($p<0.05$) than the heart rate method for EE of Group A and 12% higher values ($p<0.05$) for Group S.

Energy status was also determined for Group A and Group S. Significant difference was observed between Group A and Group S according to TDEE and TDEI at $p<0.05$. Paired sample t test showed a significant difference between TDEE and TDEI ($p= 0.028$) in Group A, but did not show a significant difference in Group S ($p>0.05$). The mean energy requirement of Group A and Group S according to the ICMR (2010) recommendations [12] was 14.4% and 20.3% less than the recommendations respectively when the heart rate method was used to estimate EE. Factorial method gave higher EE as compared to the heart rate method and thus Group A subjects had 1.0% higher energy requirement as compared to the ICMR (2010) recommendations and Group S had 7.2% lower energy requirement as compared to the recommendations. The mean energy requirement of Group A and Group S according to ICMR (1990) recommendations [13] was 14.0% and 18.7% less than the recommendations respectively when the heart rate method was used to estimate EE. When expressed as multiples of BMR, mean PAL value for Group A was 1.79 ± 0.07 and for Group S it was 1.36 ± 0.07. PAL value for Group A was nearly 32% higher as compared to Group S.

5. Discussion

The study was based on the premise that the energy requirement of Group A would be higher as compared to Group S. Further, the objective was to compare the two methods used for measuring EE and the accuracy of these two methods, namely HRM and the factorial method in the study groups. The study results showed that Group A and Group S subjects had a mean WC of 71.6 cm and 72.8 cm respectively. WHO/IASO/IOTF (2000) classification for adult women according to WC who are at risk for developing associated co-morbidities is >80 cm, [14] which indicated low risk for developing co-morbidities at this stage of life among both groups. BMI of Group S was higher as compared to the Group A by 3.8%. Asians generally have a higher percentage of body fat than white people of the same age, sex and BMI. Also, the proportion of Asian people with risk factors for type 2 DM and cardiovascular disease is substantial even below the existing WHO BMI cut-off point of 25 kg/m^2 for adults [15].

5.1. Physical Work Capacity

Physical work capacity data revealed that there was no difference among Group A and Group S. There is no clear consensus on whether cardiorespiratory fitness in youth is indicative of habitual moderate to vigorous physical activity. According to a review that included over 25 studies, there was only a small to moderate relationship between physical activity and cardiorespiratory fitness. While it is acknowledged that other factors, such as genetics, [16] contribute to individual levels of cardiorespiratory fitness, studies examining fitness and physical activity make reasonable arguments for the use of cardiorespiratory fitness as a proxy measure for habitual moderate to vigorous physical activity at the group level [17,18]. Exercise or training leads to the improvement of work capacity and a slightly higher PWC_{170} of Group A indicated that they belonged to the active group. Despite of having >2 years of training the active group engaged only for 3 months actively in sports training per year. Thus only a small difference was obtained in the physical work capacity between Group A and Group S.

5.2. Activity Diary Method for Estimating EE

Factorial method studies of TDEE are useful for understanding energy balance in living human populations, and adaptations to different environmental and nutritional circumstances [19-23]. The study results showed that the factorial method gave higher values as compared to the heart rate method. Factorial method generally suffers from an inherent disadvantage of using literature costs. Use of literature values for estimating the energy cost of activities in the diary method could result specifically in overestimation of daily EE for two reasons. First, the use of energy values derived from discrete measurements to estimate the expenditure of serial activities may fail to account for transitions in EE from one activity to the next, and may, thus, give a higher energy value than is appropriate for those transition periods. Second, literature values could be overvalued for this population. Studies comparing the diary method with continuous 24 hour measurements of EE in a respiration chamber and accelerometers found individual discrepancies, but concluded that the factorial method was adequate for predicting population EE [20,23].

5.3. Heart Rate Method for Estimating EE

In view of energy intake data, HRM gave closer estimates of TDEE than factorial method for Group A and Group S. Heart rate monitoring is a method for estimating energy expenditure that is based on the strong positive correlation that exists between heart rate and oxygen consumption. The relationship between HR and oxygen consumption (VO_2), while unique to each individual, is normally described as linear at energy expenditure above basal and below maximal output. Among the various factors posture, site of muscle activity, emotions, temperature, meal, physical training affect the heart rate/ energy expenditure relationship hence individual equations are used for computing energy expenditure from heart rate records. Heart rate is a better predictor of oxygen consumption at sub-maximal than maximal levels. The variation from this technique is probably ± 5 to 15% from continuously recorded values, depending on the amount of sedentary activity involved [5]. Figure 1 depicts

$HR\text{-}VO_2$ relationship curve for one subject belonging to Group A.

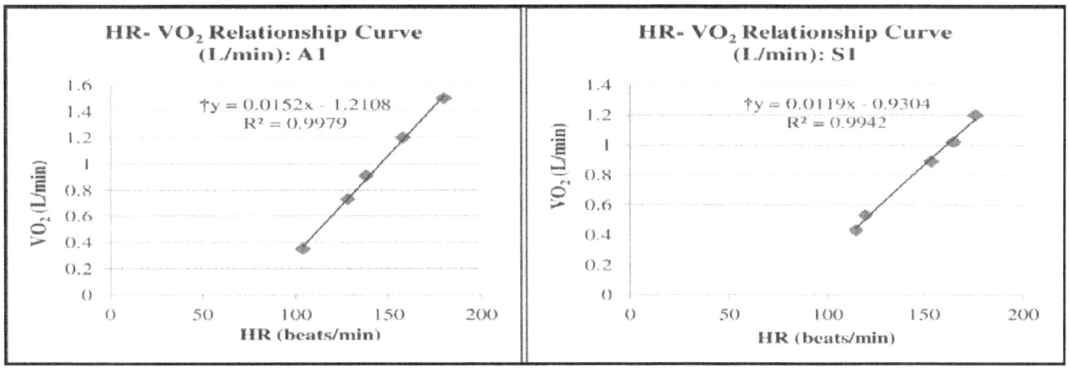

Figure 1. Individual $HR\text{-}VO_2$ relationship curve (HR- VO_2 curve for one subject showing a linear relationship between heart rate (HR) and oxygen consumption (VO_2) for one Group A and one Group S subject. † y= EE (Kcal/ minute), x= HR (beats/minute))

It is well documented that there are different HR/EE relationships for low and high levels of activity. Therefore, FHFLEX was determined, above which HR/EE relationship can be applied and below which RMR was used. BMR value given by FAO/WHO/UNU (2004) was used for duration of sleep [1]. FHFLEX i.e. the point of inflection was determined individually for all the subjects. The heart rates above FHFLEX were used to calculate VO_2 from the regression equations. Individual regression equations for Group and Group S are given in Table 4. Average of heart rates below FHFLEX was computed and used to calculate the TDEE. Mean FHFLEX values of Group A and Group S were 104.5 ± 11.35 and 105.1 ± 7.16 beats/ minute respectively. In aerobically fit subjects the lower HR FLEX seems appropriate and the resting HR during standing can be as high as, or even higher than the lowest exercising HR. Thus, regression equations were derived for the time spent in activities where heart rate was more than FHFLEX. Individual graphs between VO_2 and HR were made to estimate VO_2 from HR above FHFLEX. The equation used to determine EE was:

$$EE\ (Kcal/\min) = 5 * VO_2(L/\min) \qquad (6)$$

Table 4. Individual Regression Equations for Group A and Group S (Group A, Active; Group S, Sedentary; EE, energy expenditure. [1] y= EE (Kcal/ minute), x= HR (beats/minute).)

Group A	Regression equation[1]	Correlation Coefficient	Group S	Regression equation[1]	Correlation Coefficient
A1	y = 0.015x - 1.210	+0.99	S1	y = 0.011x - 0.930	+0.99
A2	y = 0.021x - 1.742	+0.99	S2	y = 0.012x - 0.902	+0.99
A3	y = 0.013x - 0.921	+0.99	S3	y = 0.014x - 1.427	+0.97
A4	y = 0.017x - 1.216	+0.99	S4	y = 0.010x - 0.754	+0.98
A5	y = 0.012x - 0.891	+0.97	S5	y = 0.016x - 1.512	+0.98
A6	y= 0.020x - 1.626	+0.99	S6	y = 0.012x - 0.929	+0.99
A7	y=0.012x - 0.685	+0.99	S7	y = 0.015x - 1.634	+0.99
A8	y = 0.012x - 0.913	+0.99	S8	y = 0.014x - 1.061	+0.99
A9	y = 0.009x - 0.817	+0.99	S9	y = 0.012x - 1.020	+0.98
A10	y = 0.016x - 1.319	+0.99	S10	y = 0.008x - 0.577	+0.99
A11	y = 0.031x - 4.402	+0.99	S11	y = 0.010x - 0.633	+0.99
A12	y = 0.016x - 1.538	+0.92	S12	y = 0.015x - 1.259	+0.99
A13	y = 0.014x - 1.244	+0.99	S13	y = 0.016x - 1.403	+0.95
A14	y = 0.011x - 0.677	+0.99	S14	y = 0.011x - 0.986	+0.99
A15	y = 0.018x - 1.723	+0.99	S15	y = 0.011x - 1.056	+0.97

One of the inaccuracies of the minute by minute heart rate method is giving a slow return of the heart rate to resting levels than the EE after bouts of activity. This could lead to inaccurate data. Although the heart rate technique cannot give as accurate results as given by calorimetry or DLW method, it can give a close estimate of EE even in small groups in free living conditions.

On an average the active women were spending around 2.4 kcal/min and according to European Network for Prevention and Health Promotion in Family Medicine and General Practice (EUROPREV) guide on Promoting Health through Physical Activity, the EE for basketball game accounts for 7 METs i.e. 6.4 Kcal/min which is much above the expenditure by Group A in their basketball practice (body weight = 55 Kg for adult women [24]). Therefore, the only difference between Group A and Group S was that despite both being college students, Group A was spending 1 hour in the morning basketball practice session. Sixty minutes of daily exercise has been advocated to increase the PAL of sedentary people to a value of 1.75 or greater, which assists in weight maintenance [1]. Simple efforts like this can raise the PAL from 1.36 to 1.75. If this 1 hour of physical activity is a sport or any other rhythmic exercise, the advantage of cardio-respiratory maintenance is gained additionally to weight maintenance. Such activities prevent chronic degenerative disorders and thus there is a recommendation in the society as a whole to become moderate workers by doing exercise.

6. Conclusion

Heart rate monitoring is a non-invasive technique which is ideal for the active population and allows free movement of the subjects. In view of energy intake data HRM gave closer estimates of TDEE than factorial method. The heart rate technique is a useful tool for computing energy requirement of active groups because of its simplicity and potential use in free living conditions. More research is needed on heart rate method to measure EE on India's growing sedentary population.

7. Financial Support

No source of support, including grants, fellowships, and gifts of materials.

8. Conflict of Interest

The authors have no potential conflict of interests.

9. Abstract Publication

The abstract of the paper entitled "Measurement of energy requirement by heart rate method and physical work capacity for young active and sedentary women, has been published in the 46th Annual National conference of Nutrition Society of India Scientific Proceedings (November' 2014) in the category of Young Scientist Award, Community Nutrition (Oral) and 47th Annual National Conference of Indian Dietetic Association Scientific Proceedings (December' 2014) in the category of Experimental Nutrition (Poster).

10. List of Abbreviations

1. BF%- Body fat percent
2. BMI- Body Mass Index
3. BMR- Basal Metabolic Rate
4. BP- Blood pressure
5. DIPAS- Defence Institute of Physiology and Allied Sciences
6. DLW- doubly labelled water
7. DM- Diabetes Mellitus
8. EE- Energy expenditure
9. EUROPREV- European Network for Prevention and Health Promotion in Family Medicine and General Practice
10. FAO- Food and Agriculture Organisation
11. FHFLEX- heart rate where two HR-VO_2 relation curve change
12. HC- Hip circumference
13. HR- Heart rate
14. HRM- heart rate method
15. IASO- International Association for the Study of obesity
16. ICMR- Indian Council of Medical Research
17. IOTF- International Obesity Task Force
18. MUAC- Mid upper arm circumference
19. PAL- Physical Activity Level
20. PAR- Physical Activity Ratio
21. PWC- Physical work capacity
22. PWC_{170}- Physical work capacity at heart rate 170
23. RDA- Recommended Dietary Allowance
24. RMR- Resting Metabolic Rate
25. TBW- Total body water
26. TDEE- Total daily energy expenditure
27. TDEI- Total daily energy intake
28. TEE- Total energy expenditure
29. UNU- United Nations University
30. VO_2- Oxygen consumption
31. W- watts
32. WC- Waist circumference
33. WHO- World Health Organisation

References

[1] FAO/WHO/UNU, "*Human Energy Requirements*," Food and Nutrition Technical Report series 1, 2004. [Online] Available: http://www.fao.org/docrep/007/y5686e/y5686e00.html. [Accessed on 2nd March' 2011].

[2] Silva, A.M., Santos, D.A., and Matias, C.N, et al. "*Accuracy of a combined heart rate and motion sensor for assessing energy expenditure in free-living adults during a double-blind crossover caffeine trial using doubly labeled water as the reference method*," Eur J Clin Nutr 69. 20-27. 2015.

[3] Yu, Z., Volgyi, E., and Wang, R, et al. "*Comparison of heart rate monitoring with indirect calorimetry for energy expenditure evaluation*," J Sport Health Sc 1 (3). 178-183. 2012.

[4] Liu, S., Gao, R., and Freedson, P, "*Computational Methods for Estimating Energy Expenditure in Human Physical Activities*," Med Sci Sports Exerc 44 (11). 2138-2146. 2012.

[5] Shephard, R.J., and Aoyagi, Y, "*Measurement of human energy expenditure, with particular reference to field studies: an historical perspective*," Eur J Appl Physiol 112 (8). 2785-2815. 2012.

[6] Bland, J., Pfeiffer, K., and Eisenmann, J.C, "*The PWC170: comparison of different stage lengths in 11-16 year olds*," Eur J Appl Physiol 112 (5). 1955-1961. 2012.

[7] World Health Organisation, "*Obesity: preventing and managing the global epidemic*," WHO Technical Report Series 894, 2000. [Online] Available: http://www.who.int/nutrition/publications/obesity/WHO_TRS_894/en. [Accessed on 13th March' 2011].

[8] Dirix, A, and Tittel, K, *The Olympic Book of Sports Medicine (The Encyclopaedia of Sports Medicine)*, Wiley-Blackwell Publishers, London, 1988.

[9] Gopalan, C, Sastri, B.V.R, and Balasubramanian, S.C, *Nutritive value of Indian foods*, ICMR offset Press, Hyderabad, 1989.

[10] Maxfield, M.E, "*The indirect measurement of energy expenditure in industrial situations*," Am J Clin Nutr 24. 1124-1138. 1971.

[11] Spurr, G.B., Prentice, A.M., Murgatroyd, P.R., Goldberg, G.R., Reina, J.C., and Christman, N.T, "*Energy expenditure by minute by minute heart rate recording: comparison with indirect calorimetry*," Am J Clin Nutr 48. 552-559. 1988.

[12] Indian Council of Medical Research, "*Nutrient Requirements and Recommended Dietary Allowances for Indians,*" 2010. [Online] Available: http://www.icmr.nic.in. [Accessed on 11th Februrary' 2011].

[13] Indian Council of Medical Research, "*Nutrient Requirements and Recommended Dietary Allowances for Indians,*" 1990. [Online] Available: http://www.icmr.nic.in. [Accessed on 11th Februrary' 2011].

[14] WHO/IASO/IOTF, "*The Asia-Pacific perspective: Redefining obesity and its treatment. Health communications*," 2000. [Online] Available: http://www.wpro.who.int/nutrition/documents/docs/Redefiningobesity.pdf. [Accessed on 11th Februrary' 2011].

[15] World Health Organisation, "*Appropriate body mass index for Asian populations and its implications for policy and intervention strategies*," Lancet 363. 157-163. 2004.

[16] Bouchard, C., and Rankinen, T, "*Individual differences in response to regular physical activity*," Med Sci Sports Exerc 33. S446-S451. 2001.

[17] Byrd-Williams, C.E., Shaibi, G.Q., and Sun, P, et al. "*Cardiorespiratory fitness predicts changes in adiposity in overweight Hispanic boys*," Obesity 16 (5). 1072-1077. 2008.

[18] Aleksandravičienė, R., Liaudeneckaitė, J., Liaugminienė, R., Siaurodinas, A., and Stasiulevičienė, L, "*Assessment of physical working capacity of differently trained and aged female aerobic gymnasts*," Sportas Nr 3 (86). 5-10. 2012.

[19] Leonard, W.R, "*Laboratory and field methods for measuring human energy expenditure*," Am J Hum Biol 24 (3). 372-384. 2012.

[20] Henriksson, H., Forsum, E., and Lof, M, "*Evaluation of Actiheart and a 7 d activity diary for estimating free-living total and activity energy expenditure using criterion methods in 1·5-and 3-year-old children*," Br J Nutr 111 (10). 1830-1840. 2014.

[21] Leonard, W.R., Snodgrass, J.J., and Sorensen, M.V, "*Metabolic adaptation in indigenous Siberian populations*," Annu Rev Anthropol 34. 451-471. 2005.

[22] Gamboa, J.A.A., and Garcia, F.D.G, "*Impact of seasonal scarcity on energy balance and body composition in peasant adolescents from Calakmul, Campeche Mexico*," Am J Hum Biol 19. 751-762. 2007.

[23] Geissler, C.A., Dzumbira, T.M., and Noor, M, "*Validation of a field technique for the measurement of energy expenditure: factorial method versus continuous respirometry*," Am J Clin Nutr. 44: 59. 1986.

[24] EUROPREV, "*Guide on Promoting Health through Physical Activity*," European Network for Prevention and *Health Promotion*, 2007. [Online] Available: http://www.europrev.org/documents/PhysicalActivityGuide.pdf. [Accessed on 13th March' 2011].

The Determination of the Relationship between Levels of Narcissim and Motivational Trends in the Individual Sports Branches

Ünsal Tazegül[1,*], Aytekin Soykan[2]

[1]Dumlupinar, Turkey
[2]School of Physical Education and Sports, Marmara University, Stanbul, Turkey
*Corresponding author: zegerunsal@hotmail.com

Abstract The purpose of this study is to determine the relationship between levels of narcissim and motivational trends in the individual sports branches. The sample of the study includes a total of 350 young athletes in the branches of boxing, freestyle wrestling, Greco-Roman wrestling, taekwondo and weightlifting, participated in Turkey Youth Champions in 2011. Sport-specific motive scales (SSMS) and Narcissistic Personality Inventory (NPI) was utilized in order collect the datas in this study. SPSS 15 package software was used for the data analysis. The test of Kolmogorov-Smirnov to determine whether the data had a normal distribution, the test of Levene was applied to determine the homogeneity of variances and it was determined that the datas had an homogeneous and normal distribution. Descriptive statistics and Pearson correlation analysis were used in the analysis of the data. In the result of data analysis, there was a statistically significant relationship between the motive to achieve success with exploitation dimension and the power motive with superior dimension. ($p<0,05$).

Keywords: *athlete, narcissism, motivation, relation*

1. Introduction

At the time of being looked up the dictionary meaning of Narcissistic Personality, It is found out that it is described as person's over level of admiration to his own physiological and psychological features and over self-love [1,2].

Narcissist athletes reveal hostility and skepticism for human relations in their later relationships due to their negaitve experinces with their families in early childhood. As a result, pre-conditions of social feedback and self-implications, remain uncertain manner, so that doubts arise about the value of social feedback. Narcissistic athletes feel the need for testing whether the others bear appreciative thoughts or not and keep their relations under constant pressure in order to get the desired feedback. However, due to negative experinces in their early childhood not only they have distrust but also they can not really love and care the others, at the same time underestimate them [3].

Narcissistic athletes, reveal a calm and self-confident quality in their social behaviours. The fact that they seem to be trouble-free and saturated is thought to be related with their being graceful by the others. For others, this reveals immodesty, arrogance and complacence in the human relations, snobbish manners, much self-confidence and presumption. Narcissistic athletes generally use others for their own interests, exploit them, expect them for the fulfillment of their requests without beware of anything and giving anything in return. Therefore, they are seen as far from being humble, extremely self-centered and non-giver people [4].

Narcissistic athletes are the people who admire themselves physically and mentally, see themselves above, expect continuous appreciation, interest and approval, they will meet exclusive of interest wherever they go and think that they deserve the superior place. Such intense narcissistic injuries and disappointments in expectations is also often the inevitable reality. Narcissistic self-esteem of individuals are fed from outside interests, tastes, approvals. People in question can not stand criticisms and anticipate for constant praises. For this reason, their apperances and manners are formed to grasp all these. Since they make use of the others for glorifiying, seem to be superior and reveal themselves; their friendships are just to get benefit from the others in this way. Narcissistic athletes are known as selfish, egocentric since they do not show empathy towards emotions, thoughts and needs of others [5].

Narcissism may sometimes affect the performance of the athletes positively. Narcissistic athletes themselves feel valuable, and their admiration for others to gain advantage depends on the capabilities of reveal themselves. They reveal their superiority by exhibiting the best movements that they perform in the sports field and try to attract attention. They are less interested in being loved and cared when compared to other people. Therefore, narcissistic athletes behave combatant and self assertive during the competition in order to avoid the destruction of their self-esteem due to performance failure. The most important thing for a narcissistic athlete is to win. They also apply for unethical behaviors in order to acquire the targeted objective [6].

In case of a failure, they try to prove that it occured due to mischance. They never believe that they lost the match due to their own failure and they related the defeat to the rules of the refree, mistakes of the rules, viewers and the wrong tactic given by the coach. The athletes having narcissistic features are more successful in individual sports rather than the team sports. The most of the characteristics defining narcissism put forth the reality that narcissists can not be team players. Since they are deprive of the ability to empathize they can not understand, care the emotions and thoughts of their team mates and see their team mate as a mediator to display their performance. The important thing for the narcissistic athletes is being the center of interest by displaying their capabilities rather than victory of the team. For this reason, it is hard for a team consisting of narcissistic athletes to show their skills in a coherent and coordinated way [6].

The narcissism types seen in athletes are divided in to two as dangerless and pathological:

Dangerless narcissism: Athlete's own struggle, and the resulting object is something that at the end of occupation. For example, a movement is learned from working with athletes that have achieved success, or due to a narcissistically compliment. Emerged as a result of their efforts to object, his excessive interest in the success of their own works of non-stop throughout the study, his interest in the materials used is balanced. Wherefore the factors that create dangerless narcissism self evaluate itself [7].

Pathological narcissism: Its object is not created or produced by the athlete, it is the thing owned by him. For example, his body, appearance, wealth, beauty... sickly narcissistic athletes have achieved something of a feature, not because they have also boast [7].

1.1. Extents of Narcissism Seen in Athletes

Extent of Superiority: It represents self-confidence, independence, the need to be ambitious and successful.

Extent of Exploitation: It represents rebelliousness, inadaptability, spitefulness, not to respect and show tolerance towards others.

Extent of Authority: It reflects dominance, be assertive, leadership, being critical and self-confidence.

Extent of Pretension: It decribes being ambitious, need for power, domination, spitefulness and recalcitrance.

Extent of Self-sufficiency: It is related with assertiveness, independence, self-confidence and need for success.

Extent of Exhibitionism: It is related with seeking for emotion, extroversion and not controlling of the impulses.

Extend of Self esteem: The person finds himself physically attractive and for this reason he thoughts that he is judged by the others [8].

Briefly, the motivation means ''to direct and mobilize and dispose working'' for the people. The motivation can be identified in the form ''to act with one's own desires and wishes'' to perform a certain purpose [9].

The factors affecting to continuation of the sport or gaining continuity of the sport are called as the sport-motive. Thanks to these motives, the process causing to continue the sports activity is called the motivation in the sport. There are many different ways to motivate the individuals. In the context of sport and participation, it is also very important to undertstand what the motivation is. The motivation is the process to obtain and use the resources which is possible such as the ability, time and energy [10].

How to be perceived by individuals the external factors and effects on motivation is important. So, what motivate the Athletes to sport? Each individual has different the motives directing the participation in terms of the physical fitness sport and social relations. The extrinsic motive is one of them [11,12]. The individuals are motivated with the extrinsic motives in terms of the rewarding and social appreciation [13].

1.2. Types of Motivation

Intrinsic Motivation, briefly is that person's self-motivated. People who are intrinsically motivated in order to be competent (skillful) have an internal hunger. These people have the ability to manage themselves in order to be successful [14].

Extrinsic motivation is the strengthen or reinforce, which can be appeared in the negative and positive effects through other people, and based on the material and moral values reducing or increasing the possibility of behavior's recurrence. Extrinsic rewards can be financial materials (for example: coupe, money, medals and so on extrinsic rewards). Extrinsic rewards can also come from immaterial sources. (For example, be appreciated, be praised and so on.) [15,16].

Extrinsic motivation is not a situation which is directly related to the athlete. The simplest way to understanding the motivation of the external environment is to accept it as a process and to divide into (needs, motivations, goals,)the basic parts constituting it. The basic motivation process is usually expressed as follows [17].

The purpose of this study is to reveal the relationship between the levels of narcissism and motivation levels, by determining the levels of narcissism and motivational trends of young male athletes.

2. Materıal and Method

2.1. Participants

The sample of this study constitutes a total of 350 athletes, including 70 male boxer, 70 male free-style wrestler, 70 greco-roman wrestler, 70 male weightlifters and 70 male kickboxer which is selected by random sampling method and participated in Youth championship Turkey 2011. Competition dates: Free-style wrestling is on 5-6 March in Antalya, Box is on 7-13 February in Bayburt, Kick boxing is on 27 June-2 July in Samsun, Weightlifting is on 4-6 March in Aydın, Greco-roman weightlifting is on 18-20 February in Corum.

2.2. Research Data Collection

1. The validity and reliability study in Turkey developed by Willis (1982) and Sport-Specific Success Motivation Scale made by Tiryaki ve Gödelek have been used in. The scale of Willis constitues of two sub-dimensions. The first of these sub-dimensions is the demonstration of power motive (power motive, POW), latter the motivations regarding the success. The motives regarding success; are the motive to approach success, (MAS) and the motive to avoid failure (MAF). As a result of reliability analysis made by Tiryaki and Gödelek, it was determined as r=0.81 for the power demonstration sub-scale and r=0.82 for the approach failure sub-scale and r=0.80 for the Avoidance of failure sub-scale depending on the alpha reliability coefficients. The high of scores obtained from the dimension of ''Power Demonstration "and " Approach to Success''; the motivation of athlete is high in related to motivational aspects and if score is low, it indicates the opposite situation. The high score from "Avoidance of failure'' dimensions indicates the athlete's fear of failure and having more stress [18].

2. Narcissistic Personality Inventory composed of 16 questions and translated into Turkish by Salim Atay in 2009 was used as a scale factor. NPI composed of 16 questions was arranged by Daniel R. Ames, Paul Rose ve Cameron P. Anderson in 2005 translated into Turkish by Salim Atay. After the pilot application by Atay Cronbach's Alpha value was determined as 0.57 in the first performed study. Reliability coefficient below the values expected due to the presence of each factor scale, the negative correlation is detected and evaluated and determined not provide additive scale of four, were revised statement. After the measurements performed this change Cronbach's Alpha value was raised to 0.652. The questions in 16 questions scale factor translated into Turkish by Atay also distributed in 6 factors as superiority, authority, pretension, self sufficiency and exploitation similar to the 16 questions NPI English version. The points that can be gained from NPI are: extent of authority 0-2, extent of exhibitionism 0-3, extent of explotation 0-3, extent of pretension 0-2, extent of self-sufficiency 0-3, extent of superiority 0-3, total narcissism is between 0-16 points. As the point increases the level of narcissism also increases [19,20].

2.3. Data Analyses

SPSS 15 package software was used for the data analysis. The test of Kolmogorov-Smirnov to determine whether the data had a normal distribution, the test of Levene was applied to determine the homogeneity of variances and it was determined that the datas had an homogeneous and normal distribution. Descriptive statistics and correlation analysis were used in the analysis of the datas.

3. Results

In this section, the findings reached in a result of research are evaluated.

In the correlation analysis in Table 2, it was found a statistically significant relationship in between the motive to achieve success with exploitation dimension and the power motive with superiority dimension.

Table 1. Athletes' motivation trend and descriptive statistical findings of narcissism

	N	Mean	SD
Exhibitionism	350	1.327	.908
Authority	350	.968	.760
Exploitation	350	1.456	.811
claim rights	350	.583	.705
Self-sufficiency	350	1.350	1.003
Superiority	350	1.083	.911
Total Narcissism	350	6.770	2.637
Power Motive	350	39.211	6.629
Reach to Success	350	61.220	8.605
Avoid Failure	350	33.365	7.202

Table 2. Analysis of correlation

Correlations				
		Power motive	Reach to Success	Avoid Failure
Exhibitionism	Pearson Correlation	.013	.014	.012
	P	.806	.791	.827
Authority	Pearson Correlation	-.022	-.059	.004
	P	.689	.272	.937
Exploitation	Pearson Correlation	-.025	-.113*	.039
	P	.637	.035	.469
Claim Rights	Pearson Correlation	-.001	.038	.003
	P	.987	.485	.952
Superiority	Pearson Correlation	.119*	.076	.060
	P	.026	.159	.267
Self-sufficiency	Pearson Correlation	.026	.029	.027
	P	.635	.594	.610
Total Narcissism	Pearson Correlation	.041	.000	.049
	P	.442	.997	.360

4. Discussion

When descriptive statistics findings indicating the motivational trends and narcissism and its sub-dimension are examined, the values are as follows; the exploitation of athletes in the fisrt place (1.456±.811), self-sufficiency dimension (1.350 ± 1.003) in second place, exhibitionism dimension (1.327 ±.908) in third place, superiority dimension (1.083 ±.911) in fourth, authority dimension

(0.968 ±.760) in fifth, the dimension of claim rights (0. 583 ±.705) in sixth place, total levels of narcissism (6.770 ± 2.637). The reason for being more developed of the sub-dimension of exploitation is to make the best way and they have an intensive study in order to achieve the necessary condition for the success. At the end of this intensive works, it causes to be different of people who are not athletes and they have a better physical appearance and who can make the movements difficult to obtain by people who are not athletes, depending on the development of the technical and physical characteristics of athletes. It is an important role in the development of exploitation properties in athletes. When these results are evaluated according to DSM-IV criteria, it can be said for athletes within the scope of work that they are a rebellious, have discordant relationships with their surroundings, not show any respectful and tolerant attitudes towards people and want to be superior in its relations with other people.

Tazegül, (2013a) in boxers has identified a positive relationship between narcissism and motivational orientations. This result is interpreted by the researcher according to the scale of the result is argued that the scale properties. Because the narcissist always be at the forefront athletes, want to prove themselves by demonstrating their ability, so the motivation is always high [21].

Tazegül et al. (2013b), the data wrestlers level of narcissism (6.707 ± 2.775) was set [22].

Tazegül (2013c) found that, there is a statistically significant relationship between weight lifting, and Greco-Roman wrestlers regarding age and levels of narcissism [23].

Tazegül (2011) found as follows; Weightlifters narcissism level (7.283 ± 2.786),boxers (7.216 ± 2.584) and the level of narcissism of Greco-Roman wrestlers (6.750±2.777). Tazegül (2012) found as follows; the level of narcissism of the athletes in kick boxing branch (6.533±2.849),the level of narcissism of the athlete in freestyle wrestling branch (6.333±3.578) [24].

When the descriptive statistics findings indicating the motives trends of the athletes under working are examined, they are determined as follows: ''power motive'' of the athletes (39.211±6.629), reach to success (61.220±8.605), escape from success (33.365±7.202). The power motive of the athletes under the working is more advanced, It is considered that the most important reason is due to young athletes of the study sample and due to the sport ages of the athletes are early. Young athletes are an attempt more showing and proving themselves and more desiring the success in the early years of sports lives. Çekin, Tatar, & Afyon (2001) found that the motives of athletes in the age group 14-16 engaged in individual sports are to tprove himself, to obtain a good place in society and to be healthy. Moreover, the athletes's social status to be achieved through the championship and awards are the important factors to be high of young athletes motivations(25). Rewarding is one of the most effective among the motivating factors [26].

Kuru & Abakay (2009), identified as follows in their studies; power motive of non-degree wrestlers is (38.40± 3.97), those with degree in Turkey (39.30±5.08), those with degree in the international tournament (37.42±4.59). it is identified as follows for non-degree wrestlers in the motive to escape from success ; the motive to escape from success (34.45± 5.99). Those with degree in Turkey (35.48 ±5.40). those with degree in the international tournament (35.37 ±4.57) [27].

Aktop (2002), in study, examined the sub-dimensions of success motivations and found as follows; Individual athletes's sub-dimensions of power motive is (37.89), the sub-dimension of the approach motive to success is (62.50), the sub-dimension of the motive escape from success is (28.17) [28].

Tazegül, Kalkavan, & Ersoy (2012), in their study, determined as follows; the power motive of the wrestlers that are Turkey's champion is (39.055±3.749), the power motive for the boxers that are Turkey's champion in the branch of boxing is (37.900±5.258) [29].

Soyer, et al. (2010) haven't found a significant relation between the ages and success motivations of the athletes, they found a significant relation in the gender factor [30].

In the research made by Engür (2002) for determining its effect on the success motivation in elite athletes state anxiety levels, found that the succes motivation of male athlete is higher than female athletes [31].

Aslan & Kuru (2002), in their study, found a relationship in the positive low level of significance between the motives to avoid failure and the sporting experiences of the first league footballers and also in the negatif low level of significance between the power motive and the sporting experiences in the second league footballers [32].

Turkmen (2005) found the requirement for success professional football players found higher than the requirements for success amateur soccer players [33].

As a result of the study determining the factors of the motivation influencing to the Ural (2008) 's team performance, it was determined that the motivation level of athletes engaged in sports for less than 5 years is lower than and athletes engaged in sport for less than 10 years [34].

In comparing the motivations of sport-specific success of female and male athletes made by Erman, Şahan, & Can (2004), it was not be found significant differences in terms of sub-parameters of achievement motivation between male and female athletes [35].

Karabulut, Kirazcı, & Aşçı (2000) determined the following values; the value of the power motive of experienced athletes (40.87), inexperienced athletes (39.49), and the motive approach to success of experienced athletes (64.23), inexperienced (64.41), the motive to avoid failure of experienced athletes (31,02), inexperienced (32.71). However, there was a significant difference between the two groups [36].

5. Conclusion

In correlation analysis, it was found a statistically significant correlation in a between the motive to reach success with the exploitation size and the power motive with superiority dimension. When these results are evaluated according to the scale of narcissism and motivational orientation, this result is thought as normal. The power motive and the motive to reach success represents high motivation and desire for success in athletes. The dimension of the superiority level in narcissism represents self-confidence, independence, be ambitious and the need for success. Thus, the motivation of athlete who is self-confident and successful will be high. Consequently, it was determined a relationship in between the superior dimesion of narcissism with the motivation and the athletes have a good the motivation trends levels. It was considered that the reason of the relation occurring between the superior dimesion with the motivation trends levels is to be the young of sports age and age of athletes in the study group.

References

[1] Güney, S. (1998). Davranış Bilimler ve Yönetim Psikolojisi Terimler Sözlüğü: Ankara.

[2] Hançerlioğlu, O. (1993). Ruhbilim Sözlüğü, İstanbul: Remzi kitap evi.

[3] Morf, Carolyn,C. & Rhodewalt,F. (2001). "Unraveling the Paradoxes of Narcissism: A Dynamic Self-Regulatory Processing Model", Psychological Inquiry, Vol.12, No.4, ss. 177-196.

[4] Köroğlu,E.,& Bayraktar, S. (2007). Kişilik Bozuklukları, Ankara: HYB Basım Yayın.

[5] Rozenbaltt,S. (2002). In Defence of Self: The Relationship of Self-Esteem and Narcissism to Agressive Behavior, Yayınlanmamış Doktora Tezi, New York Brookville :Long Island University, Psychology.

[6] Wallace, H. M, & Baumeister R, F. (2002). "The Performence of Narcissists Rises and Falls With Percieved OpportAunity For Glory", Journal of Personality and Social Psychology, Vol. 82,No.5, ss832.

[7] Fromm, E. (1994). Sevginin ve Şiddetin Kaynağı, İstanbul: (Çev: Y.salman,N.İçten). Payel Yayınları.

[8] Gülmez, N. (2009). Narsistik Liderlik, Yayınlanmış yüksek lisans Tezi, Marmara Üniversitesi, Sosyal Bilimler Enstitüsü, İstanbul.

[9] Koçel, T. (2003). İşletme Yöneticiliği, İstanbul: Beta Yayınları.

[10] Martin, J.J.,& Mushett, C. A. (1996). Social Support Mechanisms Among Athletes with Disabilities. Adapted Physical Activity Quarterly 13: 74-83.

[11] Brasile, F. M., Kleiber, D. A., & Harnisch, D. (1991). Analysis of Participation Incentives Among Athletes With and Without Disabilities. Therapeutic Recreation Journal, 25 (1): 18-33.

[12] Hellandsig, E.T. (1998). Motivational Predictors of High Performance and Discontinuation in Different Types of Sports Among Talented Teenage Athletes. International Journal of Sport Psychology, 29: 27-44.

[13] Hatfield, K. L. (1998). A Study of Participation Incentives Among Collegiate Athletes With and Without a Disability. Master's thesis, Southern Illinois University at Carbondale.

[14] Nicholls, J.G, & Robert G.C. (1992). The General and The Specific in the Devolopment and expression of Achievement Motivation; Motivationin Sport and Exercise, Human Kinetices Boks.

[15] Konter, E. (2004). Antrenörlük ve Takım Psikolojisi, Ankara: Palme Yayıncılık.

[16] Konter, E. (1995). Sporda Motivasyon, İzmir: Saray Tıp Kitapevi.

[17] Gülen, A. (1998). Başarı Motivasyonu ve İş Örgütlerinde Yönetim Üst ve Orta Kademe Yöneticiler Üzerinde Bir Çalışma, Yayınlanmış Yüksek Lisans Tezi, Abant İzzet Baysal Üniversitesi, Sosyal Bilimler Enstitüsü, İşletme Ana Bilim Dalı, Bolu.

[18] Tiryaki, Ş.,& Gödelek, E. (1997). Spora Özgü Başarı Motivasyonu Ölçeğinin Türk Sporcuları İçin Uyarlama Çalışması; 1. Uluslar arası Spor Psikolojisi Sempozyumu Bildirileri, Bağırgan Yayınevi.

[19] ATAY, S. (2009). Narsist Kişilik Envanterinin Türkçeye Standardizasyonu. Gazi Üniversitesi İktisadi ve İdari Bilimler Fakültesi Dergisi. 11/1, 181-196.

[20] Atay, S. (2010). Çalışan Narsist, İstanbul: Namar yayınları.

[21] Tazegül, Ü. (2013a). Investigating the Relationship Between Narcissism and Motivation Level of Boxings, The Journal of Academic Social Science Studies, Volume 6 Issue 5, p. 679-691.

[22] Tazegül, Ü., Soykan, A., Sancaklı, H. (2013b). Investigating the relationship between narcissism and motivation level of wrestlers, Global Advanced Research Journal of History, Political Science and International Relations Vo 2(2), 027-033.

[23] Tazegül, Ü. (2013c). an examınatıon of the relatıonshıp between the level of narcıssısm and socıo-demographıc status of sportsmen from varıous sport branches, Journal of Sports and Performance Researches cilt 4, sayı 1, pp. 23-3.

[24] Tazegül Ü. (2011). Comparison of narcissims Level of athletes in some branches, International Journal of Sport Studies.Vol., 1 (4), 168-179.

[25] Çekin M. D., Tatar Y., & Afyon Y. A. (2001) 14-16 Yaş Grubunu Spora Teşvik Eden Unsurlar. Selçuk Ü., Eğitim Fakültesi Dergisi., Sayı 7.

[26] Wampbell, E., & Jones, E. (1994). Psychological Well-being in Wheelchair Sport Participants and Nonparticipants. Adapted Physical Activity Quarterly 11: 404-15.

[27] Kuru, E., & Abakay, U. (2009). Güreş Grekorornen Genç Milli Takım Sporcularanın.Başarı motivlotivasyon Düzeylerinin, Sportif Tecrübe ve Antrenman Sıklığı Açısından İncelenmesi Beden Eğitimi Spor Bilimleri Dergisi cilt, 11 sayı 9, 41-50.

[28] Aktop, A. (2002). *Spora Özgü Başarı Motivasyonu İle Psikolojik ve Yapısal Özellikler Arasındaki İlişkinin İncelenmesi*, Yayınlanmamış,Yüksek Lisans Tezi, Akdeniz Üniverstesi, Antalya.

[29] Tazegül, Ü., Kalkavan, A., & Ersoy, A. (2012). Farklı Bireysel Sporlardaki Sporcuların Motivasyon Düzeylerinin Elde Ettikleri En Büyük Derece Değişkenine Göre Karşıtlaştırılması, 2ND Internatıonal Socıal Scıences ın Physıcal Educatıon and Sport Congress, May 31-June 2, Ankara /Turkey.

[30] Soyer, F., Can, y., Güven, H., Hergüner, G., Bayansalduz, M., & Tetik, B. (2010). Sporculardaki başarı motivasyonu ile takım birlikteliği arasındaki ilişkinin incelenmesi, ınternational journal of human sciencec, Vol:7 No:1, 226-239.

[31] Engür, M. (2002). Elit Sporcularda Başarı Motivasyonunun, Durumluk Kaygı Düzeyleri Üzerine Etkisi, Yayınlanmış, Yüksek Lisans Tezi, Ege Üniversitesi, İzmir.

[32] Aslan, A.,& Kuru, E. (2002). Profesyonel ve Amatör Futbolcuların Başarı Motivasyonu Farklılıkları ve Sportif Tecrübe ile İlişkisi, Gazi Beden Eğitimi ve Spor Bilimleri Dergisi. 2:29.

[33] Türkmen, M. (2005). Profesyonel Erkek Futbolcular İle Amatör Erkek Futbolcuların Başarı Motivasyon Düzeylerinin İncelenmesi (İzmir-Manisa Örneği), Yayınlanmış Yüksek Lisans Tezi, Celal Bayar Üniversitesi, Manisa.

[34] Ural, O. (2008). Futbolda Takım Performansına Etki Eden Motivasyonel Faktörlerin Belirlenmesine Yönelik Bir Uygulama (Gençlerbirliği Spor Kulübü Örneği), Yayınlanmış Yüksel Lisan Tezi, Gazi Üniversitesi Sağlık Bilimleri Enstitüsü, Beden Eğitimi ve Spor Anabilim Dalı, Ankara.

[35] Erman, A. K., Şahan, A., & Can., S. (2004). Sporcu Bayan ve Erkeklerin Spora Özgü Başarı Motivasyonlarının Karşılaştırılması, *10th ICHPER Sd European Congress*& TSSA 8th International Sport Science Congress, 17-20 November, Antalya.

[36] Karabulut, C., Kirazcı, S., & Aşçı H. F. (2000). Takım ve Bireysel Sporcuların Başarı Motivasyonu Düzeylerinin İncelenmesi; *Hacettepe Üniversitesi 6. Spor Bilimleri Kongresi,* 3-5 Kasım, Ankara.

17

Lance Armstrong's Era of Performance: Demonstrating the Post Hoc Fallacy

Hein F.M. Lodewijkx*

Department of Psychology, Open University, Heerlen, The Netherlands
*Corresponding author: Hein.Lodewijkx@ou.nl

Abstract In consequence of USADA's charges, Lance Armstrong conceded he doped during his cycling career. The logic proposed in the *post hoc fallacy* entails that Armstrong's sportive feats are therefore 'caused' by his doping use. This fallacy generalizes to the belief put forward in the doping debate that the progress in speed over time in professional cycling is determined by riders' use of progressively potent doping agents. To examine this fallacy, the current study compared Armstrong's mountain time trial wins, realized in the Tour de France (2001, 2004), to victories demonstrated by riders in similar races uphill in the French race (1958–1996, $N = 17$). The fallacy expects that riders will race faster over time and that Armstrong's achievements will be far superior to other riders. However, if these expectations are disconfirmed the fallacy will be refuted. We developed a climbing index to evaluate riders' km/h performances: Cl_I = (Corrected altitude climb / Distance trial) • 100. Higher values indicate more demanding races. Mediation regression analyses showed that, over time, the trials became less demanding, b = -.0076 ($\Delta R^2 = .201$, $p \leq .05$), and that riders raced b = 0.201 km/h faster per year ($\Delta R^2 = .234$, $p \leq .05$). The index had a robust influence on riders' speed (r = -.97) and they raced b = -2.302 km/h slower per unit of the index ($\Delta R^2 = .932$, $p \leq .0001$). The significant mediating influence of the index, b = 0.175 km/h ($p \leq .05$), subsequently reduced riders' progress in speed to a nonsignificant b = 0.026 km/h per year (p = .38, $\Delta R^2 = .003$). Furthermore, Armstrong's performances did not prove to be outliers. Findings invalidate the reasoning employed in the post hoc fallacy, since the CL_I and not the year in which riders competed constitutes the main determinant of riders' performances. They also entail that Armstrong's modern doping agents may not have given him the proposed advantage over his forerunners who won trials before the 1990s, i.e., the years in which these potent aids were not yet rampant in professional road racing.

Keywords: *archival records, epo doping, professional road cycling, time trial performance*

1. Introduction

A downpour of massive doping schemes has placed the professional cycling world in ill repute the last twenty years [1]. The most recent incident, evoking worldwide commotion, concerns American ex–professional cyclist Lance Armstrong. As a result of USADA's allegations [2] [3], in January 2013 he acknowledged the use of epo, blood transfusions, and testosterone during his active cycling career. These banned doping agents are proposed to powerfully enhance performance, thereby contributing to, or even determining, the superior cycling feats demonstrated by the disputed American racer in his seven Tour de France victories [2,3]. However, we doubt the soundness of this assertion, because we argue that it may constitute an instance of the *post hoc ergo propter hoc fallacy* (translation: after this, therefore because of this [4]). This *post hoc fallacy* reflects the erroneous belief that because there is a temporal sequence in events, one event is the cause of the other. Thus, Armstrong's winning performances ("after this") are assumed to be caused by his doping use ("because of this"). The current study aims to show that this flawed logic might apply when explaining Armstrong's achievements. To this end, we compared his winning performances, realized in mountain time trials in the Tour de France in 2001 and 2004, to victories demonstrated by riders in similar races uphill in the French race between 1958 and 1996.

1.1 Previous research

Two previous studies contrasted Armstrong's time trial wins, demonstrated on flat and rolling terrain, to victories of other riders in comparable races. Surprisingly, they yielded no solid empirical evidence that his performances were significantly faster than his counterparts. Findings of both studies are summarized in Table 1. The first study [5] compared Armstrong's performances to cyclists, who, from 1934 to 2010, won trials in the three European Grand Tours (Tour de France, Giro d'Italia, and Vuelta a España) facing distances that were equivalent to Armstrong's (50-61 km). The second study [6] contrasted his wins to time trial victories demonstrated by all former multiple Grand Tour winners (1949-1995; Coppi, Anquetil, Merckx, Hinault, Indurain) as well as all riders who won trials in the three tours from 2006 to 2011. The variation in trial distances in the latter study was much larger (8.2-137 km) than in the former. Both studies assessed riders' mean kilometers per hour (km/h) performances as the dependent variable and they yielded practically identical results on this measure. The first row in Table 1 shows that, across time trials, Armstrong's performances initially were faster than performances of the other riders, explaining 3-6.4% of the variation in speed. Only the first study yielded a significant rider main effect. Importantly, however, after statistically adjusting for the strongly confounding influence of the year in which riders competed, in both studies the speed differences between riders disappeared and the rider main effects explained trivial amounts of 0.1-1.3% of the variation in riders' achievements. The positive relationship between year of competition and km/h performances accounted for a significant 41.3-57% of the performance differences between riders, indicating that riders progressively race faster over the years. Both studies further revealed that only one of Armstrong's victories went beyond the very rigorous 68%-CI and none of them surpassed the bandwidth of the 95%-CI.

Table 1. Summary of Findings of Studies Comparing Armstrong's Time Trial Performances to Other Cyclists

	Study 1 (50-61 km) ($N = 62$)			Study 2 (8.2-137 km) ($N = 97$)		
Variables	Armstrong	Other riders (1934-2010)	ΔR^2	Armstrong	Multiple winners (1949-2011)	ΔR^2
Unadjusted mean km/h	49.37	44.67	064*	49.37	46.91	.030‡
Adjusted mean km/h	45.10	45.53	.001	47.49	47.05	.013
Year of competition			.570**			.413**

‡ $p \leq .10$; * $p \leq .05$; ** $p \leq .001$

1.2. Research Question: Demonstrating the Post Hoc Fallacy

The latter findings imply that the wins of the American ex–cyclist cannot be regarded atypical or 'abnormal.' Besides, the slight amounts of variation explained by the (un)adjusted rider main effects in the two studies suggest that the time trial achievements of all riders are quite comparable and that, therefore, Armstrong did not strongly benefit from his doping use. However, this conclusion may be criticized, since both studies revealed a significant yearly progress in riders' speed. Armstrong won his trials between 1999 and 2005. Hence, the linear relationships could lead one to conclude that Armstrong indeed raced faster than his predecessors and that the doping agents he resorted to might have strongly contributed to these achievements [2,3]. Although we rebutted this criticism extensively in foregoing papers [5,6,7,8], in the current study we will comment once more on this way of circular reasoning, because it might reflect the logic underlying the post hoc fallacy. The fallacy is illustrated in Figure 1. Armstrong's victories can be seen as winning performances (W_P) in Figure 1. He also used modern, ergogenic doping aids, labeled doping use in a certain year (D_Y) in Figure 1. The post hoc fallacy implies that W_P ("after this") is caused by D_Y ("because of this"). This reasoning generalizes to the often heard opinion in discussions about effects of doping, suggesting that the progress in speed over the years in professional road racing (W_P) can be attributed to the use of progressively powerful and advanced banned substances (D_Y) [5-10]. The current study purports to show that this reasoning may be false by examining the relationship between the year in which riders' competed (D_Y) and their winning performances in mountain time trials (W_P). If the relationship between D_Y and W_P proves to be nonexistent, than the logic employed in the post hoc fallacy is refuted.

The foregoing Armstrong studies deliberately assessed his individual time trial achievements as the criterion to appraise his performances over the years, rather than focusing on his final km/h achievements in the seven Tours he won (1999–2005). Several historic studies [7,8], which examined all first–ranking performances of riders in the Tour, Giro, and Vuelta from 1903 to 2011($N = 256$), indicated once more that the accomplishments of the American racer were not exceptional. However, these studies may suffer from a methodological flaw. Cyclists' ultimate km/h performances, realized after three weeks of competition in multi–stage cycling races, cannot be considered individual performances, because they may be strongly affected by the (often inestimable) athletic efforts exerted by the bunch of riders participating in the races (the 'peloton'). In individual time trials, riders' efforts are not influenced by these confounding, coordinated peloton forces. In a time trial riders individually race for the fastest time, making it impossible to benefit from the joint labors of cooperating riders in the race through drafting (profiting from the slipstream other riders). Thus, in a time trial riders can only rely on their own athletic capabilities [5,6,11]. Therefore, we maintain that an assessment of these individual performances will increase chances to (indirectly) explore the impact of ergogenic doping agents on Armstrong's cycling feats.

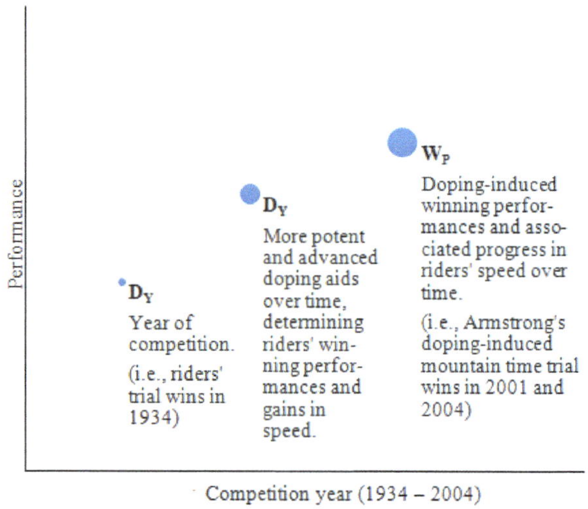

Figure 1. Illustration of the post hoc fallacy to account for riders' winning performances over time

Time trial racing constitutes one of the most demanding disciplines in professional road racing and, within this discipline, mountain time trials are a class on their own [11]. To critically evaluate findings and conclusions pertaining to the two previous Armstrong studies and to investigate the post hoc fallacy, the present research contrasted Armstrong's winning performances in these demanding races to victories of other riders. The logic of the fallacy suggests an increase in riders' speed over time. Moreover, given the proposed powerful ergogenic effects of Armstrong's doping aids [2,3], it further assumes that his km/h performances will be far superior to achievements of the other winners.

2. Method

2.1. Design and Sample

Mountain time trials are rarely scheduled in the three tours [11,12] and the archival records of Magnier and co–workers [12] revealed that all in all nineteen of these trials occurred in the Tour de France in the years following WW II (1958-2004). Records relating to the Giro and Vuelta supplied by [12] were incomplete, forcing us to restrict the examination of our research questions to riders' performances in these nineteen trials. Magnier et al. [12] provided information concerning the winners of the trials, their mean km/h and time performances, as well as the names of the mountains and their altitudes, but they did not give details relating to the slopes of the climbs. We succeeded to retrieve this information from Codifava [13] and cross–checked it with data provided by Van Lonkhuyzen [14] and Ejnes et al. [15]. Table 2 presents descriptive statistics of the variables we measured.

2.2. Measurements

We took notice of the day at which the trials were scheduled during the Tours. The mean *stage number* indicates that, on average, the trials took place at the end of the second week of the three–week races ($M = 14$, $SD = 4$). The *years of competition* ranged from 1958 to 2004. In 1958, famous climber Charly Gaul won the first trial to the top of Mont Ventoux in the Provence. As Table 2 shows, Armstrong won the last two races uphill in 2001 and 2004. The mean *distances* of the trials amounted to $M = 28.85$ km. Note that there is a large between–trial variation in these distances ($SD = 13.14$ km) of which we come to speak below. French five–time Tour winner Bernard Hinault faced the longest and Spanish climber Frederico Bahamontes the shortest trial.

The *altitudes* of the climbs varied between 0.857 km (Cote d'Engins) and 1.909 km (Mont Ventoux) with $M = 1.606$ km ($SD = 0.349$). However, reckoning our research questions, we doubted the validity of these altitudes, because cyclists faced less high elevations. Most of the trials are located at high mountains in the French Alps or Pyrenees, meaning that the riders did not start their races at sea level. However, the altitudes of the climbs are measured from sea level [14]. For instance, it is documented [15] that Charly Gaul in his 1958-trial to Mont Ventoux started his race at Bédoin, a village located at the foot of the climb with an elevation of 327 m. The altitude of Gaul's trial thus amounted to1.582 km and not 1.909 km. To validly evaluate riders' achievements, we therefore accounted for the elevation at which riders began their trial. After scrutinizing various sources relating to the history of climbs in professional road racing [12,13,14,15], we estimated the *corrected altitudes* of the climbs. They were operationalized as the difference in km between the documented base of the climb (where riders started the race) and the top (where the finish line was drawn). Table 2 indicates that the corrected altitudes are substantially lower (515 m) than the uncorrected heights ($M = 1.091$ km, $SD = 0.292$).

The average *slope* of the climbs is defined as the rise over the run: (rise of the climb / horizontal distance) • 100. The mean slopes amounted to $M = 6\%$ ($SD = 1.37$). Spanish rider and former Tour winner Pedro Delgado as well as Dutch time trial specialist Eric Breukink faced the 'easiest' climbs (Cote d'Engins, $M = 3.3\%$). In 2004, Armstrong faced the steepest climb to the top of l'Alpe d'Huez ($M = 7.8\%$).

As regards the dependent variable, across the sample riders' mean *km/h performances* amounted to $M = 28.87$ ($SD = 5.56$). On average, it took riders approximately one hour to finish the trials ($M = 58{:}01$, $SD = 18{:}20$). Note that both performance measures show a large variability, owing to the variation in the distances of the time trials to which we will attend to in the next section.

2.2.1. Climbing Index

Surprisingly, preliminary analyses revealed that larger distances of the trials are strongly associated with faster km/h performances, $r = .83$ ($p \leq .001$). This can be explained by the fact that longer races may involve extended stretches of relatively flat roads, enabling riders to maintain higher speeds compared to trials in which riders instantly have to climb. Moreover, the correlation between the corrected altitude and riders' km/h performances was significant, $r = -.56$ ($p = .01$), whilst the correlation with the uncorrected altitudes was not, $r = -.38$ ($p = .11$). The corrected altitudes thus appear to have better discriminatory value. Additionally, the strong distance–km/h performance relationship entails that we should control for this variable in order to validly address our research questions. Inspired by the research of El Helou and co–workers [9], we therefore developed a *climbing index*, also operationalized as the rise over the run. The rise concerns the corrected altitude in km and the run the total distance of the trial in km and it is expressed in percentages:

Since longer trials involve less climbing kilometers, they are (relatively) less difficult for riders to maintain higher speeds. Therefore, we assume that higher values of the CI_I designate more demanding trials in terms of riders' instant climbing efforts. Table 2 presents descriptive statistics of the index: $M = 4.36\%$, $SD = 2.26$. The strong interrelationships of the index with other variables make clear that the CI_I accounts for the influence of the variation in distances of the trials on riders' performances ($r = -.85$, $p \leq .001$) as well as for the influence of the corrected altitudes ($r = .54$, $p \leq .05$) and the slopes of the climbs ($r = .64$, $p \leq .01$). Besides, the index correlates nearly perfectly with riders' speed ($r = -.97$, $p \leq .001$) explaining 94% of the variation between riders. For these reasons, we chose to attend to our research questions using two variables: The year in which riders competed, permitting an evaluation of Armstrong's performances in 2001 and 2004, and the Cl_I.

Table 2. Descriptive Statistics of Riders' Performances in Mountain Time Trials in the Tour de France (N = 19)

Year	Rider	Climb	Stage	Dis-tance	Alti-tude	Cor. Alti-tude	Mean Slope	Cl_I	Mean Km/h	Mean Time	Pred. Km/h	Res. Km/h
1958	Gaul	M. Ventoux	18	21.5	1.909	1.582	7.1	7.36	20.76	1:02:09	21.34	-0.59
1959	Bahamontes	P. de Dome	15	12.5	1.415	1.033	7.5	8.26	20.69	0:36:15	19.28	1.41
1962	Bahamontes	S.bagnères	13	18.5	1.804	1.179	6.3	6.37	23.43	0:47:23	23.71	-0.29
1965	Gimondi	Revard (n)	18	26.9	1.538	1.292	6	4.80	26.97	0:59:50	27.41	-0.43
1977	van Impe	Avoriaz	15	14	1.833	0.873	6	6.21	24.84	0:33:49	24.49	0.35
1978	Zoetemelk	P. de Dome	14	52.5	1.415	1.033	7.5	1.97	36.69	1:25:51	34.27	2.42[a]
1979	Hinault	S.bagnères	2	23	1.804	1.179	6.3	5.13	26.56	0:53:59	27.03	-0.47
1979	Hinault	Avoriaz	15	54.2	1.833	0.873	6	1.61	34.75	1:33:35	35.12	-0.37
1983	Arroyo	P. de Dome	15	15.6	1.415	1.033	7.5	5.82	25.60	0:35:09	25.54	0.07
1983	van Impe	Avoriaz	19	15	1.833	0.873	6	6.62	22.99	0:40:43	23.69	-0.70
1984	Fignon	Ruchère	16	22	1.042	0.544	4.5	2.47	31.29	0:42:11	33.27	-1.98[a]
1987	Bernard	M. Ventoux	18	36.5	1.909	1.582	7.1	4.33	27.47	1:19:44	29.06	-1.60[a]
1988	Delgado	C. d'Engins	13	38	0.857	0.652	3.3	1.72	36.54	1:02:24	35.11	1.42
1989	Rooks	Orc.-Merlette	15	39	1.840	0.709	5.1	1.82	33.01	1:10:42	34.91	-1.81[a]
1990	Breukink	C. d'Engins	12	33.5	0.857	0.652	3.3	1.95	35.35	0:56:52	34.64	0.71
1994	Ugrumov	Avoriaz	19	47.5	1.833	0.873	6	1.84	34.34	1:22:59	34.99	-0.65
1996	Berzin	V.d'Isère	8	30.5	1.810	0.970	4.2	3.18	35.27	0:51:53	31.95	3.32[b]
2001	Armstrong	Ch.rousse (s)	11	32	1.721	1.311	6.5	4.10	28.47	1:07:27	29.98	-1.51[a]
2004	Armstrong	A. d'Huez	16	15.5	1.845	1.127	7.8	7.27	23.44	0:39:41	22.75	0.69
M			**14**	**28.85**	**1.606**	**1.019**	**6.0**	**4.36**	**28.87**	**58:01**	**28.87**	**0**
(SD)	**-**	**-**	**(4)**	**(13.14)**	**(0.349)**	**(0.292)**	**(1.37)**	**(2.26)**	**(5.56)**	**(18:20)**	**(5.37)**	**(1.41)**

Notes: Distance and (corrected) altitudes are in kilometers. [a] Performances beyond ±68%-CI. [b] Performances beyond ± 95%-CI.

2.3. Analyses

We examined our research questions using a mediation regression model (OLS, [16,17]) with riders' mean km/h performances as the criterion and competition year and the CL_I as predictor variables. The results of these analyses allow an evaluation of Armstrong's doping–induced wins: "Are his performances predicted by competition year and the Cl_I or not, and do they constitute outliers?" If competition year proves to be the main predictor variable and Armstrong's performances are statistical outliers as well, this will render the reasoning underlying the post hoc fallacy plausible. However, if these expectations are disconfirmed, the logic will be disproved. Consistent with previous studies [5,6], we further used the stringent 68%- and 95%–CIs (± 1*SD* or ± 2*SD* from the sample mean, respectively) as the criterion to determine outliers. Conventionally, however, performances beyond ±3*SD* are considered outliers [18]. Last, we assessed whether influential cases biased the regression model. Analyses were conducted using IBM–SPSS (v. 20).

3. Results

3.1. Km/h Performances

Following guidelines for mediation analyses provided by [16,17] the regression analyses we conducted, involved four steps. Figure 2 summarizes findings of the analyses. The first step in the analyses showed that the year in which cyclists competed is negatively related to the Cl_I, b = -0.076 (ΔR^2 = .201), indicating that the trials became less brutal over time. The second step revealed that competition year is positively related to riders' mean km/h performances, b = 0.201 km/h (ΔR^2 = .234). Per year riders race 201 m faster. The third step indicated that the index has a strong negative influence, showing that riders race b = -2.302 km/h (ΔR^2 = .932) slower per unit of the index. In the fourth step we simultaneously entered competition year and the index in the regression equation. This step not only allows a test of the mediation effect of the index on the competition year–performance relationship, but also permits an estimation of the degree to which the influence of competition year on riders' achievements is affected by the index. The lower panel in Figure 2 presents the results of the fourth step. The resulting unstandardized b = 0.026 km/h (ΔR^2 = .003) indicates that riders raced 26 m faster per year. This relationship is not significant (p = .38) and explains 0.3% of the variation in riders' km/h performances. The fourth step further revealed that the Cl_I fully mediated the competition year–performance relationship (z = 2.10, p ≤ .05) and accounted for a substantive part of the variation in this relationship, b = 0.175 km/h. Thus, the mediating effect of the index ultimately resulted in the adjusted, nonsignificant influence of competition year on the dependent variable, i.e., 0.201 - 0.175 = 0.026 km/h. The two variables jointly explain 92.7% of the variation in riders' performances, to which the index contributed by far the most. To conclude, as there is no solid evidence that riders race faster over time, our findings put great pressure on the logic underlying the post hoc fallacy.

3.2. Outliers and normality

The analyses further yielded information concerning riders' predicted and residual performances, which are presented in the last two columns of Table 2. The correlation between the two variables, r = .00, indicates a very good fit of the regression model. Residuals give an indication which performances are not predicted by the variables included in the regression model and, therefore, permit us to evaluate which performances may constitute outliers. Figure 3A and Figure 3B present regression plots of riders' predicted performances with 68%– and 95%–CIs. Table 2 and the figures show that one of Armstrong's wins surpassed the 68%–CI and it concerns his 2001 trial to Chamrousse in the French Alps. However, in this trial he did not perform faster, but 1.51 km/h slower than predicted. In his 2004 trial to l'Alpe d'Huez he raced 690 m faster than predicted. Yet, this performance did not even surpass the 68%–bandwidth. Hence, regarding our research questions, we conclude that the achievements of the American racer do not constitute outliers.

Table 2 and Figure 3A and Figure 3B further indicate that four other riders exceeded the 68%-CI. Three of them performed slower than predicted: French riders Laurent Fignon (1984) and Jeff Bernard (1987) and Dutch cyclist Steven Rooks (1989). In 1978, Dutch rider and former Tour winner Joop Zoetemelk performed faster than predicted on his climb of Puy de Dome in the Massif Central.

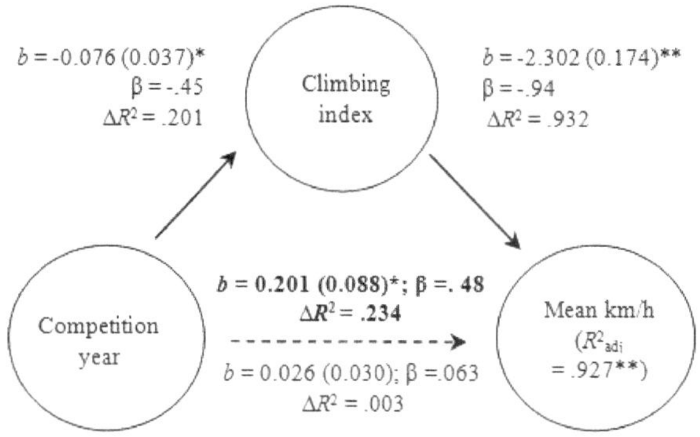

$^*p \leq .05$; $^{**}p \leq .001$

Figure 2. Mediation model of variables explaining differences in riders' km/h performances. Presented are unstandardized regression weights (*b*) and associated standard errors (SE_b) in parentheses and standardized weights (β). As to km/h performances, *b* and SE_b are in kilometers per hour per year, or in kilometers per hour per unit of the climbing index. The unadjusted relationship between year of competition and km/h performances is in bold type face. The broken arrow indicates a mediated relationship

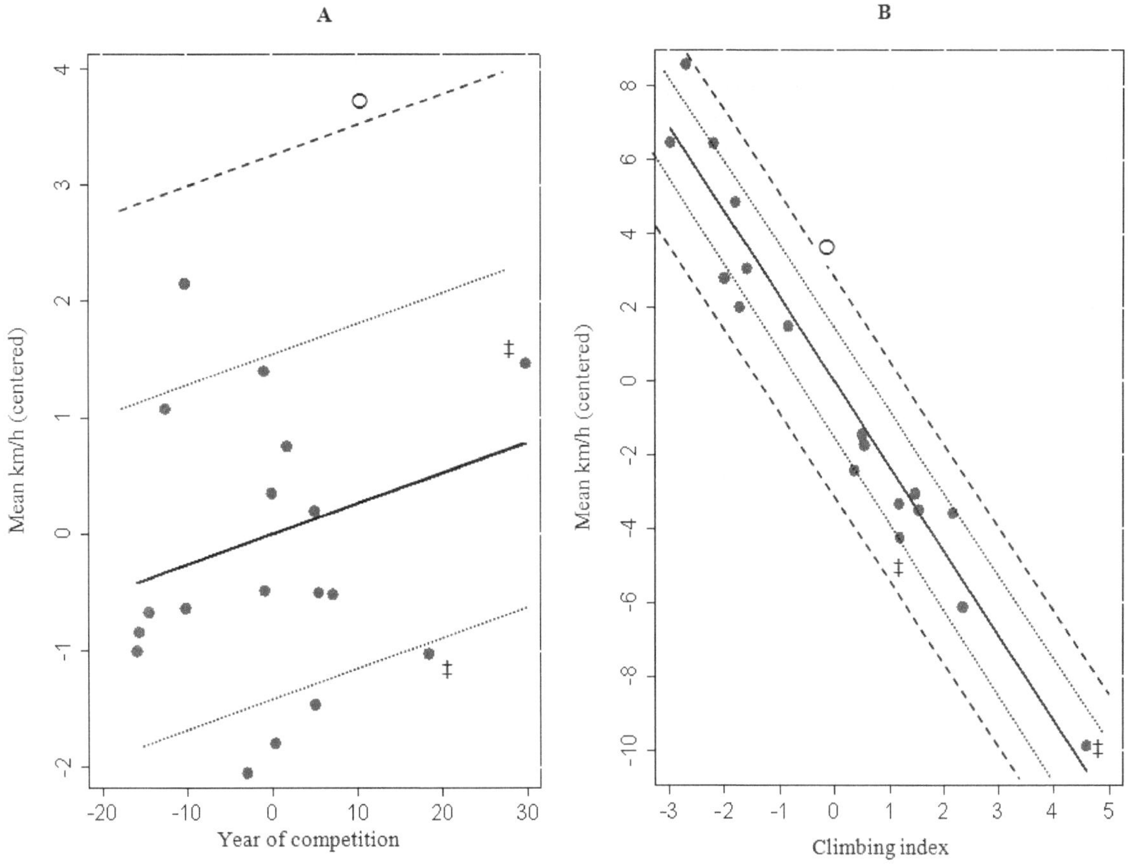

Figure 3. Plots of riders' mean km/h performances regressed on year of competition and the climbing index. Dotted lines indicate the 68%-CI and broken lines the 95%-CI. Open dots (O) present Berzin's performance beyond the 95%-CI and double daggers (‡) Armstrong's performances. Negative values of the centred mean km/h indicate slower performances

Only one of the nineteen cyclists went beyond the 95%–CI in his performance, it concerns Russian rider Yevgeni Berzin in the 1996 trial to Val d'Isère in the Alps. Although we utterly realize that the number of observation is far too low to reliably estimate whether riders' observed, predicted and residual time performances depart from normality, we did evaluate these performan-ces. They all appeared to be normally distributed (Kol-mogorov–Smirnov tests, $zs \leq 0.71$, $ps \geq .70$), indicating there are no signs of any 'abnormal' fast or slow perfor-mances among the riders, including Armstrong's. To give examples, Figure 4 illustrates the normal probability plots of riders' observed and residual performances.

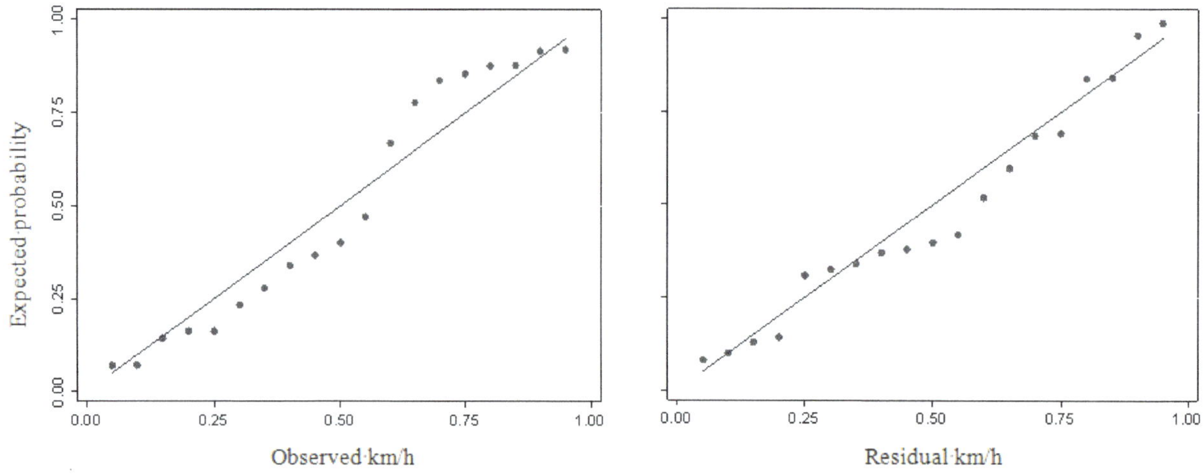

Figure 4. Normal probability plots of riders' observed and residual km/h performances

3.3. Influential Cases

Relative to the other riders, Armstrong's win of the 2004 trial to l'Alpe d'Huez yielded a large leverage value, $h = 0.44$, suggesting that this specific performance might have had an undue influence on the negative slope of the regression line, owing to the fact that his predicted speed strongly deviated from the mean predicted speed. This performance can be seen in Figure 3B (bottom right) and, again, it reveals a comparatively 'slow' achievement of the American racer. To check whether his achievements biased our findings in any way, we conducted auxiliary regression analyses and excluded Armstrong's performances. The results closely matched previous findings. The influence of year of competition ($b = 0.033$ km/h, $p = .49$) and the Cl_I ($b = -2.305$ km/h, $p \leq .001$) slightly departed from the weights presented earlier. The same is true for the total $R^2_{adj} = .928$ ($p \leq .001$). Accordingly, Armstrong's leverage on the overall regression findings appears to be very small. Moreover, we note that it involved a relatively slow and not a conspicuous fast performance, which fell within the bandwidth of the 68%-CI. Importantly, Armstrong's performances did not alter our main finding concerning the post hoc fallacy: Whether or not we included his wins in the analyses, after controlling for the robust effect of the Cl_I, competition year turned out to yield a negligible influence on riders' sportive achievements.

4. Discussion

The logic presented in the post hoc fallacy suggestedan increase in speed in riders' mountain time trial performances over the years and, given the proposed powerful ergogenic effects of Armstrong's doping aids, it further assumed that his performances would be superior to achievements of the other winners we included in our sample. Our findings, however, are inconsistent with this logic. After controlling for the influence of the Cl_I on riders' accomplishments, there is no evidence that riders raced significantly faster over time. Moreover, Armstrong's wins in 2001 and 2004 did not appear to be superior, but rather extremely comparable to the achievements of the other riders. As a matter of fact, his performances came out comparatively slow. What all these findings entail for Armstrong's doping–induced wins will be addressed in later sections, after a discussion of the validity of our study.

4.1. Validity

Although our observations revealed that our regression model is valid and stable, this does not mean to say that there are no factors that may have threatened the internal validity of the study. These factors mainly concern operationalizations and measurements of the variables we used. We already mentioned the problems relating to the altitudes of the climbs. Although one might not suspect this, there is also disagreement about the slopes. For instance, according to some sources the altitude of l'Alpe d'Huez is 1860 m and not 1845 m, and the documented slopes vary between 7.7% and 8.7%. Moreover, there is the additional problem that the corrected altitudes we estimated do not have to agree with the exact spot at which the start and finish lines were drawn in the various time trials. Whenever we encountered such problems, we decided to check at least three different sources [12,13,14,15]. In cases in which two of the three sources showed agreement on a certain value, we included this value in our measurements. If all three sources disagreed, we decided to include the value in between. Besides, the measurement of the distances of the time trials and the related mean km/h and time performances, recorded in the early years of the French race, might also be unreliable. During these years, time for example was sometimes registered by hand [15], and, obviously, this may have consequences for the computation of riders' speed. The same argument holds for the distance of the stages. Thus, in some cases our measurements may be unreliable. However, they only constitute sources of random error; they did not introduce systematic errors in our study. Then again, we have seen that the corrected altitudes predicted riders' km/h performances better than the uncorrected altitudes. Furthermore, the Cl_I, which we based on the corrected altitudes, had a robust influence on riders' performances over time. As a single variable, the index explained 94% ($r = -.97$) of the variation in riders' speed, adding validity to our findings and conclusions.

4.2. The Post Hoc Fallacy

This brings us to critically appraise Armstrong's doping–induced wins. Our regression findings designated that, in first instance, there is a significant yearly progress in riders' speed from 1958 to 2004. Since Armstrong won the last two trials in 2001 and 2004, this relationship could lead one to conclude that he indeed raced faster than the other riders did and that the doping agents he used probably contributed to his superior achievements. However, since the Cl_I fully mediated the relationship between competition year (D_Y in Figure 1) and riders' performances (W_P), it follows that the (causal?) relationship between the two variables is nonexistent. This means that competition year (with the associated doping use) is irrelevant as an explanatory variable to account for difference in riders' speed, at least where it concerns riders' individual exploits in mountain time trials in the Tour de France. Accordingly, these observations convincingly demonstrate the false way of thinking used in the post hoc fallacy — the main determinant of riders' performances is the CL_I, not the year in which riders won their trial.

After controlling for the mediating influence of the index, findings further revealed that competition year accounted for a minor and nonsignificant 26 m improvement in riders' performances per year, which explained 0.3% of the speed differences between riders. There is the possibility that these minimal improvements may have been influenced by riders' doping use over the years. However, if this assumption is valid, it would imply that Armstrong's advanced doping agents did not give him the advantage over the other riders as suggested by [2,3]. After all, 78% of the riders in our sample demonstrated their feats before the 1990s, that is, in a period in which the use of Hb-augmenting doping aids (epo and blood doping) was not yet rampant in professional road racing [7,8,9,10]. Most of the riders we investigated thus lacked the assumed benefits of the modern ergogenic doping agents, which were available to Armstrong and the other riders in the years of the 'epo epidemic' and thereafter [7,8].

Additionally, it is also conceivable that the effects of doping can be detected in the unexplained amount of variation in riders' winning performances (7.3%), which is not accounted for by competition year or the Cl_I. Yet, we argue that this is not a cogent argument either. The residuals appeared to be normally distributed, Armstrong's performances came out comparatively slow, and neither of them surpassed the 95%–CI. Moreover, there are numerous variables which may plausibly account for these unexplained differences, besides doping use. For example, meteorological conditions (wind, heat, rain) during the trials may have strongly influenced riders' speed. Furthermore, the profiles and the irregularity of the climbs vary strongly [15,19]. Compared to l'Alpe d'Huez, Mont Ventoux and Puy de Dome for instance, are known to be much more demanding climbs, characterized by regularly occurring abrupt steep ascents of 12-14% [13]. This impedes riders' efforts to maintain a steady pace while climbing, which may negatively influence their performances. Then again, improvements in the condition of the roads, and technological innovations in the weight and aerodynamics of the bikes and gearing equipment over the years, may have positively affected riders' achievements. The same argument holds for the profiles and distances of the Tours in which riders competed, which improved over the years, thereby facilitating riders' speed [7,8,11,15].

4.3. Overestimated Effects of Epo?

All these observations lead us to conclude that the performance–enhancing effects of the doping aids Armstrong resorted to might not be as powerful as assumed. This conclusion does not agree with Lundby and Olsen's study [20]. They reviewed results of laboratory studies which assessed the relationship between epo administration and participants' improvements in aerobic exercise capacity, measured by maximum oxygen uptake (VO_{2max}), defined as an estimate of cardio–respiratory, circulatory and muscular fitness that measures the fastest rate at which oxygen can be utilized by the body during intense exercise. They estimated epo effects of 8–12% on exercise capacity. As to blood doping the estimations are 5–10% [21]. Conversely, however, findings of all three Armstrong studies conducted thus far are consistent with other, more critical research which concluded that the effects of Hb-augmenting doping aids on cyclists' endurance performances are overestimated [22,23] and even lack scientific evidence [24]. To critically examine the strength of the epo doping-aerobic performance relationship, Lodewijkx et al. [25] conducted a meta–analysis on findings of seventeen laboratory studies (1991-2010) that hitherto investigated this relationship. The analysis revealed modest effect sizes of the experimental epo vs. control / placebo treatments: $d = 0.41$-0.49, $r = .19$-$.44$ and $r^2 = .04$-$.19$. These findings entail that a considerable 81-96% of the differences in performance improvement observed in the studies cannot be explained by epo administration. The largest epo-induced improvement in VO_{2max} found in the analysis equaled an increase in speed of about 1 km/h. Perneger [10] arrives at the same conclusion concerning this increase in speed. However, we emphasize that this slight increase is solely restricted to laboratory situations. It is a well–known fact that such improvements cannot be directly extrapolated to multi–stage cycling races that last three weeks [24,25,26]. All these observations imply that judgments pertaining to the strong ergogenic effects of epo on aerobic exercise capacity might be flawed. In turn, this entails that the relationship between epo doping and performances of cyclists at real contests is strongly overrated too. In our view, this constitutes the most parsimonious explanation for the null results we obtained regarding Armstrong's expected superior time trial performances.

5. Conclusion

Perhaps there remains only one variable which may plausibly explain our observations. It refers to the unique, physical propensities and related time–trial capacities of the very gifted riders we investigated, from Charly Gaul in 1958 to Lance Armstrong in 2004. Our findings illustrate that these capabilities may be underestimated, in particular where it concerns riders who demonstrated their feats in mountain time trials in the early years of the Tour de France. These capabilities make the achievements of all riders comparable, not their doping use. We also argue that our findings leave hardly any room for rival explanations, such as the use of banned substances, to account for differences in riders' performances over time. Last, our study demonstrates that false, circular logic, as put forward the post hoc fallacy, may hinder the exchange of arguments in the sometimes animated discussions about the (alleged) effects of doping in professional cycling.

References

[1] Dilger A., Frick B. and Tolsdorf F., "Are athletes doped? Some theoretical arguments and empirical evidence." *Contemporary Economic Policy,* 25 (4): 604-615, 2007.

[2] USADA, *Statement from USADA CEO Travis T. Tygart regarding the U.S. Postal Service Pro Cycling Team doping conspiracy,* 2012. Online available: http://cyclinginvestigation.usada.org.

[3] USADA, *Reasoned decision of the United States Anti-Doping Agency on disqualification and ineligibility,* 2012. Online available: http://cyclinginvestigation.usada.org

[4] Carroll R. T., *The skeptic's dictionary: A collection of strange beliefs, amusing deceptions, and dangerous delusions.* Hoboken (NJ): John Wiley & Sons, 2003.

[5] Lodewijkx H.F.M. and Verboon P., "Armstrong's era of performance-Part I: Are his time trial performances much different from other winners?" *Journal of Athletic Enhancement*, 2: 1, 2013. Online available: http://dx.doi.org/10.4172/2324-9080.1000106

[6] Lodewijkx H.F.M. and Bos A.E.R., *"Armstrong's era of performance-Part II: Too often the doping debate involves 'arguments from ignorance."* Manuscript submitted for publication. Heerlen (The Netherlands): Open University, 2013.

[7] Lodewijkx H.F.M. and Brouwer B., "Some empirical notes on the 'epo epidemic' in professional cycling." *Research Quarterly for Exercise and Sport*, 82 (4): 593-608, 2011.

[8] Lodewijkx H.F.M. and Brouwer B., "Tour, Giro Vuelta: Rapid progress in cycling performance starts in the 1980s." *International Journal of Sports Science,* 2(3): 24-31, 2012.

[9] El Helou N., Berthelot G., Thibaut V., Tafflet M., Massif H., Campion F. et al., "Tour de France, Giro, Vuelta, and classic European races show a unique progression of road cycling speed in the last 20 years." *Journal of Sports Sciences*, 28 (7): 789-796, 2010.

[10] Perneger T. V., "Speed trends of major cycling races: Does slower mean cleaner?" *International Journal of Sports Medicine*,31: 261–264, 2010.

[11] Lucia A., Earnest C. and Arribas C., "The Tour de France: a physiological review." *Scandinavian Journal of Medicine and Science in Sports*, 13: 275-283, 2003.

[12] Magnier D., Picq P., Debreilly, M., Zingoni P., Haffreingue H. and Bey J.-L., *Cycling remembered* [In French: *Memoire du cyclisme*]. Online available: http://www.memoire-du-cyclisme.eu, 2013.

[13] Codifava G., *Cycling climbs.* Online available: http://www.salite.ch, 2012.

[14] Lonkhuyzen M. van, *Cycling cols.* Online available: http://www.cyclingcols.com, 2012.

[15] Ejnès G., Bouvet P., Brunel P., Dufourq R., Laget S. et al., *Tour de France, 100 years.* [In French: *Tour de France 100 ans.* (Vol. I, II, and III)]. Paris: L'Equipe, 2002.

[16] Preacher K. J. and Hayes A. F., "Asymptotic and resampling strategies for assessing and comparing indirect effects in multiple mediator models." *Behavior Research Methods, 40*, 879-891, 2008.

[17] Hayes A. F. "INDIRECT: An SPSS-macro for estimating indirect path coefficients in regression models." Online available: http://afhayes.com/spss-sas-and-mplus-macros-and-code.html, 2013.

[18] Field A., *Discovering statistics using SPSS* (2nd editition). London: Sage, 2009.

[19] Kerckhoffs R. and Janssens R., *Triumph and tragedy on the climbs of the Tour* (In Dutch: *Triomf en tragiek op de Tourcols*). The Hague: Uitgeverij BZZtôH, 2003.

[20] Lundby C. and Olsen N. V., "Effects of recombinant human erythropoietin in normal humans*." Journal of Physiology,* 589 (6),1265-1271, 2011.

[21] Bytomski J. R., Moorman III, C. T. and MacAuley D., *Oxford American handbook of sports medicine.* Oxford: Oxford University Press, 2010.

[22] Kuipers H., "Putative effects of doping in cycling." [In Dutch: "Vermeende effecten van doping in de wielersport"]. *Nederlands Tijdschrift voor Geneeskunde*, *150*, 2643-2645, 2006.

[23] Brouwer B., Lodewijkx H. F. M. and Kuipers H., "Doping confessions of cyclists revisited." [In Dutch: "Doping-bekentenissen langs de meetlat"]. *Sportpsychologie Bulletin, 20,* 24-37, 2009.

[24] Heuberger J. A. A. C., Cohen-Tervaert J. M., Schepers F. M. L., Vliegenthart A. D. B., Rotmans J. I., Daniels J. M. A., Burggraaf J. and Cohen A. F., "Erythropoietin doping in cycling: Lack of evidence for efficacy and a negative risk–benefit." *British Journal of Clinical Pharmacology*, 2012.

[25] Lodewijkx H.F.M., Brouwer B., Kuipers H. and Van Hezewijk R., "Overestimated effect of epo administration an aerobic exercise capacity: A meta-analysis." *American Journal of Sports Science and Medicine*, 1 (2): 17-27, 2013.

[26] Hopkins W. G., Hawley J. A., and Burke L. M., "Design and analysis of research on sport performance enhancement." *Medicine and Science in Sports and Exercise*, 31: 472-485.

18

Frequency Analyses of Postural Sway during Prolonged Sitting on a Large Gymnastics Ball and Stool

Borut Kirn*, **Vito Starc**

Medical Faculty, University of Ljubljana, Ljubljana, Slovenia
*Corresponding author: borut.kirn@mf.uni-lj.si

Abstract Selected schools in Slovenia have launched an initiative to replace school chairs with large gymnastics balls (LGBs) in order to improve children's posture. The rational given was that LGB saffect posture in a way that is beneficial to the body because they mimic the frequencies of body movement during walking. To identify the influence of seating furniture on the frequency of postural sway, the postural dynamics of eight school children were studied. A comparison was made of their posture while they were sitting on a stool and on a LGB, each for 30 minutes. The lumbar lordosis (LL) and pelvicinclination (PI) angles were both studied. They were measured from the sagittal plane with a video measurement system (3 fps). From the time pattern of each angle, calculations were made to determine the frequency spectrum median and distribution of power in frequency spectra at four intervals: 1) 0.01–0.05 s^{-1}, 2) 0.05–0.1 s^{-1}, 3) 0.1–0.33 s^{-1}, and 4) 0.33–0.6 s^{-1}. It was determined that the median for LL is at a higher frequency on a LGB (LGB = 0.17 s^{-1} ± 0.03 s^{-1}, stool = 0.14 s^{-1} ± 0.03 s^{-1}, $p < 0.05$), but no differences were found in PI. Sitting on a LGB had more power in the third interval with a typical sway period of 5 s ($p < 0.05$), whereas sitting on as tool had more power in the first interval with a typical sway period of 33 s ($p < 0.05$). Sitting on a LGB influences the upper body dynamics and promotes a sitting posture with a period of sway that is closer to the sway pattern experienced during walking as compared to sitting on a stool.

Keywords: *frequency spectrum, sitting dynamics, posture, measurement, seating furniture*

1. Introduction

Selected schools in Slovenia have considered partial substitution of standard classroom chairs with large gymnastics balls (LGB). It is known that poor posture during prolonged sitting is a predictive risk factor for lower back pain [1,2,3]. To reduce this possibility, a dynamic type of chair like a balance chair or LGB [4,5,6] was introduced as an alternative to a standard chair. Dynamic chairs force users into dynamic sitting, which is characterized by continuously changing posture. The rationale behind poor posture while using these chairs is that dynamically changing the posture is beneficial for users because it periodically loads and unloads different musculoskeletal segments, which reduces overload and injury, and improves nutrition of cartilage [7,8,9].

In order to evaluate the effect of dynamic seating, the sitting posture needs to be measured continuously during prolonged periods of sitting. Furthermore, the large amount of data measured needs to be processed in order to obtain parameters that are simple to understand and express characteristics of sitting dynamics in order to distinguish between the effects of different types of seats.

Various studies have evaluated the pattern of spinal posture during prolonged sitting [10]. The lumbar flexion/extension angle was measured during sitting on a chair and analyzed to determine the preferred sitting postures that individuals changed among while sitting.

Frequency analysis is an alternative approach in analyzing human movement dynamics [11]. This kind of analysis is often used in studies of postural sway during a quiet stance [12]. Dynamic sitting requires balancing the upper body in a similar way tothat used while standing. However, frequency analysis has not yet been applied in evaluating the dynamics of sitting.

This study investigated whether frequency analyses (the median of the power frequency spectrum) of pelvic inclination and lumbar spine curvature reveal a difference between sitting on a LGB and on a stool.

2. Methods

2.1. Experiment Participants

Eight schoolchildren (10–11 years old; four male, four female) with physically normal development participated in the study. Their average height was 147.2 ± 4.0 cm and their average weight was 38.0 ± 5.1 kg. A week before the measurements, a trained physiotherapist explained to them how to sit on a LGB. After initial instruction, each child sat on a LGB during classes for at least 1 day. The study was approved by the ethics committee and parental approval was obtained for every child.

2.2. Experimental Protocol

Prior to the experiment, each child's overall height and popliteal height were measured to enable appropriate adjustment of the size of the LGB and the stool.

Children sat on a ball and on a stool during two separate sessions, each lasting 30 minutes.

The children sitting on a stool (left) and LGB (right) wore optical markers during measurements. The video was recorded in a dim environment to facilitate automatic marker position extraction.

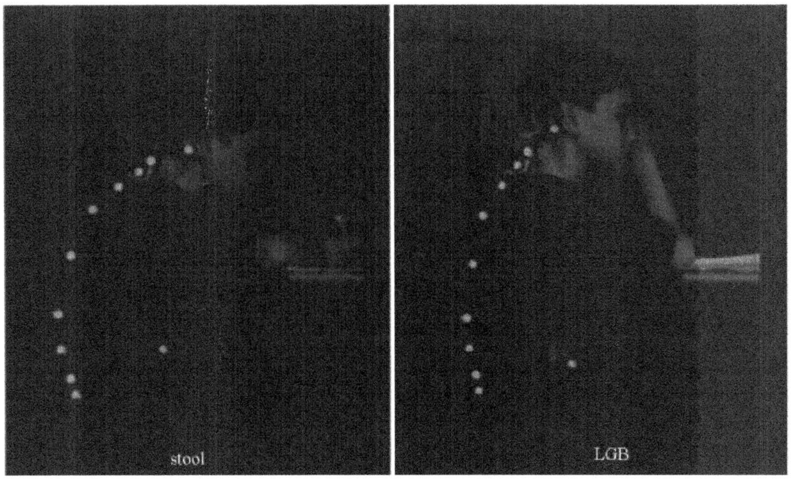

Figure 1. Optical markers in the sagittal plane

2.3. Assessment of Sitting Posture

The measurement technique has been described and evaluated in detail in previous studies [13]. In brief, the sitting posture of each child was recorded from a lateral view using a digital video camera (Figure 1). The camera was leveled on a tripod, and therefore the vertical side of the image was parallel to the direction of gravity. It was located 5 m from the child at a height of 1 m and positioned perpendicular to the plane of motion to decrease errors of perspective. Five markers constructed of a LED diode were fixed on the free end of a 2 cm long frame, as shown in Figure 2, and were positioned at the most superior parts of the spinal prominence of lumbar vertebrae L1, L3, and L5, of sacrum S2, and at the anterior superior iliac spine (ASIS).

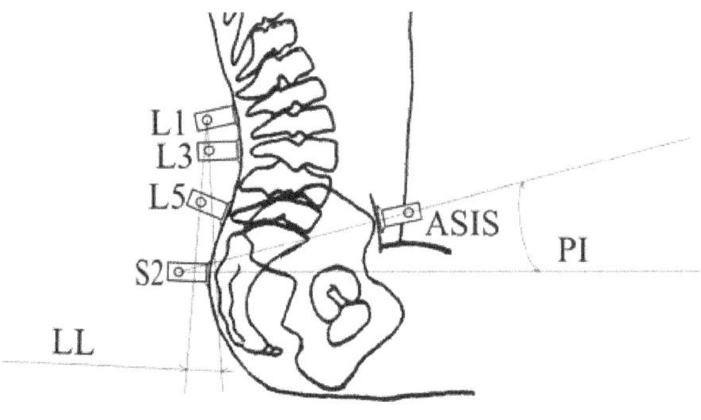

Figure 2. Definition of angles

The intensity of the light in the room was low; therefore, the optical markers were clearly visible on the recorded image. The images, which were digitized and fed into the computer with a spatial resolution of 320 × 280 pixels and with an acquisition rate of 3 frames per second, were analyzed to determine the position of each marker. For this purpose, the researchers developed motion analysis software, which found the position of the marker in the first image and traced its position during the rest of the session.

Optical skin markers L1, L2, and L3 were used to define the lumbar lordosis (LL) angle; markers ASIS and S2 together with a horizontal line were used to define pelvicinclination (PI).

2.4. Definition of Angles

The marker's coordinates were used to determine two angles, which served to describe the sitting posture. The PI angle was defined as the sharp angle between the line connecting markers S2, SAIS, and the horizontal line (Figure 2). The LL angle was defined with markers L1, L3, and L5, as shown in Figure 2. The angle was considered negative in the case of kyphotic lumbar curvature.

2.5. Data Analysis

For each session measured, the researchers determined a power frequency spectrum (PFS) for the PI and LL time courses. The frequency range between 1/90 s^{-1} and 3/5 s^{-1} was then normalized. The median split PFS into two intervals so that the power in both was equal.

The researchers then determined the fraction of the power in four intervals: 1) 1/90–1/20 s^{-1}, 2) 1/20–1/10 s^{-1}, 3) 1/10–1/3 s^{-1}, and 4) 1/3–3/5 s^{-1}. Paired *t*-test statistics were used to compare groups between sitting on a LGB and sitting on a stool and between PI and LL.

3. Results

Altogether, 5,400 consequent values of the PI and LL angles were recorded for each session (Figure 3). The LL median of the PFS on the LGB occurs at higher frequencies (Figure 4), which means that sitting on a LGB is characterized by higher frequency postural dynamics (LL median: LGB = 0.17 $s^{-1} \pm 0.03$ s^{-1}, stool = 0.14 $s^{-1} \pm$ 0.03 s^{-1}, $p < 0.05$). The difference of the PI median of the power frequency spectrum is not significant (PI median: LGB = 0.13 $s^{-1} \pm 0.01$ s^{-1}, stool = 0.13 $s^{-1} \pm 0.01$ s^{-1}, $p >$ 0.05).

Considering LL, the fraction of the power (Figure 5) in the intervals of PFS is larger in the third interval when sitting on a LGB (LGB: 4.09 ± 0.61, stool: 3.39 ± 0.44, $p < 0.05$) and in the first interval when sitting on a stool (LGB: 1.83 ± 0.61, stool: 2.67 ± 0.81, $p < 0.05$). There is no significant difference in the second and fourth intervals and there is no significant difference in PI for any interval.

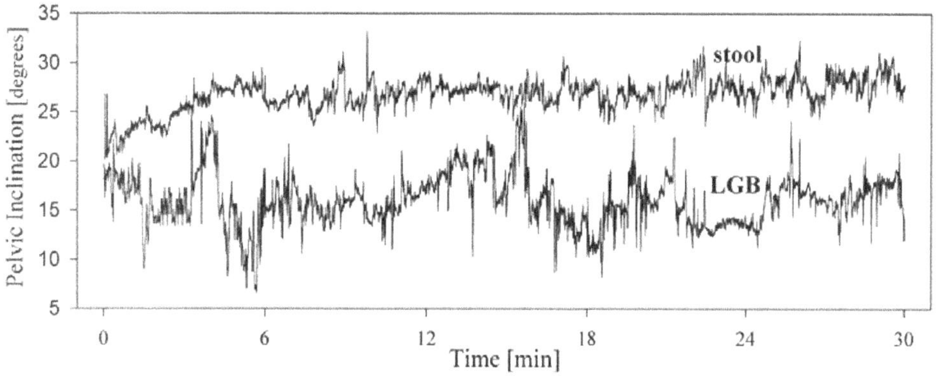

Figure 3. PI time course

The PI angle during 30 minutes of sitting on a stool (Figure 3, top line) and on a LGB (Figure 3, bottom line) was measured with an acquisition rate of 3 s^{-1}. Note that there is less fluctuation on the stool.

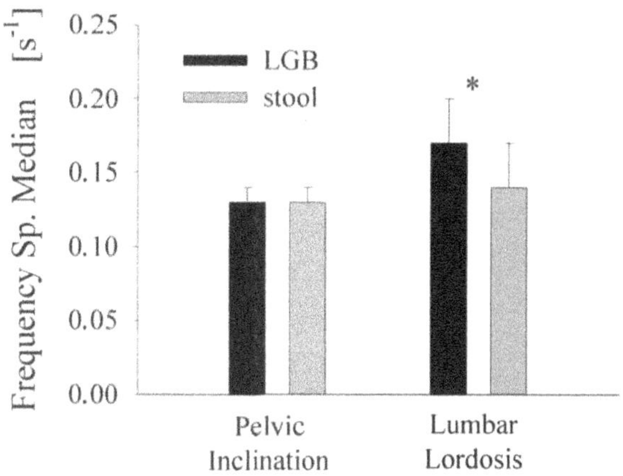

Figure 4. Frequency spectra median

Figure 4 shows that the median value of LL was found to be at significantly (*) higher frequencies when sitting on a LGB. There is no difference in PI.

Figure 5 shows the power of each interval with respect to a LGB and a stool. Intervals in units of s^{-1} are 1) 1/90–1/20, 2) 1/20–1/10, 3) 1/10–1/3, and 4) 1/3–3/5. Note the statistically significant (*) difference in the first and third intervals.

sway was found with a period of 33 s. These two periods represent a pattern of loading and unloading of tissues.

The nature of sitting on a LGB is that it requires maintenance of balance [14]. Posture balance maintenance resembles a standing or walking posture, in which balance must also be continuously maintained [12,15,16]. It is a matter of speculation whether the same mechanisms for balance maintenance are used in both cases.

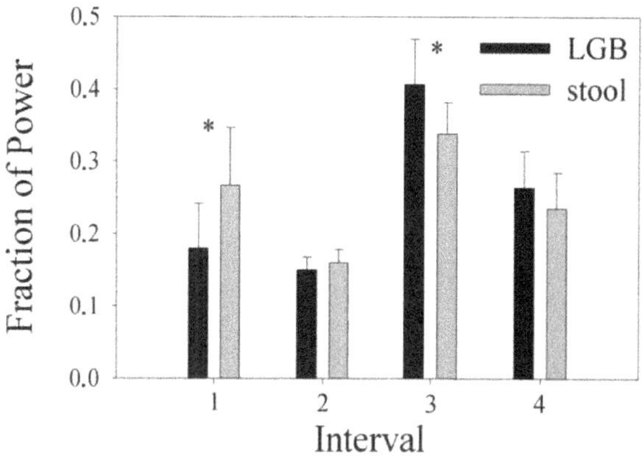

Figure 5. Four intervals of LL angle power frequency spectra4. Discussion

4. Discussion

This study showed that while sitting on a LGB only the upper part of the body adopts a more dynamic posture (as indicated by the LL median), whereas the PI dynamics remained fairly similar whether sitting on a LGB or a stool.

Regarding the sway of the upper body, this study found that while sitting on a LGB there is more sway with a typical period of 5 s as compared to a stool, where more

The human body requires movement to nourish structures such as the nucleus pulposus of the intervertebral disc and to provide periodic rest to muscles. Rotatory dynamic sitting [9,17] periodically changes the spinal load and the result is, as reported, increased spinal length.

The posture dynamics were measured from a sagittal plane, which was a limitation of this study's measurement technique. It is possible that the subjects also had sway dynamics in both the frontal and transversal plane. However, the researchers believe that dynamics in the sagittal plane demonstrate the majority of postural dynamics.

Higher frequency of sway on a LGB is associated with more frequent muscular activity. This dynamic was not pursued in this study and warrants further investigation in the future [4,5].

Recently, in rehabilitation of children with cerebral palsy, hippotherapy was introduced based on the movement of riding a horse. It seems that riding a horse decreases the spastic tension of muscles and develops proper motor reflexes. Perhaps the same mechanism is created during dynamic sitting on a LGB.

It is expected that the effect of dynamic sitting is most pronounced when the periodicity of movements while sitting is similar to the periodicity of movements during walking because the body is well adapted to it.

5. Conclusion

With regard to the selection of the type of classroom seating, this study has demonstrated that the dynamics of sitting on a LGB have some characteristics of standing or walking, which the researchers believe is beneficial as an occasional seating substitute in the classroom [4,5,18].

This study shows the importance of frequency spectra analyses in understanding postural dynamics. It enables comprehensive integration of a large quantity of measured data.

Acknowledgments

The authors would like to thank physiotherapist AlenkaPučko for her skillful acquisition of the data and the teachers and pupils at KolezijaPrimary School in Ljubljana for their participation in the study.

Statement of Competing Interests

The authors have no competing interests.

List of Abbreviations

LGB = large gymnastics ball.
PI = pelvicinclination angle.
LL = lumbar lordosis angle.
PFS = power frequency spectrum.

References

[1] Cardon G, De Clercq D, De Bourdeaudhuij I, Breithecker D: Sitting habits in elementary schoolchildren: a traditional versus a "Moving school". *Patient Educ Couns* 2004, 54 (2): 133-142.

[2] Geldhof E, De Clercq D, De Bourdeaudhuij I, Cardon G: Classroom postures of 8-12 year old children. *Ergonomics* 2007, 50 (10): 1571-1581.

[3] Furian TC, Rapp W, Eckert S, Wild M, Betsch M: Spinal posture and pelvic position in three hundred forty-five elementary school children: a rasterstereographic pilot study. *Orthop Rev (Pavia)* 2013, 5 (1): e7.

[4] Kingma I, van Dieen JH: Static and dynamic postural loadings during computer work in females: Sitting on an office chair versus sitting on an exercise ball. *Appl Ergon* 2009, 40 (2): 199-205.

[5] McGill SM, Kavcic NS, Harvey E: Sitting on a chair or an exercise ball: various perspectives to guide decision making. *Clin Biomech (Bristol, Avon)* 2006, 21 (4): 353-360.

[6] O'Sullivan K, McCarthy R, White A, O'Sullivan L, Dankaerts W: Lumbar posture and trunk muscle activation during a typing task when sitting on a novel dynamic ergonomic chair. *Ergonomics* 2012, 55 (12): 1586-1595.

[7] McGill SM, Hughson RL, Parks K: Lumbar erector spinae oxygenation during prolonged contractions: implications for prolonged work. *Ergonomics* 2000, 43 (4): 486-493.

[8] Reenalda J, Van Geffen P, Nederhand M, Jannink M, M IJ, Rietman H: Analysis of healthy sitting behavior: interface pressure distribution and subcutaneous tissue oxygenation. *J Rehabil Res Dev* 2009, 46 (5): 577-586.

[9] van Deursen DL, Snijders CJ, van Dieen JH, Kingma I, van Deursen LL: The effect of passive vertebral rotation on pressure in the nucleus pulposus. *J Biomech* 2001, 34 (3): 405-408.

[10] Zemp R, Taylor WR, Lorenzetti S: In vivo spinal posture during upright and reclined sitting in an office chair. *Biomed Res Int* 2013, 2013: 916045.

[11] Karlsson A, Norrlin S, Silander HC, Dahl M, Lanshammar H: Amplitude and frequency analysis of force plate data in sitting children with and without MMC. *Clin Biomech (Bristol, Avon)* 2000, 15 (7): 541-545.

[12] Willigenburg NW, Kingma I, van Dieen JH: Center of pressure trajectories, trunk kinematics and trunk muscle activation during unstable sitting in low back pain patients. *Gait Posture* 2013, 38 (4): 625-630.

[13] Kirn B, Starc V: The video technique developed for measuring epicardial strains on guinea pig's left ventricle. *J Biomech* 2005, 38 (1): 169-173.

[14] Dunk NM, Callaghan JP: Lumbar spine movement patterns during prolonged sitting differentiate low back pain developers from matched asymptomatic controls. *Work* 2010, 35 (1): 3-14.

[15] Mazaheri M, Coenen P, Parnianpour M, Kiers H, van Dieen JH: Low back pain and postural sway during quiet standing with and without sensory manipulation: a systematic review. *Gait Posture* 2013, 37 (1): 12-22.

[16] Willigenburg NW, Kingma I, van Dieen JH: Precision control of an upright trunk posture in low back pain patients. *Clin Biomech (Bristol, Avon)* 2012, 27 (9): 866-871.

[17] van Dieen JH, Koppes LL, Twisk JW: Low back pain history and postural sway in unstable sitting. *Spine (Phila Pa 1976)* 2010, 35 (7): 812-817.

[18] O'Sullivan K, O'Keeffe M, O'Sullivan L, O'Sullivan P, Dankaerts W: The effect of dynamic sitting on the prevention and management of low back pain and low back discomfort: a systematic review. *Ergonomics* 2012, 55 (8): 898-908.

19

Analysis of the Conducts of Elite Futsal Goalkeeper in the Different Situations of the Game

A. Paz-Franco[1,*], A. Bores-Cerezal[2], R. Barcala-Furelos[3], M. Mecias-Calvo[4]

[1]Physical Coach, Al Wahda Futsal, Abu Dhabi, UAE
[2]Physical Coach, Spain National Team, Spain
[3]Special Didactics, University of Vigo, Spain
[4]Physical Coach, Santiago Futsal, Spain
*Corresponding author: info@adrianpaz.com

Abstract The analysis of Futsal goalkeeper acquires great relevance due to the characteristics demanded by the competition that requires its position with respect to the other players and the importance that has this specific position in the game. For this reason we have analyzed the existing interactions between the conducts of the Futsal goalkeeper and different variables (actions, play area, goal-block or error-goal, game situation and team). We have used and observational methodology, because it is one the options of the scientific study of the behavior, as much in real situations as in controlled situations. The results show that in the shots made to the goal, a 76.5% of them are goalkeeper interventions, in situation of positional attack (54%), with an incidence in the game on the sidelines areas of the field (L-39%, R-33%) and being the technical action more important the cross (33.7%). Therefore, it is observed relation between the goalkeeper's action and the zone where the opponent shots, between the actions performed by the goalkeeper and the goal (success-block/error-goal), and between the action and the belonging to a specific team. Otherwise, it is not observed relation between goalkeeper's action and the diverse situations of the game.

Keywords: *indoor soccer, team sports, technique, motor action, training*

1. Introduction

Futsal is a team sport, that it is characterized by the playful-motor situation of regulated and institutionalized competition, and which it is been from the interactions of cooperation-opposition that occurs between the sportsmen and the means in which they interact (Moreno, 1994).

The elite sport is any organized physical exercise prescribed, in that the training and the competition occupy most of the time and in which the level of exigency is maximum (Coakley, 1983), and that in addition to reach and to maintain the maximum performance, the sportsman uses almost all his time training, which requires physical, mental and social dedication completely (Wylleman, De Knop, Mekenhorst, Theeboom, Annerel, 1993).

The performance in the team sports is the result of the capacity of physical and psychic skills of the different players in its collaboration and also of its capacity of cooperative acting (Konzag, Döber & Herzog, 1997), developed in conditions of individual and collective fight with the adversaries (Hernández Moreno, 1994; Teodorescu, 1984), in changing surroundings that selectively grant greater or smaller relevance to the conducts of game in the partial and final performance (Álvaro et al, 1996; Martín Acero, 1993; Seirul-lo, 1993, 1998), with a certain system of game that it is the set of norms that govern the individual, group and collective actions with the objective to obtain the maximum performance of all the equipment and players (Espar, Gerona, 2004).

Martín Acero y Vittori (1997), indicate that without sufficient, multimethodical and coordinated scientific researches that they leave from the necessities of the practice one will not advance in the elaboration of a Theory of the Collective Sport Games. And, therefore, in the validation or negation of the training routines that indeed are able to improve the levels of performance of the sportsmen (Research- Action).

Diverse publications and studies on the reality of the goalkeeper, they try to observe the variables that condition their conduct, as well as the diverse actions they make (Antúnez et al, 2010; LLopis, 2010; Medina et al, 2010; Mulqueen, Woltalla, 2011; Pascual, 2011, Edelman, 2011). Consequently, one becomes necessary to work of specific and individualized way by means of a progression adapted to the referred sport modality, so that we prepare to the goalkeeper for the competition (García, 1997; Hernández Moreno, 2001; Igea, 1997; Medina et al, 2009; Medina et al, 2010).

Like in other collective sports such as soccer, basketball, handball or the hockey, in Futsal the initial positioning of the players is made starting off with specific positions.

Those positions are a concrete space that each player in the game land occupies, based on the game system that is applied in a while certain of the game (Antón, 1993). We can consider that the specific position of each player varies mainly based on the game system but principally, if the team is in offensive or defensive phase. This does not happen in case of the goalkeeper, who will hold its position and its functions in the defensive phase is referred.

Diverse specialists talk about the Futsal's goalkeeper and its necessary and continued adaptation to make their specific tasks (Bárcenas, 1976; Bárcenas, Román, 1991; Czerwinski, 1993; Paccoud, 1990; Román, 1995), agreeing these authors in equipping with manifest singularity to this figure, accentuated by its dualidad of functions: offensive and defensive, and justified by the importance of its incidence in the outcome of the game.

The fulfillment of the tasks and own exigencies of the specific position of the goalkeeper, is developed in that medium complex and multiform, and are influenced by the circumstantial aspects of the game and the regulation (Antúnez, 2003).

Like in soccer, handball or hockey where the roll of doorman or goalkeeper exists (Sampedro, 1999), the real situation in the most of the games, it will be the last opposing to surpass by the opposite team before obtaining the goal, with the responsibility that it entails. To Palau (2002), the doorman of elite Futsal is a determining factor during the competition, because its performance to a great extent determines the success or the failure of the team. A good preparation, adapted the requirements of the competition, will arrange to the goalkeeper in situation to have greater percentage of success in its interventions.

According to Mutti (2003), the position of the goalkeeper is the most important in Futsal; no other demands that the sportsman is a specialist with respect to their position. This specificity comes marked by its positioning in the field (last player to defend the goal, observes all the game) and for being the only player who has a space of the delimited field where its behavior can be different with respect to the other players. To Fonseca (2001), difference to the goalkeeper of the rest of players because he is the only player with his own characteristics, which make him different from the other members of the team. Mutti (2003), adds that the participation of the goalkeeper in the game in relation to the success (stopped) or error (goal) has a very high incidence and consequently in the performance as much of companions as of adversaries. For that reason he deserves a special consideration and specific training, looking for the purpose of equipping it with the conditions demanded by its position and compatible with its responsibility in the game.

The goalkepeer can be considered in his double function, like the first attacker or the last defender in his collective contribution. In sequence of importance and by the transcendence of its actions, it is possible to be turned in to the most decisive player of all. To Sampedro (1993), the situation, position, the task to develop within the game and, mainly, the regulation, give a differentiating character between the remaining players. This player, as Valdano says (1997), talking about the doorman, it has the audacity to use his hands, in a sport that thinks with the head and it gambles eminently with the foot. As well, the regulation forces the goalkeeper to dress a different color shirt from its companions, adversaries and referees.

The goalkeeper is a specific position that demands special characteristics and, therefore, it must dominate all the facets of the game, own and the pertaining ones to other specific positions, depending on the functions that must fulfill; and that in addition is put under the different interpretations from the regulation, according to its location on the game field.

Therefore, the object of study of the present I articulate has been to analyze the behavior of the goalkeeper of Elite Futsal in the different situations from game, thus to be able to respond to the questions that determine the study object: How influences the diverse variables in the elite doorman? Can condition their conduct before a certain action of the game? Realize always the same motor actions before different situations from the game?

2. Material and Method

This study considers from an observational investigation (Figure 1). Having been analyzed the games corresponding to the XXII Futsal Spain King Cup celebrated in Segovia, from February 3rd to February 6th 2011, in where the 8 first teams of the First Division Spain at the end of the first part of the competition have competed: el Barcelona, El Pozo, Interviú, Manacor, Autos Lobelle, Triman Navarra, Benicarló, Caja Segovia, obtaining a sample (n=16) during the course of the competition. The studied variables are: actions of the goalkeeper, team, zone of the field, conditioners and goal.

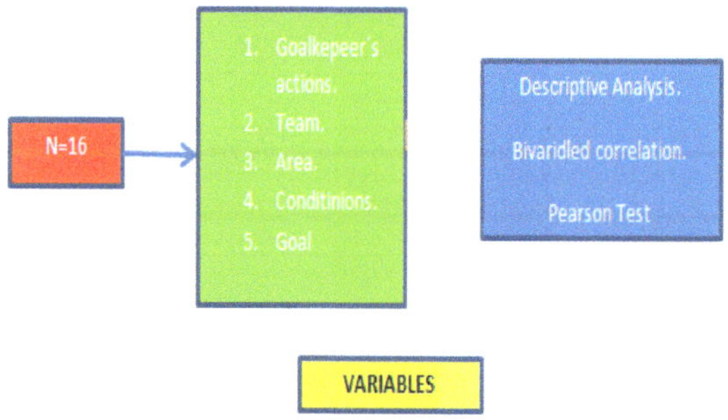

Figure 1. Investigation scheme

For the analysis of the variables has been used software ASTRO Sport Systems, whose purpose is to provide digital support to the Futsal's technicians and players. Actually, it is a common tool used in national teams or to analyze Futsal's great championships.

The procedure used has been divided into three phases. In first place, the captures of the actions required for the investigation were made. In the second phase the captures are analyzed being transferred the observation to a list ad-hoc that divides the field of game in 8 zones (Figure 2).

The third and last phase supposed the statistical treatment of the data for which the program SPSS 19.0. was used, analyzing the measures of central tendency (average, typical deviation, etc.) and, in a descriptive form, the different selected variables: actions of the Futsal's goalkeeper, zone of the field, conditioners, goals and team. Also, the test of Pearson was created for the analysis between variables, getting the correlation between variables: success, zone, conditions and actions. In order to obtain the results of this last mentioned test between variables, the test of bivaried correlations was used. The level of signification was set at 95%.

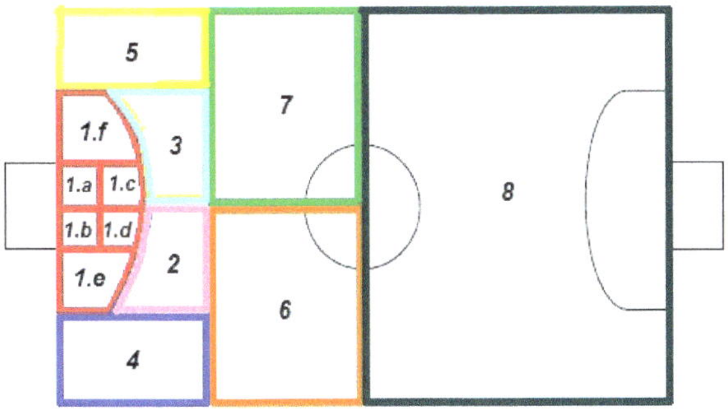

Figure 2. Futsal's field áreas

3. Results

We observed the predominant action of the goalkeeper is the cross-foot action (Figure 3), within 17.35%, followed by the action hand-deviation, within 10.2%. It is observed as most of the results appear in the initial values, range of values pertaining to cross actions (33.7%) and split (18.9%), representing a 52.6% of total actions.

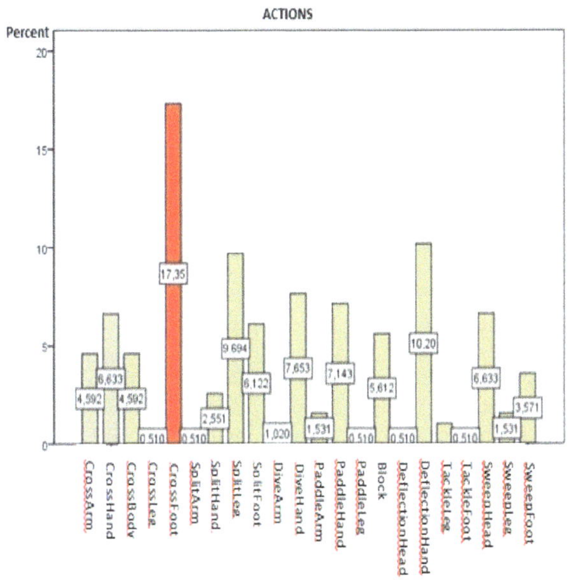

Figure 3. Variable Goalkeeper's actions

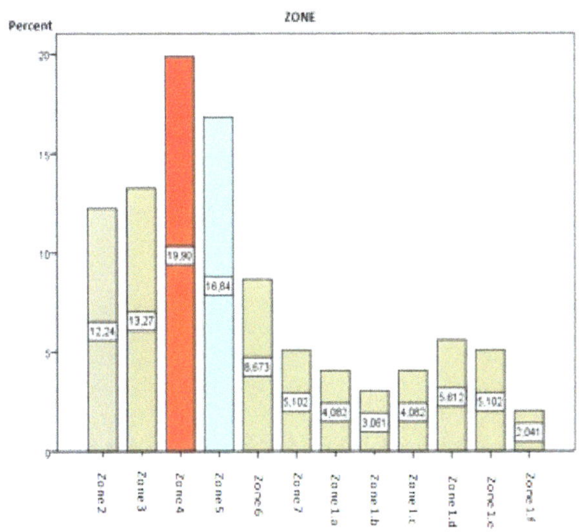

Figure 4. Variable Futsal's field areas

In the frequencies obtained for the zone variable (Figure 4), they emphasize the values obtained for zone 4 (19.9%) and zone 5 (16.84%) representing the zones with greater incidence in the game, being these two lateral zones from where the goalkeeper receives the greater amount of shots on goal. If in addition we include the central zones 2 and 3, within 12.24% and 13.27% respectively, we obtain a 62.25% of the shots on goal are made from the adjacent zones to the area, that is to say, from the periphery.

The constraint that is more repeated is the situation of 4x4 (54.08%) followed by the situation of 5x4 -known as player-goalkeeper- (7.1%), being the rest 38.82% situations of superiorities or inferiorities, both offensives and defensives (Figure 5).

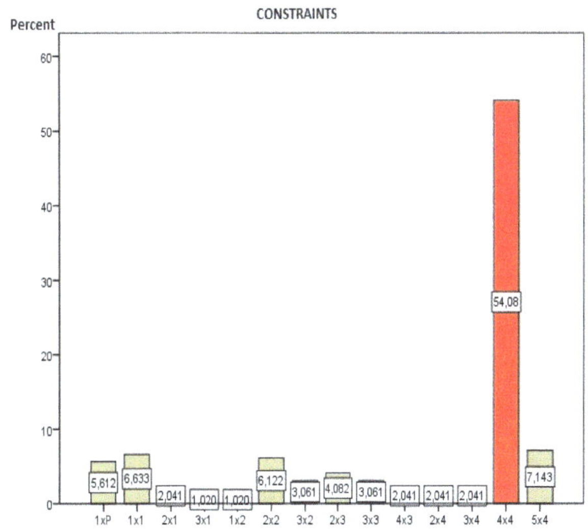

Figure 5. Variable Constraints

In the frequencies obtained for the variable Goals (Success), the save (G0), represents 76.5% from total of the sample (Figure 6), whereas 23.5% remaining one shows the conducts of the goalkeeper that finalize in goal, being the zones G1, G3 and G9 (Figure 7) those that respectively represent a greater index of getting a goal on the part of the adversary with a 4.5% each one of the zones, with respect to 23.5% total.

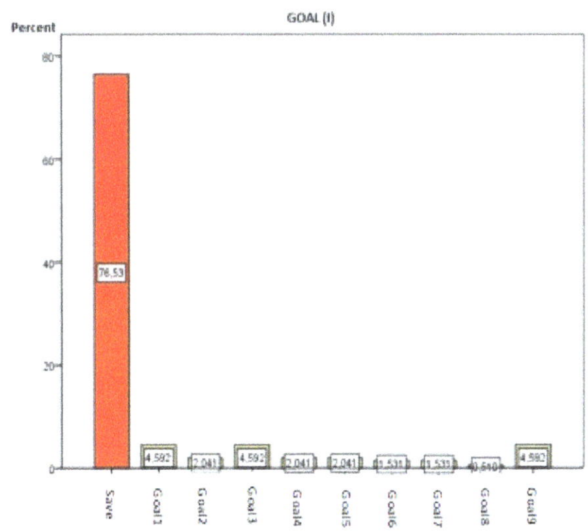

Figure 6. Variable Goals (I)

The fitted Goals represent 23.5% of the total of the interventions of the doorman, in who many of the actions are erroneous (Figure 7). In the erroneous actions, there are 3 zones of goal that have greater incidence as far as the reception of a goal: Goal Zone 1, Goal Zone 3 and Goal Zone 9, with a 4.5 % respectively, that it supposes 13.5% on 23.5% of the total of fitted goals.

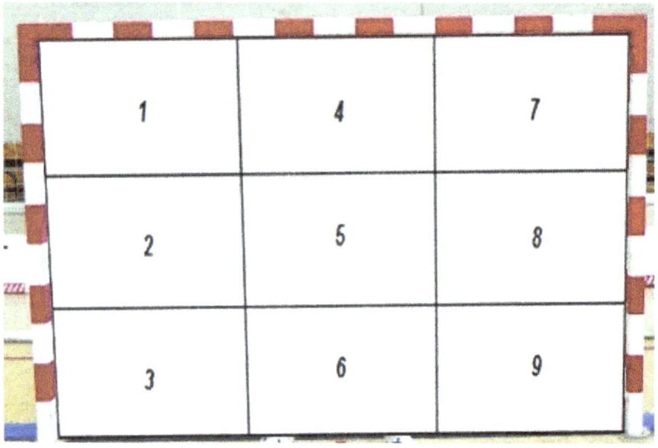

Figure 7. Variable Goals (II)

At sight of the obtained results we have made a statistical analysis between the different variables, with the objective to observe the existing relation between the same ones, determining which relations exist between the variable "Actions" and the rest of variables: Zone, Goal and Team. The level of signification has been set to (p = 0.004), (p = 0.010) and (p = 0.001) respectively, observaing that the action to perfom by the goalkeeper has a close relation with the Zone where the opponent is shooting, what will determine a certain motor action or another one, in the same way that an incorrect action of the goalkeeper is going to be negative for its team: the Goal. It is observed in the same way, as the property to a determined Team influences in the motor action to make by the Futsal's goalkeeper.

By contrast, it is not observed a relation between the variables Actions and Constraints (p=0.786), that is to say, the game situations that occur previous to any shot on goal (4x4, 3x2, 2x1...) they do not influence in the motor action of the goalkeeper.

4. Discussion

In order to know the real potential of productivity of the sportsman, it is necessary to relate it to the demands in the official games with competitive perspective, because these will be the indicators to program later training.

Van Lingen (1999), states that if one is just allowing players to run or to increase "gymnasium" training to fortify itself, then the only thing that will be obtained is to reinforce the muscle to carry out all those movements. Therefore, the factors that we must analyze and consider in a training planning are those that the player demands, according to its technical-tactical and psychological work to do during the competition. Nevertheless, another percentage to increase the performance must, by the direct influence that it has, to the sport diet, the social situation and the system of daily civic-sport life of the player. Being the situations ignored and not contemplated in the planning, and that are insofar determining for the performance. The tendency of the training system has to have an integral character taking into account the sportsman from a holistic perspective, leaving back the analytic scheme and being this decompensated (to separate technical aspect from the physical and psychological ones).

Seiru-lo (2000), maintains that the separation of body and mind no longer exists, the human being must be educated and trained as a unique process of optimization of the sportsman. When training a team, the planning is born from the individual, that is to say, according to its function and capacity it faces various game actions requiring different answers each time, as it happens in a competitive match. By automating excessively exercises are working only a portion of the athlete, both cognitively and physically. It can be valuable in psycho motor sports, but not in social motor sports.

Futsal, as a team sport provides many complex situations which pose a major challenge in terms of decision-making (Greháigne, Godbout, Bouthier, 2001). Motor skills that occur in team sports are characterized, principally, because the necessity to adapt to changing environment where they develop. Therefore, in performing this type of work, besides the technical component of motor performance, it is required by the player to employ tactical conducts that enable him to give competent performance in each stage of the game (Thomas, Thomas, 1994). Team sports involve, essentially, a series of sequences and game situations that are added to every moment, making it difficult to get an identical reproduction (Ruiz, 1994). That is why, these sports require from the player, additionally unlike individual sports, cognitive activities of perception and decision making.

In 1963, Barbara Knapp says that skill in team sports is determined by technique and decision making, understanding the technique as the ability to carry out the motor component of the action, and decision making as knowledge to choose the right technique based on the particular situation where the action is playing.

Cognitive components include knowledge and decision making, while the skill component would correspond to motor execution (Iglesias, Ramos, Fuentes, Sanz, Del Villar, 2003). Therefore, the quality of decision-making in a game situation is as important as the execution of motor skills, both being crucial to athletic performance (Thomas, 1994; Blomqvist, Luhtanen, Laakso, 2001).

The formation and maintenance of an elite athlete should be complete, avoiding as much as possible not to leave anything to chance. As we ascend to the next levels of sport's requirement, this increases the variables to be controlled and requires an increasingly scientific and technological support. These factors of performance indicate that the elite goalkeeper's profile is fitted perfectly to this profile of performance, being capable to be investigated.

Comparing the results with those of similar studies, we observed that from all of the observed actions, a 76.5%, were successful, while a 23.5% of the motor actions finished in Goal (Figure 6). Martín Rascón (2009), reflects in his study similar results to those obtained here, being 74% of motor actions successful and 26% of motor actions that ended in a goal.

Regarding to shooting zones, the results show a higher incidence in the lateral zones, 4 and 5 (Figure 2), with

19,9% and 16,84% (Figure 4) respectively of the total, while Martín Rascón (2009) highlights the central area (47%) as the highest, in terms of incidence.

By contrast, the results obtained by Ferreira (1998), are similar to ours, emphasizing the lateral areas, with 22% and 16% respectively, as the areas of greatest impact on the game.

For areas where the goalkeeper receives more goals, are G1, G3 y G9 with 19.25% respectively each (Figure 7), coinciding zones G3 y G9 with the results obtained by Martín Rascón (2009) in his study, in which further emphasizes as incident area, the right side of the goal, with 52% of total incidence, which considered a problem because most of the porters are right-handed.

5. Conclusions

The game situations before a shot on goal do not determine motor action to be performed by the Futsal goalkeeper. Regardless of the game situation (3x2, 4x4, 2x2, etc.) their are other variables that will affect their motor action. The first is belonging to a particular team. The existence of diverse methodologies combined with the idea that each professional athlete has in their area of work can cause training differences in respect to different clubs.

By contrast, motor actions are closely related to the firing on goal, since it determines that the performance by the goalkeeper in one or another way. We can say that even without driving action types exist in each area, if there are predominant motor actions in each of the same.

They, also, will determine the success or failure of launches to the rivals goal, determining largely the outcome of the action. Since the proper execution of a specific motor action and the correct choice of the same for any given game situation, will the futsal goalkeeper ready to make a save (success) in that game situation, assuming an erroneous choosing a goal against.

Sampedro (1997) says that "the keeper error as last player is hardly remediable by a teammate".

References

[1] Abernethy, B. (1996). Training the visual-perceptual skills of athletes. The American Journal of Sports Medicine, 24, 89-92.

[2] Abernethy, B., Kippers, V., Mackinnon, L. T., Neal, N. J., y Harharan, S. J. (1997). The Biophysical Foundations of Human Movement. Champain, IL., Human Kinetics, pp. 295-311.

[3] Álvaro, J.; Dorado, A.; González Badillo, JJ.; González, J.L.; Navarro, F.; Molina, JJ.; Portolés, J.; Sánchez, F. (1996). Modelo de análisis de los deportes colectivos basado en el rendimiento en competición, INFOCOES, 7, 21-41.

[4] Anguera, M.T., Blanco, A., Losada, J.L., Hernández Mendo, A. (2000): *La metodología observacional en el deporte: conceptos básicos. Lecturas: Educación Física y Deportes, 5 (24).* (http//www.efdeportes.com/efd24/obs.htm).

[5] Antón, J. L. (1993). Hacia una lógica conceptual en Balonmano. Ponencia presentada en Congreso Internacional de Especialistas en Balonmano. Madrid.

[6] Antúnez, A. (2003). La interceptación en la portera de balonmano: efectos de un programa de entrenamiento perceptivo-motriz. Madrid: C.V. Ciencias del Deporte.

[7] Antúnez, A., García, M. M., Argudo, F. M., Ruiz, E., & Arias, J. L. (2010). Resultado de un programa de entrenamiento perceptivo-motor sobre la eficacia en competición de la portera de balonmano según la oposición del lanzador. / result of a perceptive-motor trining program on the efficacy in competition from handball female goalkeeper according to the thrower opposition. Revista Kronos, 9(17), 29-37.

[8] Barbero Álvarez JC , D´Ottavio S , Granda Vera J, Castagna C. (2009). Aerobic fitness in futsal players of different competitive level. J Strength Cond, Res 23: 2163-6.

[9] Bárcenas, D. (1976). Técnica. Madrid: Federación Española de Balonmano.

[10] Bárcenas, D. y Román, J. D. (1991). Balonmano: Técnica y Metodología. Madrid: Gymnos.

[11] Blomqvist, M., Luhtanen, P., y Laakso, L. (2001). Comparison of two types of instruction in badminton. European Journal of Physical Education, 6, 139-155.

[12] Casáis Martínez, Luis. Rey Eiras, Ezquiel. Apuntes de Fundamentos de los Deportes Colectivos I: Balonmano. 2012, Facultad de las Ciencias de la educación y del deporte, Universidad de Vigo.

[13] Coakley, J. (1983). *Leaving Competitive Sport: Retirement or Rebirth?*, Human Kinetics Journals, QUEST volume 35, Issue 1, February.

[14] Czerwinski, J. (1993). El Balonmano, técnica, táctica y entrenamiento. Barcelona: Paidotribo.

[15] Dellal A, Hil-Haas S, Lago-Penas C, Chamari K. Small-sided games in soccer: amateur vs. professional players' physiological responses, physical, and technical activities. J Strength Cond Res 2011; 25: 2371-81.

[16] Edelman, B. (2011). *The goalkeeper.* Directed by S. Timoshenko, screenplay by Lev Kassil. USSR: Lenfilm, 1936 *Bob Edelman Soccer & Society*, 1743-9590, Volume 12, Issue 1, 2011, Pages 42-43.

[17] Espar y Gerona (2004). Elementos para el diseño de tareas del entrenamiento en los deportes de equipo, Master Profesional en Alto Rendimiento en Deportes de Equipo. Área Coordinativa, Barcelona. Byomedic – Fundació F.C. Barcelona.

[18] Ferreira, P. (1998). "Caracterização da finalização em equipas de Futsal". UNICAMP (SP), 1998.

[19] Fonseca, G.M.M. (2001). Futsal – treinamento para goleiros 2. ed. Rio de Janeiro: Editora Sprint Ltda, 2001

[20] García, A. R. (1997). Análisis de los gestos técnicos y acciones del juego en fútbol sala recurso electrónico (Versión 1.0 ed.). Madrid Gymnos, D.L. 1997: Gymnos.

[21] González Víllora, S., Gutiérrez, D., Pastor, C., Fernández, J. (2007). Análisis funcional de los deportes de invasión: importancia del subsistema técnico-táctico en el juego. Concreción en el Fútbol. Retos. Nuevas tendencias en educación física, deporte y recreación. 2007, nº12, pp18-28.

[22] Gréhaigne, J. F., Godbout, P., y Bouthier, D. (2001). The teaching and learning of decision making in team sports. Quest, 53, 59-76.

[23] Hernández Moreno, J. (2001). Análisis de los parámetros espacio y tiempo en el fútbol sala. la distancia recorrida, el ritmo y dirección del desplazamiento del jugador durante un encuentro de competición: Los casos de J. gay (defensa), C. marrero (cierre), J. beto (pivote), J. limones (ala) y J. clavería (portero). Apunts.Educación Física y Deportes, (65), 33-44.

[24] Hernández Moreno, J. (1994): Análisis de las estructuras del juego deportivo. Fundamentos del deporte, Barcelona: INDE.

[25] Igea, J. M., & Durán, R. (1997). El portero en el fútbol sala. Madrid Gymnos, 1997: Gymnos.

[26] Iglesias, D., Ramos, L. A., Fuentes, J. P., Sanz, D., y Del Villar, F. (2003). El conocimiento y la toma de decisiones en los deportes de equipo: una revisión desde la perspectiva cognitiva. Revista de Entrenamiento Deportivo, 17, 2, 5-11.

[27] Knapp, B. H. (1963). Skill in sport: the attainment of proficiency. Routledge and Kegan Paul, London.

[28] Konzag, I.; Döbler, H.; Herzog, H-D. (1997). Entrenarse jugando, Barcelona. Paidotribo.

[29] Lago Peñas, Carlos. Apuntes de Fundamentos de los Deportes Colectivos I: Fútbol. 2011, Facultad de Ciencias de la educación y deporte, Universidad de Vigo.

[30] LLopis, L. (2010). *Implicación y relación del portero en el juego colectivo.* Madrid 2010: Revista ABFUTBOL.

[31] Makaje N, Ruangthai R, Arkarapanthu A, Yoopat P. (2012). Physiological demands and activity profiles during futsal match play according to competitive level. J Sports Med Phys Fitness, 52(4):366-74.

[32] Martín Acero, R. (1993). Velocidad y velocidad en deportes de equipo, Colección CadernosTécnico-Pedagóxicos do INEF de Galicia, A Coruña. Centro Galego de Documentación e Edicións Deportivas.

[33] Martín Acero, R; Vittori, C. (1997). Metodología del rendimiento deportivo (I): Sentido, definición y objeto de estudio, Revista de Entrenamiento Deportivo, XI, 1, 5-10.

[34] Martín Rascón, J. (2009). *¿Dónde radica el error del gol en Fútbol Sala? Análisis del portero.* Revista Internacional de Deportes Colectivos. 2, 36-57.

[35] Milanez VF, Pedro RE, Moreira A, Boullosa DA, Salle-Neto F, Nakamura FY. (2011). The Role of Aerobic Fitness on Session Rating of Perceived Exertion in Futsal Players. Int J Sports Physiol Perform, 6; 358-66.

[36] Medina, A. A., del, M. G., Iturriaga, F. M. A., Lara, E. R., & Artero, J. L. A. (2009). Efecto de un programa de entrenamiento perceptivo-motor sobre la eficacia global de la portera de balonmano en CompeticiÓn. / effect of a perceptive-motor training program on the global efficacy from handball female goalkeeper in competition. / efeito de um programa de treinamento perceptivo-motor sobre a eficacia global da golera de handbol na CompetiÇao. Cuadernos De Psicología Del Deporte, 9(2), 31-43.

[37] Medina, A. A., del, M. G., Iturriaga, F. M. A., Lara, E. R., & Artero, J. L. A. (2010). Entrenamiento perceptivo en la portera de balonmano ante la trayectoria del tiro. Revista Internacional De Medicina y Ciencias De La Actividad Física y Del Deporte, nº37.

[38] Moreno, J.H. (1994). Fundamentos del deporte. Analisis de las estructuras del juego desportivo. 1.ed. Barcelona: Inde Publicaciones, 1994.

[39] Mulqueen, T., Woltalla, M. (2011). *The Complete Soccer Goalkeeper: Techniques and Tactics for Stopping Every Shot.* Soccer Journal May/Jun2011, Vol. 56 Issue 3, p54 2p.

[40] Mutti, D. (2003). Futsal: da iniciação ao alto nível. 2 ed. São Paulo: Phorte, 2003.

[41] Paccoud, B. (1990). L' entrainement du gardien de but. EPS, 40, 39-42.

[42] Palau, X. (2002) Apuntes de Preparación física aplicada al fútbol sala. Curso de 2º nivel de Entrenadores. Centro de Alto Rendimiento de Sant Cugat, Barcelona.

[43] Pascual, J. (2011). *Manual técnico del portero de fútbol.* Barcelona 2011: Paidotribo.

[44] Román, J. D. (1995). El portero. En Real Federación Española de Balonmano (Ed.), Clinics Deportes de Base y de Entrenadores de Élite, (pp. 15-16). Madrid: RFEBM.

[45] Ruiz, L. M. (1994). Deporte y aprendizaje. Procesos de adquisición y desarrollo de habilidades. Madrid: Visor.

[46] Ruiz-Risueño, J., De la Cruz Sanchez, E. (2008). El papel del entrenador en la capacidad decisional de los jugadores. Retos. Nuevas tendencias en Educación Física, Deporte y Recreación. 2008, nº 13, pp. 5-10.

[47] Sampedro, J. (1993). *Iniciación al Fútbol Sala.* Madrid 1993: Gymnos.

[48] Sampedro, J. (1997). "Análisis praxiológico de los deportes de equipo: una aplicación al futbol sala". Director: José Hernández Moreno. Universidad Politécnica de Madrid, 1997.

[49] Sampedro, J. (1999). Fundamentos de táctica deportiva. Análisis de la estrategia de los deportes. Madrid: Gymnos.

[50] Seirul-lo, F. (1993). Planificación del entrenamiento en deportes de equipo, Master en Alto Redimiento Deportivo. Módulo 2.1.7., Madrid. C.O.E.-Universidad Autónoma de Madrid.

[51] Seirulo, F. (1998). Preparación física en deportes de equipo, Curso de Postgrado en Preparación Física, A Coruña, no publicado.

[52] Seirul.lo, F. (2000) Una línea de trabajo distinta. I Jornadas de Actualización de Preparadores Físicos, COE, 5 de Junio.

[53] Teodorescu, L. (1984). Problemas de teoria e metodogia nos jogos desportivos, Lisboa. Livros Horizonte.

[54] Thomas, K. T. (1994). The development of sport expertise: From Leeds to MVP legend. Quest, 46, 211-222.

[55] Valdano, J. (1997). *Los cuadernos de Valdano.* Madrid. El Pais-Aguilar.

[56] Van Lingen, Bert. (1999) Captación de talentos en holanda. Nazioarteko futbol elkaraldiak. Editorial Bizkaiko Foru Aldundia, Bizkaia, 155-165.

[57] Vera, G., Pino, J., Romero, C., Moreno, I. (2007). Propuesta de valoración técnico-táctica mediante una situación de juego colectivo básico en el fútbol de iniciación. Retos. Nuevas tendencias en Educación Física, Deporte y Recreación. 2007, nº12, pp. 29-35.

[58] Wylleman, P., De Knop, P., Menkehorst, H., Theeboom, M., y Annerel, J. (1993). Career termination and social integration among elite athletes. In S. Serpa, J. Alves, V. Ferreira, & A. Paula-Brito (Eds.), Proceedings of the VIII World Congress of Sport Psychology (pp. 902-906). Lisbon: International Society of Sport Psychology.

Effect of Anthropometric Characteristics and Socio-Economic Status on Vertical Jumping Performances in Tunisian Athletic Children

C Aouichaoui[1,*], Y Trabelsi[1], Z Tabka[1], M Dogui[2], JP Richalet[3], E Bouhlel[1]

[1]Laboratory of Physiology and Lung Function Testing, Faculty of Medicine Ibn-El-Jazzar, University of Sousse, Sousse, Tunisia
[2]Laboratory of Physiology, Faculty of Medicine, Monastir, Tunisia
[3]Laboratory of Cellular and Functional Responses to Hypoxia, University of Paris 13, Bobigny, France
*Corresponding author: chirineaouichaoui@yahoo.com

Abstract The purpose of this study was to examine the effect of socioeconomic factors on vertical jumping performance as well as on anthropometric parameters in athletic Tunisian children aged 7 to 13 in both sexes.
Four hundred and seven athletic Tunisian children (218 boys and 189 girls) ranging from 7 to 13 were randomly selected to participate in our study. They were asked to perform Squat jumps (SJ) and Countermovement jumps (CMJ) and to response to a questionnaire. Jump heights and leg power were simultaneously provided by the optojump device. Correlations and regression models were calculated in order to identify which factors influenced jumping performance variables. In our population of athletic Tunisian children, the socioeconomic status did not influence vertical jumping parameters whereas morphological factors were the main predictive factors of jumping. This research may help verifying the effectiveness of a specific training program and detecting highly talented athletes.

Keywords: *squat jump, countermovement jump, athlete, child, socioeconomic status*

1. Introduction

Assessment of aerobic metabolism during growth and maturation has been extensively studied in children. However, short-term maximal anaerobic power remains relatively poorly understood [48], particularly in trained children. This could be attributed to ethical considerations and/or the difficulties to recruit young trained subjects. Anaerobic metabolism, force, velocity and peak power are determinant factors in many physical activities and sports. Most of the studies on the anaerobic metabolism have been done on sedentary children using cycle ergometer [14,29,47]. Little attention has been paid to the vertical jump test which allows the estimation of the peak power of lower limbs [7]. The vertical jump test has emerged as a consistent test in adults as well as for children [47]. Some studies showed significant correlations between the force-velocity test and the vertical jump [8,47]. This field test is easy and could be realized in a great population. Several factors could affect the performance during the test. Some of these factors are related to the tested participants (e.g differences in gender, age, body composition, growth and maturity) [10,21], while others are predominantly related to lifestyle factors such as physical activity, environmental conditions, sport selection and training [5]. Indeed, there are high correlations between jump performances and maximal anaerobic power [47]. Powerful athletes have high percentage of fast-twitch muscle fibres and high muscle performances. Specific anaerobic training, by using jumps and/or short sprints enhance ATP production by the anaerobic system (ATP-PC and anaerobic glycolysis). The mechanisms responsible for the reported improvements in anaerobic pathways are also related to improvements in aerobic fitness [4]. In addition, mechanisms responsible for jump performances enhancements are mainly related to muscle mechanical proprieties, such as contractile and elastic components [20], muscle type and architecture [15]. Repeated brief actions, such as sprints, or jumps depends essentially in both contractile and metabolic factors, such as energy supply (e.g. phosphocreatine utilisation and resynthesis), CPK enzymatic activity, calcium liberation, and improvements in H+ regulation [4].

An environmental factor, such as socioeconomic status (SES) is of great interest to those who study children's development. Indeed, some studies showed that low SES children have lower maximal anaerobic power than high SES children [6]. The authors suggested the role of negative energetic balance in the limitation of muscle power in such children.

Identification of factors influencing the development of muscle power may lead to specific strategies to select young athletes, distinguish between different performance levels, or provide normative data for various athletic or patient populations [10]. Factors which determine anaerobic performance include muscle quantity, muscle fibre type, musculoskeletal architecture, and neuromuscular activation [23,50].

During growth, a short-term performance, such as jumping, throwing and short sprinting depends essentially on the anaerobic mechanisms. In this context, the ability to produce short-term maximal anaerobic power is related in part to variation in age, sexes, body size, especially fat-free mass and muscle cross-sectional area [14,29]. For example, Buchanan & Vardaxis [10] showed that height and weight are important predictors of muscle strength in young players. However, it has suggested that development changes in muscle power cannot be explained merely by quantitative changes in growth [14]. Other factors such as altitude, socioeconomic status, and children's physical fitness levels may also influence short-term maximal anaerobic power among children [5,6].

Some studies have shown that short-term anaerobic power is significantly affected by socioeconomic and nutritional status. Blonc et al. [6] showed that socioeconomic status had significant effects on aerobic and anaerobic power in prepubertal Bolivian girls. Anaerobic power (Pmax, force-velocity test, wingate test) was reduced in low socioeconomic status (LSES) Bolivian girls at both high and low altitude. Bedu et al. [2] found also that LSES Bolivian boys have lower peak power values developed during anaerobic exercises. The authors suggested the weaker maximal power observed in LSES boys in comparison with high socioeconomic status (HSES), as a direct consequence of impaired structural and metabolic muscle function due to nutritional deprivation during childhood, especially muscle volume and enzymes activities responsible for both anaerobic glycolysis and oxidative metabolism. Moreover, Jiménez Pavón et al. [18] showed positive associations between socioeconomic status and lower body muscular strength (standing long jump, squat jump, counter movement jump and Abalakov jump) in European adolescents. The low socioeconomic status, as assessed by family affluence, influences physical fitness (upper body muscular strength) in European adolescents independently of total body fat and habitual physical activity. The family affluence scale was used as an index of socioeconomic status, which includes 4 questions answered by the child: do you have your own bedroom? How many cars are there in your family? How many PC are there in your home? Do you have internet access at home? By contrast, in elderly person, Rantanen et al. [33] demonstrated that the socioeconomic status was not associated with muscle force. Syddal et al. [40] showed also that lower social class was associated with falls in grip strength among older women only. They reported that negative social circumstances characterized essentially by material deprivation.

More recently, Trabelsi et al. [45] showed that lung function parameters in healthy Tunisian children were influenced by socioeconomic status. However, little attention has been paid to the relationship between socioeconomic status, anthropometric variables and vertical jumping parameters in Tunisian athletic children.

The majority of research studies have examined the relationships between leg power and anthropometric parameters [9,10]. To the best of our knowledge, there is no study on the effect of socioeconomic factors on vertical jumping performance as well as on anthropometric parameters in athletic Tunisian children. We hypothesized that socioeconomic factors influence age, height, weight, fat-free mass and vertical jumping performance among athletic Tunisian children. Therefore, we undertook to evaluate the effect of socioeconomic status on vertical jumping performance and anthropometric characteristics among athletic Tunisian children aged 7 to 13 in both sexes

2. Methods

2.1. Experimental Approach to the Problem

This study was designed to examine the effect of socioeconomic status on vertical jumping parameters and anthropometric variables in athletic Tunisian children. 407 subjects (218 boys and 189 girls) were asked to perform Squat jumps (SJ), Countermovement jumps (CMJ) and to response to a questionnaire. Jump height and leg power were simultaneously provided by the Optojump photocells. Non parametric analysis of variance and General Linear Model (GLM) were used to analyze the data set and to identify which factors significantly influence performance variables.

2.2. Subjects

Four hundred and seven athletic Tunisian children (218 boys and 189 girls) ranging in age from 7 to 13 were selected randomly to be the subject of our study.

The subjects were selected by a two- level cluster sampling: (a) four out of 15 clubs from central Tunisia were randomly chosen. The sample included a mix of school children, from rural and urban areas; (b) the sample involved also children practicing many sports such as gymnastics, soccer, handball, volleyball, basketball, swimming and tennis. All players passed medical examinations within 15 days prior to the tests. All subjects who participated in the study had no injury of their lower limbs.

A medical questionnaire, recommended for epidemiological research was used to assess subject characteristics such as medical and surgical histories. After answering the questionnaire, subjects were selected according to the exclusion criteria defined as follow: The history of neurological (n=2), muscular (n=13) or cardiac diseases (n = 6), and 8 children unable to perform vertical jump tests adequately. On the basis of these criteria, 29 children from 436 were excluded. Finally, 407 athletic children were included in subsequent analysis.

Prior to the study, the coach, the children and their parents/guardian had been fully informed of the aim of the research, the protocol and the procedure of the investigation before signing a written consent, which was in accordance with legal requirements and the Declaration of Helsinki, and was approved by the ministry of education and by the Research Ethics Committee of Farhat Hached Hospital (Sousse).

The athletic children are enrolled in a training program developed by their clubs, which consists of training 3 times per week for the children aged 7 to10 and 4 times per week for the children aged 11 to 13. Each training session lasted about 2 hours. During the competition season they participated each week in the official national championship.

2.3. Questionnaire

A medical questionnaire, modified from Ferris [16] and translated into the Arabic language, was distributed by the interviewer and was answered by the child with parent's assistance. This questionnaire was tested with 100 children before the study. The modified questionnaire was used previously by Trabesli et al. [45] in 756 Tunisian children. It was adapted according to the Tunisian context, and contained the essential information to assess the economic status of children, using some items proposed by the National Institute of Statistics [32]. The socioeconomic score was objectively assessed according to parental occupation which is a better indicator of the current socioeconomic status than education which can not reflect changes in social status that occur after schooling ends [13]. For example, in Tunisia, many poor families cooked and heated their home with wood until now. The social classes were assessed according to the classification used by Arshad & Hide [1] as follows: Class 1, professionals (doctors, solicitors and directors); Class 2, farmers, managers, teachers, engineers, etc.; Class 3, skilled workers, such as nurses and technicians; Class 4, low-skilled workers as factory works; Class 5, (a), unskilled workers, such as labourer, and Class 5 (b), unemployed

We group class1, 2 and 3 as high socioeconomic status (HSES) and class 4 and 5 as low socioeconomic status (LSES) [32]

2.4. Test Procedures

All subjects completed two preliminary familiarization sessions to minimize any effects of learning and to be informed about pretest instructions. The experiment was conducted during spring season in Tunisia. Ambient temperature and relative humidity values were between 18-20ºC and 35-50% respectively. In addition, the tests were performed in the afternoon (2 pm-4pm) to rule out a possible effect of the circadian rhythm on the performance [3].

Individuals were asked to sleep normally and to wear the same sportswear and shoes for all the tests. They were also asked to avoid solid food for 2 hours before the test.

The test-retest intraclass correlation coefficients of the testing procedure variables used in this study were >0.91 and the coefficients of variation ranged from 0.9 to 7.3%.

2.4.1. Vertical jumping tests

Jumping performance was evaluated with the Optojump photocell system (Microgate SRL, Italy), which consists of two parallel bars placed approximately 1 m apart and parallel to each other. Optojump bars were connected to a portable computer and the propriety software (optojump software, version 3.01.0001) allowed jump height quantification.

All subjects performed the squat jump (SJ) and countermovement jump (CMJ) in their sports clubs under the supervision of the same investigator which are two of the most used jump modalities in sport practice and testing [37].

The children were given two practice jumps before the specific jump test was conducted. Three jumps were separated by a 2 minutes rest period to ensure sufficient recovery.

For all jumps, the athletes started with their hands on their hips to eliminate the influence of the arms swing impulse [6]. For the SJ test, they were instructed to sink and hold a knee position (approximately 120º Knee angle) for three seconds. On the count of three the child was instructed to jump as high as possible without performing any countermovement before the execution of the jump. A successful trial was one where there was no sinking or countermovement prior to the execution of the jump [22].

The CMJ assessment required the child to be in a standing position and, prior to jumping, counter-moved until the knee was flexed approximately to 90º.They were then instructed to sink as quickly as possible and then jump as high as possible. Verbal encouragements were constantly given to maintain high motivation in these groups. All subjects performed 3 consecutive experimental trials for each jump. The highest value for each jump was retained for analysis [22].

2.4.2. Anthropometry

Prior to jump data collection, Standing and sitting heights were measured with an appropriate stadiometer (Harpenden Portable Stadiometer, UK) to the nearest 0.1 cm. The difference between the standing height and the sitting height allowed us to determine the leg length. Body weight was obtained with a digital scale (Harpenden Balance Scale, UK) to the nearest 0.1 Kg. Body mass index (BMI) was calculated as weight divided by the square of the height. Waist size was measured around the smallest part of his or her waistline underwear with tape measure. Skinfolds thicknesses were estimated to the nearest 0.1 mm using a Harpenden Skinfold Caliper (Holtain Ltd, Crosswell, UK). We measured biceps, triceps, subscapular and supra iliac skinfold thickness. Each was measured in duplicate on the left side of the body and the mean value was used for calculation. The errors of measurement were less than 1mm and the reliability was greater than 95% [31].

We predicted the body density from the equation of Johnston et al. [19].The conversion of body density to percent fat (% fat) was accomplished using the age-gender conversion constants of Lohman [26].

Body fat weight was calculated as follows: fat weight= %fat × (weight / 100). For determining fat-free weight, it has been calculated by subtracting fat weight from total body weight [11].

2.5. Statistical Analyses

All values were expressed as arithmetic means ± standard deviation (SD). Data from boys and girls were analyzed separately. The normality of all anthropometric and vertical jumping parameters was tested by Kolmogorov-Smirnov tests [38].

All means were compared using the Kruskal-Wallis nonparametric analysis of variance [24].

We used General Linear Model (GLM) and multiple regressions to reveal the global effect of anthropometric variables and socioeconomic status on jumping performance parameters.

Data were analyzed using the statistical software (SPSS version 17.0). Statistical significance was set at $p < 0.05$.

3. Results

3.1. Anthropometric characteristics

Frequency distributions in both genders according to socioeconomic status are shown in Figure 1. We classified class groups 1, 2 and 3 as high socioeconomic status (HSES) and class groups 4 and 5 as low socioeconomic status (LSES). The two Socioeconomic classes were homogeneous ($p < 0.05$). (Figure 1).

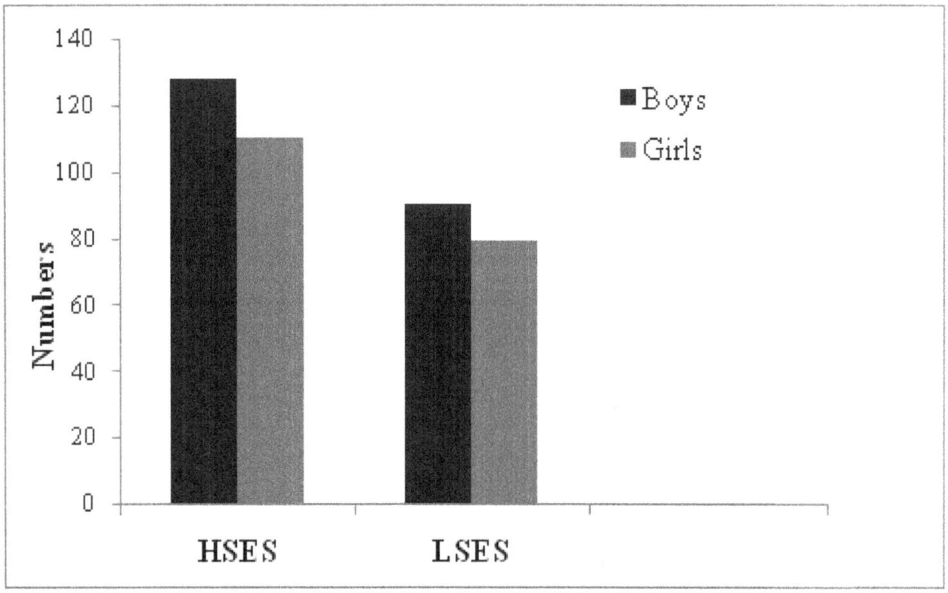

Figure 1. Frequencies distribution of athletic Tunisian children according tosocioeconomic status and gender

The anthropometric characteristics of boys and girls of high (HSES) and low socioeconomic status (LSES) are presented in Table 1. Boys and girls of HSES and LSES were statistically ($p < 0.05$) different for all anthropometric variables except for body mass index and fat-free mass. Non parametric comparison of means revealed significant effect of the socioeconomic status on body mass index and body fat only in boys. Significant differences ($p < 0.05$) were found in age, standing height, sitting height and leg length among the HSES and LSES girls.

Table 1. Mean and ± standard deviation of anthropometric variables of boys and girls of high (HSES) and low socioeconomic status (LSES)

Anthropometric characteristics	**Boys**		**Girls**	
	HSES	**LSES**	**HSES**	**LSES**
Number	128	90	110	79
Age (years)	10.1 ± 1.8 *	9.7 ± 1.9	9.6 ± 1.9	10.2 ± 1.8§
Standing height (m)	1.40 ± 0.09	1.39 ± 0.09 *	1.42 ± 0.14	1.47 ± 0.13§
Sitting height (m)	0.70 ± 0.04*	0.69 ± 0.04 *	0.71 ± 0.05	0.73 ± 0.05§
Leg length (m)	0.70 ± 0.06	0.69 ± 0.06 *	0.70 ± 0.09	0.73 ± 0.09§
Waist size (m)	0.62 ± 0.06	0.61 ± 0.06 *	0.63 ± 0.08	0.65 ± 0.08
Body mass (kg)	35.08 ± 7.21	33.46 ± 6.52 *	35.93 ± 9.02	37.67 ± 8.53
Body mass index ($kg.m^{-2}$)	17.57 ± 1.59§	17.08 ± 1.45	17.50 ± 1.84	17.21 ± 2.16
Body fat (kg)	3.01 ± 1.81 §	2.38 ± 1.51 *	4.40 ± 2.29*	5.04 ± 2.55
Fat-free weight (kg)	32.01 ± 6.01	31.06 ± 5.50	31.58 ± 7.09	32.71 ± 6.65

Significant difference between boys and girls in the same socio economic status: *$p < 0.05$
Significant difference between HSES and LSES in boys and girls : § $p < 0.05$
HSES = High Socio-economic status
LSES = Low socio-economic status

3.2. Vertical Jumping Performance: Effect of Sexes and Social Economic Status

Mean and standard deviation of vertical jumping performance in athletic Tunisian children by socioeconomic status and sex are shown in Table 2.

For the Countermovement Jump (CMJ), the HSES and LSES boys demonstrated significantly ($p < 0.05$) higher CMJ height and CMJ power than HSES and LSES girls. There were no significant differences in vertical jumping parameters between HSES and LSES in both sexes.

Table 2. Mean and ± standard deviation of jumping performance in athletic Tunisian children by socio-economic status and sex

	Boys		Girls	
	HSES	**LSES**	**HSES**	**LSES**
Number	128	90	110	79
CMJ height (m)	0.17 ± 0.03*	0.17 ± 0.03	0.16 ± 0.03	0.16 ± 0.03
CMJ power (W.Kg^{-1})	13.9 ± 2.7*	14.2 ± 2.86*	13.1 ± 2.9	13.2 ± 2.6
SJ height (m)	0.16 ± 0.03	0.16 ± 0.03	0.16 ± 0.04	0.16 ± 0.03
SJ power (W.Kg^{-1})	13.2 ± 2.7	13.2 ± 2.6	13.5 ± 2.9	13.6 ± 2.6

Significant difference between boys and girls in the same socio economic status: *$p < 0.05$.
CMJ = Counter-Movement Jump**HSES** = High Socio-economic status
SJ = Squat Jump.**LSES** = Low socio-economic status

3.3. Univariate Liaisons between Anthropometric Variables and Vertical Jumping Performance

Spearman correlations coefficients were calculated to check the influence of interaction between anthropometric and vertical jumping parameters. Spearman correlations of anthropometric variables and socioeconomic status with vertical jumping parameters in HSES and LSES athletic children are displayed in Table 3 and Table 4. Anthropometric variables were correlated significantly with CMJ power, CMJ height, SJ power and SJ height in HSES and LSES children. HSES children presented statistically significant correlations coefficients with standing height (Figure 2), sitting height, leg length (Figure 3), waist size, body mass (Figure 4) , fat-free mass (Figure 5). However, LSES children presented only statistically correlations with age, standing height, leg length and fat free mass. Similar results were observed with SJ power.

Table 3 .Spearman correlation coefficients (r) between vertical jumping parameters and anthropometric measures in HSES athletic Tunisian children (n=238)

	CMJ power (W.Kg-1)	CMJ height (m)	SJ power (W.Kg-1)	SJ height (m)
Age (years)	0.35**	0.48**	0.25**	0.39**
Standing height (cm)	0.30**	0.39**	0.24**	0.36**
Sitting height (s)	0.24**	0.30**	0.21**	0.28**
Leg length (cm)	0.28**	0.39**	0.22**	0.36**
Waist size	0.17**	0.24**	0.11*	0.23**
Body mass (Kg)	0.23**	0.36**	0.18**	0.33**
Body mass index (kg.m^{-2})	0.01	0.10*	0.003	0.11*
Body fat	-0.006	0.08	0.02	0.09*
Fat-free mass	0.28**	0.41**	0.22**	0.38**

* $p < 0.05$, ** $p < 0.01$.

Table 4. Spearman correlation coefficients (r) between vertical jumping parameters and anthropometric measures in LSES athletic Tunisian children (n=238)

	CMJ power (W.Kg^{-1})	CMJ height (m)	SJ power (W.Kg^{-1})	SJ height (m)
Age (years)	0.25**	0.45**	0.25**	0.31**
Standing height (cm)	0.16*	0.32**	0.19**	0.23**
Sitting height (s)	0.13	0.26**	0.22**	0.19**
Leg length (cm)	0.15*	0.32**	0.14	0.23**
Waist size	0.12	0.28**	0.11	0.23**
Body mass (Kg)	0.15	0.34**	0.14	0.20**
Body mass index (kg.m^{-2})	0.02	0.09	-0.06	-0.08**
Body fat	-0.09	0.08	0.02	0.021
Fat-free mass	0.21*	0.38**	0.18	0.24**

* $p < 0.05$, ** $p < 0.01$.

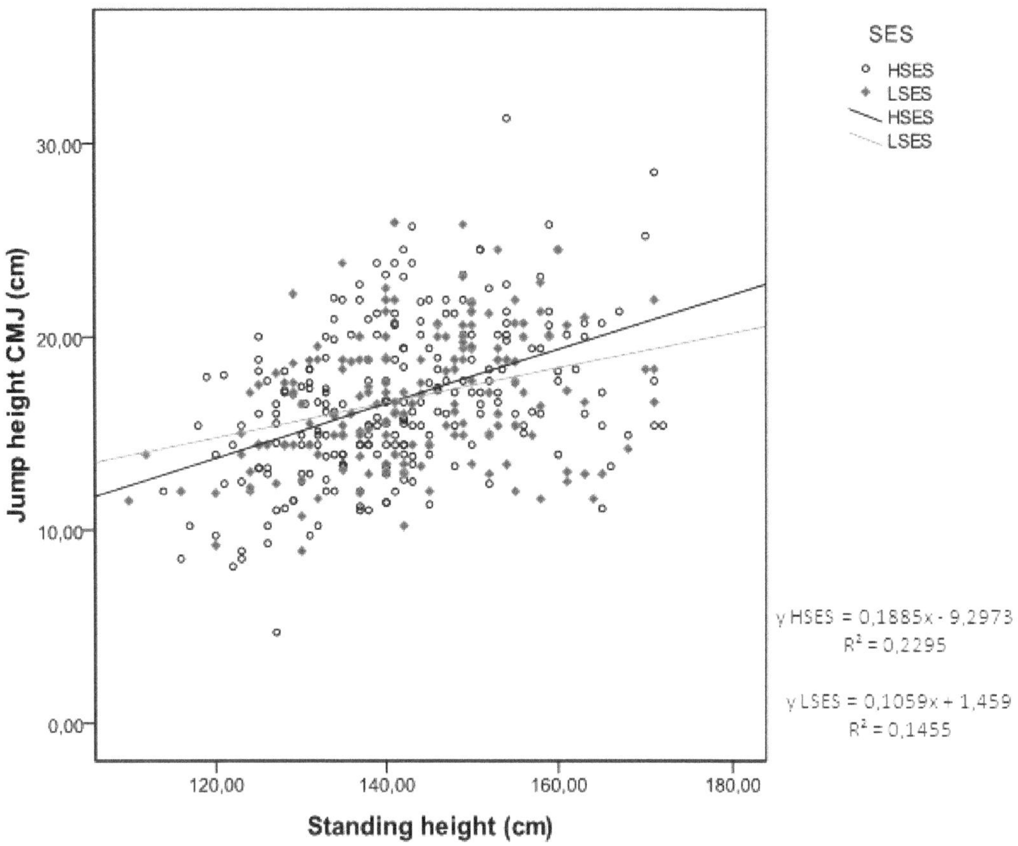

Figure 2. Relationships between jump height and standing height in the children of high (HSES) and low (LSES) socioeconomic status during the countermovement jump (CMJ)

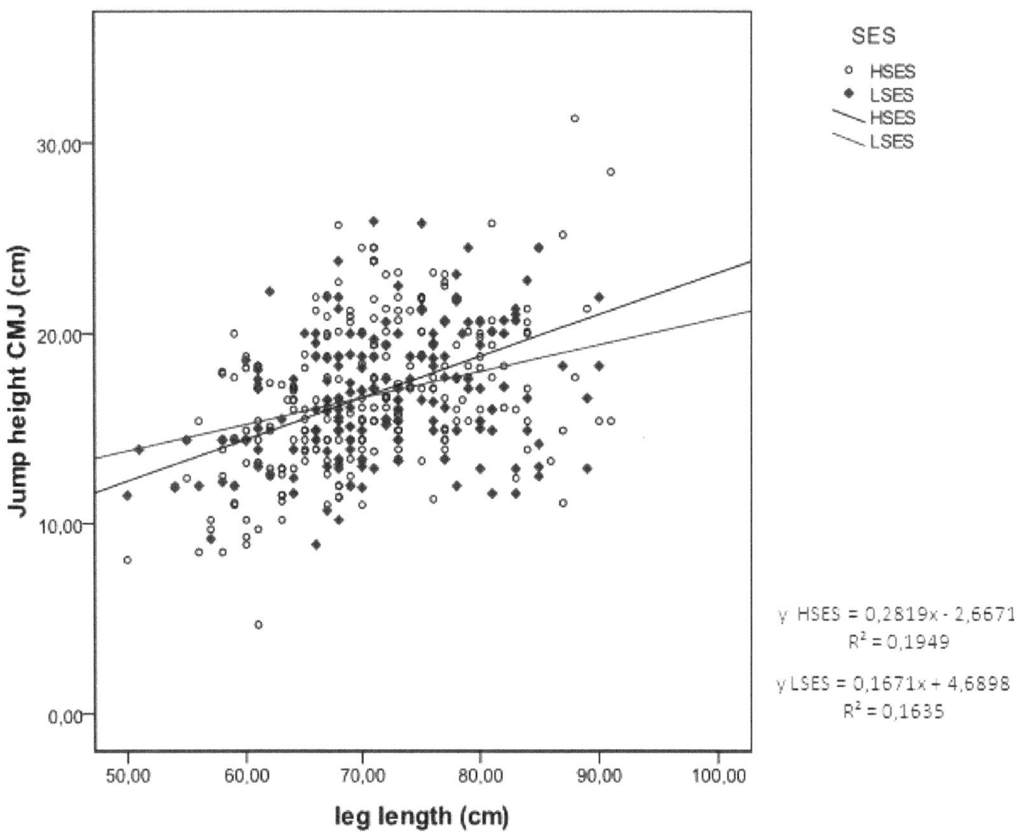

Figure 3. Relationships between jump height and leg length in the children of high (HSES) and low (LSES) socioeconomic status during the countermovement jump (CMJ)

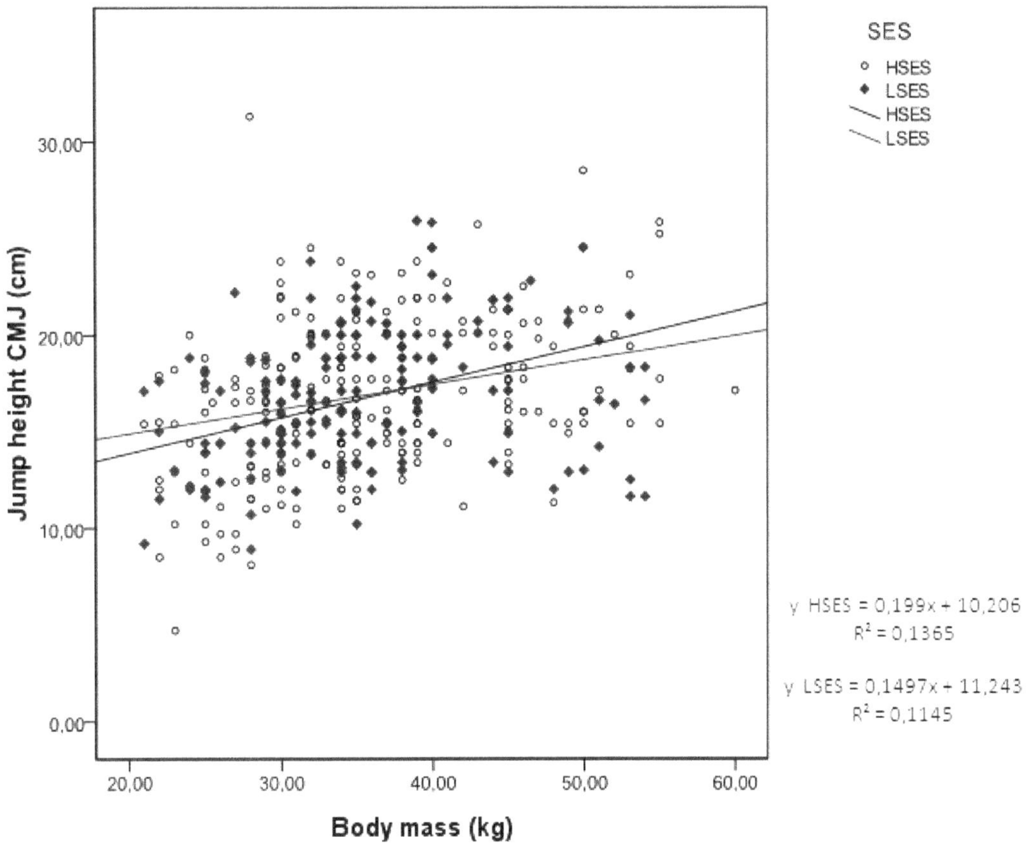

Figure 4. Relationships between jump height and weight in the children of high (HSES) and low (LSES) socioeconomic status during the countermovement jump (CMJ)

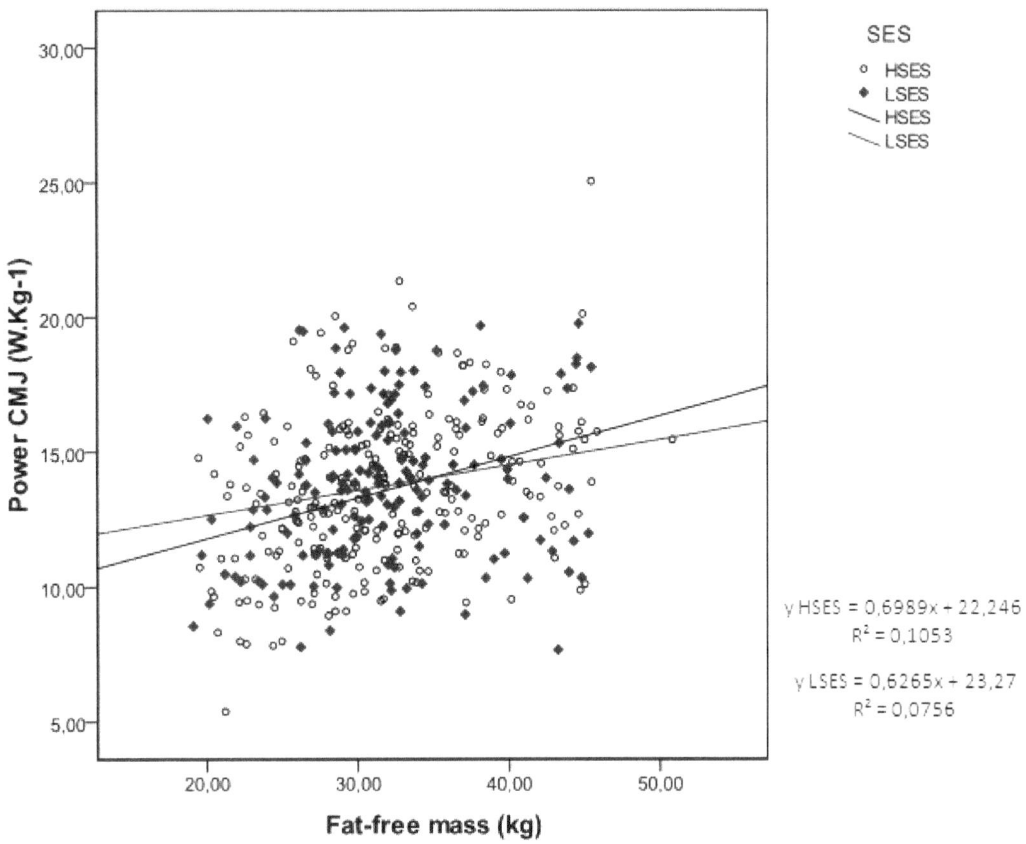

Figure 5. Relationships between power and fat-free mass in the children of high (HSES) and low (LSES) socioeconomic status during the countermovement jump (CMJ)

Only body fat was inversely correlated with CMJ power in HSES children (r= -0.006). Body mass index was also inversely correlated with SJ power (r = -0.06) and SJ height (r = -0.08, $p < 0.01$) in LSES children.

3.4. Relationships between Anthropometric Characteristics, Socioeconomic Status and Vertical Jumping Performance in Athletic Tunisian Children

Correlations between dependent vertical jumping performances and anthropometric parameters in HSES and LSES children were significant (Table 3 and Table 4).

Results of general linear model analyzing the multiple predictors (independent variables) of vertical jumping parameters were shown in Table 5. In this global way, waist size, sitting height, body mass index, leg length, body fat, socioeconomic status, had no significant correlations with vertical jumping parameters. However, for the other anthropometric parameters significant correlations were found for sex, age, height, body mass and fat-free mass for CMJ height, CMJ power, SJ height and SJ power ($P < 0.05$). The multiple linear regressions showed that age and sex were the major explanatory variables for jumping performances (R^2= 0.26, R^2=0.15; R^2=0.16; R^2=0.06; $p < 0.05$ respectively), whereas the socioeconomic status and the others anthropometric measurements (Height, body mass, fat-free mass, waist size, sitting height, body mass index, leg length, body fat) were excluded from the predictive equations (data not shown).

Table 5. General linear model analyzing the multiple predictors (independent variables) of vertical jumping performance variables in athletic children. Tests of global effects

	Dependent variables			
Predictors	**CMJ height**	**CMJ power**	**SJ height**	**SJ power**
Sex	P=0.876	P=0.167	P=0.014	P=0.008
Age	P=0.000	P=0.001	P=0.000	P=0.018
Height	P=0.190	P=0.597	P=0.199	P=0.048
Body mass	P=0.195	P=0.014	P=0.865	P=0.006
Fat-free mass	P=0.101	P=0.005	P=0.320	P=0.005
Waist size	P=0.455	P=0.526	P=0.753	P=0.629
Sitting height	P=0.196	P=0.860	P=0.114	P=0.122
Body mass index	P=0.721	P=0.696	P=0.514	P=0.417
Leg length	P=0.247	P=0.758	P=0.160	P=0.094
Body fat	P=0.542	P=0.412	P=0.046	P=0.542
Socioeconomic status	P=0.876	P=0.970	P=0.898	P=0.614

4. Discussion

The main findings of the present study that the socioeconomic status did not influence vertical jumping parameters in our athletic Tunisian children.

The measurements of performance in vertical jump are objectively provided by the optojump system which is valid and reliable for jump height estimation [17].

The CMJ and SJ were chosen because they have been found to be the most reliable and valid field tests for assessing the explosive power output of the lower limbs in physically active subjects [27]. We only selected athletic children whose jumping performance was found to be reproducible.

The socioeconomic score was objectively assessed according to parental occupation which is a better indicator of the current socioeconomic status than education which can not reflect changes in social status that occur after schooling ends [13]. The association between vertical jumping performance and anthropometric parameters with each of the four classes were difficult to interpret because of the insufficient size of socioeconomic classes. Therefore we divided the whole sample into two categories the High (HSES) and low (LSES) socioeconomic status as suggested by Blonc et al. [6]

4.1. Anthropometric Characteristics

Anthropometric differences found between boys and girls from the same socioeconomic status may be explained by the growth and mature processes [34]. Our study included children aged between 7 and 13 years, and the onset of puberty corresponds classically to a biological age of ≈ 11 years in girls and 13 years in boys [42]. Under the influence of testosterone, which is a potent anabolic hormone, boys have a significant increase in lean body mass exceeds the total gain in weight because of the concomitant loss of adipose tissue [41]. Sex differences could occur previously in children [43,44].

Differences between HSES and LSES of girls in anthropometric parameters could be explained by the growth.

4.2. Vertical Jumping Performance

We found that boys jumped higher than girls in HSES and LSES. Hormonal secretion plays a key role. Indeed, testosterone, Growth Hormone (GH), Insulin-like Growth Factor I (IGF-I) and insulin influence muscle hypertrophy during growth and maturation. Testosterone concentration, starts increasing at puberty, this is associated with significant muscle hypertrophy in prepubertal trained subjects [49]. Moreover, increasing levels of testosterone induce differentiation of muscles fibers in boys compared to girls, especially fast-twitch fibers [20].

We found no significant differences in vertical jumping performances between two HSES and LSES classes in athletic Tunisian children. However other studies reported by Doré et al. [14], Jiménez Pavón et al. [18], and Bedu et al.[2] revealed that power output were significantly affected by socioeconomic status. Others studies demonstrated that LSES children had significantly lower anaerobic performance than HSES children [14].We paid attention that these studies were interested in untrained subject.

Indeed, the low socioeconomic class (LSES) is a complex reality composed by several interrelated factors of which under nutrition is only one. Malnutrition could lead to a reduction in physical growth [39] and thereafter to the peak muscle power. In our study, the lack of differences in jump performances between HSES and LSES athletic children could be explained by an adequate daily dietary intake. Indeed, our children trained regularly in sport clubs, they could have free equilibrated meals. This could attenuate the effect of socioeconomic status on performance. Furthermore, they are well attended by pediatrician, who must alert for signs and symptoms of under nutrition and/or overtraining. So, sports clubs provided similarly adequate attention to their high (HSES) and low (LSES) athletic Tunisian children.

Moreover, Training programmes may contribute improving strength [35] which is another explanation for the lack of differences in vertical jumping performance between HSES and LSES children. In fact, each training programme affects muscle differently depending on recovery time and exercise intensity. However, in general, short periods of high muscle load with long recovery periods induce an adaptative response of anaerobic metabolism such as increases in phosphocreatine (PCr) kinase activity, while longer periods of effort have no effect on PCr metabolism, but induce a greater adaptative response in glycolytic metabolism [12,36].

Linossier et al. [25] revealed that sprint training caused a large increase in maximal power, mainly due to an increase in strength. However, the ability to develop strength in training seemed to be related more to intrinsic fibre properties (% fast twitch b fibre area and adenylate kinase activity). Indeed, increases in the proportion of type II muscle fibres with sprint training connected with the transformation of slow twitch fibre and fast twitch b fibres into fast twitch a fibres.

4.3. Relationship between Vertical Jumping Performance and Anthropometric Characteristics

In agreement with recent studies, we found correlations between power jump height and age in HSES and LSES athletic children [43,46]. Tsubaki et al. [46] found a high correlation between age and maximum power in physically active Japanese males and females under 20 years old. Taylor et al. [43] showed that Jump height and peak power increased progressively year by year for males between 10 and 15 years. Some investigators have suggested that sex- and age-related differences in anaerobic performance may be attributed to differences in the ability to recruit and activate muscle during exercise [50]. Vandewalle et al. [47] reported correlations between body mass, vertical jump and peak power measured during force-velocity test. The authors suggested that athletes with high jump performances or peak power have high percentage of type II muscle fibres.

We also found that height, weight, leg length and lean body mass were correlated with leg power and jump height. This could be explained by the increase in muscle length during growth which contribute to power, since the power of a muscle is determined by its volume, as the product of the mean cross-sectional area and length [43]. This data is in agreement with study reported by Markovic & Jaric [28], who suggested that power calculated from the ground reaction force recorded during different types of maximum vertical jumps, was strongly related to body size.

In our study, we found high correlation between fat-free mass and leg power in trained children. This is an agreement with the study of Mercier et al. [30] who reported that lean body mass explained 88% of the total variance of maximal anaerobic power.

Jump weight measurements is a simple practical tool helping to identify talented children in explosive sports that require movement of body mass or the manipulation of an external mass [43].

4.4. Multiple Regression Equations of Jumping Performances Predicted in Healthy Tunisian Children

The general linear model and analysis of multiple regression equations allowed us to study the interrelation between the various liaisons with the vertical jumping performance globally and within each predictive factor. Using this statistical method we were able to determine that, in HSES and LSES Tunisian athletic children, the main factors affecting the vertical jumping performance were the sex, age, height, weight and fat-free mass ($P < 0.05$). The multiple stepwise regressions also indicated that sex and age were the major explanatory variables of jumping performances in HSES and LSES athletic Tunisian children.

In conclusion, using multivariate analysis in the whole population and by socioeconomic status, we have shown that morphologic parameters; sex, age, height, body mass and fat-free mass were the main factors affecting vertical jumping performance. These findings are important because identification of factors affecting vertical jumping performance may help to improve muscular performance by evaluating individual athletes, detecting talented young athletes and protecting trained children from possible injury.

Acknowledgments

This study was supported by the Tunisian Ministry of Higher Education and Scientific Research.

Conflict of Interest

There is no conflict of interest regarding the information provided in this study.

References

[1] Arshad, S.H., & Hide, D.W. (1992).Effect of environmental factors on the development of allergic disorders in infancy. *Journal of Allergy and Clinical Immunology*, 90,235-241.

[2] Bedu, M., Falgairette, G., Van Praagh, E., & Coudert, J. (1994). Effect of Chronic Hypoxia and socioeconomic status on anaerobic power of 10- to 12-year-old Bolivian Boys. *International Journal of Sports Medicine*, 15, S84-S89.

[3] Bernard, T., Giacomoni, M., Gavarry, O., Seymat, M., & Falgairette, G. (1998).Time-of-day effects in maximal anaerobic leg exercise. *European Journal of Applied Physiology*, 77,133-138.

[4] Bishop, D., Girard O., & Mendez-Villanueva A. (2011). Repeated-Sprint ability-Part II. Recommendations for training. *Sports Medicine*, 41(9), 741-756.

[5] Blimkie, C.J.R. (1989). Age and sex associated variation in strength during childhood: Anthropometric, morphologic, neurologic, biomechanical, endcrinologic, and physical activity correlates. In C.V. Gisolfi, & Lamb. D.R, (Eds.). Perspectives in exercise science and sports medicine. Indianapolis: Benchmark (pp. 99-163).

[6] Blonc, S., Fellmann, N., Bedu, M., Falgairette, G., De Jonge, R., Obert, P., Beaume, B., Spielvogel, H., Tellez, W., Quintela, A., San Miguel, J.L., & Coudert, J. (1996). Effect of altitude and socioeconomic status on VO_{2max} and anaerobic power in prepubertal Bolivian girls. *Journal of Applied Physiology*, 80, 2002-2008,

[7] Bosco, C., Luhtanen, P., & Komi, P.V. (1983) .A simple method for measurement of mechanical power in jumping. *European Journal of Applied Physiology*, 50, 273-282.

[8] Bouhlel, E., Bouhlel, H., Chelly, M.S., & Tabka, Z. (2006).Relation entre la puissance maximale anaérobie mesurée lors de l'épreuve charge-vitesse, la détente verticale et le 5-jump test chez le garçon entraîné. *Science & Sports*, 21, 1-7.

[9] Buchanan, P.A., & Vardaxis, V.G. (2009).Lower-extremity strength profiles and gender-based classification of basketball players ages 9-22 years. *Journal of Strength and Conditioning Research*, 23, 406-419.

[10] Buchanan, P.A., & Vardaxis, V.G. (2003).Sex-related and age related differences in knee strength of basketball players ages 11-17 years. *Journal of Athletic training*, 38, 231-237.

[11] Buskirk, E.R., & Mendez, J. (1984) .Sports science and body composition analysis: emphasis on cell and muscle mass. *Medicine and Science in Sports and Exercise*, 16,584-593.

[12] Cadefau, J., Casademont, J., Grau, J.M., Fernandez, J., Balaguer, A., Vernet, M., Cusso, R, & Urbano-Marquez, A. (1990). Biochemical and histological adaptation to sprint training in young athletes. Acta Physiologica Scandinavica 140, 341-351.

[13] Demissie, K., Ernst, P., Hanley, J.A., Locher, U., Menzies, D., & Becklake, M.R. (1996). Socioeconomic status and lung function among primary school children in Canada. *American Journal of Respiratory and Critical Care Medicine*, 159,719-723.

[14] Doré, E., Diallo, O., França, N., Bedu, M., & Van Praagh, E. (2000). Dimensional changes cannot account for all differences in short-term cycling power during growth. *International Journal of Sports Medicine*, 21, 360-365.

[15] Earp, J.E., Joseph, M., Kraemer, W.J., Newton, R.U., Comstock, B.A., Fragala M.S., Dunn-Lewis, C., Solomon-Hill, G., Penwell, Z.R., Powell, M.D., Volek, J.S., Denegar, C.R., Häkkinen, K, & Maresh, C.M. (2010). Lower-body muscle structure and its role in jump performance during squat, countermovement, and depth drop jumps. *Journal of Strength and Conditioning Research*, 24(3), 722-729.

[16] Ferris, B.G. (1978).Epidemiology standardisation project II. Recommended respiratory disease questionnaire for use with adults and children in epidemiological research. *American Review of Respiratory Disease*, 118, 7-53.

[17] Glatthorn, J.F., Gouge, S., Nussbaumer, S., Stauffacher, S., Impellizzeri, F.M., & Maffiuletti, N.A. (2011) .Validity and reliability of optojump photoelectric cells for estimating vertical jump height. *Journal of Strength and Conditioning Research*, 25, 556-560.

[18] Jiménez Pavón, D., Ortega, F.B., Ruiz, J.R., España Romero, V., García Artero, E., Moliner Urdiales, D., Gómez Martínez, S., Vicente Rodríguez, G., Manios, Y., Béghin, L., Répasy, J., Sjöstrom, M., Moreno, L.A., González Gross, M., & Castillo, M.J. (2010).Socioeconomic status influences physical fitness in European adolescents independently of body fat and physical activity: the HELENA Study. *Nutrición Hospitalaria*, 25, 311-316.

[19] Johnston, J.L., Leong, M.S., Checkland, E.G., Zuberbahler, P.C., Conger, PR, & Quinney, HA. (1988) .Body fat assessed from body density and estimated from skinfold thickness in normal children and children with cystic fibrosis. *American Journal of Clinical Nutrition* 48, 1362-1366.

[20] Kanehisa, H., Ikegawa, S., Tsunoda, N., & Fukunaga, T. (1994). Strength and cross-sectional area of Knee extensor muscles in children. *European Journal of Applied Physiology*, 68, 402-405.

[21] Katzmarzyk, P.T., Malina, R.M., & Beunen, G.P. (1997). The contribution of biological maturation to the strength and motor fitness of children. *Annals of Human Biology*, 24, 493-505.

[22] Komi, P.V., & Bosco, C. (1978). Utilization of stored elastic energy in leg extensor muscles by men and women. *Journal of Medicine and Science in Sports* 10: 261-265.

[23] Korff, T., Horne, S.L., Cullen, S.J., & Blazevich, A.J. (2009). Development of lower limb stiffness and its contribution to maximum vertical jumping power during adolescence. *Journal of Experimental Biology*, 212, 3737-3742.

[24] Kruskal, W.H., & Wallis, W.A. (1952). Use of ranks in one criterion variance analysis. *Journal of the American Statistical Association*, 47,583-621.

[25] Linossier, M.T., Dormois, D., Geyssant, A., & Denis, C. (1997). Performance and fibre characteristics of human skeletal muscle during short sprint training and detraining on a cycle ergometer. *European Journal of Applied Physiology*, 75, 491-498.

[26] Lohman, T.G. (1989) .Assessment of body composition in children. *Pediatric Exercise Science*, 1, 19-30.

[27] Markovic, G., Dizdar, D., Jukic, I., & Cardinale, M. (2004).Reliability and factorial validity of squat and countermovement jump tests. *Journal of Strength and Conditioning Research* 18, 551-555.

[28] Markovic, G., & Jaric, S. (2007). Is vertical jump height a body size-independent measure of muscle power. *Journal of Sports Sciences* 25, 1355-1363.

[29] Martin, R. J., Doré, E., Hautier, C. A,. Van Praagh, E., & Bedu, M. (2003). Short-term peak power changes in adolescents of similar anthropometric characteristics. *Medicine & Science in Sports & Exercise*, 35, 1436-1440.

[30] Mercier, B., Mercier, P., Granier, P., Gallais, DLe., & Prefaut C.(1992).Maximal anaerobic power: relationship to anthropometric characteristics during growth. *International Journal of Sports Medicine*, 13, 21-26.

[31] Moreno, L.A., Joyanes, M., Mesana, M.I., González-Gross, M., Gil, C.M., Sarría, A., Gutierrez, A., Garaulet, M., Pérez-Prieto, R., Bueno, M., Marcos, A., & the AVENA Study Group. (2003). Harmonization of anthropometric measurements for a multicenter nutrition survey in Spanish adolescents. *Nutrition*, 19:481-486.

[32] National Institute for Statistics and Economic Studies. Socioprofessional category guideline. Paris: INSEE; 1993.

[33] Rantanen, T., Era, P., Kauppinen, M., & Heikkinen, E. (1997). Maximal isometric muscle strength and socioeconomic status, health, and physical activity in 75-year old persons. *Journal of aging and physical activity*, 2, 206-220.

[34] Rogol, A.D., Clark, P.A., & Roemmich, J.N. (2000) .Growth and pubertal development in children and adolescents: effects of diet and physical activity. *American Journal of Clinical Nutrition*, 72, 521S-8S.

[35] Rowland, T. (2005). Children's Exercise Physiology. Human Kinetics, Champaign.

[36] Sahlin, k. (1978). Intracellular pH and energy metabolism in skeletal muscle of man. *Acta physiological Scandanavian supplementum*, 455, 1-56.

[37] Slinde, F., Suber, C., Suber, L., Edwen, C.E., & Svantesson, U. (2008) .Test-retest reliability of three different countermovement jumping tests. *Journal of Strength and Conditioning Research*, 22, 640-644.

[38] Smirnov, N. V. (1939). Estimate of deviation between empirical distribution functions in two independent samples, Bull Moscow University, 2, 3616.

[39] Spurr, G.B., Reina, J.C., Dahners, H.W., & Barac-Nieto, M. (1983).Marginal malnutrition in school- aged Colombian boys: functional consequences in maximum exercise. *American Journal of Clinical Nutrition*, 37, 834-847.

[40] Syddal, H., Evandrou, M., Cooper, C., & Sayer, A.A. (2009).Social inequalities in grip strength, physical function, and falls among community dwelling older men and women: findings

from the Hertfordshire cohort study. *Journal of Aging and Health*, 21, 913-939.

[41] Tanner, J.M. (1989) .Fetus into man: physical growth from conception to maturity. Cambridge, MA: Harvard University Press.

[42] Tanner, J.M., Whitehouse, R.H., Marshall, W.A., & Carter, B.S. (1975). Prediction of adult height, bone age, and occurrence of menarche, at age 4 to 16 with allowance for midparental height. *Archives of Disease in Childhood*, 50, 14-26.

[43] Taylor, M.J.D., Cohen, D., Voss, C., & Sandercock, G.R.H. (2010).Vertical jumping and leg power normative data for English school children aged 10–15 years. *Journal of Sports Sciences*,28, 867-872.

[44] Temfemo, A., Hugues, J., Chardon, K., Mandengue, S.H., & Ahmaidi, S. (2009). Relationship between vertical jumping performance and anthropometric characteristics during growth in boys and girls. *European Journal of Pediatrics*, 168, 457-464.

[45] Trabelsi, Y., Pariès, J., Harrabi, I., Zbidi, A., Tabka, Z., Richalet, J.P, & Buvry, A. (2008). Factors affecting the development of lung function in Tunisian children. *American Journal of Human Biology*, 20, 716-725.

[46] Tsubaki, A., Kubo, M., Kobayashi, R., Jigami, H., & Takahashi, H.E. (2009) .Normative values for maximum power during motor function assessment of jumping among physically active Japanese. *Journal of Musculoskeletal and Neuronal Interactions*, 9: 263-267.

[47] Vandewalle, H., Peres, G., Heller, J., Panel, J., & Monod, H. (1987).Force-velocity relationship and maximal power on a cycle ergometer : Correlation with the height of a vertical jump. *European Journal of Applied Physiology*, 56, 650-656.

[48] Van Praagh, E., & Doré, E. (2002). Short-term muscle power during growth and maturation. *Sports Med*icine, 32, 701-728.

[49] Vrijens, D. (1978). Muscle strength development in the pre-pubescent and post-pubescent age. *Medicine and Science in Sports*, 11, 152-158.

[50] Wakahara, T., Takeshita, K., Kato, E., Miyatani, M., Tanaka, N.I., Kanehisa, H., kawakami, Y., & Fukunaga, T. (2010).Variability of Limb Muscle Size in Young Men. American Journal of Human Biology, 22, 55-59.

21

Effects of Repeated Training on Controlled Force Exertion and Retention in Dominant and Nondominant Hands

H. Kubota[1,*], S. Demura[2], M. Uchiyama[3], K. Takahashi[4]

[1]Faculty of Education, Gifu University, Gifu, Japan
[2]Graduate School of Natural Science & Technology, Kanazawa University, Ishikawa, Japan
[3]Research and Education Center for Comprehensive Science, Akita Prefectural University, Akita, Japan
[4]Faculty of Community Health Care, Department of Judo Physical Therapy, Teikyo Heisei University, Chiba, Japan
*Corresponding author: hkubota@gifu-u.ac.jp

Abstract This study aimed to examine the effects of repeated training on the controlled force exertion (CFE) test and retention in dominant and nondominant hands. The subjects were 10 young males (mean age, 21.8 ± 1.4 years). The CFE test was used as the repeated training task and performed 5 days per week over 3 weeks (a total of 15 times). The exertion value of the subjects' handgrip strengths was matched to constantly changing demand values for 40 s. Three trials were performed after one practice trial. The difference between the demand value and the grip exertion value was used as the evaluation parameter, referred to as the CFE error, and the mean of the second and third trials was used for analysis. The initial and final values for the dominant and nondominant hands and those taken one month after the repeated training task were used for analysis. A two-way analysis of variance revealed that the final CFE errors for both hands were significantly smaller than the initial CFE errors, and no significant difference was found between the dominant and nondominant hands in the final tests. In addition, after one month, the CFE errors for both hands were significantly smaller than the initial CFE errors and were significantly smaller in the dominant hand than in the nondominant hand. Repeated training in controlled force exertion improves CFE in both the dominant and nondominant hands, but the dominant and nondominant hands differ in retention of the effects.

Keywords: *laterality, motor control, motor learning*

1. Introduction

The functional right-left difference in body parts with bilateral symmetry in humans is called "laterality" [1,2,3,4]. In laterality, either the right or left side in a body with bilateral symmetry is superior to the other side in achievement of motor or cognitive task. The dominant hand is generally superior in muscle strength, quickness, accuracy, and dexterity. Laterality appears from infancy because of the influence of inherited factors [5]. The difference between the dominant and nondominant hands becomes more pronounced because of the preferential use of the dominant hand in activities of daily life such as writing or using chopsticks. Laterality also influences the coordination ability. Noguchi et al. [6] reported that laterality is found in the Moving Beans with Tweezers test and the Purdue Pegboard test, which are used to evaluate dexterity, an element of coordination; their results indicated that the dominant hand is superior to the nondominant hand. Ohtsuki et al. [7] found that laterality in grading ability becomes more pronounced with the influence of an acquired factor.

Controlled force exertion (CFE) refers to the ability to properly adjust force exertion values to demand values. To evaluate CFE, Nagasawa et al. [8,9] developed a test in which the subjects match their submaximal grip strengths to changing demand values presented as a bar chart or a waveform on the display of a personal computer. Kubota et al. [11,12] examined laterality of CFE in young males and females using the CFE test and reported that it is found in both males and females. In addition, they examined and reported laterality in young and elderly females.

As mentioned above, lateral dominance appears in motor tasks that demand dexterity of the hands, fingers, and upper limbs, and the dominant hand is superior [13]. Taylor and Heilman [14] examined the differences between the right and left hands in motor task proficiency using a complex key-pressing task and reported that the motor task proficiency period is shorter in the right hand than in the left hand. It can be inferred that the dominant hand, which is preferentially used in the activities of daily life, becomes more proficient at functions that involve a series of movements than the nondominant hand. The dominant hand is also superior in functions involving the peripheral and central nervous systems; thus, the movements improve smoothly with repetition of the appropriate feedback.

Regarding the retention of motor learning, Shea and Kohl [15,16] examined constant and variable practice using the handgrip task and reported the latter superior for retention of motor learning. However, retention of motor learning in the dominant and nondominant hands and retention of the effects of repeated CFE training have not previously been examined. Because the dominant hand is superior to the nondominant hand in motor learning [14], a difference between the two hands may be found in retention of motor learning.

It was therefore hypothesized that laterality would be found in retention of motor learning in addition to the training effect of the CFE test. This study aimed to examine the effects of repeated CFE test training and the retention of the effects in the dominant and nondominant hands.

2. Methods

2.1. Subjects

Subjects were 10 healthy young males (mean age 21.8 ± 1.4 years; height 171.8 ± 5.8 cm; weight 65.2 ± 4.7 kg). Mean values for height and body mass were similar to the Japanese normative values (Laboratory Physical Education in Tokyo Metropolitan University, 1989). Before the experiment, all subjects were judged to be right-handed by a Demura et al. [17] handedness inquiry. No subject had any disability of the upper limbs. Each subject could observe the computer display without difficulty; therefore, it was judged that individual vision did not affect the measurements. Prior to measurement, the purposes and procedures of this study were explained in detail to each subject, and consent for participation in this study was obtained from all subjects. The protocol for this study was approved by the Ethics Committee on Human Experimentation of the Faculty of Human Science, Kanazawa University (Ref. No. 2012-02).

2.2. Measurement

2.2.1. Experimental Procedure

The subjects performed repeated training (a total of 15 times) of controlled force exertion (4 trials per day by the dominant and nondominant hands) 5 days per week for 3 weeks. Repeated training in controlled force exertion was conducted according to the same procedure as the CFE test, and CFE errors were recorded each time. The subjects were not restricted to perform activities of daily life.

2.2.2. Controlled force exertion test

We measured maximal handgrip strength and CFE using a Smedley's handgrip mechanical dynamometer (Sakai, Tokyo, Japan) with a range of 0.0–99.9 kg and a hand biofeedback system (EG-100; Sakai, Tokyo, Japan). The information from the handgrip device was transmitted at a sampling rate of 20 Hz to a computer through a data output cable after A/D conversion. The subjects exerted grip strength using a handgrip device while sitting on a chair in front of the computer display, with the elbow straight and close to the body, without contact between the dynamometer and the body or the chair. The size of the grip was set such that they felt comfortable squeezing it. They performed the CFE test while attempting to minimize the differences between the demand and grip values that were being presented on the computer. A bar chart was used to represent the data according to the criteria established by Nagasawa et al. [9]. The demand values increased and decreased from 5% to 25% of the maximal grip strength at a constant frequency of 0.2 Hz. Relative values based on the maximal handgrip strength, but not absolute values, were used as the demand values. First, the maximal handgrip strength was measured twice with a 1-min interval to set the demand values, and the greater value was used in this study. The program was designed to present the demand values within a constant range on the display regardless of differences in each participant's maximal handgrip strength. The duration of the CFE test was 40 s, and the CFE was estimated using the data, excluding the first 15 s of each trial, considering a stable time of performance. The sum of the differences between the demand value and the grip exertion value was used as the estimates of the CFE error. Smaller errors in CFE were interpreted to indicate superior CFE. The subjects performed the CFE test 3 times after one practice trial, and the mean of the second and third trials was used as a representative value.

2.3. Statistical Analysis

The data were reported using ordinary statistical methods, including mean and standard deviation [± standard deviation (SD)]. A two-way analysis of variance (dominant/nondominant hands and measurement period) was used to examine significant differences between the means of the CFE errors in the dominant and nondominant hands. When a significant interaction or a primary effect was found, a multiple comparison test was performed using Tukey's Honestly Significant Difference method. The level of significance was set a priori to 0.05. An effect size (ES) was calculated to examine the size of the mean difference. ES was interpreted as follows: <0.2 as small, >0.5 as intermediate, and >0.8 as large.

3. Results

Table 1 shows the means and SD of the CFE errors for the dominant and nondominant hands at the initial and final times and one month after repeated training. Two-way analysis of variance revealed a significant primary effect in the dominant/nondominant hands and the measurement period. Multiple comparisons showed that the dominant hand had smaller CFE errors than the nondominant hand at the initiation of the experiment (ES = 0.46). No difference was found between both hands at the time of the final measurement. One month after the repeated training, the CFE errors in the dominant hand were smaller than that in the nondominant hand (ES = 0.56). In both hands, the errors at the initial measurement were larger than those at the final measurement (dominant hand: ES = 2.34, nondominant hand: ES = 2.92). Similarly, in both hands, the errors at the initial time were larger than those one month after the end of repeated training (dominant hand: ES = 2.04, nondominant hand: ES = 2.35).

Table 1. Means of the CFE errors in the dominant and nondominant hands and testresults (two-way analysis of variance)

	Dominant hand			Nondominant hand						Post hoc
	Mean	SD	CV	Mean	SD	CV		F-value	Partal η^2	HSD
Initial time	569.1	150.1	26.4	632.3	126.7	20.0	F1	22.03*	0.71	Initial, One month: Dom < Nondom
Final time	296.6	67.7	22.8	327.0	76.8	23.5	F2	74.98*	0.89	Dom, Nondom: Initial > Final, One month
One month after training	326.7	75.2	23.0	372.9	90.8	24.3	F3	0.37	0.04	

unit: %,*: $p < 0.05$, F1: dominant and non-dominant hand, F2: time, F3: intaraction, SD: standard deviation, CV: coefficient of variance, CV = SD/mean × 100, Dom: Dominant hand, Nondom: Nondominant hand, Initial: Initial time, Final: Final time, One month: One month after training

4. Discussion

The results of the present study showed that in both the dominant and nondominant hands, the CFE errors improved by repeated training. Nakamura et al. [18] reported that the learning effect in tracking tasks is related to both comprehension of target trajectory (declarative memory) and improvement of the target tracking procedure (procedural memory). It can be inferred that improvement of these two types of memory promotes learning, thereby decreasing the CFE errors, because the CFE test performed in this study used the same relative load and the same speed in each trial during training. In the CFE test, visual and perceptual information from peripheral tissues is processed in the brain, and muscle strength is exerted in response to motor commands from the brain. In short, the subjects consider the size of the error between the demanded and exerted values based on visual feedback and coordinate force output via motor commands [12]. Thus, the accuracy of cognitive information processing, motor commands, and force output improved with repeated training.

The present results indicate that the difference between the dominant and nondominant hands detected at the initiation of the experiment was lost by 3 weeks period of the repeated training. Lateral dominance generally appears in motor tasks that require dexterity in the hands, fingers, and upper limbs and the dominant hand is superior [13]. Kubota and Demura [11,12] reported that laterality was found in young males and females and also in young and elderly females. In the present study, the CFE errors at the initiation of the experiment were also smaller in the dominant hand than in the nondominant hand.

However, the difference between the dominant and nondominant hands was lost after 3 weeks from the initiation of the experiment. Noguchi et al. [19] reported that lateral dominance is found in the practice effect in the Moving Beans with Tweezers test from results showing that the practice effect is found only in the nondominant hand. They reasoned that the practice effects was not found in the dominant hand because it is frequently used in movements similar to those in the Moving Beans with Tweezers test in daily life, and therefore did not develop. For motor tasks similar to movements in daily life, the practice effect may not be evident in the dominant hand after related coordination skills improve to a certain level. From the above, it can be inferred that the difference between the dominant and nondominant hands reduced because the performance of the nondominant hand improved, while the performance of the dominant hand reached an upper limit.

The CFE error reduced in the dominant and nondominant hands by repeated training over a 3-week period and the effects remained one month after training. However, the difference between the CFE of the two hands at the initiation of the experiment reappeared one month after the training, perhaps because the practice effect may fade more easily in the nondominant hand than the dominant hand.

5. Conclusion

In both the dominant and nondominant hands, CFE is improved by repeated training in controlled force exertion. The dominant and nondominant hands may retain the effects of training differently because the training effect erases the difference in CFE between the two hands and it reappears one month after the task.

References

[1] Geshwind, N., Behan, P., “Left-handedness: Association with immune disease, migraine, and developmental learning disorder,” *Proc Natl Acad Sci*, 79. 5097-5100. 1982.

[2] Gur, R. C., Turetsky, B. I., Matsui, M., Yan, M., Bilker, W., Hughett, P., Gur, R.E., “Sex differences in brain gray and white matter in health young adults: Correlations with cognitive performance,” *J Neurosci*, 19. 4065-4072. 1999.

[3] Dolcos, F., Rice, H.J., Cabeza, R., “Hemispheric asymmentry and aging: right hemisphere decline or asymmetry reduction,” *Neurosci Biobehav Rev*, 26. 819-825. 2002.

[4] Roy, E.A., Bryden, P., Cavill, S., “Hand differences in pegboard performance through development,” *Brain Cogn*, 53. 315-317. 2003.

[5] Chi, J.G., Dooling, E.C., Gilles, F.H., “Left-right asymmetry of the temporal speech areas of the human fetus,” *Arch Neurol*, 34. 346-348. 1977.

[6] Noguchi, T., Demura, S., Aoki, H., “Superiority of dominant and nondominant hands in static strength and controlled force exertion,” *Percept Mot Skills*, 109. 339-346. 2009.

[7] Ohtsuki, H., Hasebe, S., Okano, M., Furuse, T., “Comparison of surgical results of responders and non-responders to prism adaptation test in intermittent exotropia,” *Acta Ophthalmol Scand*, 75. 528-531. 1997.

[8] Nagasawa, Y., Demura, S., Yamaji, S., Kobayashi, H., Matsuzawa, J., “Ability to coordinate exertion of force by the dominant hand: comparisons among university students and 65-to 78-year-old men and women,” *Percept Mot Skills*, 90. 995-1007. 2000.

[9] Nagasawa, Y., Demura, S., “Development of an apparatus to estimate coordinated exertion of force,” *Percept Mot Skills*, 94. 899-913. 2002.

[10] Nagasawa, Y., Demura, S., Kitabayashi, T., “Concurrent validity of tests to measure the coordinated exertion of force by

computerized target pursuit," *Percept Mot Skills*, 98(2), 551-560. 2004.

[11] Kubota, H., Demura, S., "Gender differences and laterality in maximal handgrip strength and controlled force exertion in young adults," *Health*, 3(11). 684-688. 2011.

[12] Kubota, H., Demura, S., Kawabata, H., "Laterality and Age-level Differences between young women and elderly women in controlled force exertion (CFE)," *Arch Gerontol Geriatr*, 54. e68-e72. 2012.

[13] Demura, S., Yamaji, S., Goshi, F., Nagasawa, Y., "Lateral dominance of legs in maximal muscle power, muscular endurance, and grading ability," *Percept Mot Skills*, 93. 11-23. 2001.

[14] Taylor, H. G., Heilman K. M., "Left-hemisphere motor dominance in right-handers," *Cortex*, 16. 587-603. 1980.

[15] Shea, C.H., Kohl, R.M., "Specificity and variability of practice," *Res Q Exerc Sport*, 61. 169-177. 1990.

[16] Shea, C. H., Kohl, R. M., "Composition of practice: Influence on the retention of motor skills," *Res Q Exerc Sport*, 62. 187-195. 1991.

[17] Demura, S., Sato, S., Nagasawa, Y., "Re-examination of useful items for determining hand dominance," *Gazz Med Ital-Arch Sci Med*, 168(3). 169-177. 2009.

[18] Nakamura, M., Ide, J., Sugi, T., Terada, K., Shibasaki, H., "Method for studying learning effect on manual tracking of randomly moving visual trajectory and its application to normal subjects," *IEICE, J78-D-II*, (3). 547-558. 1995.

[19] Noguchi, T., Demura, S., Nagasawa, Y., Uchiyama, M., "An examination of practice and laterality effect on the purdue pegboard and moving beans with tweezers," *Percept Mot Skills*, 102. 265-274. 2006.

Importance of Anthropometric Characteristics in Athletic Performance from the Perspective of Bangladeshi National Level Athletes' Performance and Body Type

Adhikari Anup[1,*], Pervin Nahida[2], Rumy Nazrul Islam[2], Ali Kitab[3]

[1]Anthropmetrica, Toronto, Canada
[2]Bangladesh Institute of Sports (BKSP), Dhaka, Bangladesh
[3]Bangladesh Athletic Federation, Dhaka, Bangladesh
*Corresponding author: dranupadhikari@yahoo.com

Abstract The significant role of anthropometric characteristics in sport performance besides other factors is well known. Requirement of specific physique for good performance in specific sports has been established in different studies. The athletic performance of Bangladesh is not that much well and that might be due to different physiological or psychological or skill level aspects. A physical and physiological study was conducted to find out the reason for poor performance of the Track and Field athletes as athletic performance was more dependent on physiological demands besides skill and techniques. Body composition, somatotype and VO_{2max} of twenty-eight national level athletes (15 male and 13 female) were studied at Bangladesh Institute of Sports (BKSP). Average height and weight of the female athletes of the present study were 157.6 cm (± 5.4) and 50.6 kg (± 4.5) respectively with an average age of 17.8 yr (± 1.6). The stature ranged between 149.0 cm and 166.2 cm whereas that of body weight was between 44.0 kg and 60.3 kg. Similarly their male counterparts possessed an average height of 171.2 cm (SD ± 7.5, range 157.4.cm - 181.4 cm) with an average body mass of 62.7 kg (SD ± 8.2, range 47.2 kg– 73.5 kg). A slightly high body fat% of 18.4 (SD ± 2.3, range 14.1% - 22.0%) was observed for the female athletes whereas that of their male counterparts was 7.9% (SD ± 1.5, range 5.7% - 11.3%). Average balanced mesomorph with less mesomorph component was observed for the female athletes (2.7±0.5–3.4±0.9–2.7±0.9) while that of their male counterparts was ectomorphic mesomorph with less mesomorph component (1.5±0.4–4.0±1.1–3.0±1.1). Normal range of body fat% was observed both in male and female athletes with slightly higher in females. An average VO_{2max} of 45.3 $ml.kg^{-1}.min^{-1}$ (SD ± 6.6, range 34.1-56.1) was observed for female athletes whereas that of their male counterparts was 59.1 $ml.kg^{-1}.min^{-1}$ (SD ± 5.3, range 50.3- 68.4). Anthropometric characteristics in terms of Somatotype of the Bangladeshi athletes were poor compare to Olympians and other international athletes though the physiological aspects in terms of VO_{2max} were more considerable compare to international athletes. Hence, poor performance of Bangladeshi athletics might be due to poor anthropometric characteristics which support the importance of Anthropometric characteristics in athletic performances.

Keywords: *body composition, somatotype, athlete, bangladesh*

1. Introduction

Body composition and somatotype of a sportsman has a significant role in sports performance besides other factors like physiological and physical fitness, psychological aspects, skills etc. Requirement of specific physique for good performance in sports had been supported by different studies [1]. Various studies had been attempted to relate performance level with body type and body composition [2,3,4,5,6]. Relationship between the leg length and performance level during running had been established by different studies [5,6,7,8]. Similarly, physiological aspects in terms of VO_{2max} had an important role in athletic performance which was revealed by different studies [9-16]. Track and Field games (except Long distance and Marathon running) required a moderate and good aerobic power (VO_{2max}) besides good anaerobic power and muscle strength. Especially in Throwing and Jumping events, need more muscle strength with good muscularity. The athletic performance of Bangladesh was very poor. There might be different reasons but poor physical structure might be one of them. Lack of anthropometric studies on Bangladeshi athletes could not establish the influence of anthropometric characteristics on their performance level. The present study was aimed to evaluate the anthropometric characteristics of the Bangladesh national athletic squad and establish the importance of anthropometric characteristics on performance level.

2. Method

2.1. Subjects

The national athletic squad came to Bangladesh Institutes of Sports (BKSP) campus for a month long training program. Twenty-eight national level athletes (15 male and 13 female) were tested for their body composition and somatotype as a part of their Physical and Physiological evaluation.

2.2. Anthropometric Measurements

Anthropometric measurements were measured on a same day for each player in same session to avoid technical error with a criterion anthropometrist accredited by ISAK [17]. Method described in the International Society for The Advancement of Kinathropometry manual [18] was followed. Stature was measured with an Anthropometric Rod (GPS) up to 1 mm and body mass was measured with an electronic weighing machine. Skin fold thickness were measured with a Harpenden Skinfold caliper. Anthropometric tape was used for measuring girth while sliding caliper was used to measure bone diameter.

2.3. Somatotype

Heath – Carter [19] method was followed for Somatotype rating. The following equations were uses for calculating somatotype.

Endomorphy = $-0.7182 + 0.1451 \times \sum SF - 0.00068 \times \sum SF^2 + 0.0000014 \times \sum SF^3$ where $\sum SF$ = (sum of triceps, subscapular and supraspinale skinfolds) multiplied by (170.18/height in cm). This is called height-corrected endomorphy and is preferred method for calculating endomorphy)

Mesomorphy = $0.858 \times$ humerus breadth $+ 0.601 \times$ femur breadth $+ 0.188 \times$ corrected arm girth $+ 0.161 \times$ corrected calf girth $-$ height $\times 0.131 + 4.5$

Three different equations are used to calculate ectomorphy according to the height -weight ratio (HWR):

If HWR is greater than or equal to 40.75 then, Ectomorphy = $0.732 \times \text{HWR} - 28.58$.

If HWR is less than 40.75 and greater than 38.25 then, Ectomorphy = $0.463 \times \text{HWR} - 17.63$.

If HWR is equal to or less than 38.25 then, Ectomorphy = 0.1

2.4. Body Fat%

Durnin and Womersley [20] technique was followed for body density. Body fat % was derived from the equation of Brozek et al [21].

2.5. $VO_{2\,max}$ (Maximum Oxygen Consumption Capacity)

The Bruce maximal graded exercise test protocol [22] was followed to measure the VO_{2max}. The subject ran on a Treadmill (LE 200, Viasys, German) with a initial speed of 1.7 mph at 10% grade. The inclination of the Treadmill was increased by 2% after every 3min interval. The speed was increased from 1.7 mph to 2.5mph, 3.4mph, 4.2mph, 5.0 mph, and 5.5 mph with an interval of 3min at each stage upto exhaustion. RQ more than 1 also considered as a criteria for measuring VO_{2max}. Expired gas was analyzed breath by breath technique with a metabolic analyzer (Oxycon Pro, Eric Jager, Viasys, Germany).

Table 1. Anthropometrical characteristics and VO_{2max} of Bangladeshi male national athletes

Players ID	Event	Age (yr)	Height (cm)	Weight (kg)	Fat %	Somatotype			VO_{2max} ($ml.kg^{-1}min^{-1}$)
						Endo	Meso	Ecto	
01 MA	Triple Jump	32	168.5	54.7	10.1	1.2	3.3	3.9	68.4
02 MB	100 m	29	167.7	52.9	8	1.6	3.3	4.2	64.4
03 MC	100 m	26	170.9	55.3	5.8	1.1	3.2	4.3	68.0
04 MD	100 m	35	168.4	63.6	8	1.6	4.2	2.3	66.7
05 ME	Hurdles	25	171.5	75.4	9.8	1.9	7	1.2	52.3
06 MF	400 m	26	160.6	59.2	6.9	1.5	4.9	1.6	50.3
07 MG	400 m	19	157.4	47.2	5.9	1.2	3.6	3.3	58.9
08 MH	Triple Jump	22	162.7	60.1	11.3	2.4	5.1	1.9	59.3
09 MI	100, 200 m	23	172.9	55.5	5.7	1.2	2.4	4.6	58.5
10 MJ	100,200 m	23	178.3	71.3	7.4	1.3	3.6	2.9	58.4
11 MK	Hurdles	24	172.8	66.9	8.1	1.5	4.6	2.6	57.6
12 ML	Triple Jump	23	181.4	70.2	7.7	1.3	4	3.7	55.6
13 MM	100 m	23	173.2	68.2	8	1.5	4.4	2.5	58.8
14 MN	100 m	22	175.3	66.5	8.6	1.6	4	3.1	56.5
15 MO	100 m	19	187	73.5	7	1.1	3.4	4.1	55.6
16 MP	100 m	20	169.6	63	8.2	2.5	5	2	56.0
mean		24.4	171.1	62.7	7.9	1.5	4.1	3.0	59.1
SD		4.4	7.5	8.2	1.5	0.4	1.1	1.1	5.3

Table 2. Anthropometrical characteristics and VO_{2max} of Bangladeshi female national athletes

Players ID	Event	Age (yr)	Height (cm)	Weight (kg)	Fat%	Somatotype			VO_{2max} (ml.kg^{-1}min^{-1})
						Endo	Meso	Ecto	
01 FA	High Jump	16	166.2	53.7	22	3.2	2.2	3.7	34.1
02 FB	High Jump	22	163.5	50.6	19.8	2.9	1.8	3.8	35.0
03 FC	Long Jump	19	159.3	48.5	18.6	2.6	2.4	3.4	48.8
04 FD	Hurdles	16	161.7	54.8	18	2.3	3.3	2.6	48.7
05 FE	800 m	17	162.5	51.3	19.2	2.7	3.4	3.5	52.5
06 FF	400 m	18	149	46.3	18.7	2.7	3.9	1.8	41.0
07 FG	100,200 m	16	150.3	47.6	16.8	2.4	4	1.8	42.3
08 FH	800,1500 m	18	155.9	45	14.1	1.7	3.3	3.5	56.1
09 FI	Throwing	18	156.2	60.3	23	4	4.9	1	46.0
10 FJ	High Jump	19	153	44	16.8	2.4	3.3	3.2	48.5
11 FK	100, 200 m	17	152.9	51.2	17	2.7	4.4	1.6	48.5
12 FL	100 m	17	161.7	54.8	16.6	2.3	3.8	3	48.7
13 FM	100 m	18	156	49.3	18.5	2.7	3.2	2.6	39.1
mean		17.8	157.6	50.6	18.4	2.7	3.4	2.7	45.3
SD		1.6	5.4	4.5	2.3	0.5	0.9	0.9	6.6

3. Results

Table 1 showed the anthropometrical characteristics and VO_{2max} of the male athletes whereas the Table 2 showed that of the female counterparts. The male athletes were 24.4 yr old in average with a range between 19 yr and 32 yr. The average stature obtained for these male Bangladeshi athletes was 171.1 cm (± 7.5) with a range between 157.4 cm and 181.4 cm. The body weight of these male athletes varied from 47.2 kg to 72.5 kg with an average body weight of 62.7 kg.

Table 2 showed the anthropometrical characteristics and VO_{2max} of the female counterparts. Most of the female athletes were very young with an average age of 17.8 yr (± 1.6) with a range between 16 yr and 22 yr. Their average height was 157.6 cm (± 5.4). The tallest girl of the group was 166.2 cm compare to the shortest stature of 149.0 cm. Average body weight was comparatively low which was 50.6 kg with a standard deviation of 4.5 where the highest value was 60.3 kg and the lowest was 44 kg.

A slightly high body fat% of 18.4 (SD ± 2.3, range 14.1% - 22.0%) was observed for the female athletes whereas that of their male counterparts was 7.9% (± 1.5) with a range between 5.7% and 11.3%. Poor muscularity with less mesomorph component were observed for most of the athletes while considering the male and female both. The female athletes were balanced mesomorph in average whereas the male athletes were ectomorphic mesomorh in average. The obtained components were 2.7-3.4-2.7 with a standard deviation of ± 0.5-0.9-0.9 for endo-meso-ecto components for the female athletes whereas those of male athletes were 1.5-4.1-3.0 with a standard deviation of ± 0.4-1.1-1.1.

Average VO_{2max} for the male athletes was 59.1 ml.kg^{-1}.mim^{-1} with a range between 50.3 and 68.4. The standard deviation was 5.3 ml.kg^{-1}.min^{-1}. Similarly, that of their female counter parts was 45.3 ml.kg^{-1}.mim^{-1} with a range between 34.1 and 56.1 (SD ± 6.6 ml). In both cases the aerobic power in terms of VO_{2max} were moderate and in some cases they were in good category (Table 1 and Table 2).

4. Discussion

Physical characteristics of a sportsman has a tremendous influence on the performance level besides personal skill and mental ability and a range of studies had been done on sportsman about their morphological evaluation along with their performance related morphological issues [23-28]. These studies revealed that height can play a significant role in contributing to success in some sports by offering certain natural advantages. For those sports where this could be a contributing factor, height can be useful (although certainly not in all cases, and is not the only factor) since in general it affects the leverage between muscle volume and bones towards greater speed of movement and power, depending on overall build, fitness and individual ability. However, there can also be significant disadvantages posed by size and resultant mass that could prove to be a hindrance to success. But in Track and Field athletics, most of the events required a good height and weight for better performance [23-28].

In the present study, most of the female athletes were very young and some of them were under 19 yr except one with 22 yr. But their male counterparts were more senior to them and all were more than 19 yr. The average height was comparatively less than their international counterparts but very close to average height of Bangladeshi women. Average height of Bangladeshi women was comparatively less. According to the recent study, the average Bangladeshi women possessed an average height of 147.9 cm with a standard deviation of 5.2 where the range was between 119.5-165.4 cm [29]. Similarly, the average height of Bangladeshi male squad was also less than their international counterparts but very similar to the average height of Bangladeshi male population [29].

Negative relationship between sports performance especially sprinting events and adiposity in terms of body Fat% were revealed by different studies though some of the studies showed less relationship of body fat% with endurance activity in term of maximum oxygen consumption [30,31,32]. However, a range between 3.3% and 18.4 was reported for male athletes whereas that of the female was observed to be in between 8.4% and 28%. These included Track and Field, Soccer, Basketball, Football, Ice Hockey, Body building, Wrestling,, Cross-Country skiing, Baseball, Tennis and Power lifting. However, Track and field athletes possessed as low as

3.3% body fat for the marathon runners whereas the male sprinters and discus throwers reported to be with a higher value of 16.4%. Similarly, the female Pentatheletes reported to have lowest value of 11% whereas the Track and field jumpers and hurdlers were performing with 20.7% fat. Highest values were observed for the female Discus throwers and Shot-putters, which were 25% and 28% respectively [33,34]. For the Bangladeshi female athletes, an average value of 18.4% was observed which seemed to be satisfactory when compare to their other international counterparts. The long distance runners possessed low value of 14.1% whereas that of jumping event players was 22%. While the Bangladeshi male athletes were considered they possessed an average value of 7.9 percent. Sprinters possessed a low value of 5.7 in contrary to the 11.3 for the jumpers.

Body type in terms of somatotype is an important factor for enhancement of performance besides other factors, which has been supported by various studies [23,35,36,37]. Recent studies showed that body mass index (BMI), reflecting greater muscle mass rather than greater adiposity, is the important factor associated with best performance for the world-class sprinters. The study also revealed that in track and field athletes, the reciprocal ponderal index (RPI) was an important indicator of best performance with tall and lean body type. However the study supported the decade long hypothesis for encouraging the ectmorphic mesomorph body type for the of Track and Field athletes with higher reciprocal Ponderal index [38]. Other studies also showed that mesomorphic component was a dominant characteristic of somatotype for Track and Field athletes compare to other two components [4,5,6,7,8,37,38].

Bangladeshi male athletes of the present study were ectomorphic-mesomorph in average with a endo-meso-ecto components of 1.5-4.1-3.0 whereas the female athletes were balanced mesomorph with endo-meso-ecto components of 2.7-3.4-2.7. Most of the male athletes were very poor in muscularity, which were less than 4. Only two of the whole squad possessed mesomorphic components more than 5. Similarly in female squad, most of the athletes were with less than 4.0 mesomorphic component whereas only three were more than 4.0 mesomorphic components. In both cases the mesomorphic components were very less indicating poor muscularity for the Bangladeshi athletes irrespective of gender. Bangladeshi male track and field athletes possess less mesomorph components while comparing with the average 5.0 ($\pm$ 0.9) mesomorph component of the Olympic athletes compiled by Carter [32]. The male Olympic athletes, compiled by Carter [32] possessed an average somatotype of 1.8- 5.0-3.0 with a standard deviation of $\pm$ 0.5-$\pm$0.9-$\pm$0.8. Interestingly, the average somatotype of the Bangladeshi male athletes were very similar with somatotype value observed for the neighboring Indian rural athletes which was 2.6-3.3-3.4 studies by Bhatnagar and Grewal [2]. Similar observations were also observed for the female track and field athletes too. The average somatotype for the female Track and Field athletes, compiled by Carter [32] for the 1968 and 1976 Olympics, were 2.8-3.7-3.2 which was higher than the average somatotype of Bangladeshi female athletes.

Maximum oxygen consumption capacity (VO_{2max} is one of the most important characteristics for cardio-vascular fitness, especially for the long distance events in athletic field. In sprinting events and in Throwing & Jumping events, anaerobic power is more dominant than aerobic power or VO_{2max} and require a moderate VO_{2max} rather than a high VO_{2max} [17,18,19,20,30,31,32]. In the present study all the athletes were from sprinting events or from Throwing & Jumping events and require a moderate level of VO_{2max}. Both male and female athletes possessed a moderate value for VO_{2max} compared with international standard, which did not reflected in their sports performance.

The performance level of Track and Field events for Bangladesh was not good enough compare to other countries even when compare with South Asian athletes. Most of the athletes in Bangladesh are from low socio-economic status. Only few athletes were from middle-income group. This poor socio economic status causes unavailability of proper nutrition required for the athletes' growth and development during their adolescent stage, absence of which hinder the growth and development of muscle along with other physical characteristics, though they had a moderate of high level of aerobic power sufficient for showing good performance in their own events which they did not. Thus, good performance in their own events might be hampered by their poor physical characteristics though they had a moderate to good aerobic power compare to international athletes. Hence, it could be concluded that anthropometrical characteristics were one of most influential factors in determining good athletic performances besides other physiological characteristics.

References

[1] Carter, J.E.L, Heath, B.H., Somatotyping – development and application. Cambridge, Cambridge University Press, 1990.

[2] Bhatnagar,. D.P., Grewal, R., A comparative study of rural athletes of four states of India, Brit. J. Sports Med., 18 (1): 34-37, 1984.

[3] Bayios, I.A., Bergeles, N.K., Apostolidis, N.G., Noustsos, K.S., Koskolou, M.D., Anthropometric, body composition and somatotype differences of Greek elite female basketball, volleyball and handball players, J. Sports Med Phys Fitness, 46 (2): 271-280, 2006.

[4] Artioli, G.G., Gualano, B., Franchini, E., Batista, R.N., Polacow, V.O., Jr. Lancha, A.H., Physiological, performance, and nutritional profile of the Brazilian Olympic Wushu (kung-fu) team, J Strength Cond Res, 23 (1): 20-25, 2009.

[5] Hagberg, J.M., Rankinen, T., Loos, R.J., Perusse, L., Roth, S.M., Wolfarth B., Bouchard, C., Advances in exercise, fitness, and performance genomics in 2010, Med. Sci. Sports Exerc., 43 (5): 743-752. 2011.

[6] Kim, J., Cho, H.C., Jung, H.S., J.D. Yoon, J.D., Influence of performance level on anaerobic power and body composition in elite male judoists, J Strength Cond Res, 25 (5): 1346-1354, 2011

[7] Kyriazis, T., Terzis, G., Karapatsos, G., Kavouras, S., Georgiadis, G., Body composition and performance in shot put athletes at preseason and at competition, Int J sports Physiolo Perform, 5 (3): 417-421, 2010.

[8] Potteiger, J.A., Smith, D.L., Maier, M.L., Foster, T.S., Relationship between body composition, leg strength, anaerobic power, and on-ice skating performance in division I men's hockey athletes, J Strength Cond Res, 24 (7): 1755-1762, 2010.

[9] Conley, D.L., Krahenbuhl, G.S., Running economy and distance running performance of highly trained athletes, Med. Sci. Sports. Exerc, 12: 357, 1980.

[10] Hoffman, J.R., Physiological Aspects of Sport Training and Performance, Champaign, IL, Human Kinetics, 25-26, 2002.

[11] Brook, G.A., Fahey, T.D., Baldwin, K.M., Exercise Physiology: human Bioenergetics and its application, 4th ed, New York, McGraw-Hill, 2005.

[12] Astrond, P.O., Rodahl, K., Dahl, H.A., Stromme, S.B., Textbook of work physiology: Physiological basis of Exercise, 4th ed, Champaign, IL, human Kinetics, 2003.

[13] John, E. H., Guyton and Hall Textbook of Medical Physiology, 12th Ed., Saunders, 2012.

[14] Hagerman, F.C., Applied physiology of rowing, Sports Med. 1 (4) (4): 303-26, 1984.

[15] Bassett, D. R., Howley, E.T., Maximal oxygen uptake: "classical" versus "contemporary" viewpoints, Med Sci Sports Exerc, 29 (5): 591-603, 1997.

[16] Bassett D.R Jr. & Howley E.T., Limiting factors for maximum oxygen uptake and determinants of endurance performance, Med Sci Sports Exerc. 32 (1): 70-84, 2000.

[17] ISAK, International Society for the Advancement of Kinanthropometry, 1986, www.isakonline.com

[18] ISAK manual, International standards for Anthropometric Assessment, edited by Michael Marfell-Jones, Tim Olds, Arthur Stewart and L.E. Lindsay Carter, Published by International Society for the Advancement of Kinanthropometry, 2012

[19] Heath, B.H., Carter, J.E.L, A modified somatotype method, American Journal of Physical Anthropology, 27: 57-74, 1967.

[20] Durnin, J.V.G.A., Womersly, J., Body fat assessed from total from total body density and its estimation from skinfold thicknesses. Brtish Journal Nutrition, 32: 77-79, 1974.

[21] Brozek. J., Grande, F., Anderson, J.T., Keys, A., Densitometric analysis of body composition: revision of some quantitative assumptions. Annals of the New York Academy of Sciences, 110: 113-140, 1963.

[22] Bruce, R.A., Kusumi, F., Hosmer, D., maximum oxygen intake and nomographic assessment of functional aerobic impairment in cardiovascular disease, American Heart Journal, 85: 546-562, 1973.

[23] Carter, J.E.L., Physical Structure of Olympic athletes, Part II, Kinanthropometry of Olympic Athletes, Ed Karger, Basel,1984.

[24] Sidhu, L.S., Kansal, D.K., Kanda, B.S., Anthropometric and roentgenogrammetric assessment of physique and body composition of athletes specialising in throwing events, J Sports Med Phys Fitness, 115 (3): 192-198, 1975.

[25] Novak, L.P., Bestit, C., Mellerowicz, H., Woodward, W.A., Maximal oxygen consumption, body composition and anthropometry of selected Olympic male athletes, J Sports Med Phys Fitness,18 (2): 139-151, 1978.

[26] Cureton, K.J., Sparling, P.B., Distance running performance and metabolic responses to running in men and women with excess weight experimentally equated, Med Sci Sports Exerc, 12 (4): 288-294, 1980.

[27] Bhatnagar, D.P., Some morphological measures in athletes, volleyball and Kabbadi players of rural areas of Madhya Pradesh, J Sports Med Phys Fitness, 20 (1): 102-109, 1980.

[28] Slaughter, M.H., Lohman, T.G., An objective method for measurement of musculo-skeletal size to characterize body physique with application to the athletic population, Med Sci Sports Exerc, 12 (3): 170-174, 1980.

[29] Hosegood, V., Oona, R., Campbell Body mass index, height, weight, arm circumference, and mortality in rural Bangladeshi women: a 19-y longitudinal study, American Journal of Clinical Nutrition, 77 (2): 341-347, 2003.

[30] Goran, M., Fields, D.A., Hunter, G.R., Herd, S.L., Weinsier, R.L., Total body fat does not influence maximal aerobic capacity, International Journal of Obesity, 24, 841-848, 2000.

[31] Sporis, G., Jukic, I., Bok, D., Vuleta, D. Jr., Harasin, D., Impact of body composition on performance in fitness tests among personnel of the Croatian navy, Coll Anthropol, 35 (2): 335-339, 2011.

[32] McArdle, A.D., Katch, F.I., Katch, V.L., Exercise Physiology, 5th Ed, Lippincot Williams & Wilkins, 794-819, 2001.

[33] Franchini, E., Del, Vecchio, F.B., Matsushigne, K.A., Artioli, G.G., Physiological profiles of elite judo athletes, Sports Med, 41 (2): 147-166, 2011.

[34] Aitken, A., Clarke, P.T., Brown, I.J., Kay, D., The relationship between body shape (somatotype) and body satisfaction (cathexis) in male physical educators, Scottish Journal of Physical Education, 8 (3): 30-33, 1980.

[35] Bale, P., Colley, E., Mayhew, J., Size and somatotype correlates of strength and physiological performance in adult male students, Australian Journal of Science and Medicine in Sport, 16: 2-6,1984.

[36] Watts, A.S., Coleman, I., Nevill, A., The changing shape characteristics associated with success in world-class sprinters, J Sports Sci, 14: 701-718, 2011.

[37] Vucetic, V., Matkovi, B.R., Sentija, D., Morphological differences of elite Croatian track-and-field athletes. Coll Anthropol, 32 (3): 863-868, 2008.

[38] Nande, P., Mudafale, V., Vali, S., Anthropometric profile of female and male players engaged in different sports disciplines, The Internet Journal of Nutrition and Wellness, 8 (1), 2009, available at http://yester.ispub.com/journal/the-internet-journal-of-nutrition-and-wellness/volume-8-number-1.

Questionnaire: Loss of Entertainment in Spanish Futsal (PEFSE)-Results Analysis

J. Cachón-Zagalaz[1,*], P. Valdivia-Moral[2], A. Lara-Sánchez[1], M. L. Zagalaz-Sánchez[1], D. Berdejo-del-Fresno[3,4]

[1]University of Jaén, Jaén, Spain
[2]University of Huelva, Huelva, Spain
[3]The Football Association, London, England
[4]Sheffield FC Futsal
*Corresponding author: jcachon@ujaen.es

Abstract In the absence of questionnaires addressing the analysis of the rule's change in futsal and the need to find an instrument that is capable of carrying out this objective, the aim of this study is to design and develop a questionnaire to assess the loss of entertainment in futsal. To do this, the sample consisted of 279 subjects with roles as a coach, player, physiotherapist, amateur referee and journalist since all of them are part of the sport. The instrument is based on the new rules imposed by FIFA in the kick-in and corner and their impact on the show. This descriptive cross-sectional study where is designed and implemented a closed-responses ad hoc questionnaire to subjects related with futsal in the first category to obtain objective information was undertaken. The analysis of data showed satisfactory results in terms of reliability and validity. It can be concluded that this scale is valid and reliable instrument to analyze changes in the rules of futsal.

Keywords: *futsal, rules of the game, spectacle, subjects, questionnaire*

1. Introduction

The fast football, indoor soccer or ice football, as it is known in the United States, has its home in Canada almost two centuries ago [1,2]. It was developed as an alternative in places with harsh winters to allow soccer practitioners to continue playing. They did in a wooden floor over the ice hockey court [3]. However, as currently known, futsal (FS) originated in Uruguay in schools, developing the modern version from 1930 onwards, when Professor Juan Carlos Ceriani defines the times and rules. It was played on a basketball court with 5 players on each team. This version will be adopted as the official by the FIFA and, in the opinion of most experts, offers the best conditions for the football development of children.

This research is situated within the social sciences and sports. It has analytical and descriptive nature of socio-metric data, such as Rincón, Arnal, Latorre and Sans [4] point, it fits into the constructivist paradigm, within the scope of collective contact sports that aims to demonstrate that subjects related with Futsal such as spectators, fans, players, coaches, referees, journalists, managers and physiotherapists, saying that the show is no longer as attractive as it was before 2006 [5]. At this point it should be noted that Spain has been 2 times World Champion (Guatemala'00, China Taipei'04) 6 times European Champion (Spain'96, Russia'01, Czech Republic'05 , Portugal'07 , Hungary '10 , Croatia'12), 7 times IV Nations Tournament Champion (Italy'91, Belgium'93, Holland'94, Spain'95, Holland'97, Spain'98, Spain'10), 2 times FIFA Champions (Singapore 1997 and 2001); 1 time Grand Prix Champion (Brasil'10) 2 times Runners up in the World Championships (Spain'96, Brasil'08) and 1 time Runners up in the European Championships (Spain'99).

According to Cachón [6], the publication of the Laws of FS by the Royal Spanish Football Federation (RFEF), the President thereof, Ángel María Villar Llona states that [7]:

> *For many years, the FIFA (Fédération Internationale de Football Association) has allowed that the FS were practiced with different game rules in order to promote its development and not to hinder its progress. Currently, it has reached a stage of development such that the most suitable for its future is permanently unify and thus help the sport to be played under the same Game Rules. With the unification of the Laws, recognition and dissemination of this activity between the media and the public will be improved, and the training of coaches, players and referees will be optimized as they will not have to adapt to variations when participating in international competitions.*
>
> *For all the above, FIFA decided that the 2006-2007 season, all member associations, began their FS competitions under the FIFA FS Laws of the Game.*

Due to rules change imposed, this research is justified by the comparative study of the futsal rules prior to 2006 and the rules applied since then until now (2013) in Spain, the so-called "FIFA rules". The application of the new rules in Spain, involves a comparison and further analysis as global rules (FIFA) did not apply in Spain and the game had its own characteristics that made it more dynamic and spectacular.

In the literature review, studies in this field have not been found. However, the Teseo Database, only three doctoral theses analyzing the FS appear, but none of them refers to the rules, before or after 2006. In the first, Bortoli [8] discusses the cognitive abilities in futsal, indispensable for the development of a team sport and to implement strategies for throw-ins. The second, Jiménez-Jiménez [9], takes a praxeological study of the structure of the teaching situations in cooperation/opposition sports with common space and simultaneous participation: handball and FS. Finally, the study of Barbero Álvarez [10] explains the development of a photogrammetric system and its synchronization with the heart rate records for the analysis of competition in team sports.

In specialized sport journals, particularly in the futsal expert magazine, *Revista Fútbol-Táctico*. A football and futsal professional journal, there are three papers that could in any way relate to this study. The first two signed by the Departmento Técnico [7] and the FIFA FUTSAL [11], state about the futsal rules review. Both are completely consistent, except the first paragraph of the first study dating back to 1999. The content says the review is subject to the approval of the member associations, provided that the principles of these Laws are respected. In the same magazine, it highlighted for the interest of this research the article of López Hierro [12] dealing with set-pieces of El Pozo Murcia Futsal Team (Spanish first division). Referred to the set-plays of 2006-07, the article focuses on three sections: the first one on the corners, the second with the throw-ins/kick-ins and third one on free kicks with wall, although the analysis of the throw-ins is purely technical and does not address the social impact of these rules.

Summaries were revised up to ten years ago, of the scientific, academic and sports content journals, often used in our Spanish community whose most recent numbers collected large amount of articles on football, which could be a reference to our study. However they do not devote any attention to the regulations or allude to futsal. The few articles talking about futsal, relate to sports training and fitness. There are also countless articles for futsal on the internet; however, none of them refers directly to our research problem.

Among the rules that were modified to adapt our rules to the international one, highlight two that are considered as the most determining factors of game development and the loss of its dynamic and spectacular character. These are the kick-ins and corner kicks.

Thanks to the theoretical review the importance of rules change in futsal can be seen. Thus, the existence of a tool that enables to measure the opinions of the leading subjects of the sport is essential for further analysis. Therefore, the aim of this study is to design and develop a questionnaire to assess the loss of entertainment in futsal. This instrument will be useful to all subjects involved in this sport (players, referees, coaches, managers, physiotherapists and spectators).

2. Methods

2.1. Research Design

The context is the Spanish futsal and the changes that it has suffered in Spain by following the Laws of the Game imposed in 2006. The study is located within the ex post facto or experimental methods and seeks the views of the subjects involved. A quantitative methodology has been used, because the characteristics research –descriptive method– is suited to the subject matter. It has been completed with qualitative techniques whose exposure has been elsewhere [13]. The phases that were followed were:

1. Project design/preparation and goal setting.
2. Design ad validation of the instrument: "Loss of Entertainment in Spanish Futsal: change of the corner and throw-in/kick-in rules" (in Spanish: Pérdida del espectáculo en fútbol sala español: cambio de regla en saque de banda y córner (PEFSE)).
3. Information collection, data analysis and issuance of findings and conclusions.
4. Writing report.

2.2. Participants

The subjects of this study has been the participants (players, fans, coaches, managers, referees, physiotherapists and journalists) of the XX Spain Futsal Cup Championship, held in Granada during the months of February and March 2009. The sample was randomly selected according to a probabilistic extraction procedure [14]. Specifically, the random cluster sampling was use since the sampling unit is a group of elements of the population.

The following table shows the subjects' characteristics, the corresponding sample and the percentage of the population involved.

Table 1. Percentage distribution of samples

Participants	Population	Sample	%
Coaches	9	9	100,0
Players	104	67	64,4
Managers	10	1	10,0
Referees	16	9	56,3
Fans	740	185	25,0
Physiotherapists	8	2	25,0
Journalists	15	6	40,0
Total	902	279	30,9

Due to the instability of the populations and the difficulties of access to them, we have tried to obtain the representation of the population by percentages rather than mathematical formulas, as indicated by Bugeda [15]. In this sense it is clear the following incidents:

- The population of coaches coincides. However there is a first technical coach per team having 8 teams, plus an assistant coach in one team, representing a total of 9.
- Players were given the questionnaire at the hotel. The questionnaire was taken back the day after.
- The questionnaire was given to 4 managers, however only one filled in it as they did not have time to help with the project.

- The competition lasted 4 days. The questionnaire was given to the fans at half time during the quarter final games.
- The questionnaire was given to 6 (12 referees) out of 8 pairs of referees. Only 9 of them participated in the study, as the other 3 did not give it back.
- The questionnaire was given to 2 out of 8 (1 per team) physiotherapists. They were continuously working after the matches.
- There were 15 accredited journalists, 6 of them foreign. The questionnaire was given to those who had the Spanish language as mother tongue. Only 6 gave it back.

2.3. Variables

The variables of this study are shown in the Table 2.

Table 2. Types of variables used in the study

Type of variable	
Categorical/Attributive	• Gender • Occupation • Qualification • Educational Qualification
Quantitative	• Age
According dimensions	• Review about rules changes Throw-in before 2006 • Kick-in after 2006 • Corner before 2006 • Corner after 2006

2.4. Questionnaire Design

The instrument must meet two basic requirements of validity and reliability. To Latiesa [16] validity refers to "the process used really measures what is intended to measure and purpose refers to the property of the instrument that produces the same results in different tests." In this sense Morales Vallejo [17] states that occurs when "an instrument is valid when it measures what it purports to measure him." As for reliability, "A collection instrument completely reliable data is one that if used twice the same circumstance, produce identical data" [18]. In particular, for the study of the psychometric properties of the questionnaire have proceeded to calculate the reliability and validity by:

A. Items Analysis
   a. Homogeneity Index
   b. Validation Study
   c. Literature Review
   d. Validation by Experts
   e. Pilot Study
   f. Factor Analysis
B. Reliability of the questionnaire
   a. Cronbach's alpha test

The instrument has 30 items (without those that relate to socio-demographic variables) that are answered with a Likert scale. The guidelines described by Valdivia-Moral, Molero, Campoy and Zagalaz [19] were followed to study the validity. Thus, the scale was sent to a group of expert reviewers to achieve the validity of its content who evaluated the degree of understanding of the items and their suitability to the study. These experts were PhD university professors from both Spanish and international agencies. Then we proceeded to the completion of a pilot study which allowed us to evaluate the validity and reliability of understanding of the instrument. Once administered the instrument, we proceeded to score and analyze using the statistical package for Windows SPSS.19. Likewise, the statistical tests necessary to achieve the construct validity and reliability were performed. The characteristics of this study do not make it possible for reliability through a test-retest-test, therefore the Cronbach's alpha test [20] was used.

Different statistical tests to achieve validity were performed, highlighting the KMO test and Bartlett's test of sphericity, 2) Model of principal component 3) Varimax rotation. These tests, in addition to eliminating those items that decreased the Cronbach alpha coefficient, led to the dimensions and variables shown in Table 3.

Table 3. Questionnaire design "Loss of Entertainment in Spanish futsal: rules changes in Throw-ins and Corners" (PEFSE)

VARIABLES	TYPE
Gender	1 closed question
Age	1 closed question
Occupation	1 closed question
Opinions generated with the rules changes	7 closed questions
Throw-in (hands) before 2006	7 opened questions
Kick-ins (feet) after 2006	7 opened questions
Corner before 2006	7 closed questions
Corner after 2006	7 closed questions

3. Results

3.1. Items Analysis

All items were answered with minimum values of 1 and maximum of 5. Likewise items with larger standard deviation were numbered 1, 2, 3, 11 and 27. Those who have submitted lower standard deviation were 7, 8, 10 and 13.

3.2. Analysis of Reliability

To carry out the calculation of the reliability or internal consistency we used the coefficient α of Cronbach. The reliability coefficients are interpreted as a correlation, considering that higher values than 0.70 indicate high reliabilit [21]. Likewise, considering that according to Fox [18] acceptable correlations are those from 0.70 and even 0.60, when critical review estimates are made.

Initially, the questionnaire consisted of 35 items. After application of the coefficient α of Cronbach, a value of .668 was obtained. It was proceeded to remove those items whose score was below .025 and negative correlation. So, we proceeded to remove a total of 5 items. This resulted in the coefficient increased to a score of .705.

3.3. Validity Analysis

Apart from the different tests that are performed to obtain the different types of validity (e.g. PhD expert reviewers), a factor analysis was performed. Although the KMO indicator and Bartlett's test of sphericity obtained scores (.881 and .000, respectively) indicating that you can proceed to its completion, it was decided to maintain the initial number of dimensions and distribution of the items in each dimension, since it is a questionnaire that attempts to gather information from "before" and "after", of changes in the rules of futsal after 2006 and how they affect the game. Likewise, following Valdivia-Moral et al. [19], it can be highlighted that the validity rates achieved were: 1) Content validity through literature review and experts' test, 2) Educational validity, by experts' test, 3) Validity of understanding, by pilot study and, finally, 4) Construct validity, thanks to the KMO indicator and Bartlett's sphericity test.

3.4. Analysis of Sociodemographic Variables

The distribution of respondents in relation to the gender variable was 73.4% men and 26.6% women. As for the age of respondents, 75% of respondents were between 20 and 30 years old, 14.1% were over 30 and under 40 and finally, 10.9% were more than 40 years old. Regarding occupation, 66.3% were fans, 24% players, 3.1% were coaches, with the same percentage for the referees, journalists were 2.2%, 0.8% physiotherapists and finally 0.4% of the respondents were managers.

4. Discussion

In recent years it has investigated the changes of rules in different sports to advance the educational aspects of sport or, as in this case, to support the game. For this, the use of instruments to establish an analysis of the change of the rules is necessary. Therefore, given the lack of specific tools to analyze in futsal, it is necessary to design and develop a questionnaire to assess the loss of entertainment in futsal. This instrument will be useful to all involved in this sport (players, referees, coaches, managers, physiotherapists and spectators).

Following the later, one of the main problems of this discussion is that it is not possible to compare this study with others of the same sport. Hence, this paper can shed light on this scientific field.

The structure of the instrument has five dimensions which allow further analysis of the changes included in the regulations because each dimension corresponds to a significant change in the rules of the futsal. This detailed analysis of the rules would not have been possible if we had set the dimensions based on the statistical tests.

Regarding the psychometric properties of the instrument it is important to highlight that has a Cronbach's alpha of .705, following the recommendations of Nunnally [21] and Fox [18]. That is why it can be said that this questionnaire has high reliability. Regarding the validity, was achieved in various ways. First, the review of expert reviewers, which improved the instrument based on the contributed comments. Furthermore, the Bartlett's test of sphericity and the KMO indicator gave optimal results. Finally, the literature review and pilot test provided different types of validity to the instrument already discussed above.

As the most significant aspects obtained in the answers given by the respondents noted that the variable "change" was valued positively all rule changes: the mean was 3.57 and the mode 5, which indicated a gap between the two values. The data confirmed that there are more subjects that disagree rather than agree on this item. Furthermore, the variable "play" said that it was harder for the player to take the kick-in than the throw-in. The results shown an of average 4.03 and a mode of 5. The data supported the conclusion that there were more subjects in disagreement with the statement of the item. Finally, the variable "player" which indicated that it was more difficult for the player to take the kick-in rather than the throw-in. The mean was 3.98 and the mode 5. Therefore, the most called options were "disagree" and "strongly disagree".

Finally, despite not having found similar instruments in futsal, in this discussion the aim is to compare the data found with those of other authors. Thus, the study of Barbero [10], which highlights the need for reliable data on the futsal competition that may contribute to greater specificity of training and performance improvement, the instrument developed is used to compare different game situations and thus encourage training activities. On the other hand, regarding the study of Juárez, Andrés and Navarro [22], the results found are consistent with these authors about the importance of the explosive actions in futsal players, also Juárez, González and Navarro [23] highlight the sport entertainment when the maximal speed displacements in futsal players are analyzed.

5. Conclusions

Depending on the purpose and the results obtained it can be concluded that it has achieved a good tool to evaluate the new changes of the futsal rules. Likewise, the instrument meets the criteria of reliability and validity types. Ultimately the PEFSE has the appropriate and required psychometric properties needed in this type of surveys. Therefore, the scientific community has an instrument which allow to assess the impact of the rules introduced in the sport of futsal.

References

[1] Cachón, J., Morente, H. and Lara, A.J., "Antecedentes del fútbol sala", *Quadriceps,* 1 (4). 2007.

[2] Cachón, J., Lara, A.J., Cuadrado, V. and Morente, H., "Fútbol sala escolar I. Antecedentes", In *Actas del IV Congreso Internacional y XXV Nacional de Educación Física*, Universidad de Córdoba. Córdoba, 2-5 April, 2008.

[3] Rivarola, M. Fútbol Rápido o "Indoor": Guía de Canchas Locales. *El Sol de Sonoma.* 2007. Available: http://elsolsonoma.com/2007/020107/Deportes. 14 Agosto 2013.

[4] Rincón, D. el, Arnal, J., Latorre, A. and Sans, A. *Técnicas de investigación en Ciencias Sociales*, Dykinson, Madrid, 1995.

[5] Cachón-Zagalaz, J., Rodrigo-Conde, M., Campoy-Aranda, T., Linares-Girela, D. and Zagalaz-Sánchez, M.L., "Fútbol Sala y educación. Aprendizaje de un deporte colectivo para los escolares", *Journal of Sport and Health Research,* www.journalshr.com, 4(3), 145-254, 2012a.

[6] Cachón Zagalaz, J. *Análisis de la incidencia en el espectáculo deportivo del nuevo reglamento del FS (2006) en España.* Tesis Doctoral. Universidad de Jaén, 2010. www.micinn.es/teseo:https://www.educacion.es/teseo/mostrarRef.do?ref=923580.

[7] Departamento Técnico, "Reglamento del Fútbol Sala", *Fútbol-Táctico. Revista profesional de Fútbol y Fútbol Sala*, 5, 2007.

[8] Bortoli, R. *Estudio de las capacidades cognoscitivas en el fútbol sala.* Tesis doctoral, s/p. Universidad de León, 2000.

[9] Jiménez Jiménez, F. *Estudio praxiológico de la estructura de las situaciones de enseñanza en los deportes de cooperación/oposición de espacio común y participación simultánea: balonmano y fútbol sala.* Tesis doctoral, s/p. Universidad de Las Palmas de Gran Canaria. 2000.

[10] Barbero Álvarez, J.C. *Desarrollo de un sistema fotogramétrico y su sincronización con los registros de frecuencia cardíaca para el análisis de la competición en los deportes de equipo. Una*

aplicación práctica para el fútbol sala. Tesis doctoral, s/p. Universidad de Granada, 2002.

[11] FIFA FUTSAL. "Reglamento FIFA FUTSAL", *Fútbol-Táctico. Revista profesional de Fútbol y Fútbol Sala,* 19, noviembre, 2008. Available: http://www.futbol-tactico.com/futbolsala/articulo.php?idedi=6&cat=0&id=20.

[12] López Hierro, J.V. "Jugadas a balón parado El Pozo Murcia", *Fútbol-Táctico. Revista profesional de Fútbol y Fútbol Sala, 4.* 2007. Available: http://www.futbol-tactico.com/futbolsala/articulo.php?idedi=6&cat=0&id=20.

[13] Cachón, J., Campoy, T., Rodrigo, M., Linares, D. and Zagalaz, M.L. "Análisis cualitativo del cambio de las reglas de juego del fútbol sala (2006) en España", *Ágora para la EF y el Deporte,* 14 (3), 332-347, 2012b.

[14] Heinemann, K. *Introducción a la metodología de la investigación empírica en las ciencias del deporte*, Paidotribo, Barcelona, 2003.

[15] Bugeda, J. *Manual de técnicas de investigación social.* Instituto de Estudios Políticos, Madrid, 1974.

[16] Latiesa, M. Validez y fiabilidad de las observaciones sociológicas. En M. García Ferrando, J. Ibáñez and F. Alvira (edts.). *El análisis de la realidad social. Métodos y técnicas de investigación*, Alianza, Madrid, 1994.

[17] Morales Vallejo, P. *Medición de actitudes en psicología y educación*, Comillas, Madrid, 2000.

[18] Fox, D. *El Proceso de Investigación en Educación.* Universidad de Navarra, Pamplona, 1981.

[19] Valdivia-Moral, P.A., Molero, D., Campoy, T. J. and Zagalaz, M.L. "Pensamiento coeducativo del profesorado de Educación Física: Propiedades psicométricas de una escala", *Revista Internacional de Medicina y Ciencias de la Actividad Física y del Deporte.* 2013.

[20] Garrido, M.E., Zagalaz, M.L., Torres, G. and Romero, S. "Validación de un cuestionario para el análisis del comportamiento y actuación de los padres y madres en el deporte", *Retos. Nuevas tendencias en Educación Física, Deporte y Recreación,* 18, 71-76, 2010.

[21] Nunnally, J.C. *Psychometric theory,* McGraw-Hill, New York, 1978.

[22] Juárez Santos-García, D., Andrés Moreno, M. and Navarro Valdivieso, F. "Relaciones entre diferentes desplazamientos en carrera a la máxima velocidad en jugadores de fútbol sala", *Red: revista de entrenamiento deportivo*, 22 (1), 23-26, 2008a.

[23] Juárez Santos-García, D., González Ravé, J.M. and Navarro Valdivieso, F. "Diferencias en las medidas de diversas acciones explosivas entre futbolistas de campo y futbolistas de sala", *Red: revista de entrenamiento deportivo*, 22 (1) 11-16. 2008b.

Recovery & Regeneration Behaviours in Elite English Futsal Players

D. Berdejo-del-Fresno[1,2,*], M. W. Laupheimer[1,3,4]

[1]The Football Association, London, England
[2]Sheffield FC Futsal, England
[3]Queen Mary, University of London, England
[4]Sports & MSK Physician BUPA, London, England
*Corresponding author: daniberdejo@gmail.com

Abstract Futsal is a high-intensity, intermittent sport where accelerations and short sprints are performed at maximal or almost maximal intensity, interspersed by brief recovery periods, during a period of time relatively long. The aim of this study was to analyse the recovery and regeneration, as well as the hydration status of the futsal players in a 1-week period (3 days out, 1 travelling day and 3 days in a camp). Twenty elite level male futsal players from a national team that compete internationally, volunteered to participate in this study. Anthropometric measures, TQR questionnaires and Urine Osmolality status were analysed. The TQR questionnaire showed that there are statistical differences ($p < 0.05$) between both periods; in and out the training camp. Also, the hydration status of the players was not the desirable. The TQR questionnaire and the analysis of the urine with a refractometer might be two good methods to give feedback to the players about the categories where they should implement an action plan with the main aim to educate them.

Keywords: *hydration, TQR, urine osmolality, team sport, indoor soccer, indoor five-a-side football*

1. Introduction

Futsal is a high-intensity, intermittent sport where accelerations and short sprints (usually with a duration of 1 to 4 seconds) are performed at maximal or almost maximal intensity, interspersed by brief recovery periods (activities of low intensity or pauses), during a period of time relatively long (75-80 minutes) [1-6]. From this, it is deduced that, in order to improve their futsal performance, players must arrange specific futsal conditioning with some additional resistance and sprint and agility training.

Although futsal is a relatively new sport, there is a large amount of articles analysing and studying the anthropometry of futsal players, the parameters of futsal, its physiological demands and the fitness level of the teams [1-7]. However, to our knowledge, there is no study that analyses the recovery and regeneration behaviours in futsal players. This aspect is of great importance for the optimal construction of physical and sport-specific conditioning programmes to improve futsal performance and avoid the overtraining syndrome. Since the main objective for a coach is to optimise athletic performance [8], the best performance improvements come from prescribing an optimal amount of physical training with proper recovery periods to allow for the greatest adaptation before competition [8,9].

There are many methods used to measure the training process or the training load performed but few to monitor and control the recovery process. One such framework for this is referred to as the total quality recovery (TQR) process and was developed by Kenttä & Hassmén [10]. The TQR is a recovery and regeneration points system that helps the athletes to assess their own recovery and give them feedback about which aspect must be improved. Several authors have emphasised the need to identify the probable causes of staleness and the need to match these with sufficient rest, sleep, relaxation, nutrition or other needed interventions [11,12]. Among the different approaches directed towards such recovery, the 4 main categories stated by the TQR were: nutrition and hydration, sleep and rest, relaxation and emotional support, and stretching and active rest.

Furthermore, it is well known that the replenishment of glycogen and fluid stores is necessary to tolerate frequent, intense bouts of training. This might be the most important factor in maintaining high intensity training. Fluid is necessary for more than maintaining performance capacity alone; each gram of carbohydrate requires 3g of water to bind to muscle glycogen. Insufficient fluid intake will thus inhibit performance by allowing less glycogen to be stored. To utilise an individual's carbohydrate limit (approximately 1000g), 3000g of water is needed for it to bind to muscle glycogen [13].

An easy way to know the dehydration level of a sportsman is to weigh the subject before and after practising sport. In intermittent sports that are practised for less than 3 hours and under no extreme weather conditions, the water loss through breathing is relatively low compared to the water loss through sweating [14]. A weight loss percentage higher than 1% causes a decrease in the physical performance [15,16,17,18]. When that percentage is superior to 2%, the subject's cognitive functions, such as perceptive discrimination and reaction time, start to worsen [15,16,19,20,21]. Reaction time has special relevance in futsal, since futsal is a team sport where performance is affected by both the physical capacity of the players and their cognitive skills used to solve some play demands. Therefore, the control of the hydration status of the athletes can help them to increase their recovery and regeneration and hence their performance.

Thus, the aim of this study was to analyse the recovery and regeneration, as well as the hydration status of the futsal players in a 1-week period, when players are in and out of a training camp. The hypothesis was that an exhaustive control of the recovery and regeneration together with the hydration status applied over a consecutive 7-day period would increase the self-care of the players and hence their performance.

2. Material and Methods

2.1. Subjects

Twenty elite level male futsal players from a national team that compete internationally, volunteered to participate in this study after having signed the corresponding informed consent. The anthropometric values of the futsal players participating in this study are indicated in Table 1. The TQR questionnaire (Table 2) was administrated to each player every day. Finally, the hydration status was assessed through the players' urine osmolality (U_{osm}). The study was conducted in accordance with the Declaration of Helsinki (2008) and all procedures were approved by the Research Ethics Committee at the institutional University relative to human or animal research.

Table 1. Anthropometric characteristics of the team

n	20
Age (years)	25.39 ± 4.05
Age Range (years)	19.34 ± 4.05
Height (cm)	179.75 ± 5.69
Weight (kg)	73.93 ± 7.87
BMI (m/kg2)	22.88 ± 1.88

Table 2. TQR questionnaire and guidelines given to the players (RECOVERY & REGENERATION POINTS SYSTEM)

RECOVERY STRATEGY	Possible Points	Mon	Tues	Wed	Thurs	Fri	Sat	Sun	SCORING GUIDE ADJUSTMENTS
NUTRITION	8								
Breakfast	1								Give ½ a point for a less than full breakfast
Lunch	2								Give 1 point for a less than full lunch
Dinner	2								Give 1 point for a less than full dinner
Pre-workout snack	1								
Post-exercise refueling within 60 minutes	2								Give 1 point for delaying more than 60 min
HYDRATION	2								
Pre-exercise urine: clear or light colour	1								
Post-exercise urine: clear or light colour	1								
SLEEP & REST	4								
8 hours of restful sleep	3								Give 2 points for 7 to <8 hours Give 1 point for 6-7 hours
Nap during the day	1								
RELAXATION & EMOTIONAL STATUS	3								
Fully relaxed 60 minutes post-workout or 30 minutes of feet-up relaxation post workout	1								
No daily psycho-social stress	2								Give 1 point for mild stress
COOLDOWN/STRETCHING	3								
Adequate cooldown after exercise	2								Give 1 point for partial cooldown
Stretching & foam roller for at least 10 minutes	1								
TOTALS	20								

Fill out this guide over the course of a week to assess your recovery behaviours. The daily total reveals whether you are paying adequate attention to your physical and mental recovery needs.

2.2. TQR Questionnaire

The questionnaire (Table 2) was filled in by the players every day before bedtime. The recovery and regeneration point system grades and monitors actions (i.e. individual proactive recovery interventions) which, potentially, optimise and accelerate the recovery process. Futsal players simply scored their actions and accumulate recovery "points" over a 24-hour period from the main 4 recovery categories: nutrition and hydration, sleep and rest, relaxation and emotional support, and stretching and active rest. Nutrition and hydration allow the accumulation of a maximum of 10 recovery points; sleep and rest a maximum of 4 points; relaxation and emotional support a maximum of 3 points; and stretching and active rest a maximum of 3 points. Thus, the maximum overall score were 20 points. The daily total revealed whether players were paying adequate attention to their physical and mental recovery needs. The overall score of the players was classified in the following three categories: 17-20 daily points is optimal; 15-16 points is good but shows room for improvement; 14 or fewer points means you need to evaluate your recovery behaviours. These three categories were not given to the players, therefore they were not able to know their classification and therefore manipulate their score.

2.3. Urine Osmolality

Players were issued with a graduated beaker every night before bedtime and instructed to record the first morning urine of the following day. An Osmocheck refractometer (Vitech Scientific Ltd, West Sussex, UK) was used to provide an indicative reading of urine osmolality (U_{osm}) pre training. The Osmocheck is a thermally compensated, digital hand-held refractometer that is calibrated from 0 to 1500 mOsml·kg^{-1}H$_2$O with a manufacturer's reported measurement accuracy of ± 20 mOsml·kg^{-1}H$_2$O [22]. The unit measures the refractive index of the urine which is directly related to specific gravity (the mass concentration of urinary solutes). It calculates osmolality (the molecular concentration) based on the empirical relationship between specific gravity and osmolality [22,23]. The manufacturer reports a correlation of 0.99 [22]. U_{osm} was measured in accordance with the manufacturer's guidelines: prior to each measurement the zero-setting procedure was performed, and the prism of the refractometer was cleaned and calibrated against distilled water. Players were instructed to collect a sample of mid-stream urine (first urine in the morning) in a small beaker before the training session. Using a Pasteur pipette 0.3 mL of urine was placed onto the prism surface of the Osmocheck and a reading was taken. Lord [23] notes that the relationship between specific gravity and osmolality may vary if glucose and protein are present in the urine. Medi-Test Combi-8 (Macherey-Nagel, Düren, Germany) reagent strips were used to assess the urine for the presence of glucose and protein. A reagent strip was briefly dipped into the beaker of urine and any excess urine was removed. A reading was taken after 45 seconds by comparing to a colour chart 8 (Macherey-Nagel, Düren, Germany). The remaining urine in the beaker was included in the participant's voided urine total. U_{osm} concentrations greater than 1200 mOsml·kg^{-1}H$_2$O are consistent with severe dehydration [24]. However, according to the manufacturer's guidelines the U_{osm} concentrations of the players were classified in three groups: good between 200-600 mOsml·kg^{-1}H$_2$O, warning if the U_{osm} was more than 600 mOsml·kg^{-1}H$_2$O and danger if the U_{osm} was higher than 1000 mOsml·kg^{-1}H$_2$O. Players were not given feedback about their hydration status.

2.4. Period analyzed

The study was carried out through 7 consecutive days (1 week) in January. The weekly schedule was as follows: the first 3.5 days (Monday, Tuesday, Wednesday and Thursday morning) players were out of the training camp. The next 3.5 days (Thursday evening, Friday, Saturday and Sunday) players were in the training camp. The urine samples were taken and analyzed on Friday, Saturday and Sunday morning.

2.5. Statistical Analyses

Descriptive statistics were performed for all the variables in order to check for the assumptions of normality. Mean ± standard deviation of the data was calculated. Normal distribution and homogeneity of the parameters were checked with Shapiro–Wilk, and Levene's test. The statistical differences were assessed using Student's t test. A P value of 0.05 or lower was considered as being statistically significant. An analysis was performed using SPSS version 16.0 (Chicago, IL, USA).

3. Results

All the variables were normally distributed. Levene's test showed no violation of homogeneity of variance. The general group characteristics were the following: they were aged 25.39 ± 4.05, had a Body Mass Index (BMI) of 22.88 ± 1.88, a weight of 73.93 ± 7.87 kg, and a height of 179.75 ± 5.69 cm. The anthropometric results for the team participating in this study are presented in Table 1.

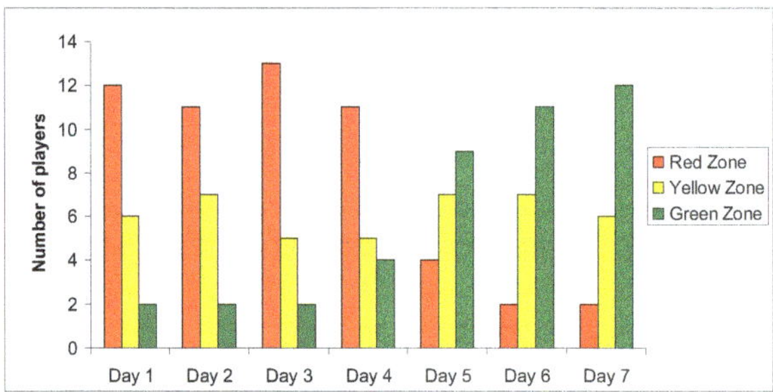

Figure 1. Number of players in each zone every day according to the TQR questionnaire. Green zone (GZ) (optimal) is 17-20 points, Yellow zone (YZ) (good but shows room for improvement) is 15-16 points and Red zone (RZ) (recovery behaviours need to be reviewed) is <14 points. Day 1: 12 players in RZ, 6 players in YZ and 2 players in GZ; Day 2: 11 in RZ, 7 in YZ and 2 in GZ; Day 3: 13 in RZ, 5 in YZ and 2 in GZ; Day 4: 11 in RZ, 5 in YZ and 4 in GZ; Day 5: 4 in RZ, 7 in YZ and 9 in GZ; Day 6: 2 in RZ, 7 in YZ and 11 in GZ; and Day 7: 2 in RZ, 6 in YZ and 12 in GZ

Figure 1 shows the results of the TQR questionnaire. The number of player in the green zone (17-20 points) and yellow zone (15-16 points) tended to increase through the week, while on the contrary the number of players in red zone (<14 points) tended to decrease. Table 3 shows the average points achieved every day in the whole team (n=20). The points in the days 5, 6 and 7 obtained statistical differences with the points from all the others days (day 1, 2, 3 and 4) ($p<0.05$). Table 4 shows the points and the percentage obtained every day in the 4 main categories stated by the TQR: nutrition and hydration, sleep and rest, relaxation and emotional support, and stretching and active rest. The players improved their recovery and regeneration behaviours when they were in the camp compared to when they were out the camp in all the categories. However, nutrition, relaxation and emotional support and stretching and active rest obtained the highest improvements (approximately 30% more points) (Table 4). Furthermore, day four (travelling day) was the day with the lowest total score. All the categories obtained the lowest number of points of the week as well.

Table 3. Average points, standard deviation (SD), maximum points, and minimum points obtained in each day by the players in the TQR questionnaire when they were in and out the training camp

	Camp (in / out)	Mean (points)	SD	Max (points)	Min (points)
Day 1	Out	12.36	3.24	18.00	5.50
Day 2	Out	12.39	3.09	18.00	7.00
Day 3	Out	12.13	3.02	18.00	8.00
Day 4	Out/In*	9.57	5.41	18.00	2.00
Day 5	In	16.08	1.98	19.00	13.00
Day 6	In	16.85	1.82	19.00	12.00
Day 7	In	15.42	2.02	18.00	12.00

* The meeting up for the players in the hotel was on Thursday at 19:00 to take dinner.

Table 4. Points and percentage of the total points (20) obtained every day in each category of the TQR questionnaire

Categories and possible points	Day 1		Day 2		Day 3		Day 4		Day 5		Day 6		Day 7	
	Points	%	Points	%	Points	%	Points	%	Points	%	Points	%	Points	%
Nutrition (8)	5.75	71.88	6.14	76.79	5.53	69.17	4.70	58.75	7.31	91.35	7.54	94.23	7.17	89.58
Hydration (2)	1.07	53.57	1.14	57.14	1.07	53.33	0.67	33.33	1.23	61.54	1.15	57.69	1.50	75.00
Sleep & Rest (4)	2.50	62.50	2.07	51.79	2.80	70.00	2.07	51.67	2.46	61.54	3.00	75.00	2.42	60.42
Relaxation & Emotional Status (3)	2.07	69.05	2.07	69.05	2.07	68.89	1.47	48.89	2.62	87.18	2.62	87.18	2.42	80.56
Cooldown/Stretching (3)	0.96	32.14	0.96	32.14	0.67	22.22	0.67	22.22	2.46	82.05	2.54	84.62	1.92	63.89
TOTAL (20)	**12.36**	**61.79**	**12.39**	**61.96**	**12.13**	**60.67**	**9.57**	**47.83**	**16.08**	**80.38**	**16.85**	**84.23**	**15.42**	**77.08**

Figure 2 shows the results in the urine tests. The players were classified according to the U_{osm} in the three zones (danger, warning and good) given by the manufacturer. Approximately, the 50% of the squad was in the warning or danger zone every day, therefore their hydration status was not adequate. Table 5 shows the mean U_{osm}, standard deviation (SD), maximum U_{osm}, and minimum U_{osm} obtained in each day. In general, it can be stated that approximately the 50% of the players were in an inadequate hydration status, and the average U_{osm} in the team was above 600 $mOsml \cdot kg^{-1}H_2O$ (warning zone) every day.

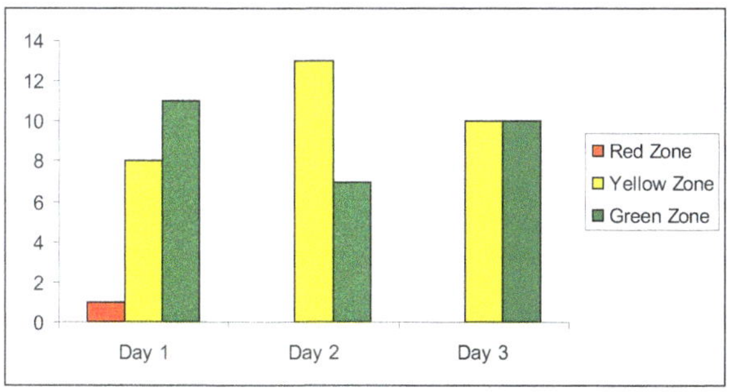

Figure 2. Number of players in each zone every day according to the U_{osm}. Red zone (RZ) (danger) is a U_{osm} more than 1000 $mOsml \cdot kg^{-1}H_2O$, Yellow zone (YZ) (warning) is a U_{osm} higher than 600 $mOsml \cdot kg^{-1}H_2O$ and Green zone (GZ) (good) is a U_{osm} between 200-600 $mOsml \cdot kg^{-1}H_2O$. Day 1: 1 player in RZ, 8 players in YZ and 11 players in GZ; Day 2: 13 in YZ and 7 in GZ; and Day 3: 10 players both YZ and GZ

Table 5. Mean U_{osm} ($mOsml \cdot kg^{-1}H_2O$), standard deviation (SD), maximum U_{osm} ($mOsml \cdot kg^{-1}H_2O$), and minimum U_{osm} ($mOsml \cdot kg^{-1}H_2O$) obtained in each day

	Mean $mOsml \cdot kg^{-1}H_2O$	SD	Max $mOsml \cdot kg^{-1}H_2O$	Min $mOsml \cdot kg^{-1}H_2O$
Day 1	619.50	202.18	1050.00	230.00
Day 2	655.00	246.10	980.00	280.00
Day 3	606.50	127.37	850.00	280.00

4. Conclusions

The purpose of this paper was to research into the recovery and regeneration, as well as the hydration status of the futsal players in a 1-week period, when players are in and out of a training camp with their national team. The hypothesis was that an exhaustive control of the recovery and regeneration together with the hydration status applied over a consecutive 7-day period would increase the self-care of the players and hence their performance.

The TQR questionnaire showed that there are statistical differences ($p<0.05$) between both periods; in and out the training camp. Basically, the data showed that the players' recovery and regeneration behaviours are very different when they are training with their own clubs compared to when they are in a camp with the national team. Camp days (day 5, 6 and 7) showed a totally different trend (Figure 1); since the number of players with poor behaviours is decreasing significantly. Furthermore, the futsal players of this study obtained their lowest daily score (9.57) on day 4 (travelling day) (Table 3). They obtained the lowest number of points in all categories (nutrition and hydration, sleep and rest, relaxation and emotional support, and stretching and active rest) of the week as well. Therefore, the training sessions planned and the training load for the next day (day 5) should take that into account.

Analysing the scores obtained in this study in each of the 4 categories stated by the TQR, it may be highlighted the following (Figure 3 and Figure 4):

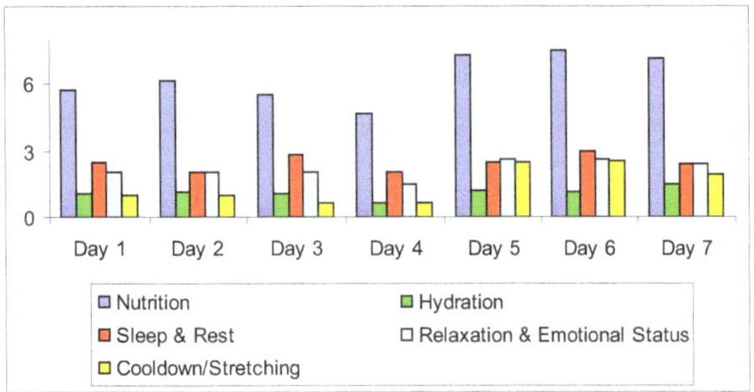

Figure 3. Points out of 20 obtained every day in each category of the TQR questionnaire

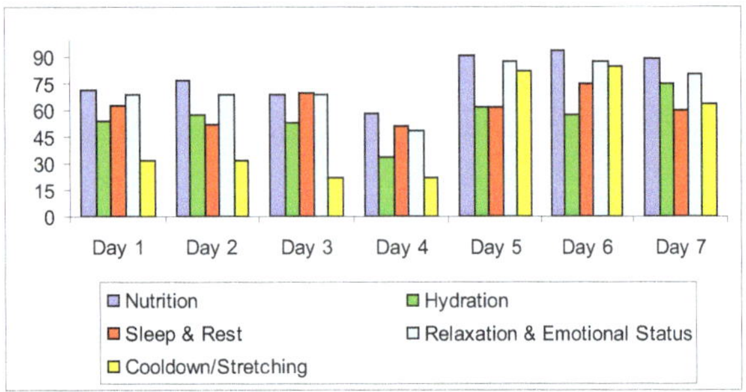

Figure 4. Percentage of the total points (20) obtained every day in each category of the TQR questionnaire

Nutrition and hydration: the futsal players of this study improved their nutrition behaviours throughout the week. They obtained between the 90-95% of the points of this category when they were in the camp compared to the 70-75% of the points when they were out of the national camp. The main reasons for these differences are: a) players used to miss any food, especially breakfast or lunch; b) players were not consistent taking the pre-workout snack; and c) players not always refueled post-exercise within 60 minutes. Following Morgan et al. [25] and Costill et al. [26] individuals failing to ingest sufficient carbohydrates to match the energy demand of heavy training have been shown to develop signs of staleness. A poor diet with an insufficient caloric and fluid intake, particularly one lacking in carbohydrates, will decrease the capacity to tolerate physiological stress (training). Kenttä & Hassmén [10] stated that the replenishment of glycogen and fluid stores is necessary to tolerate frequent, intense bouts of training. This might be the most important factor in maintaining high intensity training. Also, ingesting protein and/or amino acids are required to promote growth, repair damaged cells and tissue, synthesize hormones, and for a variety of metabolic activities. Recent evidence indicates that ingesting protein and/or amino acids can enhance recovery, immune function, and growth and maintenance of lean body mass [27].

The players in this study (90%) gave themselves the maximum points (2) in the hydration category each day. However, the U_{osm} values showed (Table 5) the opposite. The hydration status was not adequate. They were over 600 $mOsml \cdot kg^{-1} H_2O$ every day. This fact, also, showed that the players in this study were not really conscious about their fluid intake needs and urine analysis. Fluid is necessary for more than maintaining performance capacity alone; each gram of carbohydrate requires 3g of water to bind to muscle glycogen. Insufficient fluid intake will thus inhibit performance by allowing less glycogen to be stored [10,13]. Besides, a weight loss percentage higher than 1% causes a decrease in the physical performance [15,16,17,18]. When that percentage is superior to 2%, the subject's cognitive functions, such as perceptive discrimination and reaction time, start to worsen [15,16,19,20,21]. Since reaction time might have special relevance in futsal, the control of hydration status can help them to increase their recovery and regeneration and hence their performance.

Sleep and rest: Kenttä & Hassmén [10] stated that the most frequently mentioned factor for enhancing recovery is most obvious one: rest. In this sense, rest means engaging in no physical activity (passive recovery during the daytime) and obtaining sufficient sleep [13]. In this study, the results obtained showed that the futsal players' sleep and rest behaviours did not improve significantly throughout the week. Recently [28], it has also been showed that lack of sleep appears to be associated with injury risk in an adolescent athletic population. Adolescent may benefit from additional sleep as they get older to help reduce the risk of injury during sports. The science has shown that with a proper sleep tennis players get a 42% boost in hitting accuracy during depth drills, sleep extension provides swimmers a 17% improvement in reaction time off the starting block, sleep improves split-second decision making ability by 4.3%, american football players drop 0.1 seconds off their 40-yard dash times by sleeping more, and a 20-30 minutes power nap improves alertness by 100% [29].

On the contrary, the scientific studies has also shown that a chronic sleep loss can lead to a 30-40% reduction in glucose metabolism and an 11% reduction in time to exhaustion, 2 days of sleep restriction can lead to a 3x increase in lapses of attention and reactivity, the maximum bench press drops 20 lbs after 4 days of restricted sleep and perceived exertion increases 17-19% after 30 hours without sleep [29].

Relaxation and emotional support: Kenttä & Hassmén [10] insured that mental training might help to prevent staleness [30,31,32]. This effect has been explained by an increased recovery capacity or increased stress tolerance [31]. Relaxation techniques, the use of flotation tanks, massages and saunas have also been suggested by Marion [33] as proactive recovery interventions. The players who participated in this study increased significantly their % of points in this category because the facilities and equipment in the national camp allow the technical staff to plan massages' sessions, recovery sessions in the swimming pool, sauna or spa. The learning and practice of relaxation and visualisation techniques by athletes is also recommended [31,32].

Stretching and active rest: active rest, meaning low volume and low intensity training, may accelerate the recovery process [33]. Stretching has effects similar to massage and active rest, in that it increases the blood flow thorough the muscle. Also, foam rolling has been showed to improve muscular function, performance, overuse, and joint range of motion. Recently, MacDonald at al. [34] have demonstrated that an acute bout of self-myofascial release increases range of motion without a subsequent decrease in muscle activation or force. This category showed significant improvements in the players' behaviours when they are in the national camp compared to when they are training with their own clubs. This category is where players in this study had more room to improve, as they did not have as a habit to perform a structured and organised cold-down.

To sum up it can be concluded that the players of this study had very different recovery and regeneration behaviours depending on if they are training with their own clubs or with the national team. Furthermore, their hydration status was not the desirable to recover and regenerate between training sessions. The TQR questionnaire and the analysis of the urine with a refractometer might be two good methods to give feedback to the players about the categories where they should implement an action plan. This would allow us to educate our players about their needs to recover and regenerate properly between training sessions and competitions.

Acknowledgement

The authors of this study wish to acknowledge the players who participated in this study.

References

[1] Álvarez-Medina, J., Serrano, E., Giménez, L., Manonelles, P. and Corona, P. "Perfil cardiovascular en el fútbol-sala: adaptaciones al esfuerzo". *Archivos de Medicina del Deporte*, XVIII(82): 143-148. 2001.

[2] Álvarez-Medina, J., Serrano, E., Giménez, L., Manonelles, P. and Corona, P. "Perfil cardiovascular en el fútbol-sala: respuesta inmediata al esfuerzo". *Archivos de Medicina del Deporte*, XVIII(83): 199-204. 2001.

[3] Álvarez-Medina, J., Serrano, E., Giménez, L., Manonelles, P. and Corona, P. "Necesidades cardiovasculares y metabólicas del fútbol sala: análisis de la competición". *Apunts: Educación Física y Deportes*, 67: 45-53. 2002.

[4] Barbero-Álvarez, J. C., Soto, V. and Granda, J. "Temporary analysis during match play in futsal (indoor soccer) with photogrametric system". *Book of abstract: Science and Football*, 5: 266. 2003.

[5] Barbero-Álvarez, J. C., Soto, V. and Granda, J. "Análisis de la frecuencia cardiaca durante la competición en jugadores profesionales de fútbol sala". *Apunts de educación física*, 77: 71-78. 2004.

[6] Barbero-Álvarez, J. C., Soto, V. and Granda, J. "Effort profiling during indoor soccer competition". *Journal of Sports Sciencse*, 22: 500-501. 2004.

[7] Castagna, C. and Barbero-Álvarez, J. C. "Physiological demands of an intermittent futsal-oriented high-intensity test". *Journal of Strength and Conditioning Research*, 24(9): 2322-2329. 2010.

[8] Coutts, A. J. and Aoki, M. S. "Monitoring training in team sports". *Olimpyc Laboratory: Technical Scientific Bulletin of the Brazilian Olympic Committee*, 9(2): 1-3. 2009.

[9] Gamble, P. "Periodization of training for team sports athletes". *Strength and Conditioning Journal*, 28(5): 56-66. 2006.

[10] Kenttä, G. and Hassmén, P. "Overtraining and recovery. A conceptual model". *Sports Medicine*, 26(1): 1-16. 1998.

[11] Harre, D. Principles of sport training. Berlin: Sportverlag, 1982.

[12] Kuipers, H. and Keizer, H. A. "Overtraining in elite athletes. Review and directions for the future". Sports Medicine, 6(2): 79-92. 1988.

[13] Brooks, G. A. and Fahey, T. D. Exercise physiology: human bioenergetics and its applications. New York (NY): Macmillan, 1985.

[14] Maughan, R. J., Shirreffs, S. M., Leiper, J. B. "Errors in the estimation of sweat loss and changes in hydration status from changes in body mass during exercise". *Journal of Sports Sciences*, 25: 797-804. 2007.

[15] Coyle, E. F. "Fluid and fuel intake during exercise". *Journal of Sports Sciences*, 22: 39-55. 2004.

[16] Sawka, M. N., Burke, L. M., Eichner, E. R., Maughan, R. J. and Montain, S. J. "Exercise and fluid replacement". *Medicine and Science in Sports and Exercise*, 39(2): 377-390. 2007.

[17] Wilmore, J. H. and Costill, D. L. Physiology of Sport and Exercise. Champaign, IL:Human Kinetics. 2007.

[18] Murray, R. "Hydration and physical performance". *Journal of the American College Nutrition*, 26(5 Suppl): 542-548. 2007.

[19] Cheuvront, S. N., Carter III, R. and Sawka, M. N. "Fluid balance and endurance performance". *Current Sports Medicine Reports,* 2: 202-208. 2003.

[20] Casa, D. J., Clarkson, P. M. and Roberts, W. O. " American College of Sports Medicine roundtable on hydration and physical activity: consensus statements". *Current Sports Medicine Reports,* 4(3): 115-127. 2005.

[21] Montain, S. J. "Hydration recommendations for sport 2008". *Current Sports Medicine Reports,* 7(4): 187-192.2008.

[22] Vitech. "Instruction manual digital hand-held 'pocket' urine osmolality refractometer". Vitech Scientific Ltd., West Sussex, UK.

[23] Lord, R. C. "Current concepts: osmosis, osmometry and osmoregulation". *Postgraduate Medical Journal*, 75:67-73, 1999.

[24] Smith, M. S. "Physiological profile of senior and junior England international boxers". *Journal of Sports Science and Medicine*, CSSI: 74-89, 2006.

[25] Morgan, W. P., Costill, D. L., Flynn, M. G., Ranglin, J., S., O'Connor, P. J. "Mood disturbance following increased training in swimmers". *Medicine and Science in Sports and Exercise*, 20: 408-414. 1988.

[26] Costill, D. L., Flynn, M. G., Kriwan, J., P., "Effects of repeated days of intensified training on muscle glycogen and swimming performance". *Medicine and Science in Sports and Exercise*, 20:249-54. 1988.

[27] Kreider, R. B., Campbell, B. "Protein for exercise and recovery". *The Physician and Sportmedicine Journal*, 37(2): 13-21. 2009.

[28] Milewski, M. D., Pace, J. L., Idrahim, D. A., Bishop, G., Barzdukas, A., Skaggs, D. L. "Lack of sleep is associated with increased risk of injury in adolescent athlestes". *American Academy of Pediatrics National Conference & Exhibition Proceedings*. 20-23 October 2012.

[29] Mah, C. "Sleep to be an all-star" (Infographic). Zoe, Inc. 2011.

[30] Unestahl L-E. Integrerad mental training (Integrated mental training) [Swedish]. Malmo, Sweden: Skogsgrafiska AB, 1995.

[31] Veale D. M. W. "Psychological aspects of staleness and dependence on exercise". *International Journal of Sports Medicine*, 12: 19-22. 1991.

[32] Weinberg R., Gould, D. Foundations of sport and exercise psychology. Champaign (IL): Human Kinetics, 1995.

[33] Marion, A. "Overtraining and sport performance". *Coaches Report*, 2: 12-19. 1995.

[34] MacDonald, G. Z., Penney, M. D. H., Mullalley, M. E., Cuconato, A. L., Drake, C. D. J., Behm, D. G., Button, D. C. "An acute bout of self-myofascial release increases range of motion without a subsequent decrease in muscle activation or force". *Journal of Strength and Conditioning Research*, 27(3): 812-821. 2013.

25

Anthropometric and Physical Fitness Characteristics of Elite Futsal Tunisian Players

Trabelsi Y[1,2], Aouichaoui C[1,2,3,*], Richalet JP[4], Tabka Z[1]

[1]Université de Sousse, Laboratoire de Physiologie et des Explorations Fonctionnelles, Faculté de Médecine de Sousse, Sousse, Tunisie
[2]Université de Sfax, Institut Supérieur du Sport et de l'Education Physique de Sfax, Sfax, Tunisie
[3]Université de Gafsa, Institut Supérieur du Sport et de l'Education Physique de Gafsa, Gafsa, Tunisie
[4]Université Paris 13, Laboratoire "Réponses Cellulaires et Fonctionnelles à l'hypoxie" EA 2363, Bobigny, France
*Corresponding author: chirineaouichaoui@yahoo.com

Abstract The purposes of this study are to establish the relationships among vertical jumping parameters, aerobic fitness and sprint running performance and to examine the anthropometric and physiological profile in elite Futsal Tunisian players. Twenty-six elite Tunisian Futsal players (age 26 ± 3 years, height 1.77 ± 0.75 m, weight 69.3 ± 8.5 Kg) volunteered to participate in this study. On separate days, all participants were asked to perform physical performance tests (Squat jump (SJ), countermovement jump (CMJ), sprint and aerobic power test (20-m shuttle run). Pearson's correlation coefficient and multiple regression analysis were used to analyze the data set and to identify which variables significantly influence sprint performance variables. We have found in the current study a negative association between 10 m sprint time and maximal oxygen uptake ($r = -0.44$, $p<0.05$). Leg anaerobic power characteristics were inversely related to 20 m ($r = -0.46$) and 10 × 5 m sprint time ($r = -0.41$). Therefore, muscle power and maximum oxygen uptake seem to be important physiological characteristics for sprinting performance in elite Futsal Tunisian players. This study could help practitioners and coaches to better design training by emphasizing the importance of combining adapted leg muscular power training with sprint running training programs for improving short-distance sprint performance.

Keywords: *indoor soccer, sprint performance, vertical jumps, maximal oxygen uptake*

1. Introduction

Futsal is the official five-a-side indoor soccer game and the only indoor soccer recognized by soccer's international governing body (Federation Internationale de Football Association, FIFA). Il is an intermittent high-intensity strenuous team sport played worldwide that places heavy emphasis on running speed and endurance and requires substantial strength levels to kick, tackle, turn, change pace and sprint during actions. The game is growing in popularity all over the world (12 million players in more than 100 countries) and since 1989 the world championships have been contested by 16 national teams every 4 years [13].

Futsal is a small-sided game (5v5 including the goalkeepers) that requires high physical, technical, and tactical capacity from the players. It is played on a 38-42 m × 20-25 m pitch during two 20-min clock time halves, with the clock stopped for some events that can result in a total duration game of 70-80 min. Teams can request one time out (1 min) in each half and there is a break of 10 min between halves and an unlimited number of substitutions are permitted [3]. However, it has its own character using aspects of different sports (basketball, handball, and football). Barbero-Alvarez et al. [3] revealed that Futsal is a multiple sprint sport presenting more high-intensity phases than soccer and other intermittent sports.

The mean heart rate and the percentage of maximum heart rate recorded during Futsal play were generally higher than those recorded in football, handball, and basketball matches [3]. It has been proven that Futsal players develop quicker reflexes, faster thinking and pinpoint passing [3]. Consequently the physical demands might be very high [3]. Doğramaci and Watsford [11] estimated that during competitive matches, Futsal players cover at high intensity 26% of total game distance or time. Moreover, indoor football requires a cardiovascular demand of 85 to 90% of maximal heart rate, in most matches reaching maximum heart rate [1]. Recently, Castagna and Barbero-Álvarez [9] showed that Futsal played at professional level is a high intensity exercise, heavily taxing the aerobic and anaerobic pathways.

Futsal requires physical and physiological demands on its participants, which become more pronounced with high level of competition. The physical demands are related both to technical aspects of the game and its physical contact elements. The physiological demands are linked to the intensity at which the game is played. Success in a team sport such as Futsal depends on how individual characteristics are blended within the team to form a coherent playing system. This makes the interpretation of physiological profiles of individual players more difficult than in individual sports such as athletics, cycling and swimming where the relationship between physiological capacities and sport performance can be outlined more precisely [9]. Nevertheless, the determination of the physical and physiological profiles of the Tunisian elite Futsal players can provide useful information for both the team as a whole and for the individuals who comprise it. It can also help in identifying strengths and weaknesses in individual players within the team compared to the profile of professional Futsal players. Anthropometric profile is an important selective factor for success in sport [28].

Only a few studies have analyzed some anthropometric [3,10,13] and aerobic power [3,4,10,13] characteristics of elite Futsal players among European and South American countries.

Despite its popularity and its competitive status, it is somewhat surprising to find only little information concerning the muscle power, aerobic capacity and association between muscle power and sprint running performance of current world class elite Futsal players. Knowledge of the anthropometric and physiological characteristics of elite Futsal players is of great importance since it should allow Futsal coaches to control strength/power and endurance training programs in order to adapt their players to the physiological requirements of their sport [9].

An important question is how are the sprint variables related to vertical jumping ability and aerobic fitness in elite Futsal Tunisian players? We hypothesized that vertical jumping parameters and aerobic fitness influence sprinting performance among elite Futsal Tunisian players. Therefore, the first aim of the present study is to determine the possible relationships between aerobic power (maximal oxygen uptake), anaerobic power (vertical jumping test) and sprint running performance. The second aim is to examine the anthropometric and physiological profile of elite Futsal Tunisian players.

2. Methods

2.1. Experimental Approach to the Problem

To quantify the relationship between vertical jumping performance, aerobic fitness and sprint performance and to examine the anthropometric and physiological profile of elite Futsal Tunisian players, 26 Futsal players were asked to perform 20 m shuttle run, sprint, Squat jumps (SJ) and Countermovement jump (CMJ) tests. Pearson's correlation coefficient and multiple regression analysis were used to analyze the data set to determine the possible relationships among aerobic fitness, anaerobic power and sprint running performance. The dependent variables were sprint performance parameters. The independent variables were jump performance measures and maximal oxygen uptake ($VO_{2\ max}$).

2.2. Subjects

Twenty-six elite Futsal players from Tunisian National team took part in this study. Their mean age, height and weight were 26.1±3 (21-36) years, 177±0.07 (164-197) cm and 69.3± 8.5 (56.9-87.0) kg, respectively. The players, with an active playing career of about 6 years, trained five times per week for 90 minutes per training session and participated in Tunisian Futsal Championship once a week.

Before starting the study, players had a physical examination and they answered to a medical questionnaire. Tests were performed in 31 Futsal players, some players did not perform adequately the vertical jumping (n = 2) and the sprint (n = 3) tests. Finally, 26 Futsal players were included in the subsequent analysis.

Prior to the study, the coach and the subjects had been fully informed of the aim of the experimental procedure of the investigation before signing a written consent, which was in accordance with legal requirements and the Declaration of Helsinki, and was approved by the Tunisian Ministry of Youth and Sports and by the Research Ethics Committee of Farhat Hached Hospital (Sousse).

2.3. Test Procedures

All subjects completed two preliminary familiarization sessions to minimize any effects of learning and to be informed about pretest instructions.

All the tests were performed during March 2010 in the afternoon, in the same order and in the same facilities. Testing was conducted over 4 separate sessions, separated by at least 2 days. During the first testing session, each subject was subjected to anthropometrical measurements. In the second test session, each subject was subjected to vertical jumping test. In the third testing session, sprint tests were measured and finally in the fourth session each subject was subjected to graded 20-m shuttle run test.

Players were told to refrain from heavy training, alcohol, caffeine, and tobacco usage for the 2 days preceding testing sessions. Only drinking water was allowed 2 hours before the test. As for heavy meals, the players were asked to stop taking in any foods before 3 hours of the testing sessions. The subjects were not taking any medications that would have an impact on the results of the current study. A comfortable average air temperature of about 20°C existed in all tests. Before each test, subjects performed a standard 15- to 20-minute warm-up. The test-retest intraclass correlation coefficients of the testing procedure variables used in this study were >0.91 and the coefficients of variation ranged from 0.9 to 7.3%.

2.4. Physical characteristics

The anthropometric measurements included height, weight and circumferences such, waist, upper-thigh, lower-thigh and calf girth. Subjects were weighed in minimal clothing using a digital scale (Harpenden Balance Scale, UK) to the nearest 0.1 kg. Standing and sitting heights were measured with an appropriate stadiometer (Harpenden Portable Stadiometer, UK) to the nearest 0.1 cm and the circumferences were measured to the nearest 0.1 cm using a non-elastic measuring tape. The difference between the standing height and the sitting height allowed us to determine the leg length. Body mass index (BMI) was calculated as weight (kg) divided by the square of the height (m).

Lower body impedance was measured with a Tanita TBF-604 Body Fat Monitor/Scale (Tokyo, Japan). This device requires the input of data describing the body mass, standing height, and sex of the subject who then stands on the scale, which contains the source and detector electrodes in the areas that contact the plantar surfaces of both feet. It measures lower body impedance and then calculates the body fatness (fat percentage).

Absolute body fat weight was calculated as follows: fat weight (kg) = %fat × (weight / 100). For determining fat-free weight (kg), it has been calculated by subtracting fat weight from total body weight [8].

2.5. Performance Tests

2.5.1. Vertical Jumping Test

Jumping performance was evaluated with the Optojump device (Microgate SRL, Italy) connected to a portable computer where data were recorded (Jump height, power, flight and contact times).

On an indoor court, vertical jumps were measured with both squat jump (SJ) and countermovement jump (CMJ) protocols. The Futsal players were given two practice jumps before the specific jump test was conducted. The best of three attempts to the nearest within a centimeter was recorded. The jumps were separated by a two- minute rest period to ensure sufficient recovery.

For all jumps, Futsal players retained their hands on their hips to eliminate the influence of the arms swing impulse. For the SJ test, they were instructed to go down and hold a knee position (approximately 120° Knee angle) for three seconds. On the count of three, the player was instructed to jump as high as possible without performing any countermovement before the execution of the jump. A successful trial was one where there was no sinking or countermovement prior to the execution of the jump [15].

The CMJ assessment required the player to be in a standing position and, prior to jumping, counter-moved until the knee was flexed approximately to 90°. They were then instructed to go down as quickly as possible and then jump as high as possible in the ensuing concentric phase. Verbal encouragements were constantly given to maintain high motivation in these groups [15]. All subjects performed 3 consecutive experimental trials for each jump. The best values for each jump were retained for further analysis. Players performed jumps in comfortable clothing and running shoes.

2.5.2. Sprint Tests

The sprint tests were preceded by standardized warm-ups which started with a low-intensity run followed by stretching exercises supervised by coaches. Dynamic exercises aimed at improving suppleness of muscle groups, essential in sprints: flexors and extensors of the hip, knee and ankle joints [22].

The times for 10 m, 20 m and 10 × 5 m sprint tests of players were measured using photocell gates (Brower Timing Systems, Salt Lake City, UT, USA; accuracy of 0.01 seconds). When ready to sprint, the subjects commenced the sprint from a standing start, 0.5 m behind the start. Stance for the start was consistent for each subject. The time was automatically activated as the subject passed the first gate at the 0 m mark and split times were recorded at 10 m, 20 m and 10 × 5 m. Each participant had 3 trials separated by at least 5 minutes of rest, and the fastest time, measured to the nearest 0.01 s, was used as the speed score.

Athletes performed sprints in tight fitting clothing and track spike shoes. Participants were given verbal encouragement to perform maximally during sprints.

2.5.3. Aerobic Power Test-Twenty-Meter Shuttle Run Test

The maximal multistage 20-m shuttle run test, described by Léger and Lambert [19] and modified by Léger et al. [20], was used to evaluate maximal aerobic capacity from maximal aerobic speed. Participants were required to run between two lines 20 m apart. The pace was dictated by a cassette tape emitting tones at prescribed intervals. The initial speed was set at 8.5 km. h^{-1} for the first minute and was increased 0.5 km. h^{-1} for each subsequent minute.

When runners could no longer keep up the pace by reaching the line at the time of the tone, participation was terminated and the number of laps completed was recorded [19]. Scores of the last stage number were converted to predict maximal oxygen uptake ($VO_{2\ max}$) [20]. $VO_{2\ max}$ was expressed in ml of oxygen consumed per kilogram of body weight and per minute (ml. kg^{-1}. min^{-1}).

Maximal Aerobic Speed (MAS) is the lowest speed enabling you to obtain the $VO_{2\ max}$ which the level of maximum aerobic power for a subject. During the test, the participants were verbally, encouraged to run as long as possible.

2.6. Statistical Analyses

Results are expressed as the mean ± standard deviation (SD). Data were screened for normality using the Kolmogorv-Smirnov test and summarized using descriptive statistics. Pearson's correlation coefficient and multiple regression analysis (forward stepwise) were conducted to determine the relationships between vertical jumping performance, sprint performance, maximal aerobic power and anthropometric parameters. The level of significance was set a $p<0.05$. The Statistical Package for Social Sciences (SPSS) (version 17.0) software package and STATISTICA 6.0 package were used to analyze all data.

3. Results

3.1. Physical Characteristics and Body Composition of Elite Futsal Tunisian Players

Twenty-six Futsal Tunisian players were included in the present study. Mean ± standard deviation, minimum and maximum of physical characteristics and body composition in elite Futsal Tunisian players are presented in Table 1.

3.2. Jumping and Sprinting Performance

Mean ± standard deviation, minimum and maximum for sprint performance and jump performance variables of elite Futsal Tunisian players are presented in Table 2.

Jump height and average power of Futsal players during the Countermovement Jump (CMJ) test were significantly higher ($p<0.05$) than during squat Jump test (SJ) (Table 2).

Table 1. Mean ± standard deviation, minimum and maximum of physical characteristics and body composition in elite Futsal Tunisian players

Futsal players (n=26)			
	Mean ± SD	Minimum	Maximum
Age (y)	26 ± 3	21	36
Standing height (m)	1.77 ± 0.07	1.64	1.97
Sitting height (m)	0.92 ± 0.03	0.87	0.99
Weight (kg)	69.3 ± 8.5	56.9	87.0
Body mass index (kg.m-^{2})	21.8 ± 1.6	19.3	25.5
Leg length (m)	0.85 ± 0.05	0.77	0.98
Waist size (m)	0.78 ± 0.04	0.73	0.89
Upper thigh girth (m)	0.54 ± 0.03	0.49	0.62
Lower thigh girth (m)	0.44 ± 0.02	0.41	0.49
Calf girth (m)	0.34 ± 0.02	0.31	0.38
Percent body fat (%)	12.20 ± 3.41	7.0	16.9
Absolute body fat (kg)	8.65 ± 3.08	3.98	12.62
Fat-free weight (kg)	60.70 ± 6.15	51.75	74.39

Table 2. Mean ± standard deviation, minimum and maximum of aerobic fitness, sprint and jump performance measures in elite Futsal Tunisian players

Futsal players (n=26)			
	Mean ± SD	Minimum	Maximum
Sprint performance measures			
10 m sprint time (s)	1.79 ± 0.08	1.54	1.90
20m sprint time (s)	3.19 ± 0.15	2.83	3.50
10× 5m sprint time (s)	14.52 ± 0.27	14.11	14.99
Maximal aerobic power			
$VO_{2\,max}$ (ml. min^{-1}.kg^{-1})	54.21 ± 3.41	48.30	61.90
MAV (km.h^{-1})	13.62 ± 0.56	12.60	14.90
Squat Jump measures			
Height (m)	0.30 ± 0.04	0.22	0.40
Average power (w.kg^{-1})	19.12 ± 3.21	15.31	25.59
Contact time (s)	1.04 ± 0.32	0.52	1.68
Flight time (s)	0.48 ± 0.10	0.24	0.83
Countermovement jump measures			
Height (m)	0.33* ± 0.03	0.26	0.38
Average power (w.kg^{-1})	22.82* ± 5.47	16.03	33.85
Contact time (s)	1.06 ± 0.35	0.41	1.71
Flight time (s)	0.50 ± 0.04	0.40	0.58

* Significant difference between jump height and average power during Countermovement jump and Squat jump ($p<0.05$)
$VO_{2\,max}$ Maximum oxygen uptake
MAV Maximum Aerobic Velocity

Table 3. Pearson correlation coefficients between vertical jumping parameretrs, aerobic fitness and sprint performance measures in elite Futsal Tunisian players

	1	2	3	4	5	6	7	8	9	10	11	12	13
(1) CMJ power (W.Kg-1)	1,00												
(2) CMJ height (m)	0.11	1,00											
(3) CMJ contact time (s)	**-0.38***	-0.17	1.00										
(4) CMJ flight time (s)	0.05	0.37	0.08	1.00									
(5) SJ power (W.Kg-1)	0.16	0.00	-0.31	0.20	1.00								
(6) SJ height (m)	0.23	0.10	-0.16	**0.42***	**0.39***	1.00							
(7) SJ contact time (s)	-0.32	-0.35	**0.48***	-0.12	0.00	0.04	1.00						
(8) SJ flight time (s)	0.15	-0.09	-0.17	0.20	**0.58****	**0.59****	0.07	1.00					
(9) $VO2_{max}$ (ml. min-1.kg-1)	0.00	-0.00	0.04	0.25	0.34	0.13	-0.19	0.04	1.00				
(10) MAV (km.h-1)	0.03	0.01	0.02	0.25	0.35	0.14	-0.21	0.05	**0.99****	1.00			
(11) 10 m Sprint time (s)	-0.31	0.30	-0.02	0,02	-0.06	-0.07	0.08	-0.00	**-0.44***	**-0.44***	1.00		
(12) 20 m sprint time (s)	-0.16	0.22	-0.24	**-0,46***	-0.21	**-0.46***	-0.38	-0.21	-0.29	-0.29	0.31	1.00	
(13) 10*5 m Sprint time (s)	-0.18	-0.06	0.04	-0,20	**-0.41***	-0.12	0.09	-0.06	-0.06	-0.09	-0.03	0.18	1.00

* $p<0.05$ ** $p<0.01$
$VO_{2\,max}$ = Maximum oxygen uptake
MAV = Maximum Aerobic velocity
CMJ = Counter-Movement Jump
SJ = Squat Jump

3.3. Relationships between Vertical Jumping Parameters and Sprint Performance in Tunisian Futsal Players

3.3.1. Correlations

The Pearson correlations coefficients of all jump performance variables with sprint performance measures were summarized in Table 3.

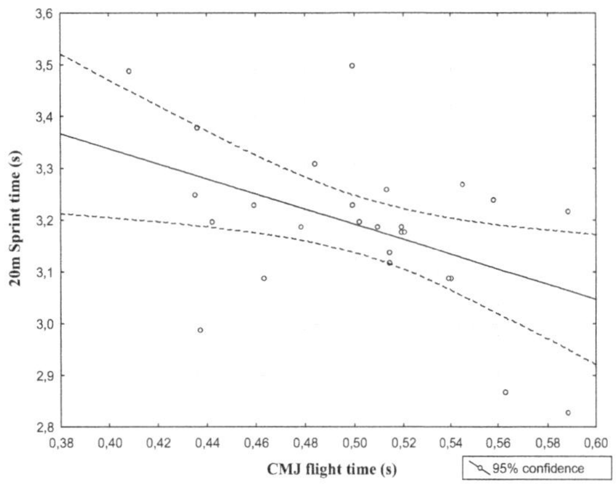

Figure 1. The relationship between 20 m sprint time and CMJ flight time in Tunisian Futsal players (r= -0.46, p<0.05).Dotted lines represent 95% estimation interval

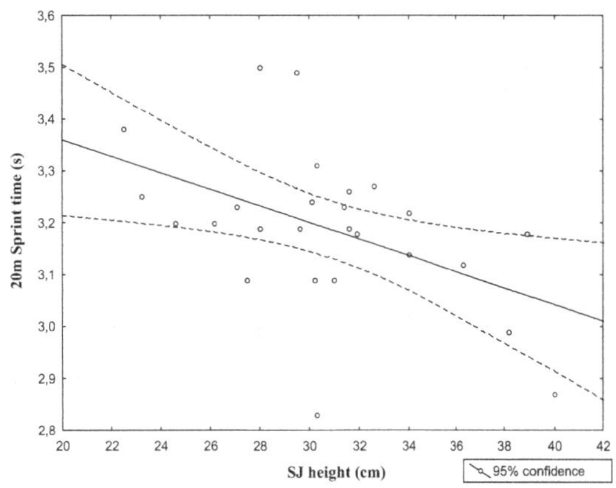

Figure 2. The relationship between 20 m sprint time and SJ height in Tunisian Futsal players (r= -0.46, p<0.05). Dotted lines represent 95% estimation interval

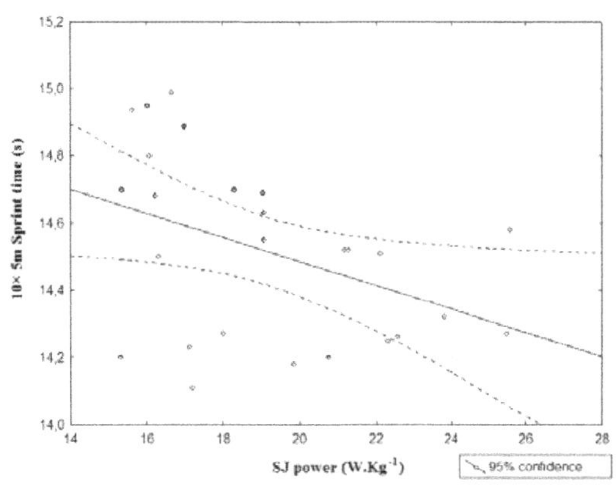

Figure 3. The relationship between 10×5 m sprint time and SJ power in Tunisian Futsal players (r= -0.41, p<0.05). Dotted lines represent 95% estimation interval

Correlation coefficients were calculated to check the influence of interaction. 20 m sprint time was correlated significantly with both CMJ flight time and SJ height (r= -0.46, p<0.05) (Figures 1 and 2). 10×5 m sprint time was correlated inversely with SJ power (r= -0.41, p<0.05) (Figure 3).

3.2. Predictors of Sprint Performance

A stepwise multiple regression analysis was used to determine the best predictors of 10 m, 20 m and 10×5 m sprint performance. Our result showed a negative association between 10 m sprint performance and $VO_{2\,max}$ in elite Tunisian Futsal players (r= -0.44, p<0.05). SJ height and SJ contact time were significant predictors of 20 m sprint performance.

The following equation explained 35% of the 20 m sprint performance variability:

20 m sprint time = 3.836 - (0.366× SJ contact time) - (0.450× SJ height).

Likewise, SJ power was the strongest predictor of 10×5 m sprint performance:

10 × 5 m sprint time = 15.198 - (0.413 ×SJ power)

3.2.1. Relationships between Aerobic Performance, Vertical Jumping Variables and Anthropometric Parameters in Tunisian Futsal Players

The analysis of stepwise multiple regression showed that the percentage of fat was negatively associated with $VO_{2\,max}$ (r= -0.41, p<0.05). The weight appeared to be a determinant of CMJ height jump (r= -0.41, p<0.05).

The anthropometric dimensions measured in this study revealed poor, insignificant relationships with sprinting performance (data not shown).

4. Discussion

The aims of the present study were to determine the relationships between vertical jumping parameters, aerobic fitness and sprint running performance and to examine the anthropometric and physiological profile of elite Futsal Tunisian players.

The measurements of performance in vertical jump are objectively provided by the Optojump system, which is valid for jump height estimation [12]. The CMJ and SJ were chosen because they have been found to be the most reliable and valid field tests for assessing the explosive power output of the lower limbs in active subjects [23]. We only selected Futsal players whose jumping performance was found to be reproducible. The times for 10 m, 20 m and 10 × 5 m sprint tests of players were provided by photocell gates device which was very often the only device for the reliable measuring sprint performance [7,27]. Aerobic fitness was considered as evaluated by maximal oxygen uptake ($VO_{2\,max}$), which is a widely used parameter in sports medicine, especially for planning and monitoring training season [3]. The maximal multistage 20-m shuttle run test was designed by Léger and Lambert in order to assess a Futsal player's aerobic capacity. This test incorporates a number of activity patterns thought to reflect the intermittent activity profile of a Futsal match. It has previously been found to be a valid and reliable method of estimating the velocity associated with $VO_{2\,max}$ [5,16,18].

4.1. Physical Characteristics

To the best of our knowledge, only few studies simultaneously analyzed anthropometric, muscle power output and sprint performance in elite Futsal players [2,3,10]. Age and height observed in the present study showed similar average values compared to those reported in Spanish male elite indoor soccer players [13], whereas there were some differences between groups in body weight, body mass index, percent body fat and fat free mass. On the contrary, it is difficult to compare results of physical fitness, sprinting and vertical jumping data among elite Futsal players with other studies due to age group differences, variability in procedures and methodologies. In order to better describe the physiological profile of Futsal Tunisian players, we presented some variables not measured in other Futsal studies such as sitting height, leg length, waist size, upper thigh girth, lower thigh girth and calf girth.

4.1.1. Relationships between Aerobic Power and Sprint Performance

Sprint performance, measured as the mean sprint time in seconds, is an indicator of Futsal performance. We have found in the current study a negative association between 10 m sprint time and maximal oxygen uptake ($VO_{2\ max}$) ($r= -0.44$, $p<0.05$). In this regard, Impellizzeri et al. [14] showed that small-sided games (i.e., 5-a-side drills) promote $VO_{2\ max}$ improvements similar to what is observed in interval running. As a consequence, Futsal training may be a plausible argument to explain the association between $VO_{2\ max}$ and 10m sprint performance. Similarly, Wisløff et al. [30] considered that the increase in distance covered, the intensity of play and the number of sprints performed and ball involvements were associated with an elevated VO_{2max} in soccer players.

The mean $VO_{2\ max}$ of 54.2 ml. min^{-1}. kg^{-1} observed in the elite Tunisian Futsal players can be compared to values reported in similar studies. Barbero Alvarez et al. [2] found in Italian semi-professional and in Spanish professional Futsal players a mean $VO_{2\ max}$ of 55.2 ml. min^{-1}. kg^{-1} and 62.8 ml. min^{-1}. kg^{-1}, respectively. Lima et al. [21] evaluated 13 professional Futsal players with a mean age of 18.6 years, and observed a $VO_{2\ max}$ of 62.8 ml. min^{-1}. kg^{-1} (direct measurement through ergospirometry) and 58.5 ml. min^{-1}. kg^{-1} (indirect measurement through a 3200 m field test). Leal Junior et al. [17] observed in 12 professional players with a mean age of 20.9 years, a mean $VO_{2\ max}$ of 55.7 ml. min^{-1}. kg^{-1}. Additionally, Castagna et al. [10] evaluated 8 professional Futsal players with a mean age of 22.4 years and found a $VO_{2\ max}$ of 64.8 ml. min^{-1}. kg^{-1}. This discrepancy in results could be due to differences in the methods of analysis, as well as the different standards of participants taking part in the studies (professional, semi- professional, elite,..). A recent study showed that $VO_{2\ max}$ was considered as a discriminative physiological variable in Futsal players of different levels [2]. This is in line with what was previously reported by several authors for soccer players [29]. Differences may be the result of genetic factors, player selection and training participation [2].

4.1.2. Relationships between Leg Power and Sprint Performance

In order to determine the profile of Tunisian Futsal player, we also analyzed the relationships between vertical jumping and sprint performance which is an indicator of Futsal performance. In the current study, power qualities were inversely related to 20 m ($r= -0.46$) and 10×5 m sprint time ($r= -0.41$). The negative correlations between leg anaerobic power characteristics and sprint performance in the Tunisian Futsal players suggest that those with higher vertical jump performance tend to have lower sprint times which are in line with the study by Bosco et al. [6] concerning the elite male soccer players. The result of the present study is in accordance with the study of Maulder et al. [24] who revealed that CMJ and SJ were predictive of 10 m sprint performance. Not only was the power generated during a CMJ important to sprint performance but the power generated during SJ also was identified as a predictor of sprint ability which is in line with our study. Strong correlations of $r= -0.72$ to $r= -0.73$ were revealed between SJ average power, SJ peak power and 10 m sprint time in the study of Maulder et al. [24]. This indicates the importance of power production from the leg musculature in sprint performance.

Especially, we found that jump height and contact time were correlated moderately with 20 m sprint time in Squat Jump (SJ). These findings are in contrast with Maulder and Cronin [25] who found a strong relationship between 20 m sprint performance and horizontal jumps in male sprinters. In addition, we revealed a negative correlation between SJ power and 10×5 m sprint time. Findings of this study emphasise the important association between concentric power and sprint performance. In a Squat Jump, the jumper starts from a stationary semi-squatted position then vigorously extends the knees and hips to jump vertically up off the ground [15]. This suggests that an athlete's relative explosive ability of the hip and knee extensors is critical for sprint performance. In fact, the elastic energy has been suggested to be necessary for sprint performance [26]. Taken together these relationships suggest a possible transfer from the gain in leg muscle power during squat jump into enhanced sprint performance. Indeed, a number of studies have previously reported that Futsal players have a significantly lower sprint running performance (10-15 m) and knee extension strength or power than soccer players. This could be probably related to a number of factors including lower globalization and international player recruitment, lower financial and social incentives, and fewer advances in nutrition, ergogenic aids, training methods or medical and kinesiological development techniques due to lower financial and social incentives [13]. Although making comparisons with research in other sports has its limitations due to differences in rules, play field, and duration, Futsal is a multiple sprint sport in which high-intensity exercise constitutes a greater proportion of match time than in football and other multiple-sprint sports.

4.1.3. Multiple Regression Equations of Vertical Jumping and Sprinting Measures

The multiple regressions showed that ($VO_{2\ max}$), jump height, power and contact time during squat jump were the determinants of sprinting performances in elite Futsal Tunisian players.

In summary, the relationships observed in our study between sprint performance measures, vertical jumping and aerobic fitness in elite Futsal Tunisian players suggest that those with higher aerobic fitness ($VO_{2\ max}$) and anaerobic power (vertical jump height, contact time and power during squat jump) tend to have a higher sprint performance. Therefore, muscle power and maximum oxygen uptake seem to be important physiological characteristics for sprinting performance in Tunisian Futsal players.

5. Practical Applications

The present study may be used as a base of comparison for further studies and help coaches to analyze the physical and physiological profiles of their teams. The data presented in this article will help practitioners and coaches to better design training by emphasizing the importance of combining adapted leg muscular power training with sprint running training programs for improving short-distance sprint performance. Elite Futsal players require a well developed aerobic fitness and repeated sprint ability to play successfully.

Acknowledgments

This study was supported by the Tunisian Ministry of Higher Education and Scientific Research.

There is no conflict of interest regarding the information provided in this study.

Special thanks to Professor Fethi Chehata for English correction.

References

[1] Álvarez, J., Gimenez, L., Corona, P., & Manonelles, P. (2002). Necesidades cardiovasculares y metabólicas del fútbol-sala: análisis de la competición. *Apunts. Medicina de l'Esport,* 67, 45-53.

[2] Barbero Álvarez, JC., D'Ottavio, S., & Granda-Vera, J. (2009). Aerobic fitness in futsal players of different competitive level. *Journal of Strength and Conditioning Research*, 23, 2163-2166.

[3] Barbero-Alvarez, JC., Soto, VM., Barbero-Alvarez, V., & Granda-Vera, J. (2008). Match analysis and heart rate of futsal players during competition. *Journal of Sports Sciences*, 26, 63-73.

[4] Baroni, BM., & Leal Junior, ECP. (2010). Aerobic capacity of male professional futsal players. *Journal of Sports Medicine and Physical Fitness,* 50, 395-399.

[5] Berthoin, S., Pelayo, P., Lensel-Corbeil, G., Robin, H., & Gerbeaux, M. (1996). Comparison of maximal aerobic speed as assessed with laboratory and field measurements in moderately trained subjects. *International Journal of Sports Medicine,* 17, 525-529.

[6] Bosco, C., Tihanyi, J., & Viru, A. (1996). Relationships between field fitness test and basal serum testosterone and cortisol levels in soccer players. *Clinical Physiology,* 16, 317-322.

[7] Bravo, DF., Impellizzeri, FM., Rampinini, E., Castagna, C., Bishop, D., & Wisloff, U. (2008). Sprint vs. interval training in football. *International Journal of Sports Medicine,* 29, 668-674.

[8] Buskirk, ER., & Mendez, J. (1984). Sports science and body composition analysis: emphasis on cell and muscle mass. *Medicine & Science in Sports & Exercise*, 16, 584-593.

[9] Castagna, C., and Barbero-Álvarez, JC. (2010). Physiological demands of an intermittent Futsal-oriented high-intensity test. *Journal of Strength and Conditioning Research*, 24, 2322-2329.

[10] Castagna, C., D'Ottavio, S., Vera, JG., & Álvarez, JC. (2009). Match demands of professional Futsal: a case study. *Journal of Science and Medicine in Sport*, 12, 490-494.

[11] Doğramaci, SN., & Watsford, ML. (2006). A comparison of two different methods for time-motion analysis in team sports. *International Journal of Performance Analysis in Sport*, 6, 73-83.

[12] Glatthorn, JF., Gouge, S., Nussbaumer, S., Stauffacher, S., Impellizzeri, FM., & Maffiuletti, NA. (2011). Validity and reliability of optojump photoelectric cells for estimating vertical jump height. *Journal of Strength and Conditioning Research,* 25, 556-560.

[13] Gorostiaga, EM., Llodio, I., Ibáñez, J., Granados, C., Navarro, I., Ruesta, M., Bonnabau, H., & Izquierdo, M. (2009). Differences in physical fitness among indoor and outdoor elite male soccer players. *European Journal of Applied Physiology,* 106, 483-491.

[14] Impellizzeri, FM., Marcora, SM., Castagna, C., Reilly, T., Sassi, A., Iaia, FM., & Rampinini, E. (2006). Physiological and performance effects of generic versus specific aerobic training in soccer players. *International Journal of Sports Medicine,* 27, 483-492.

[15] Komi, PV., & Bosco, C. (1978). Utilization of stored elastic energy in leg extensor muscles by men and women. *Medicine & Science in Sports,* 10, 261-265.

[16] Lacour, JR., Padilla-Magunacelaya, S., Chatard, JC., Arsac, L., & Barthelemy, JC. (1991). Assessment of running velocity at maximal oxygen uptake. *European Journal of Applied Physiology,* 62, 77-82.

[17] Leal Junior, EC., Souza, FB., Magini, M., & Lopes Martins, RAB. (2006). Comparative study of the oxygen consumption and anaerobic threshold in a progressive exertion test in professional soccer and indoor soccer players. *Revista Brasileira de Medicina do Esporte,* 12, 323-326.

[18] Leger, A., & Boucher, R. (1980). An indirect continuous running multistage field test: the University de Montreal Track Test. *Canadian journal of sport sciences,* 5, 77-84.

[19] Leger, A., & Lambert, J. (1982). A maximal multistage 20-m shuttle run test to predict VO_2 max. *European Journal of Applied Physiology,* 49, 1-12.

[20] Léger, A., Lambert, J., Goulet, A., Rowan, C., & Dinelle, Y. (1984). Capacité aérobie des Québécois de 6 à 17 ans. Test navette de vingt mètres avec palliers d'une minute. *Canadian journal of sport sciences,* 14, 21-26.

[21] Lima, AMJ., Silva, DVG., & Souza, AOS. (2005). Correlation between direct and indirect $VO_{2\ max}$ measurements in indoor soccer players. *Revista Brasileira de Medicina do Esporte,* 11, 164-166.

[22] Makaruk, H., Makaruk, B., & Kędra, S. (2008). Effects of warm-up stretching exercises on sprint performance. *Physical Education and Sport,* 52, 23-26.

[23] Markovic, G., Dizdar, D., Jukic, I., & Cardinale, M. (2004). Reliability and factorial validity of squat and countermovement jump tests. *Journal of Strength and Conditioning Research,* 18, 551-555.

[24] Maulder, PS., Bradshaw, EJ., & Keogh, J. (2006). Jump Kinetic determinants of sprint acceleration performance from starting blocks in male sprinters. *Journal of Sports Science & Medicine,* 5, 359-366.

[25] Maulder, P., & Cronin, J. (2005). Horizontal and vertical jump assessment: reliability, symmetry, discriminative and predictive ability. *Physical Therapy in Sport,* 6, 74-82.

[26] Mero, A., Komi, PV., & Gregor, RJ. (1992). Biomechanics of sprint running. *Journal of Sports Medicine,* 13, 376-392.

[27] Rampinini, E., Bishop, D., Marcora, SM., Ferrari Bravo, D., Sassi, R., & Impellizzeri, FM. (2007). Validity of simple field tests as indicators of match-related physical performance in top-level professional soccer players. *International Journal of Sports Medicine,* 28, 228-235.

[28] Rienzi, E., Drust, B., Reilly, T., Carter, JE., & Martin, A. (2000). Investigation of anthropometric and work-rate profiles of elite South American international soccer players. *Journal of Sports Medicine and Physical Fitness,* 40, 162-169.

[29] Stølen, T., Chamari, K., Castagna, C., & Wisløff, U. (2005). Physiology of soccer: An update. *Sports Medicine,* 35, 501-536.

[30] Wisløff, U., Castagna, C., Helgerud, J., Jones, R., & Hoff, J. (2004). Strong correlation of maximal squat strength with sprint performance and vertical jump height in elite soccer players. *British Journal of Sports Medicine,* 38, 285-288.

Impact of an Oriented Resistance Exercise and Endurance Training on the Health of Elderly Men

Rafael Reimann Baptista*, **Luis Felipe Silveira, Fábio Rodrigo Suñé, Fernanda Martins Marquesan, Gustavo Sandri Heidner, Mariana Kloeckner Pires Dias, Luciano Castro**

School of Physical Education, Pontifical Catholic University of Rio Grande do Sul, Porto Alegre, Brazil
*Corresponding author: rafael.baptista@pucrs.br

Abstract The purpose of this study was to evaluate the effects of a resistance exercise training versus an endurance training on the morpho-functional aspects of elderly men. The sample was made of 31 elderly men, divided into two groups, where 17 subjects (66.35±3.82 yrs) performed resistance exercise training (RET) and 14 subjects (69.21±6.90 yrs) performed endurance training (ET), for 12 weeks. The variables assessed were muscle thickness, body composition, electromyographic muscle activity (EMG), force production and functional mobility. A two-way ANOVA (by group and by intervention) for repeated measurements (pre- and post-) was used for the comparison of EMG. The remaining variables were analyzed intra-group (pre- and post-) using paired Student's t-test. The significance level adopted was of 5%. The ET showed significantly higher reduction in total body mass and body mass index (BMI) in comparison to the RET group. The RET group showed significantly greater gains in force production and muscle thickness when compared to the ET. Our results suggest that the combination of RET using Swiss balls and rubber bands, in other words, low cost materials, in addition to easy adherence ET, as walking, can improve the neuromuscular system and body composition.

Keywords: *aging, resistance exercise, endurance exercise, sarcopenia, body composition*

1. Introduction

The advances in medicine and the relatively recent incentives to the prevention of diseases on the population have caused an increased longevity and life expectancy of the individuals. On the other hand, the technological advances have facilitated the adoption of a sedentary lifestyle, which makes it so that these individuals not always reach old age with the expected health and quality of life.

So, it is necessary to study the Brazilian elderly person, that in 2012 already accounted for over 20 million people [1]. Specially, to study the phenomenon that may incapacitate the elderly individuals making them functionally dependent of other people is particularly important, not only to the older adults autonomy but also to the Brazilian Health Care System.

Several evidences have pointed to the fact that ageing is associated with a phenomenon known as Sarcopenia [2], that according to the European Consensus on Definition and Diagnosis involves a decrease in muscle mass and muscle function, causing loss of force production and physical performance [3].

Sarcopenia affects the muscle architecture directly, decreasing the anatomical cross sectional area (ACSA), muscle fiber length, volume and penation angle, in addition to reducing the specific force production capacity, in other words, the amount of force produced by each unit of muscle mass [4].

According to Hepple [2], the Sarcopenia process begins approximately at 50 years of age. Individuals, specially the elderly, when submitted to a strength training program, present attenuation of the atrophy effects of aging, indicating that sedentary behavior is associated with the loss of muscle mass [5,6,7,8,9].

The analysis of the influence of physical activity on the loss of muscle mass in the elderly may elucidate a more effective course of action when planning physical training programs for elderly individuals. The objective of this study was to evaluate the effects of a resistance exercise training (RET) versus an endurance training (ET) on muscle thickness, force production, muscle activity, body composition and functional mobility in elderly men.

2. Material and Methods

2.1. Ethical Aspects

This study was approved by the Research Ethics Committee of the PUCRS, protocol number 09/04696.

2.2. Sample

The sample was voluntary, composed of 31 male subjects, calculated using the following equation:

$$N = \frac{4\sigma^2 (Z_{crit} + Z_{pwr})^2}{D^2}$$

This equation indicates the sample size according to the significance level, statistical power, expected difference between groups and standard deviation of previous studies that used a similar methodology [10,11]. The subjects were divided in two groups: RET and ET. The RET group was composed of 17 elderly men, with average age of 66.35±3.82 years and the ET group was composed of 14 elderly men with average age of 69.21±6.90 years.

Table 1. Periodization of the RET program

Variable month	1	2	3	4	5	6	7	8	9	10	11	12
Series	1	1	2	2	3	3	4	4	4	5	5	5
Repetitions	15	15	12	12	10	10	8	8	6	5	5	5
Rubber band	UL, L e M	AI	AI	I	I	MI	SI	SI	SI	UI	UI	UI
Interval (s)	30	60	120	120	120	120	180	180	300	300	300	300

Key: Ultra Light (UL), Light (L), Medium (M), Average Intense (AI), Intense (I), Very Intense (MI), Super Intense (SI) and Ultra Intense (UI).

2.3. Exercise Program

The RET program consisted of training sessions using Swiss balls and rubber bands, and was overseen by one of the researchers at all times. The duration of the training program was of 12 weeks, 3 days per week (Monday, Wednesday and Friday) and the training sessions had an increasing duration of 30 to 60 minutes, depending on which phase of the program the subjects were in. The training sessions were preceded by a 5 minutes warm-up, made of active and static stretching for the main muscle groups, each performed for 10-20 seconds. By the end of the training sessions, subjects performed a cool-down made of the same stretching exercises performed on the warm-up. The training program was made of exercises for the following muscle groups: horizontal shoulder flexors, shoulder extensors, elbow flexors, elbow extensors, spine flexors, hip extensors, knee flexors and extensors. The evolution of the training program during the 12 weeks can be seen on Table 1, where the volume and intensity of training are controlled by series, repetitions, rest intervals between series and the rubber band's intensity.

The subjects that composed the ET received a program composed of a stretching routine and a protocol of endurance training that should be performed 3 days per week, preferable with a 48 hours interval between days, during the 12 weeks of the study, without direct overseeing of the researchers.

The program predicted active static stretching for the main muscle groups, with indications to be performed at the beginning and in the end of the ET sessions. The ET protocol was composed of an interval walking program, alternating moments of light and vigorous intensity, predicting gradual increase in time, from 30 minutes on week 1 to 100 minutes on week 12. The subjects were oriented to control their intensity using a perceived exertion scale of faces [12], which had a key for their interpretation.

2.4. Measurement of Muscle Thickness

The subjects were assessed while seated, with the knees and hips at 90 degrees of flexion. An ultrasound (M5, Mindray Bio-Medical Eletronics Co.) with a linear array transducer was used to measure muscle thickness of the vast lateral at rest [13,14,15]. The protocol was performed according to previous studies [16,17]. Anthropometric measurements were performed to guarantee the proper repositioning of the transducer at the post- assessments.

2.5. Measurement of Force Production

Muscle force production was measured using a load cell (Miotec Equipamentos Biomédicos LTDA) fixed on one extremity and attached to the tibia of the subjects with Velcro straps. The subjects were oriented to try to extend their knees exerting maximum force while in static contraction of the knee at 90 degrees of flexion. Corrections were made using video recordings to calculate force production through identification of the joint angles and lines of power.

2.6. Measurement of EMG

A 4 channels surface EMG system (*Miotool, Miotec* Equipamentos Biomédicos LTDA) was used to acquire EMG signal from the vast medialis, vast lateral, rectus femoris and biceps femoris muscles using bipolar electrodes arrangement (*Ag/AgCl, Meditrace*) and analyzed using the root mean square (RMS) of the signal. The placement of the electrodes and the preparation of the skin was done according to the recommendations of the *Surface ElectroMyoGraphy for the Non-Invasive Assessment of Muscles* [18]. During the first session of data gathering, notes on the anatomical points were taken to ensure that the electrode placement was the same during pre- and post- assessment.

2.7. Measurement of Functional Mobility

Functional mobility was assessed using the Timed up and go test (TUG) [19].

2.8. Statistical Analysis

Statistical analysis was done with the GraphPad Instat 3.06 (*GraphPad Software, San Diego, California, USA*). A two-way ANOVA (by group and by intervention) for repeated measurements (pre- and post-) was used for the comparison of EMG. The remaining variables were analyzed intra-group (pre- and post-) using paired Student's t-test. The significance level adopted was of 5%. Based on Altman [20], values of p between. 05 and. 10 were considered borderline. The data is showed as mean ± standard deviation.

3. Results

After the pre- tests, we have observed no statistically significant differences between groups on anthropometric measurements as total body mass, height, body fat percentage and lean body mass, as well as age.

No statistically significant changes were observed on the RET group in functional mobility (TUG test), total body mass, and vast lateral maximal and average activation.

Table 2. Pre-training results

Variable	RET group (n=17)	ET group (n=14)	p
Age	66.35±3.82	69.21±6.90	p>0.05
Total Body Mass (kg)	84.06±14.14	83.75±12.23	p>0.05
Height (cm)			p>0.05
Body Fat (%)	39.62±9.30	39.59±12.07	p>0.05
Lean Body Mass (kg)	49.93±6.81	49.81±9.37	p>0.05

Resistance Exercise Training (RET); Endurance Training (ET)

Table 3. Resistance Exercise Training Group

Variable	Pre-	Post-	p
Total Body Mass (kg)	84.06±14.14	83.82±14.27	0.0116*
BMI (kg/m²)	28.26±3.94	28.22±3.91	>0.10
TUG test (seg)	7.02±1.34	6.33±0.96	0.0210*
Abdominal circumference (m)	1.02±0.11	1.02±0.11	0.64
∑Skin folds (mm)	142.26±31.36	138.12±33.63	>0.10
Lean Body Mass(kg)	49.93±6.81	55.09±7.05	0.0024**
Fat Mass (kg)	34.13±12.10	28.73±12.14	0.0027**
Body fat (%)	39.62±9.30	33.14±10.06	0.0013**
Muscle Thickness (mm)	19.64±3.43	20.98±3.01	0.0714[1]
Force (N)	420.94±117.28	486.25±108.66	0.0044**
Vast Lateral Max	1198.60±455.90	1181.44±337.63	>0.10
Vast Lateral Average	168.45±92.15	179.15±61.14	>0.10
Vast Medial Max	988.21±401.92	1253.57±623.79	0.0395*
Vast Medial Average	144.02±69.40	197.64±121.35	0.0267*
Biceps Femoris Max	282.53±149.83	358.59±162.64	>0.10
Biceps Femoris Average	56.29±40.38	71.90±4419	>0.10

[1] p<0.10; *p<0.05; **p<0.01; Σ= sum

Table 4. Resistance Exercise Training Group

Varible	Pre-	Post-	p
Total Body Mass (kg)	83.75±12.23	82.20±11.10	0.0116*
BMI (kg/m²)	28.44±3.03	27.93±2.70	0.0155*
TUG test (seg)	6.79±1.24	6.42±1.26	0.2871
Abdominal circumference (m)	1.04±0.08	1.02±0.08	0.0407*
∑Skin folds (mm)	141.32±39.42	130.54±31.89	0.0185*
Lean Body Mass (kg)	49.81±9.37	55.92±5.57	<0.001**
Fat Mass (kg)	33.94±14.61	26.28±10.75	<0.0001**
Body fat (%)	39.59±12.07	31.14±9.22	<0.0001**
Muscle thickness (mm)	19.06±2.39	19.45±2.30	0.3575
Force (N)	447.37±177.17	443.98±148.44	0.8165
Vast Lateral Max	1041.47±352.30	1103.77±348.32	>0.05
Vast Lateral Average	142.04±44.53	153.63±41.58	>0.05
Vast Medial Max	1056.41±425.97	819.39±304.28	>0.05
Vast Medial Average	151.10±51.88	124.63±34.27	>0.05
Biceps Femoris Max	258.98±170.90	310.43±195.03	>0.05
Biceps Femoris Average	48.73±24.79	67.86±42.12	>0.05

*p<0.05; **p<0.01; Σ= sum.

We have observed changes in lean body mass, fat mass, body fat percentage and force production during maximal isometric voluntary extension of the knee. Muscle thickness of the RET group showed an average increase of 1,34 mm, which suggests that there was an increase in muscle mass, with a borderline statistical significance (p=0.07). No changes were observed on the vast lateral and biceps femoris activation, skin fold sum and BMI.

The ET group showed statistically significant reduction in total body mass, BMI, abdominal circumference and skin folds sum. A reduction in lean body mass, fat mass and body fat percentage was observed with great statistical power.

4. Discussion

When analyzing the effects of the two proposed exercise programs, we have observed that the variables related to force production, muscle thickness and knee extensor muscles were the ones that showed the biggest difference between groups, suggesting an advantage towards RET using rubber bands.

The increment in force production related to RET using rubber bands has already been demonstrated in other studies and reflects the morpho-functional adaptations of the musculo-skeletal system with the increase of the muscle fibers and penation angle, indicating an increase in the number of in-line and parallel sarcomeres, besides the increased of the maximal voluntary activation capacity and neural conduction, indicating a higher number of motor units recruited, or an increase of the frequency of stimulation of the motor units [21,22,23,24]. These adaptations are justified by the systematical use of the muscle groups, which induces alterations on the musculo-skeletal system, modifying its function and augmenting the capacity to produce force in young [25,26,27] and elderly subjects [28].

These same changes were not observed on the ET group, suggesting that this kind of activity would not be adequate to counteract the effects of Sarcopenia.

The results shown in this study elucidate the contribution of the RET on the increment of functional ability on the TUG test, probably related to the increased muscle force production in the lower limbs. Skelton, Young [29] verified that after 12 weeks of RET of moderate intensity with rubber bands, elderly subjects of ages 76-93 years showed mean increases of extension force and flexion force on the knees and hands grip strength. The authors observe that these strength gains determined the improvement of the functional ability of these elderly subjects.

The evaluation of force and power of the knee flexors and extensors is an important factor that must be taken into account when assessing functional capacity for several daily living activities, as walking, running, cycling and climbing stairs [30]. This way, the results found on the RET group seem to contribute to allow an increased functional independence in the elderly.

The ET group showed positive morphological adaptations related to body composition. These changes on the ET group, as well as on the RET group, have happened due to the insertion of physical exercises in a regular and systematic manner. These changes in body composition can be justified by the specificity of the proposed activity. Because the sample was of previously sedentary individuals, even with the execution of only endurance training, we have found significant changes on the lean body mass of the ET group.

Comparing the results obtained by the two groups, we have observed that the total body mass variation was not so big on the RET group because, as we can see on the comparison of measurements, this group suffered a bigger increase in lean body mass than the ET group. This was expected as a specific adaptation of RET [31].

The increase in lean body mass on both groups showed very close values, with a smaller change on the RET group. We believe that a 12 weeks period is too short to suggest that the results indicate that RET yields lesser lean body mass adaptations once the starting condition of sedentary individuals suggests they will have faster initial adaptations to training, in a way that it is expected that any systematic physical activity will produce lean body mass gains.

5. Conclusion

We have concluded that the RET group showed improvements in force production, muscle thickness and muscle activation, as well as in functional mobility. The ET group, on the other hand, showed positive results mostly on the anthropometric aspects. Our results suggest that the combination of RET using Swiss balls and rubber bands, in other words, low cost materials, in addition to easy adherence ET, as walking, can improve the neuromuscular system and body composition. Therefore, this combined strategy can be of great advantage to the Brazilian Health Care System, once it is of great effectiveness and easy to implement.

Acknowledgement

We would like to thank FAPERGS and PUCRS for the support to this work. The authors have no competing interests

References

[1] IBGE. *Atlas do Censo Demográfico*. 2010 [cited 28/08/2013]; Available from: http://www.ibge.gov.br/home/estatistica/populacao/censo2010/default_atlas.shtm.

[2] Hepple, R.T., "Sarcopenia--a critical perspective", *Sci Aging Knowledge Environ*, 2003 (46). pe31. 2003.

[3] Cruz-Jentoft, A.J., et al., "Sarcopenia: European consensus on definition and diagnosis: Report of the European Working Group on Sarcopenia in Older People", *Age Ageing*, 39 (4). 412-23. 2010.

[4] Narici, M.V., et al., "Effect of aging on human muscle architecture", *J Appl Physiol*, 95 (6). 2229-34. 2003.

[5] Kraemer, W.J., et al., "Effects of heavy-resistance training on hormonal response patterns in younger vs. older men", *J Appl Physiol*, 87 (3). 982-92. 1999.

[6] Kalapotharakos, V.I., et al., "Effects of a heavy and a moderate resistance training on functional performance in older adults", *J Strength Cond Res*, 19 (3). 652-7. 2005.

[7] Izquierdo, M., et al., "Effects of strength training on muscle power and serum hormones in middle-aged and older men", *J Appl Physiol*, 90 (4). 1497-507. 2001.

[8] Hunter, G.R., J.P. McCarthy, and M.M. Bamman, "Effects of resistance training on older adults", *Sports Med*, 34 (5). 329-48. 2004.

[9] Hakkinen, K., et al., "Changes in agonist-antagonist EMG, muscle CSA, and force during strength training in middle-aged and older people", *J Appl Physiol*, 84 (4). 1341-9. 1998.

[10] Rosner, B., *Fundamentals of biostatistics*. 5th ed2000, Pacific Grove, California: Duxbury

[11] Eng, J., "Sample size estimation: how many individuals should be studied?", *Radiology*, 227 (2). 309-13. 2003.

[12] Costa, M.G.D., E.H.M.; Marques, M.B.; Novaes, J.S., "Percepção subjetivo do esforço. Classificação do esforço percebido: proposta de utilização da escala de faces.", *Fitness & Performance Journal*, 3 (6). 305-313. 2004.

[13] Narici, M.V., "Human skeletal muscle architecture studied in vivo by non-invasive imaging techniques: functional significance and applications", *J Electromyogr Kinesiol*, 9 (2). 97-103. 1999.

[14] Fukunaga, T., et al., "Muscle architecture and function in humans", *J Biomech*, 30 (5). 457-63. 1997.

[15] Esformes, J.I., M.V. Narici, and C.N. Maganaris, "Measurement of human muscle volume using ultrasonography", *Eur J Appl Physiol*, 87 (1). 90-2. 2002.

[16] Kubo, K., et al., "Muscle architectural characteristics in young and elderly men and women", *Int J Sports Med*, 24 (2). 125-30. 2003.

[17] Kubo, K., et al., "Muscle architectural characteristics in women aged 20-79 years", *Med Sci Sports Exerc*, 35 (1). 39-44. 2003.

[18] SENIAM. *Surface ElectroMyoGraphy for the Non-Invasive Assessment of Muscles*. 2009 [cited 27/08/2013]; Available from: http://www.seniam.org/.

[19] Steffen, T.M., T.A. Hacker, and L. Mollinger, "Age- and gender-related test performance in community-dwelling elderly people: Six-Minute Walk Test, Berg Balance Scale, Timed Up & Go Test, and gait speeds", *Phys Ther*, 82 (2). 128-37. 2002.

[20] Altman, D.G., "Statistics in medical journals: developments in the 1980s", *Stat Med*, 10 (12). 1897-913. 1991.

[21] Melchiorri, G. and A. Rainoldi, "Muscle fatigue induced by two different resistances: Elastic tubing versus weight machines", *J Electromyogr Kinesiol*, 21 (6). 954-9. 2011.

[22] Andersen, L.L., et al., "Muscle activation and perceived loading during rehabilitation exercises: comparison of dumbbells and elastic resistance", *Phys Ther*, 90 (4). 538-49. 2010.

[23] Fahlman, M.M., et al., "Effects of resistance training on functional ability in elderly individuals", *Am J Health Promot*, 25 (4). 237-43. 2011.

[24] Krebs, D.E., A.M. Jette, and S.F. Assmann, "Moderate exercise improves gait stability in disabled elders", *Arch Phys Med Rehabil*, 79 (12). 1489-95. 1998.

[25] Kitai, T.A. and D.G. Sale, "Specificity of joint angle in isometric training", *Eur J Appl Physiol Occup Physiol*, 58 (7). 744-8. 1989.

[26] Moritani, T. and H.A. deVries, "Neural factors versus hypertrophy in the time course of muscle strength gain", *Am J Phys Med*, 58 (3). 115-30. 1979.

[27] Caiozzo, V.J., J.J. Perrine, and V.R. Edgerton, "Training-induced alterations of the in vivo force-velocity relationship of human muscle", *J Appl Physiol Respir Environ Exerc Physiol*, 51 (3). 750-4. 1981.

[28] Reeves, N.D., M.V. Narici, and C.N. Maganaris, "Effect of resistance training on skeletal muscle-specific force in elderly humans", *J Appl Physiol (1985)*, 96 (3). 885-92. 2004.

[29] Skelton, D.A., et al., "Effects of resistance training on strength, power, and selected functional abilities of women aged 75 and older", *J Am Geriatr Soc*, 43 (10). 1081-7. 1995.

[30] Neder, J.A., et al., "Reference values for concentric knee isokinetic strength and power in nonathletic men and women from 20 to 80 years old", *J Orthop Sports Phys Ther*, 29 (2). 116-26. 1999.

[31] Folland, J.P. and A.G. Williams, "The adaptations to strength training : morphological and neurological contributions to increased strength", *Sports Med*, 37 (2). 145-68. 2007.

27

Circadian Cycle and Its Influence on Parameters of Aerobic Training

Ramon Cruz[1], Francisco de Assis Manoel[2], Bruno Pereira Melo[2], Sandro Fernandes da Silva[3,*]

[1]Faculdade de Educação Física e Desporto, Universidade Federal de Juiz de Fora, Juiz de Fora, Brazil
[2]Departamento de Educação Física, Universidade Estadual de Maringá, Maringá, Brazil
[3]Departamento de Educação Física, Universidade Federal de Lavras, Lavras, Brazil
*Corresponding author: sandrofs@gmail.com

Abstract **Objectives:** This study aims to evaluate the Influence of two distinct Periods of the day on maximal aerobic power in young Athletes mountain bike. Volunteers are the mountain bike Athletes, 37.83 ± 8.87 years, and underwent two progressive maximal exercise test on a cycle Ergometer at two times of day. Gauging the behavior glucose and heart rate. The verification of normality of data was performed by the Shapiro-Wilk test for analysis of variables was Adopted t test for paired samples. Statistical we Adopted an evidence for $p < 0.05$. Results: Were the glucose threshold results not statistically significant. However trends indicating were there a better outcome in the evening. The maximal workload, maximal heart rate and glycemic load threshold. Conclusions: The results show trends on performance and circadian rhythm, and yet, the routine or team chosen for sensivity training appears to the circadian cycle.

Keywords: *circadian cycle, training and cycling*

1. Introduction

The performance variables physiological and psychological suffers interference of biological rhythms, which are cyclic changes that are regularly repeated in a given time interval generated in periods of 24 hours [1]. Some studies had been made identifying the influence of circadian cycle in determining variables on performance, as cardiovascular function [8], metabolic [9] and respiratory [2].

Physiological control of the circadian cycle is determined by changes in frequency environmental, and the light / dark cycle is one of the main synchronizers. Another way for the body to control their circadian mechanisms is necessary external and internal stimuli, acting as guides. These two pieces of information are transmitted to a biological oscillator, located in the suprachiasmatic nucleus of the hypothalamus, which acts as an integrator [3].

The interferon Consistency of the circadian cycle in human performance seems to follow the rhythm of body temperature [4,5]. Body temperature is often used as a marker rhythm, ease of measurement and its strong endogenous component. The minimum body temperature curve occurs during sleep, around 4:00 [7]. From this point, it starts increasing which increases upon awakening. After noon, there is a slight decrease, a phenomenon called *post-lunch dip,* then rise again, which leads to the occurrence of higher values at about 18:00 [9]. Similar to body temperature, heart function has also changes according to time of day, consistently lower at evening, independent of load, with a difference between day and night for 5-10 bpm.

The HR_{max} has been studied by different researchers [1,6]. In the literature we apply the cycle ergometer exercise at various times, such as: 2:00, 6:00, 10:00, 2:00pm, 6:00pm and 10:00pm and has been found that significant circadian variation in the Fc_{max} [10]. Moreover, also the use of cycling were their used the time, 4:00, 8:00, 12:00, 3:00pm, 6:00pm, 9:00pm and 24:00 h [11], and in another study that found no significant differences between the different periods [5], used four times (8:00, 12:00, 4:00pm and 8:00pm) [5].

For best response to training, it is necessary to control some markers of performance. An important marker of human performance, VO_{2MAX} shows a circadian cycle of the interference [6] as well as other markers performance aerobic and anaerobic most [1,6] such as lactate, and the critical velocity (CV) [12].

The anaerobic threshold (AT) is a parameter widely used for exercise prescription and research in exercise physiology [13]. The AT can be determined by the behavior of blood lactate, which is a body's metabolic response to stress and that means a gradual transition between the energy systems [11]. Yet another method has been highlighted in order to identify the AT, which is the blood glucose response during progressive exercise [5]. But the blood glucose response has yet been the focus of many studies seeking its new relationship with other existing parameters, especially the blood lactate response to exercise [5]. The literature is still scarce in checking the influence of circadian cycle in glycemic threshold (GT).

This study presents an interesting practical application for the prescription of cyclists training, checking the best period for the implementation of training and performance in different periods.Thus this work aims to evaluate the influence of circadian cycle in GT and physiological variables determined in a progressive maximal test.

2. Methodology

2.1. Sample

There were 8 subjects in the study used adult, 37.83 ± 8.87 years, 174.7 cm ± 8.01, 71.52 ± 11.87 kg, 20.26 ± 2.56% fat men, athletes mountain bike, with activities other than sport. All were competitive period of training, participating in regional and state exams. All subjects were pre-informed about the risks of the project and they all signed the Informed Consent approved by the ethics committee of the University of Itaúna number of protocol 002/09, following the Brazilian regulations for research on human beings, which are in accordance with the norms proposed by the treaty of Helsinki

2.2. Procedures

Subjects came to the laboratory three times, first for two days before the start of testing, for explanation of the study, signing the WIC and evaluation of body composition. The second visit occurred 48 hours after the 1st, where the subjects performed a maximal exercise test on a cycle ergometer, the ú last visit occurred at an interval of 96 hours of a first visit. Assessments were made on two moments in the morning between 7:00 and 10:00 hours and at evening from 7:00pm to 10:00pm hours. The subjects randomly performed stress tests subject to a maximum 48-hour interval between assessments for the full recovery of muscle glycogen stores and liver.

2.3. Protocol to the Maximal Exercise Test

A progressive test was used which consisted of an initial load of 15W then by increments of 30 watts every 2 minutes until exhaustion, with the frequency being maintained between 80 and 90 revolutions per minute (rpm). The test was interrupted with the exhaustion of the individual, with the impossibility of sustaining the pace of pedaling or pre-established with the detection of any event which could cause possible damage to the volunteer. At the end of each stage was performed to collect blood samples for analysis of glucose in a glucose meter Acutrend Roche ®.

2.4. Collection of Blood Glucose

The collection of blood glucose was performed in three stages in this study: 30 minutes before the test immediately before the test and each stage.

At such times, 25 mL were collected blood from the right ear lobe of individuals and then this drop was placed on a strip for analysis of specific Acutrend Roche ® Plus, which measures the concentration of glucose in plasma by strips reagentes® by *Roche* metering method of reflection in order to obtain the blood glucose concentration in these moments.

2.5. Statistical Analysis

For the analysis of all variables obtained was used descriptive statistics to deter nation of mean and standard deviation. The verification of normality of data was performed by the Shapiro-Wilk. To identify the statistical differences between the predictor variables, $_{Gluc}$ Fc, Fc $_{max}$ load and $_{max}$ load $_{Gluc,}$ we adopted the t test for paired samples. For statistical evidence we adopted a $p < 0.05$.

3. Results

The first graphic shows the average in all subjects reached the GT, these values are distinct threshold presented in Figure 2 and Figure 3, because here we consider the average of the entire group, not the average of each load. With these results we find relative values for the threshold glycemic load, as follows: 73.78% of the maximum load for the morning and 73.05% for the evening time. The charges glycemic threshold showed no significant difference ($p > 0,05$).

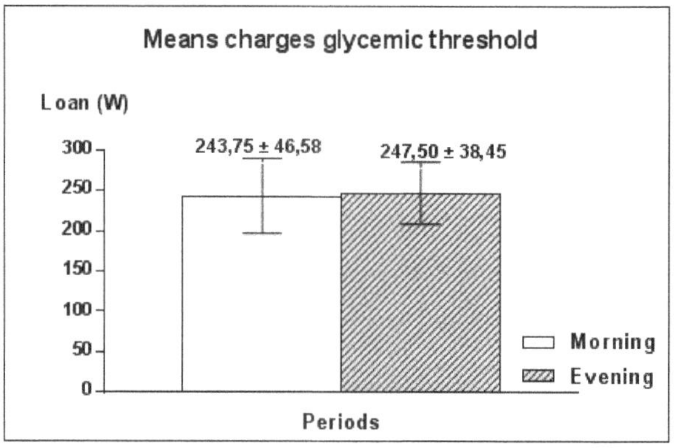

Figure 1. Mean and SD results in loads when the volunteers reached the glycemic threshold

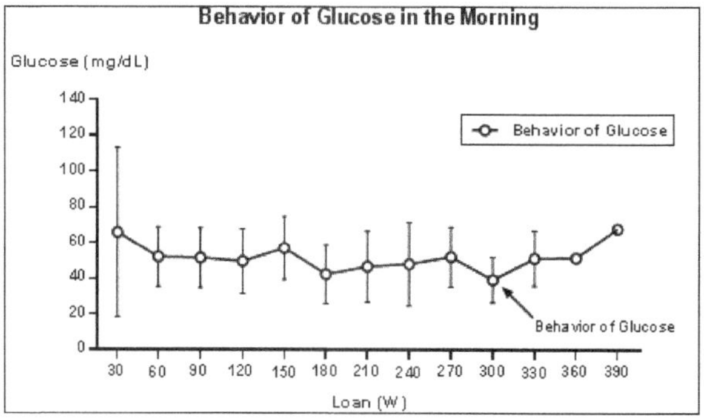

Figure 2. Behavior of glucose in the morning, with mean and SD of the volunteers on each charge, and identification of the glycemic threshold. The curve was smoothed by the software Excel

Figure 2 and Figure 3 show the average values at each load in 2 periods of study evaluation, and have identified the glycemic thresholds at every turn. These graphs are paradoxical when compared to a chart, they show different charges for the GT [13], however, remember that the glycemic curves presented show the values of the volunteers at each stage, which does not necessarily reflect the the load at which individuals reached their GT. The curves (lines) have been smoothed for better visualization of the graph tool available in Excel ® software.

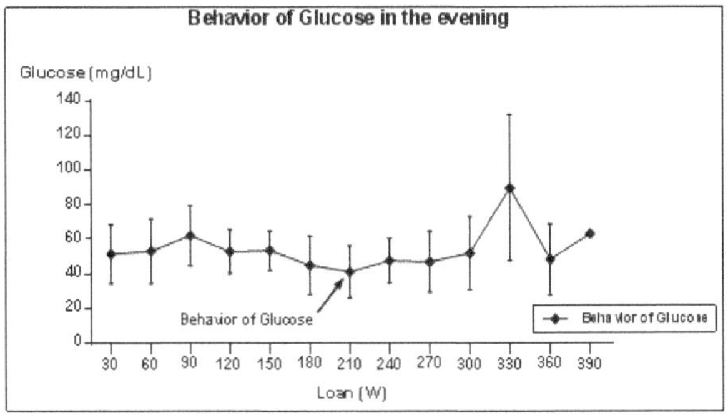

Figure 3. Behavior of glycemic during the evening, with mean and SD of the volunteers on each charge, and identification of the glycemic threshold. The curve was smoothed by the software Excel

Figure 4 shows the mean values of the loads that were achieved in both periods. Nah it was a statistically significant difference; however there is a behavior that indicates best performance at evening. The maximum load showed no significant difference (p>0,05).

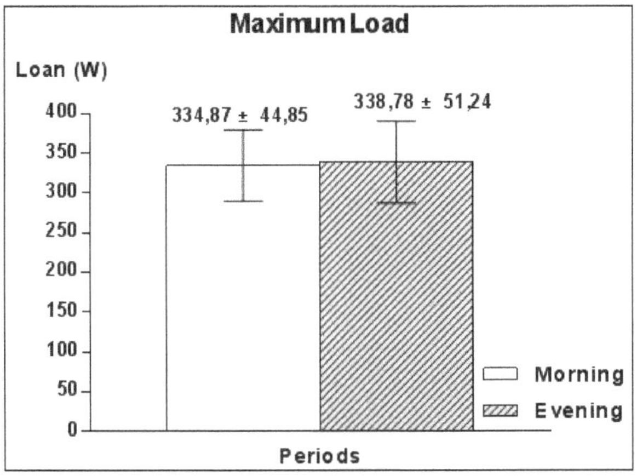

Figure 4. Mean and SD results observed in the analysis of the maximum load obtained in the tests in both periods

Table 1 contains the values of body temperature, observed in both periods. The evening the average temperature was higher, which corroborates with the literature[2]. The mean body temperature showed no significant difference (p>0,05).

Table 1. Mean and SD of the temperature in the times of the test

	Mean body temperature (°C)
Morning	35,55 ± 0,62
Evening	35,9 ± 0,4

The Figure 5 and Figure 6 bring the curves of the values m s edition of HR and blood glucose levels by goodwill of the progressive test. The heart rate values are displayed on each of the graphic marker. Being that at night it was lower in the first 7 stages, and higher in the last six.

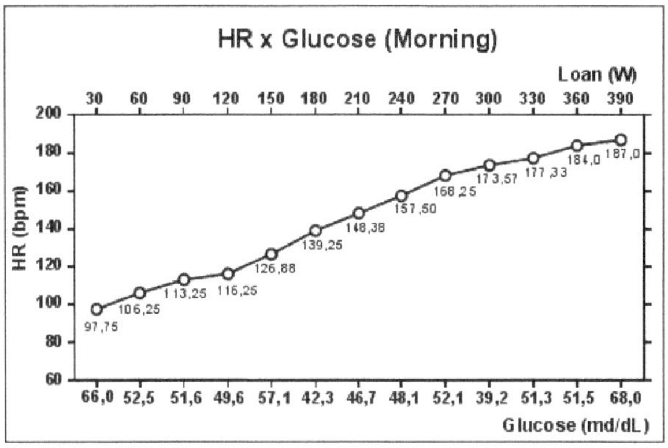

Figure 5. Describes the mean values of HR in each stage with the average values of glycemic at each stage in the morning

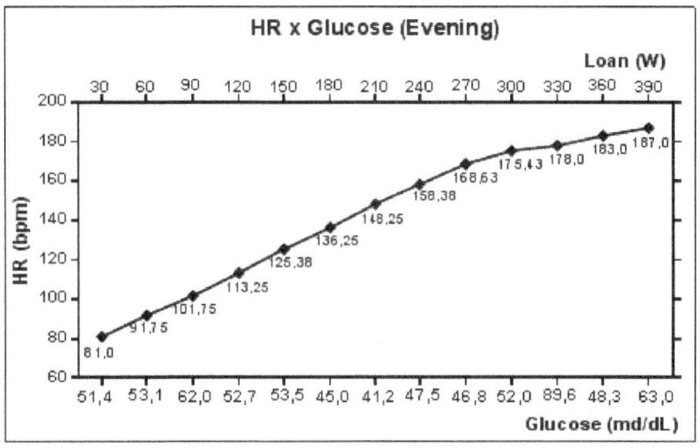

Figure 6. This graph depicts the mean values of HR in each stage with the average values of glycemic at each stage during the evening.

Table 2 shows that the average maximum HR attained in both tests was higher at evening. During this period the volunteers were great physiological responses to athletic performance (HR, Temperature, GT). The HR máx (morning and evening) showed no significant difference (p>0,05).

Table 2. Mean and SD results observed in the analysis of maximum HR obtained in the tests in two periods

	HR máx (Mornng and Evening)
Morning	179,75 ± 5,17 bpm
Evening	181,25 ± 8,71 bpm

4. Discussion

The aim of this study was to investigate the interference of the circadian cycle in GT and physiological variables determined in this metabolic transition point, the current literature there are no studies that evaluate this important predictor of performance, what about the proposed work extremely attractive.

The results of this study showed no statistically significant difference, similar to other studies with this population and research problem [4,6,14], however these variables showed an average trend, which indicates better performance on tests used at evening. In a previous study by checking the variable speed, showed the same trend of results on the behavior of physical performance on the circadian cycle [12], which we believe that the habits of the volunteers are influential in the final results of the tests.

The literature suggests that the best moments of peak performance are related to body temperature [15] with a worse performance in the morning and a better outcome in the afternoon / evening [16]. In our study we found a 2% increase in body temperature, which leads us to think that this increased tendency to perform better during the night can be directly related to the increase in body temperature, in corroborates with other studies which indicate values larger afternoon / evening [16,17,18].

The choice of two periods for evaluations of the study was based on the times when the population in general performs physical activity, not including the time of the afternoon was because we believe that the difference between the hours of the night chosen (from 7:00pm h) and afternoon hours (2:00pm to 6:00pm) would be close, and also the results were not significant between afternoon and evening, observed in a study that preceded this [12].

Maintaining or increasing rates of glucose during exercise can be explained both by the greater needs of glucose by the body as the increased intensity of exercise, promoting greater release of hyperglycemic hormones such as catecholamines, ACTH, glucagon, cortisol and growth hormone [4,13]. In our findings there was no interference of the circadian rhythm in blood glucose concentration which led to the charges in Liglic.

The concept arose with Liglic inferences that proposed the identification of anaerobic threshold by comparing the behavior of blood glucose with the behavior of lactate minimum, where similarity was found between these two variables [20]. The GT is identified by the kinetics of glucose concentration [gluc], being found in exercise intensity corresponding to the lowest [gluc] during the test, representing the point in time when the activation hiperglicemic secretion of hormones such as cortisol and that glucagon will maintain the blood glucose concentration during the entire test [20,21]. During exercise maintenance of plasma glucose levels are governed by the liver through *feeedback* signals, with increased glucose availability [21] these signals are inhibited, which could probably alter the kinetics of glucose at different times of day that could influence the performance of the workload achieved in Liglic.

Studies evaluating the effect of circadian cycle in anaerobic threshold (AT) show contradictory results similar to ours, in which there are differences in AT different times of day [22,23], these studies serve as a parameter in our study since the Liglic presents a metabolic transition, we can infer that the interference of the cycle would continue regardless of the form to determine the Lan

One hypothesis as a possible explanation for the findings in our study is that more than circadian variation, which interferes with physical performance rhythmicity is the time when the subjects performed their usual physical activities, which induce an adaptation of performance and thus would be possible to find differences in the charges assessed in the AT. This study had the limitation that no monitoring of athletes for more hours of the day, as their feed in the moments before the test. Further studies on this topic may further elucidate the influence of time of day on the variables that determine sporting performance.

5. Conclusion

The results of this study showed no interference of the circadian cycle in certain variables in the GT. It is noteworthy that there is a tendency for results to be better at evening. What sustains speculated, that the training time of the selected sample is fundamental to happen to a better performance during training and evaluation of physical abilities.

Acknowledgement

FAPEMIG- Fundação de Amparo à Pesquisa do Estado de Minas Gerais.

References

[1] Afonso L.S, Dos Santos J.F.B, Lopes J.R, Tambelli R, Santos E.H.R, Back F.A, Menna-barreto L, Lima J.R.P.: Maximal heart rate on treadmill at different times. Rev. Bras. Med. Esporte. 2006, 12 (6): 318-322.

[2] Atkinson G, Jones H, Ainslie PN. Circadian variation in the circulatory responses to exercise: relevance to the morning peaks in strokes and cardiac events. Eur J Appl Physiol 108: 15-29, 2010.

[3] Atkinson G, Todd C, Reilly T, Waterhouse J. Diurnal variation in cycling performance: influence of warm-up. J Sports Sci. 2005, 23(3): 321-329.

[4] Back FA et al. Non-photic synchronization: the effect of aerobic physical exercise Rev Bras Med Esporte. 2007, 13(2).

[5] Bessot N, Nicolas A, Moussay S, Gauthier A, Sesboüé B, Davenne D. The effect of pedal rate and time of day on the time to exhaustion from high-intensity exercise. Chronobiol Int. 2006, 23(5): 1009-1024.

[6] Cruz R Melo BP Manoel FA Castro PHC da Silva SF. Pacing Strategy and Heart Rate on the Influence of Circadian Rhythms. *JEP online*. 2013; 16(4):24-31.

[7] Cruz R, Silva SF. Indicators Of Control Parameters Of Training And Circadian Cycle. Rev. Acta Bras. Movimento Hum 2011, 1(1): 33-41.

[8] Drust B, Waterhouse J, Atkinson G, Edwards B, Reilly T. Circadian rhythm in sports performance- An update. Chronobiol Int. 2005, 22: 21-44.

[9] Frank AS et al. Impact of the human circadian system, exercise, and their interaction on cardiovascular function. Proc Natl Acad Sci. 2010, 107(4).

[10] Forsyth J, Reilly T. Circadian rhythms in blood lactate concentration incremental During Ergometer rowing. Eur. J. Appl. Physiol. 2004, 92 (1-2): 69-74.

[11] Hayes LD, Bickerstaff GF, Baker JS. Interactions of cortisol, testosterone, and resistance training: influence of circadian rhythms. Chronobiol Int. 2010, 27(4): 675-705.

[12] Hill DW. Effect of time of day on aerobic power in exhaustive high-intensity exercise. J. Sports Me Phys. Fitness 1996, 36: 155-160.

[13] Jones H, George K, Edwards B, Atkinson G. Effects of time of day on post-exercise blood pressure: circadian or sleep-related influences? Chronobiol Int. 2008, 25(6): 987-998.

[14] Racinais S, Connes P, Bishop D, Blonc S, Huel O. Morning versus evening power output and repeated-sprint ability. Chronobiol Int. 2005, 22(6): 1029-1039.

[15] Reilly T, Atkinson G, Gregson W, Drust B, Forsyth J, Edwards B, Waterhouse J. Some chronobiological considerations related to physical exercise. Clin Ter. 2006, 157(3): 249-264.

[16] Sedliak M, Finni T, Cheng S, Kraemer WJ, Häkkinen K. Effect of time-of-day-specific strength training on serum hormone concentrations and isometric strength in men. Chronobiol Int. 2007, 24(6): 1159-1177.

[17] Simões HG, Campbell CSG, Kushnick MR, Nakamura A, Katsanos CS, Baldissera V, Moffatt RJ. Blood glucose threshold and the metabolic responses to incremental exercise tests with and without prior lactic acidosis induction. Eur. J. Appl. Physiol. 2003; 89: 603-11.

[18] Simões HG, Campbell CSG, Kokubum E, Denadai, BS, Baldissera V. Blood glucose response in humans mirror lactate responses for

individual anaerobic threshold and for lactate minimum in track test. Eur. J. Appl. Physiol. 1999, 80 (1): 34-40.

[19] Souissi N, Driss T, Chamari K, Vandewalle H, Davenne D, Gam A, Fillard JR, Jousselin E. Diurnal variation in wingate test performances: influence of active warm-up. Chronobiol Int. 2010, 27(3): 640-652.

[20] Kline EC, Durstine JL, Davis JM, Moore TA, Devlin TM, Zielinski MR, Youngstedt SD. Circadian variation in swim performance. J. Appl. Physiol. 2007, 102: 641-649.

[21] Souissi N, Souissi M, Souissi H, Chamari K, Tabka Z, Dogui M, Davenne D. Effect of time of day and partial sleep deprivation on short-term, high-power output. Chronobiol Int. 2008, 25(6):1062-1076.

[22] Waterhouse J, Drust B, Weinert D, Edwards B, Gregson W, Atkinson G, Kao S, Aizawa S, Reilly T. The circadian rhythm of core temperature: origin and some implications for exercise performance. Chronobiol Int. 2005, 22(2): 207-225.

[23] Waterhouse J, Edwards B, Bedford P, Hughes A, Robinson K, Nevill A, Weinert D, Reilly T. Thermoregulation during mild exercise at different circadian times. Chronobiol Int. 2004, 21(2): 253-275.

A Talent Development Perspective on the Olympic Athlete

Rita R. Culross*

Louisiana State University, School of Education, 301 Peabody Hall, Baton Rouge, LA
*Corresponding author: acrita@lsu.edu

Abstract Using an integrated biopsychosocial approach, this paper examines the influences of physical ability, mental and emotional aspects, and the influences of home, school, and culture on the talent development of the elite athlete. The paper will also go beyond characteristics of individual Olympians to discuss how athletic performance can be enhanced through executive coaching, cognitive behavioral therapy, attention to aspects of health psychology, instruction, and neuropsychological interventions. A final section will address issues association with underperformance. The primary focus of the paper will be on Summer Olympians from the U.S., although similar examples could be provided from throughout the full range of countries competing in the Games.

Keywords: *Olympic athletes, talent development, talent enhancement*

1. Introduction

From the very beginning of the Olympic movement in ancient Greece, development of the athlete in both body and mind was seen as the route to achievement at the Games [19] The development of powers and talents through training were important responsibilities of participants in the Games that were expected by the gods and the aim of Greek educational system.

Today's modern Olympic athletes embody this same tradition through their pursuits of their sports. While many spectators view the Olympian as an individual of exceptional physical talent, the reality of the road to the Games is quite different. Innate talent may be a factor in involvement in sport, but the trajectory from God-given talent to Olympic medal winner is filled with deliberate practice and powerful external influences.

As the world turns its attention to Rio de Janeiro and the opening of the 2016 Summer Olympics August 5, the talent development literature offers a lens through which to explain the exceptional athlete. Using an integrated biopsychosocial approach, this paper examines the influences of physical ability, mental and emotional aspects, and the influences of home, school, and culture on the talent development of the elite athlete. The paper will also go beyond characteristics of individual Olympians to discuss how athletic performance can be enhanced through executive coaching, cognitive behavioral therapy, attention to aspects of health psychology, instruction, and neuropsychological interventions. A final section will address issues association with underperformance. The primary focus of the paper will be on Summer Olympians from the U.S., although similar examples could be provided from throughout the full range of countries competing in the Games.

2. Talent Development as a Frame of Reference

Historically, American conceptions of talent originated in the attention to intelligence as measured by IQ tests (e.g. [24]). Over time the view of talent broadened both from an emphasis on mental ability to one of talent within different domains, including physical performance, artistic ability, and applied domains such as entrepreneurship; as well as from a view of talent as fixed [9] to talent as the growth of ability through the support of others and the psychosocial development of the individual [16]. Although psychomotor ability was included in the 1972 definition promulgated by the U.S. Department of Education, Piirto [23] was one of the first within the field to write at length about the development of physical performers, including athletes.

Piirto postulated a model of talent development to explain talent development in various fields from the perspective of person, process, and product, as well as environmental factors. Table 1 below shows the model.

The model postulates that talent development builds upon the individual's genetic makeup. Contributing to the individual's talent are the emotional and cognitive aspects of their being; that is, individuals within a certain domain share cognitive abilities and personality traits that contribute to their success within the domain. The talent itself is largely specific to a certain domain, in this case athletic performance. Finally, the individual persons (or athletes) are influenced by what she calls environmental "suns;" i.e. the influence of the home, school, community or culture, gender, and chance in the development of their talents.

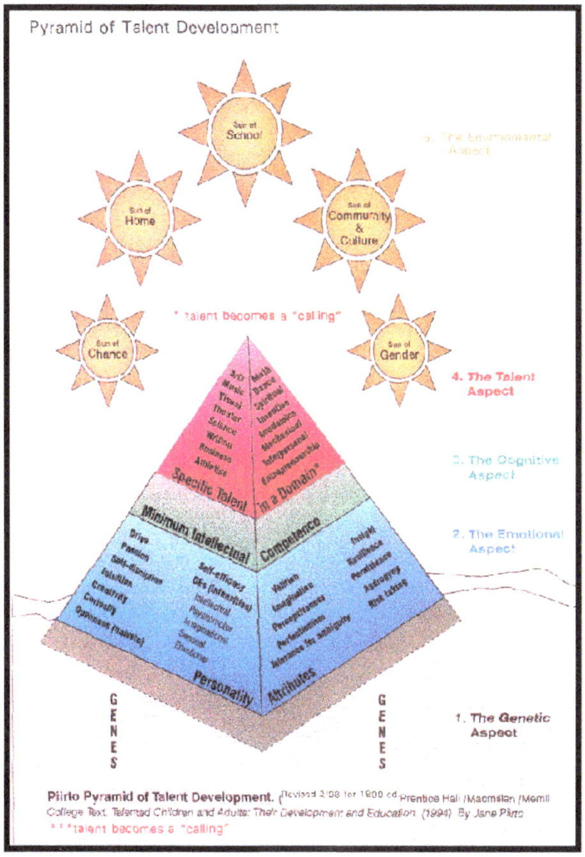

Figure 1. Piirto Model of Talent Development Copyright 2001 Jane Piirto [23] (Used with Permission)

For Olympic athletes how might this look? While athletes are popularly viewed as being born with their talents, in fact, research shows that the genetic components are more likely to be quite specific traits that in and of themselves are not sufficient to lead to high-level performance. For example, female Olympic gymnasts (think Gabrielle Douglas) are usually quite short in stature with small hips and broad shoulders [1]. While there is some evidence that this is due to the increased force required to propel longer limbs through various apparatuses, the advantage also arises from the bias in the scoring system toward acrobatic talent. Similarly, swimmers can be advantaged through body type. Michael Phelps' superior swimming ability is attributed in part to his unique body type [12]. Phelps' wingspan stretches 80 inches, more than 10 inches greater than his total height. (A typical person's height and length of outstretched arms are virtually the same length.) His size-14 feet bend 15 inches farther than typical swimmers, turning them into what Hadhazy calls virtual flippers. Regardless, as we shall see later in this paper, these physical attributes of athletes, while assets, are only part of what is required for Olympic success.

Cognitively, bodily-kinesthetic intelligence in combination with visual learning, provide the Olympic athlete with the ability to learn skilled movements and to adjust their performance based on feedback from visual images such as videotapes of their past performance. Former LSU athlete and Olympic hurdler Lolo Jones benefits from videotaped images of her training runs, in which more than 1500 images per second are taken of her runs [18]. Afterward she and her coach analyze the minute details of her performance and make adjustments for future training runs. Outside of the pool Olympic diver David Boudia is fluent in American Sign Language. "I'm a visual learner. Sign language is a visual foreign language. So I struck right into it, and, uh, it's pretty easy now" [22].

Emotionally, Olympic athletes must deal with a multitude of distractions as well as regulating their emotions in competition. Naturally physically expressive, athletes must often learn to regulate their emotions through techniques to control breathing, concentrate on the task at hand, and address fears about past failures.

As Karen Cogan, U.S. Olympic Committee senior sport psychologist, has said, "For the most part, the body knows what to do. Athletes just have to turn off their minds." ([6], p. 36) Brady Ellison, US Olympian and one of the elite archers in the world, has a tattoo of the Olympic rings on his forearm. The tattoo serves as a constant reminder of his 2008 Olympic achievement and as a motivating tool for a repeat performances in future Games. In general, Olympic athletes are highly competitive, exhibit adaptive perfectionism, and maintain mental toughness during competition [11].

Equally important to the specific abilities and aspects of the individual athlete are the environmental influences that surround the athlete's talent development. As Bloom's [2] studies have shown, talent development for athletes begins at home through the encouragement of parents to participate in recreational activities through their enrollment of the child in classes or teams, through their transportation of the child to sporting events, and even to the family's relocation close to a professional coach. The current Proctor & Gamble commercial shows three (fictional) mothers waking their children for early morning training sessions, sitting in the stands as their children perform, and cheering them on to winning performances at the Olympics. Taylor Phinney, a top U.S. cyclist, is the offspring of Connie Carpenter and Davis Phinney, both former cycling champions. Parents, particularly those who were themselves competitors, may also serve as the Olympian's coach. Valery Liukin, father and coach of 2008 U.S. Olympic gymnast, NastiaLiukin, was a famous Russian Olympian before the split up of the Soviet Union.

While schools in Piirto's model typically refer to the formal academic training received by talented individuals, with athletes education often includes specialized camps, organized team sports, and personal coaches. Virtually every single member of the U.S. Men's Basketball team has been involved in basketball since early in their youth. Most played high school, college and professional basketball and participated in summer leagues at all levels. The U.S. culture is also quite supportive of organized sports. High schools and colleges offer an array of sports teams, and hours upon hours of broadcast time are devoted to watching competitive sporting events.

Finally, according to Piirto's model chance plays a role in the talent development of Olympic athletes. Boyd Martin, a member of the U.S. Olympic equestrian team and the son of an Australian father and an American mother, bought Neville Bardos, his mount in the 2012 Olympics, for $850, a pittance in a sport where horses may cost several hundred thousand dollars. Neville Bardos was on his way to the slaughterhouse. His appeal to Martin? The horse, too, was half Australian, half

American. In a freak Memorial Day fire, Martin saved Neville Bardos' life a second time when the stable in which he was housed caught on fire, killing all the other horses inside. A chance encounter and quick sale have lead to one of the most successful partnerships in U.S. Olympic history [10].

3. The Enhancement of Talent Development in the Olympic Athlete

What really separates Olympians from lesser athletes, however, is not just the physical, cognitive and emotional characteristics of the athlete. Nor is it the solely the influence of community and culture, school, parents, or other external factors. What really separates the very best from the rest is the intense preparation and careful application of techniques from the fields of nutrition, sport psychology, and sports medicine.

Consider first nutrition. Top athletes pay careful attention to their diet, working with the advice of nutritional experts. Olympians focus on maintaining proper hydration, choosing appropriate foods for training and competition, and selecting appropriate supplements to maximize performance without risking consuming banned supplements. Male cyclists appear to meet these challenges with the support of medical and nutritional support crews [3].

With respect to sport psychology, Olympians draw upon several established techniques to maximize their performance in competition. Through the application of coaching techniques, psychologists work with athletes to manage the pressure of competition, handle distractions, and deal with loss or underperformance [13]. Athletes learn to visualize successful performance, to visualize the desired performance in advance of competition, and even to visualize standing on the medal stand. Upon winning the Ladies' Singles title at Wimbledon for the fifth timein 2012, Serena Williams said that challenging for a fourth Gold Medal at the 2012 London Olympics was a major motivator for her in overcoming her recent health problems.

More than any other single factor, however, deliberate practice is a key element in successful athletic achievement [7]. Deliberate practice is a type of practice designed to improve performance. It isn't simply repeating a sports skill over and over; it's repetition in the presence of feedback and mental concentration to improve performance. Olympic soccer players play in games where split-second decisions as much as physical skill can determine the outcomes of games. In such an atmosphere the ability to make wise choices is honed over thousands of hours of competition, where choices become second nature. Equally important, however, is that during those hours of practice the athlete is able to consciously make note of the results of a choice and receive feedback from an objective third party in the form of a coach.

Other techniques learned through sport psychology include goal-setting, perfectionism, and relaxation. Olympic athletes obviously have set major goals; e.g. to qualify for the team, to win a medal, etc. But many goals revolve around "besting" their prior records; in effect, they are competing against themselves. A visitor to a typical US Olympic Track and Field Trial will see personal record after personal record fall, as athletes seek to better their previous best performances. Relaxation is achieved by Olympic athletes through such techniques as deep breathing, imagery, or self-talk. Kayla Harrison, 2012 Olympic Gold Medalist in Judo, has discussed at length how she uses visualization, deep breathing, and, yes, even crying to mentally prepare for her matches [17]. One of the newer techniques being utilized by Olympic athletes to achieve these goals is neurofeedback. Beach volleyball star Kerri Walsh-Jennings has employed neurofeedback to improve her mental edge in training. Neurofeedback allows athletes to receive feedback through displays of brain wave that measure focus and concentration [21].

4. Underperformance: Talent in Trouble

In spite of tremendous talent, deliberate practice, and effective coaching, elite athletes can and do exhibit underperformance in competition and in their careers as a whole. This final section will discuss the impact of eating disorders, substance abuse, life/work balance issues, physical injury, and post-career transitions in the performance of Olympic athletes.

Eating disorders may affect any athlete but are more prevalent in female athletes. Because women are sensitized throughout life to focus on body image, sports such as gymnastics, in which the athlete's body is on display in revealing uniforms, may provoke the athlete to reduce caloric consumption or over-exercise to avoid gaining weight. There is some evidence that eating disorders increase over the length of the season in a sport. In the case of Olympic athletes who train year-round, this can be an even greater concern. Kim Soldati, a 2004 U.S. Olympic diver has chronicled her battle with bulimia in her quest for Olympic gold [15]. While today's Olympic organization is aware of the dangers eating disorders present, it is often difficult to identify athletes who need help because athletes hide their behavior from family and coaches.

The use of performance-enhancing drugs has cost more than one Olympian a Gold Medal. Track and field athlete Marion Jones of the U.S. lost her Olympic medals when she became tainted by a steroids scandal and eventually ended up imprisoned (Toptenz.net, n.d.). Although testing is extensive and banned substances are clearly delineated for all Olympic competitors, the pressure to excel often drives some athletes to utilize unapproved substances.

Life/work balance issues represent another area of concern for Olympians. In the U.S. sponsorships are now available to allow Olympians to dedicate large blocks of time to training without regard for financial obstacles, the pressure to balance school, family, and other aspects of life remain. U.S. Olympian Candace Parker (basketball) and Christie Rampone (soccer) have taken leaves from their sports, only to return with children in tow to practices and games [20].

Leaves from competition may also occur due to injuries sustained in practice or competition. McKaylaMaroney, U.S. women's gymnast, suffered a concussion just weeks before the U.S. Trials (NBC Olympics, 2012). Shawn Johnson, 2008 Olympic gymnast, withdrew from the same trials when she failed to heal in time from a knee injury sustained in a skiing accident while taking a break from competition.

Finally, athletes must cope with the end of a competitive career. While U.S. Olympic swimmer Dara Torres won twelve Olympic medals in five different Games, most Olympians have a much shorter lifespan as an elite athlete. Bruce (now Caitlyn) Jenner, U.S. Olympic decathlon champion, began competition in his sport in 1970 and finished his career a mere six years later. Although it can be argued that the competitive rules on compensation in the 1970's precipitated the end of Jenner's career, most Olympians compete for a relatively short period of time [4]. When their identity as an athlete wanes, they must search for a new identity through coaching, celebrity spokesperson, or an entirely new vocation. Rulon Gardner, U.S. Olympic wrestler in the Beijing Games, achieved an epic upset of a Russian champion to claim Gold in his sport. However, after returning to the U.S., his weight ballooned, and he was involved in motorcycle, snowmobiling, and archery accidents. Returning to his life as a farmer in the West, he never again regained his competitive form [5].

5. Conclusion

As we all settle in months from now to cheer our Olympic favorites on to victory, it would be wise to remember that the performances we will see represent a lifetime of work, developing talent and overcoming challenges. For the less than 10 seconds it takes to complete a 100-meter dash, it takes years of training, both mental and physical to achieve victory. The 60 seconds John Orozco competes during floor exercise represent the completion of 12 years of training, tremendous sacrifice by his family, and months of rehabilitation from a torn Achilles tendon.

Acknowledgments

The author acknowledges the support of funding from the Jo Ellen Levy Yates Professorship in the preparation of this manuscript.

Statement of Competing Interests

The author has no competing interests.

References

[1] Bale, P. &Goodway, J. (1990). Performance variables associated with the competitive gymnast. Sports Medicine, 10(3), 139-145.

[2] Bloom, B. (1985). Talent development in young people. New York, NY: Ballantine.

[3] Burke, L. (2001). Nutritional practices of male and female endurance cyclists. Sports Medicine, 31(7), 521-532.

[4] Carey, B. (2008). After glory of a lifetime, asking "What now?" New York Times. Posted on August 8, 2008 Athttp://www.nytimes.com/2008/08/18/sports/olympics/18psych.html.

[5] Cazeneuve, B. (2012). Despite failed comeback Rulon Gardner is not done wrestling. Sports Illustrated. Posted April 26, 2006 at http://www.si.com/more-sports/2012/04/26/rulon-gardner-olympic-bid.

[6] Clay, R. (2012). Gold-medal psychology. APA Monitor, 43(7), 34-38.

[7] Colvin, G. (2010). Talent is overrated. New York, NY: Penguin.

[8] Csikszentmihalyi, M. (1990). Flow. New York, NY: Cambridge.

[9] Dweck, C. (2006). Mindset: The new psychology of success. New York, NY: Ballantine.

[10] Forgrave, N. (2012). Martin, saved horse have special tie. Fox Sports. Posted June 20, 2012 at http://msn.foxsports.com/olympics/equestrian/story/Boyd-Martin-and-Neville-Bardos-the-horse.

[11] Gould, D., Dieffenbach, K. & Moffatt, A. (2002). Psychological characteristics and their development in Olympic champions. Journal of Applied Sport Psychology, 14(3), 174-204.

[12] Hadhazy, A. (2008). What makes Michael Phelps so good? Scientific American, August 18, 2008.

[13] Harmon, K. (2012). Sports psychologists extend their training to athletes' coaches and families. Scientific American. Posted August 1, 2012 at http://www.scientificamerican.com/article/olympics-sports-psychology/.

[14] Hayes, K. (2009) Performance psychology in action. Washington, DC: American Psychological Association.

[15] Helmich, N. (2006). Athletes' hunger to win fuels eating disorders. USA Today. Posted March 5, 2006 at http://www.usatoday.com/sports/2006-02-05-women-health-cover_x.htm .

[16] Horowitz, F., Subotnik, R., and Mathews, D. (2009). The development of giftedness and talent across the lifespan. Washington, DC: American Psychological Association.

[17] Humintell. (2012). Olympians and their emotions: Kayla Harrison. Posted July 10/2012 at http://www.humintell.com/2012/07/olympians-and-their-emotions-kayla-harrison/.

[18] McCluskeyM. (2012). One one-hundredth of a second faster: Building better Olympic athletes. Wired.Posted July 25, 2012 at http://www.nytimes.com/2008/08/18/sports/olympics/18psych.html.

[19] Mechikoff, R. (2010) A history and philosophy of sport and physical education: From ancient civilizations to the modern world. New York, NY: McGraw-Hill.

[20] Moscatello, C. (2012). Hey, London, the Moms are calling! Redbook. Posted July 22, 2012 at http://www.redbookmag.com/life/mom-kids/a14072/female-olympic-athletes-who-are-moms/.

[21] Murphy, J. (2012). Mental, physical training for Olympic volleyball. Wall Street Journal, July 10, 2012.

[22] NBC Olympics (2012).Profiles of David Boudia and Kayla Maroney. Posted at http://www.nbcolympics.com/athletes/athlete-david-boudia/library and http://www.nbcolympics.com/athletes/athlete-kayla-maroney/library.

[23] Piirto, J. (2004). Understanding creativity. Scottsdale, AZ: Great Potential Press.

[24] Terman, L. & Oden,M. (1959) Genetic studies of genius. Vol. V. The gifted group at mid-life. Stanford, CA: Stanford University Press.

[25] Toptenz.net (n.d.) http://www.toptenz.net/top-10-athletes-who-lost-their-olympic-medal.php.

The Effect of Listening to Brain Waves' Relaxing and Exciting Music during Intense Endurance Training on Blood Cortisol Levels of Adult Men

Saeed Rahmaty[1], Pooneh Dehghan[2,*], Keivan Khoramipour[1], Mostafa Saboory[1]

[1]Department of Sports and Physical Education, Tehran University
[2]Imaging Department, Taleghani Hospital Research Development Unit, Shahid Beheshti University of Medical Sciences
*Corresponding author: Poonehdehghan@yahoo.com

Abstract **Objectives:** Listening to music during exercise could be used to counteract reduced immune function in endurance athletes. The aim of this study was to determine the effect of listening to music, with relaxing and stimulating effect on the brain waves, during intense endurance exercise on blood cortisol levels of adult men. **Methods:** In this study, eight healthy men (n=8) with mean age of (23.25±1.83 years) were asked to perform four different protocols in a crossover design, after pre-test determination of their cortisol levels. Protocols included: intense endurance training (control) (A), intense endurance training with relaxing music (B), intense endurance training with exciting music (C), and intense endurance training with music stimulating their brain waves in four non-consecutive days (D). Their post-test cortisol levels were determined. To analyze data, the statistical tests ANOVA R.M and LSD were used. **Results:** A significant increase was observed in cortisol levels in protocols A and B, compared to pre-test ($P \leq 0.05$). While changes of the other two protocols, C and D, were not significant. ($P > 0.05$). **Conclusion:** The findings show that listening to exciting music and music stimulating brain waves counteracts cortisol rise during intense endurance exercise.

Keywords: *hypothalamic-pituitary-adrenal axis, immune system, vitality, stress*

1. Introduction

Studying the correlation of music and medicine is rapidly growing. Previously, music as a complementary therapy was the focus of many researches. It has been shown that music has a positive effect on variables such as stress, relaxation, pain, neurological cognition, cardiac function, etc. [1-5]. Recently, attention has been driven to understanding the physiologic mechanisms related to the effect and role of music on metabolic responses. Research has proven the regulatory effect of music on Hypothalamic-Pituitary-Adrenal axis (HPA), Sympathetic Nervous System (SNS), and the immune system; all of which with key functions in the regulation of metabolism and energy balance. New findings have also shown the role of music in metabolic recovery from stress, increasing lipid metabolism, and lactic acid elimination after physical activity.

Recent studies focus on a deeper understanding of the impact of music on complex human stress response by the HPA, SNS, and immune system. HPA axis activity is monitored by measuring the serum level of cortisol, adrenocorticotropic hormone, growth hormone (GH), insulin-like growth factor, and oxytocin. Cortisol is released from adrenal glands in response to adrenocorticotropic hormone, an anterior pituitary gland hormone. Cortisol initiates metabolic response by stimulating gluconeogenesis, both general and hepatic. It also suppresses the immune system secondary to the negative feedback of cytokine production. Increased catabolic state through metabolism of proteins, fats, and carbohydrates in muscle, fat tissue, connective tissue, and lymphatic tissue is another effect of this hormone. Thus, the HPA axis plays an important role in the regulation of metabolic responses and balance of energy.

Several studies have shown the role of music in reducing cortisol levels in surgical environments. Patients who had listened to music after surgery had significantly reduced cortisol levels, compared to control group (patients without music exposure) [6,7,8]. In a study by Nilsson et al [8], patients who received postoperative music therapy revealed 206 mmol per liter reduction of cortisol levels after two hours in intensive care unit, while the reduction in the control group was 72 mmol per liter. Similarly, Lord and his colleagues reported decrease in cortisol levels in patients receiving music before and after surgery. A significant reduction was observed in post-surgical cortisol levels of patients who were able to choose their music type. Koolesh and colleagues [9] demonstrated that patients who listened to music during surgery had lower cortisol levels than patients who received no such intervention. In another study, performed to determine the relaxing effect of peaceful music after stressful work, salivary cortisol ceased to increase in the group who listened to music, while its' increment continued for 30 minutes in the control group [10]. Hajizadeh and colleagues [11] found that cortisol levels in a group of patients who had music intervention during surgery did not increase, unlike the other groups. Foucault and Yamashita [12] also concluded that regardless of the gender differences, listening to music for thirty minutes reduces levels of cortisol in saliva.

Endurance training leads to cortisol secretion, which can reduce the number and function of white blood cells [13]. Stressful situations such as intense training, long training sessions, attending athletic competitions, low carbohydrate food intake, and carbohydrate deprivation during training, or lack of adequate sleep are all factors that can increase cortisol levels [14]. Cortisol affects the late leukocytosis (neutrophilia) induced by physical activity [15,16]. Neutrophilia is often caused by increased neutrophil release from bone marrow [17,18] also reduced neutrophil outflow from the blood, however, some believe that release of the attached leukocytes is considered the most important mechanism of neutrophilia induced by glucocorticoids [19]. During short-term exercise activity, if the intensity exceeds 60 to 70% of maximal oxygen uptake, concentrations of plasma cortisol increase [15,20], while intensities lower than 50% of maximal oxygen uptake decrease cortisol concentrations [20]. Long-term activity, also, increases cortisol concentrations, as it increases gluconeogenesis and maintains blood glucose concentrations.

Intense athletic activities reduce the innate immune cell function and increases secretion of cortisol. Physiological concentration of cortisol improves the immune system function, while high physiological concentrations suppress the immune system. Intravenous administration of a small amount of cortisol decreases lymphocytes by inhibiting the entry of lymphocytes to the blood and facilitates the movement of lymphocytes into the tissue [21]. Long-term exercise increases plasma cortisol levels and depletes neutrophil storage of the bone marrow. The individual uses bone marrow neutrophil storage during endurance training faster than a normal person, thus neutropenia is common in endurance athletes.

Due to the influence of music on reducing levels of the blood's cortisol and also increase of this hormone during long-term and intense exercises and its harmful effects on reducing the number of bone marrow's neutrophils and immune system suppression, it is theoretically expressed whether music can reduce the stress on the immune system during long-term and intense activity by reducing plasma levels of cortisol.

Stressful situations, physically and mentally, lead to high plasma concentrations of cortisol with suppressive effect of this hormone on immune system. On the other hand it has been shown that music could balance the incremental elevation of plasma cortisol level, theoretically counteracting its' detrimental effect on the immune system in athletes. In this study we tried to prove this theory while trying to understand whether different kinds of music had the same effect or not.

2. Materials and Methods

The current study is a developmental quasi-experimental cross design study. Researchers have compared changes of independent variables on the dependent variables in post-test stage of four groups of physical activity (control), physical activity with relaxing music (relaxing), physical activity with exciting music (exciting), physical activity with music stimulating brain waves (brain wave exciting).

After preliminary studies, sampling, determining the intervention group, determining and providing research data collection tool, a sample of eight students of Khwarizmi Sports University of Karaj entered the study. Subjects characteristics are presented in Table 1.

Table 1. characteristics of subject's (N=8)

Statistics / Index	mean	SD	maximum	Minimum
age	23/25	1/83	26	21
height	179/5	7/03	190	170
weight	75/25	6/36	92	71

Participants were advised to sleep six to eight hours the night before the test exercise. In addition, they were asked to drink plenty of liquids 24 hours before the test exercise and avoid eating, smoking, and taking caffeine three hours before the exercise. Required trainings for the test exercise were explained to them. Then, before the exercise protocol (exercise protocol is described below), blood samples were taken from volunteers to determine their pre-test cortisol levels and all participants underwent four intense endurance training protocols in non-consecutive days as following: control group, physical activity with relaxing music, physical activity with exciting music, and physical activity with music stimulating brain waves and their blood samples were taken after each exercise protocol. The interval of each exercise was one week. All participants were meanwhile released from daily pressures and stress by 15 minutes listening to Brain Refresher music before the exercise protocol. Subjects listened to music for 15 minutes before the test also during exercise the music was played continuously.

The Repeated High-Intensity Endurance Test (RHIET) test was used as the training protocol; the executive model includes eight cones placed in two rows of fours with two meters distance between each two four-rows and five meters distance between each cone in rows of four. Each participant started test with the "start" command, ran and returned the first five meters from cone A to B and then again from cone A to C, which is ten meters, and finally, from cone A to D, which is 15 meters. They ran a total distance of 60 meters (two five meters, two ten meters, plus two fifteen meters) in 30 seconds. Each participant must complete the test six times without break in a period of 30 seconds that ultimately makes the total test time 180 seconds (three minutes). If any participant ran sooner than 30 seconds during the test, he should wait and begin the next stage after 30 seconds. The test is repeated with the total time of three minutes several times. The time in each repetition of the test: 30 seconds, the distance in each repetition of the test: 60 meters, the time period of each test: 180 seconds (6 repetitions of 30 seconds), the rest time between each period of the test (rest time between each three minutes of physical activity): 30 seconds, the total number of test periods at one training session (work-rest): 43 repetitions of each test period with rest intervals of 30 seconds, and the total time of one training session: 2.5 hours.

2.1. Blood Sampling

Before the training protocol and after 12 hours of fasting, 5 mL blood was taken from the right antecubital vein of each subject in the sitting position and at rest to determine the baseline cortisol level. After activity, another blood sample was taken to evaluate cortisol level. Blood was centrifuged for 10 minutes at 3000 rpm and the serum was separated. The isolated blood serum samples were kept in the freezer at −80°C. ELISA kits (Biospes Company, China) were used to measure cortisol level.

2.2. Statistical Methods

To analyze the data, descriptive and inferential statistical methods were used. Descriptive statistics was used for mean, standard deviation, distribution, graphs, and tables and for testing research hypotheses, analysis of variance with repeated measure (ANOVA R.M) was used. As each of the four groups underwent all four training types in non-consecutive days, according to the crossover type of study, there was no need to synchronize the groups. But normal distribution of data was evaluated through Kolmogorov-Smirnov test and as data distribution was normal, parametric tests were used. Decision measurement about all of the variables was within the alpha level of five hundredths ($P<0.05$). To draw charts, Excel 2013 Software and to calculate mean, standard deviation, and repeated measurements of variance SPSS 21 was used.

3. Results

The inter-group results showed that the exciting music group (during physical activity) and brain waves stimulating music group (during physical activity) revealed no statistically significant change in cortisol compared to pre-activity ($P<0.05$), but relaxing music group (during physical activity) and control group (only physical activity) had increased cortisol level (Figure 1). The between-groups results are shown in Table 2, demonstrating significant difference in cortisol levels between exciting music group (during physical activity) and brain waves stimulating music (during physical activity), compared to relaxing music group (during physical activity) and control group (only physical activity) ($P<0.05$) and these two groups had no increased cortisol levels than pre-activity, compared with relaxing music (during physical activity) and control group (during physical activity). For the coupled comparison of mean variables, LSD test was used. Table 2 presents the results of the statistical analysis.

Table 2. Coupled comparison of mean differences of blood cortisol levels in different groups

Between-group comparison	Inferential statistics	Differences in means	Standard deviation	P value
Control group (only physical activity)	relaxing music group (during physical activity)	18/708	19/275	0./364
	exciting music group (during physical activity)	88/528	14/474	0/016 ★
	brain waves stimulating music (during physical activity)	80/474	15/279	0/027 ★
relaxing music group (during physical activity)	exciting music group (during physical activity)	69/820	23/160	0/02 ★
	brain waves stimulating music (during physical activity)	61/766	13/146	0/036 ★
exciting music group (during physical activity)	brain waves stimulating music (during physical activity)	8/054	15/251	0/614

★: Significant difference between groups by coupled comparison ($p<0.05$).

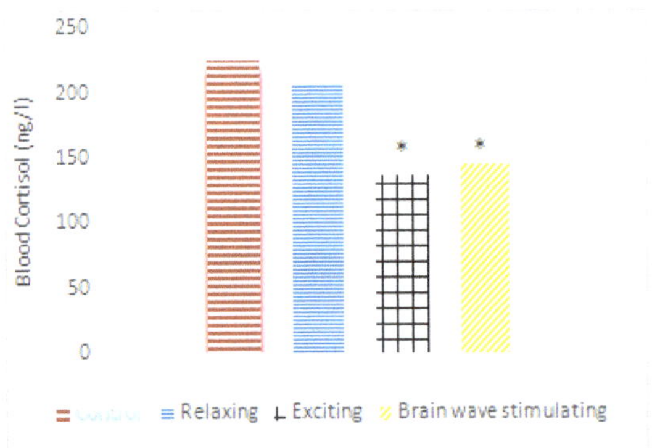

Figure 1. Between-group comparison of blood cortisol levels' variation

*: No change in cortisol amount, compared to pre-activity in the exciting music group and brain waves stimulating music, compared to control and relaxing music groups ($p<0.05$).

4. Discussion and Conclusion

The results of the current study represent a huge increase in blood cortisol levels after exercise in the control group (those who did not listen to any music) and relaxing music group (the group listening to relaxing music during intense endurance exercise), while less increase was observed in the groups listening to exciting music and brain waves stimulating music, compared tocontrol and relaxing groups. Also, the increase in blood cortisol concentrations after intense endurance training was insignificant in exciting music and brain waves stimulating music groups, which indicates minor increase in cortisol levels than pre-test values. While, significant difference was observed between cortisol levels of control and relaxing music groups than pre-test values. Although the participants had listened to music during intense endurance training in three groups, exciting music and brain waves stimulating music were more effective in preventing severe increase in blood cortisol after intense endurance training. Unfortunately, there is no similar research on the effects of music on blood cortisol levels during intense endurance training available, but in other areas of research (medicine, psychology, and neurology) some researches have been conducted with different training protocol, research methods, and statistical analysis. Despite the differences mentioned, we outline some studies conducted.

Gra and colleagues (1998) found that listening to relaxing music reduces blood levels of cortisol, while exciting music increases it [22], also, the study of Yamamoto et al. (2007) showed that listening to relaxing music after being placed in stressful conditions decreases blood cortisol concentrations [23]. The results of the current study, against Graand Yamamoto, showed significant decrease in cortisol levels immediately after intense endurance training in the group who had listened to exciting music during exercise, compared to those who had listened to relaxing music. Also Koolesh et al (2011) and Field et al (1998) reported that listening to music, regardless of the selected music tempo (fast or slow), reduces blood levels of cortisol [24,25]. Also Hajizadeh et al (2012) concluded in their study on three groups of patients: a)headset with music, b) headset without music, and c) without intervention that listening to music reduces the levels of cortisol and blood sugar after surgery [11]. Oddo et al (2003) also concluded in their study that listening to music causes less increase in cortisol levels, compared to the state of without music [26]. In the present study, also, listening to exciting and stimulating music during intense endurance training led to less increase in cortisol concentrations than the control and relaxing music groups immediately after exercise; this difference might be due to the different effectiveness of music types on the nervous system and hypothalamic-pituitary-adrenal axis adjustment that reduces cortisol secretion during intense endurance training.

Secretion of cortisol can be adjusted through rest, nutrition, music, and training supplements. 32 studies have examined the effect of music on hormones. Among these, 29 studies measured the amount of cortisol. Among these studies, 18 studied the effects of music on the reduction in cortisol, either actively or by recorded music. Only two studies had opposite trends, but in both studies cortisol increased less in the music group than in the control group. Ascher and colleagues (1993) found that this pattern of cortisol reflect ACTH secretion levels, reduced in the music group than the control group. When the researchers chose music for the participants, studies including cortisol have focused on the effects of relaxing music (n=11). But four studies that have assessed the effects of stimulating music have obtained different results. Movakkel and colleagues (1995) found similar decline by relaxing and stimulating music. While Yamamoto et al (2007) observed a decrease in cortisol only by relaxing music [23]. Also, Gra and colleagues (1998) observed increased cortisol only with stimulating music [22]. These results reveal the noticeable sensitivity of this hormone to stimulating music. Another variable is only assessed in .Leardi et al's study (2007), in which patients' cortisol level was investigated against the music selected by participants, which showed the maximum cortisol response to music selected by participants [6]. However, since this study only examined this variable with cortisol, more studies are needed to confirm these findings [6]. Of other hormones tested, Nilsson (2009) showed increased oxytocin, when participants were listening to relaxing music recordings [27]. Bateman (2001) showed increase in the proportion of dehydroepiandrosteronedion ratio to cortisol when participants had participated in the drama group [28], while Conrad et al (2007) have shown reducing cortisol levels with increasing growth hormone when the participants had listened to the recorded relaxingmusic. [29]. When participants listened to their own recorded music, Migneault (2004) showed increase in testosterone levels in men and decrease in women and insignificant changes in four other biological markers evaluated in this study, including cortisol, ACTH, epinephrine, and norepinephrine [30]. Generally, no research has studied the effect of music during intense endurance training on blood cortisol levels.

In conclusion, the current study showed that listening to exciting music and music with stimulating effect on brain waves during intense endurance training, in comparison to relaxing music or no music exposure during the same activity, can prevent blood cortisol level elevation in relation to the pretest situation. Due to the negative effects of high cortisol concentration on immune system, bone marrow storage, and other negative effects of cortisol in intense endurance training, listening to music with stimulating effect during exercise can reduce the negative effects of cortisol on the body. This effect has not been shown to appear with relaxing music.

References

[1] Bernatzky G, Presch M, Anderson M, Panksepp J. Emotional foundations of music as a non-pharmacological pain management tool in modern medicine. Neuroscience & Biobehavioral Reviews 2011; 35(9):1989-99.

[2] Cervellin G, Lippi G. From music-beat to heart-beat: a journey in the complex interactions between music, brain and heart. European Journal of Internal Medicine 2011; 22(4):371-4.

[3] Nilsson U.The anxiety-and pain-reducing effects of music interventions: a systematic review. AORN journal 2008; 87: 807-780.

[4] THAUT MH.The future of music in therapy and medicine. Annals of the New York Academy of Sciences 2005; 1060(1):303-8.

[5] Yehuda N.Music and stress. Journal of Adult Development 2011; 18(2):85-94.

[6] Leardi S, Pietroletti R, Angeloni G, Necozione S, Ranalletta G, Del Gusto B. Randomized clinical trial examining the effect of music therapy in stress response to day surgery. British journal of surgery 2007; 94(8):943-7.

[7] Lepage C, Drolet P, Girard M, Grenier Y, DeGagné R. Music decreases sedative requirements during spinal anesthesia. Anesthesia & Analgesia 2001; 93(4): 912-6.

[8] Nilsson U, Unosson M, Rawal N.Stress reduction and analgesia in patients exposed to calming music postoperatively: a randomized controlled trial. European journal of anaesthesiology 2005; 22(02): 96-102.

[9] Koelsch S, Fuermetz J, Sack U, Bauer K, Hohenadel M, Wiegel M, et al. Effects of music listening on cortisol levels and propofol consumption during spinal anesthesia. Frontiers in psychology (2011); 2.

[10] Khalfa S, Bella SD, Roy M, Peretz I, Lupien SJ. Effects of relaxing music on salivary cortisol level after psychological stress. Annals of the New York Academy of Sciences 2003; 999(1):374-6.

[11] Hajizadeh E, Lak M, Mottahedian Tabrizi E, Movahhedi Rad S, Sahraei. H. The effect of music on the level of cortisol, blood glucose and physiological variables in patients undergoing spinal anesthesia 2012. Excli - Experimental and Clinical Sciences; Vol:11.

[12] Fukui H, Yamashita M.The effects of music and visual stress on testosterone and cortisol in men and women. Neuro endocrinology letters 2003; 24(3-4):173.

[13] Khansari DN, Murgo AJ, Faith RE. Effects of stress on the immune system. Immunology today 1990; 11:170-5.

[14] Gleeson M. Immune function in sport and exercise. Journal of applied physiology 2007;103(2):693-9.

[15] Gabriel H, Schwarz L, Steffens G, Kindermann W. Immunoregulatory Hormones, Circulating Leucocyte and Lymphocyte Subpopulations before and after Endurance Exercise of Different Intensities*. International journal of sports medicine 1992;13(05):359-66.

[16] McCarthy D, Macdonald I, Grant M, Marbut M, Watling M, Nicholson S, et al. Studies on the immediate and delayed leucocytosis elicited by brief (30-min) strenuous exercise. European journal of applied physiology and occupational physiology 1992;64:607-513.

[17] Allsop P, Peters A, Arnot R, Stuttle A, Deenmamode M, Gwilliam M, et al. Intrasplenic blood cell kinetics in man before and after brief maximal exercise. Clinical Science 1992; 83 (Pt 1):47-54.

[18] Athens J, Haab O, Raab S, Mauer A, Ashenbrucker H, Cartwright G, et al. Leukokinetic studies. IV. The total blood, circulating and marginal granulocyte pools and the granulocyte turnover rate in normal subjects. Journal of Clinical Investigation 1961;40(6):989.

[19] Nakagawa M, Terashima T, D'yachkova Y, Bondy GP, Hogg JC, van Eeden SF. Glucocorticoid-induced granulocytosis contribution of marrow release and demargination of intravascular granulocytes. Circulation 1998;98(21):2307-13.

[20] Galbo H. Hormonal and metabolic adaptation to exercise: Georg Thieme Verlag 1983.

[21] Tønnesen E, Christensen N, Brinkløv M. Natural killer cell activity during cortisol and adrenaline infusion in healthy volunteers. European journal of clinical investigation 1987;17(6):497-503.

[22] Gerra G, Zaimovic A, Franchini D, Palladino M, Giucastro G, Reali N, et al. Neuroendocrine responses of healthy volunteers totechno-music': relationships with personality traits and emotional state. International Journal of Psychophysiology 1998;28(1):99-111.

[23] Yamamoto M, Naga S, Shimizu J. Positive musical effects on two types of negative stressful conditions. Psychology of Music 2007;35(2):249-75.

[24] Koelsch S, Fuermetz J, Sack U, Bauer K, Hohenadel M, Wiegel M, et al. Effects of Music Listening on Cortisol Levels and Propofol Consumption during Spinal Anesthesia. Frontiers in psychology 2011; 2:58.

[25] Field T, Martinez A, Nawrocki T, Pickens J, Fox NA, Schanberg S. Music shifts frontal EEG in depressed adolescents. Adolescence 1998;33(129):109-16.

[26] Uedo N, Ishikawa H, Morimoto K, Ishihara R, Narahara H, Akedo I, et al. Reduction in salivary cortisol level by music therapy during colonoscopic examination. Hepato-gastroenterology 2003;51(56):451-3.

[27] Nilsson U. Soothing music can increase oxytocin levels during bed rest after open-heart surgery: a randomised control trial. US National Library of Medicine National Institutes of Health. 2009; vol: 15 pp:2153-61.

[28] Bittman BB, Berk LS, Felten DL, Westengard J, Simonton OC, Pappas J, Ninehouser M. Composite effects of group drumming music therapy on modulation of neuroendocrine-immune parameters in normal subjects. US National Library of Medicine National Institutes of Health. 2001 Jan;7(1):38-47.

[29] Conrad C, Niess H, Jauch KW, Bruns CJ, Hartl W, Welker L. Overture for growth hormone: requiem for interleukin-6? Critical care medicine. 2007;35(12):2709-13.

[30] Migneault B, Girard F, Albert C, Chouinard P, Boudreault D, Provencher D, Todorov A, Ruel M, Girard DC. The effect of music on the neurohormonal stress response to surgery under general anesthesia. US National Library of Medicine National Institutes of Health. 2004 Feb;98(2):527-32.

30

The Comparison of Elite Wrestlers' State of Anxiety Before-after Weighing

Veysel Küçük[1], Ünsal Tazegül[2,*], Hamdi Sancaklı[1], Mehmet Haşim Akgül[3], A. Serdar Yücel[4]

[1]Marmara University, School of Physical Education and Sports, İstanbul, Turkey
[2]GaziUniversity, School of Physical Education and Sports, Ankara, Turkey
[3]Mehmet Akif Ersoy, University, School of Physical Educationand Sports, Burdur, Turkey
[4]Fırat University, Faculty of Sports Sciences, Elazig, Turkey
*Corresponding author: unsaltazegul@hotmail.com

Abstract Anxiety is one the significant factor which affects performance of athletes in a negative way. The purpose of this research is to compare elite wrestlers' state of anxiety before-after weighing. A state of anxiety inventory developed by Spielberg and adapted to Turkishby Ömer and Le Compte has been used in order to detect wrestlers' state of anxiety before-after weighing. SSPS 20 package software has been used while analyzing the data on this research. After it has been stated that datum has both an homogenous and normal distribution; it has been decided that parametric test method should be used in statistic analysis. In statistic analysis, diagnostic statistic and co-sample t test has been implemented. On the consequence of these analyses, the wrestlers' state of anxiety before weighing has been higher than the state of anxiety that wrestlers have after weighing.

Keywords: *state of anxiety, wrestlers, weighing*

1. Introduction

Anxiety, in terms of dictionary meaning, is a negative feeling that it is felt while facing with either a dangerous or unexpected condition [1,2,3].

The state of anxiety is subjective fear that an individual feels it due to a stressful situation [4].

Stress and anxiety can affect ability of making right decisions negatively in athletes' attitude. An athlete, who is under anxiety and stress, is unable to make right decisions and to perform his/her ability however S/he desires. Athletes, who are under extreme pressure, might have inappropriate behaviors. Not only stress makes athletes forget the actions which is well known and performed by athletes many times in trainings but also it causes athletes to perform negative actions while raising a chaos in athletes' feelings [5].

Today, it has been mentioned that there are many factors affecting athletes' sportive efficiency level. While some parts of these factors are evaluated under the name of environmental factors; some other parts of these factors are evaluated as internal factors. Athletes' psychological preparations are significant factors to be successful in performing sports. Athletes' psychological conditions and their performances are in a close relation with their level of anxiety [6,7].

As long as the researches which show relation between athletes' psychological state and their performance progress; sportive actions has gained a different dimension and it has been detected that mental activitiessuch as intelligence, attention, memory, self control, judgment, comparison, analyzing, anxiety are included in all these sportive activities [8].

It has been adopted that Anxiety affects performance in the researches which are carried out in the field of sport psychology. It should be taken care of that anxiety will not affect performance in a negative way and there should be techniques in order to cope with these situations [9].

Presence of external reinforcement and punishments, uncertainty of conclusion, dominance of opponent, scores athletes have in latest competitions, at what degree of importance of these scores have according to athletes, how athletes comprehend their physical, technique, tactic physiological capabilities as compared to their opponents' capabilities, stress and anxiety are definitive in all competitive environment and especially researches which are carried out in high level sports [10].

Every competition has a great deal of significance for athletes in terms of social and economical factors. In accomplishing success, the ability of coping with anxiety an extremely important criterion no matter how perfect an athlete is in terms of physical features and no matter how perfect training duration is. Psychological preparation should be different in accordance with fundamentals of different sports. Team sports have different dynamics compared to individual sports. It has been thought that individual athletes have more intense anxiety level than team sport athletes [11,12].

Scientists have developed new training systems in order to increase athletes' performances to the top level. Researches carried out by scientists shows that not only physical trainings is not merely significant to increase athletes performances but also psychological factors have a significant place in athletes progress [13,14].

The world's most successful athletes believe that the hardest athlete to dominate is athletes themselves. If an athlete learns to dominate his/her previous success; s/he learns easily how to dominate other athletes. For this reason, athletes should know what retains him/her from his/her goals [15].

The purpose of this research is to compare elite wrestlers' state of anxiety before-after weighing.

2. Material and Method

2.1. Samples

Samples of this study consist of 40 elite wrestlers who attended Young wrestlers' Turkey Championship in 2012. 95 wrestlers were met and 40 wrestlers out of these were decided to be in this research.

2.2. The Purpose of Gathering Information of the Research

A state of anxiety inventory developed by Spielberg (1970) and adapted to Turkishby Ömer and Le Compte (1985) has been used in order to detect wrestlers' state of anxiety before-after weighing. This inventory is a self-evaluation questionnaire that consists of short statements. It has been declared that Alpha reliability is between .83 and .87. Repetition of test reliability is between .71 and .86. Article reliability is between .34 and .72 [16].

2.3. Analysis of Data

SPSS 20 package software has been used for the analysis of data. Kolmogorov-Smirnov test has been used in order to have whether data had a normal distribution or not. Therefore, it has been found that data has had a normal distribution. Later on, Anova-Homogenety of variance test has been used in order to evaluate whether data has not had a homogeneous. After that, it has been found that data has had a homogeneous result. After the first examination; parametric test technique has been decided to be used in the statistical analysis of examined data. Diagnostic statistic and co-sample t test has been used.

3. Results

In this section, results which have been found at the end of statistical analysis have been given in 2 different charts and graphics.

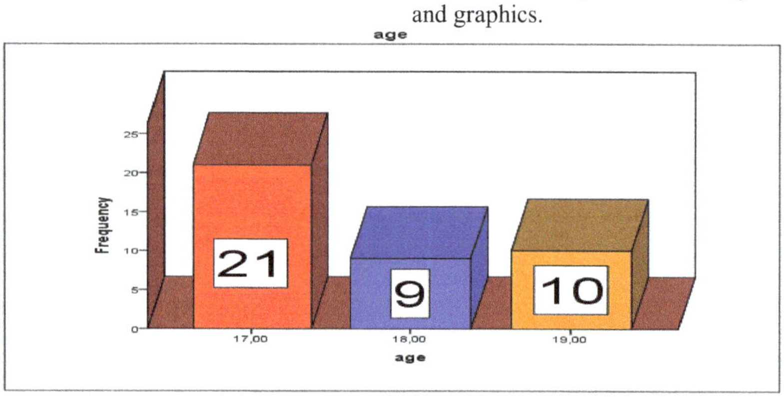

Graphic 1. Distribution of athletes' age who have attended this stud

On this chart, the data and distribution of athletes who have attended in this research have been given above. 21 wrestlers who are 17, 9 wrestlers who are 18, 10 wrestlers who are 19 have attended. 40 wrestlers attend this study in total.

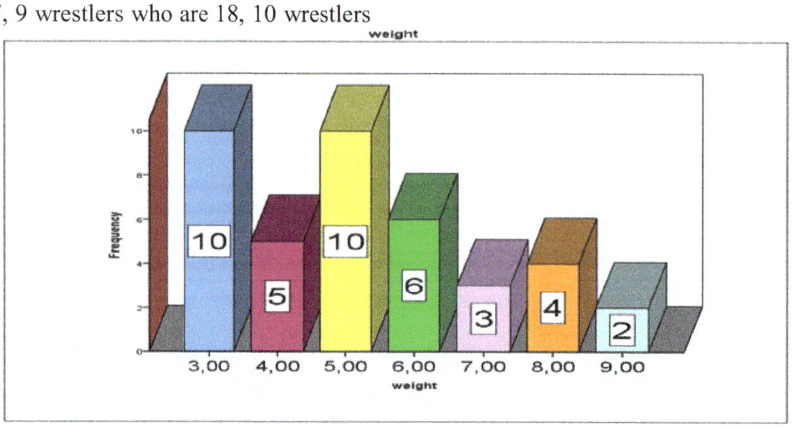

Graphic 2. The frequency distribution that shows wrestlers' pre-match weight loss

Reviewing graphic above, it has been determined that 10 wrestlers have lost 3 kilos, 5 wrestlers have lost 4 kilos, 10 wrestlers have lost 5 kilos, 6 wrestlers have lost 6 kilos, 3 wrestlers have lost 7 kilos, 4 wrestlers have lost 8 kilos, 2 wrestlers have lost 9 kilos.

Chart 1. The results of diagnostic statistic of state of anxiety

	N	$\overline{X}$	±
Level of anxiety at pre-weighing	40	48,850	6,228
Level of anxiety at post-weighing	40	37,400	11,160

Reviewing diagnostic statistics which have shown the wrestlers' level of anxiety on chart 1, it has been determined that pre-weighing has been (=48,850±6,228) and post-weighing has been (=37,400±11,160).

Chart 2. The Results of co-sample t test

Mean	Std. Deviation	T	p
11,45000	8,42448	-8,596	,000

As a consequence of comparison of wrestlers' pre-weighing and post-weighing state of anxiety points on chart 2, a reasonable difference has been found statistically ($p<0,05$).

4. Discussion

Reviewing elite athletes' pre-weighing and post-weighing state of anxiety scores, it has been understood that measure score which has been carried out 30 minutes before weighing is higher than the score which has been carried out 1 hour after weighing. In addition to the consequence of comparisons of anxiety scores at pre-weighing and post weighing; a reasonable difference has been found statistically ($p<0,05$). After analyzing results, many studies covering wrestlers and other branches have been attained. However, the study which compares level of anxiety at pre-weighing and post-weighing has not been found. Özbay compares national professional wrestlers' state of anxiety at pre-game and post-game. As a result of this comparison, he has determined that there is a reasonable difference statistically. Özbay has determined (2012)that post-game state of anxiety of wrestlers who are over-weight is lower than the ones who have both less over-weigh problems and none over-weigh problems.

Morgan (1970) apply 3 types of IPAT parallel anxiety test to 7 university wrestlers at Missouri university. The first test has been given before the season starts. The second test has been given before the game that is considered as an easy game by the coach. The third test has been given before the game that is considered as a hard game by the coach. Surprisingly, anxiety results that have been identified before games have been lower than the ones that are during pre-season anxiety results. However, there is no difference between easy games and hard games in terms of anxiety results. Afterwards, Morgan and Hammer have applied same IPAT anxiety test to four wrestlers who are from different colleges. Anxiety test have been given orderly at the beginning of the season, during the tournament, after wrestlers prepared (4 hours before the tournament), 1 hour before the first game and 15 minutes after tournament. It has been observed that anxiety has been increased 1 hour ago before the game.It has been noticed that anxiety has been decreased after tournament. It has been identified that anxiety level in real conditions have been lower compared to previous tests at later tournaments [17].

Morgan and Hammer have found that pre-game state of anxiety have been higher than post-game state of anxiety in the research on 29 wrestlers [18].

Screiber (2004)statedthat an increase might be seen on wrestlers' performances by preventing negative influences and state of anxiety [19].

Tazegüland his friends stated in their studies which were carried out in 2015 that wrestlers' anxiety score was lower than boxer, kick boxers were [20].

Çoksevimand his friends observed pre-game, post-game state of anxiety of kick boxers and short-time tempo. They found (2008) found a reasonable difference in statistical analysis [21].

In the meetings when wrestlers have weighed, it has been asked some questions about wrestlers' condition and how wrestlers have felt themselves. As a result of these questions, wrestlers' biggest concern is whether they are on the right weigh that they are expected to or not. Therefore they generally don't eat anything until the weighing time. In addition to meetings having been carried out, wrestlers have experienced some kind of anxiety on their mind that they think their performance level would decrease according to their weight loss. Rather than that wrestlers want to eat something as soon as they finish weighing. Therefore, the biggest reason why wrestlers have high anxiety scores is not being able to reach aimed weigh in accordance with their performance level. According to Martens, the state of anxiety during pre-game might affect both in-game performance and result of the game [22]. Jones and his friends (1993) stated that anxiety has a significant impact on performance [23].

A meeting with Dr Hamdi who was a grek romen national team coach once states his thoughts on his observation below:

Weight loss that is planned both by athlete and by coach, weight loss duration and amount of lost weight might affect the state of anxiety at pre-game. If an athlete decides to lose weight by his own will not obeying what coach says, an increase will be seen in athlete's performance. Also, Wrestlers who lost weight because of coach's will had an unpleasant situation while weighing. They did not even want to be weighed.

It has been believed that power decrease related to weight loss increases the state of anxiety. An athlete who feels powerless might be affected his/her state of anxiety in a sport branch that is based on power and advanced performance such as wrestling. Koral J. and Dosseville F. (2009) have found as a result of their studies that wrestlers who have sudden weight loss have low performance conditions [24]. Roemmich and Sinning (1997) have stated as a result of their studies that wrestlers who have lost weight have low performance conditions [25].

Civan and his friends (2010) compared state of anxiety and continuous anxiety of individual athletes and team athletes at pre-game and post-game. As a result of this comparison, it was found that average state of anxiety scores had different results in different sport types. Average score of state of anxiety had the highest score in individual sports. Team athletes' state of anxiety average score was found that it had a lower score than individual athletes had ($P<0, 05$). It was found that continuous anxiety at post game between individual athletes and racket based sport had no reasonable relation. However, it was found that team sport athletes' continuous anxiety average score had a higher score than individual athletes and racket based sport athletes had.

Consequently, it has been found that wrestlers have a high state of anxiety at pre-weighing. Meetings with national team athletes and national team coach result in that one of the significant reason why wrestlers have thoughts on their mind that they will not be able to lose weight they desire along with their performance level.

References

[1] Güney, S., Terminology dictionary of behavioral sciences and management psychology, Ankara, 1998.

[2] Gürgün O.A., Psychology dictionary İnkilap Book Store, İstanbul 1991.

[3] Hançerlioğlu, O., Mental science dictionary, 2nd press. Remzi Book Store, Istanbul, 1993.

[4] Türkçapar Ü (2012). Analysis of wrestlers continuous anxiety levels in terms of different variables, GEFAD / GUJGEF 32 (1): 129-140.

[5] Tazegül Ü.(2012). Comparison of handling styles with stress in individual sport, of Sports and Performance Researches, 3(2), 13-22.

[6] Gülşen, D. (2008). Analysis of problem solving ability of players who play at different leagues in terms of their positions, education status and their age, Published Master Degree Thesis, Çukurova University: Adana.

[7] Karabulut A. (2013). Analysis of 13-15 aged football players' state of anxiety in different conditions, Ahi Evran Universty Kırşehir Education faculty Journal, 14,(1), 243-253.

[8] Erbaş MK. Relation between state of anxiety andperformance of advanced basketball players, Dumlupınar University, Social Science Institution, Master DegreeThesis, Kütahya, 2005.

[9] Koy F, (1999). Comparison of state of anxiety of optimum level with perform ancen basketball players, Hacettepe Journal of SportScience, (10), 1, 30-40

[10] Gümüş M. analysis of the state of anxietys cores of professional football clubs, Sakarya University, Social Science Institution, Master Degree Thesis, Sakarya, 2002.

[11] Civan, A.,Arı,R., Görücü, A., Özdemir, M. comparison of team athletes' and individual athletes state of anxiety and continuous anxiety at pre-game and post-game, International Journal of Human Science, 2010,193-206.

[12] Konter, E., theory of psychological preparation in sport. Bağırgan Publishing Center, Ankara, 1998.

[13] Tazegül Ü. (2012). Comparison of the style of coping with stress of athletes in the individuals ports branches in sociodemographicrespectbranchesinsociodemographicrespe*InternationalJournalof Sport Studies*. Vol., 2 (2), 89-94.

[14] Tazegül Ü. (2013). The Determination of the Relationship Between Motivational Trends and the Style of Coping with Stress, *World Applied Sciences Journal*21 (1): 08-14.

[15] Biçer T. Top Performance, Beyaz Publications, Istanbul, 1998.

[16] Öner, N., Le Compte, A. 81998). Discontionary and contionary anxiety inventory book (2nd Pres) Boğaziçi University Publishing center, İstanbul.

[17] Özbay, S. (2012). Comparison of adult national wrestlers' state of anxiety at pre-game and post-game, Karamanoğlu Mehmetbey University Social Science Institution, Physical education department Master Degree Thesis

[18] Artok F.(1994). *The effect of state of anxiety on interuniversity basketball tournament players at pre-game* .Master degree thesis, Adana.

[19] Screiber, D.S. (2004). To get rid of stress, anxiety and depression, İstanbul: Elipsis Publishing, 2004.

[20] Tazegül, Ü,. Küçük, V., Tuna, G., Akgül, M.H. (2015).Comparison of Continuous Anxiety Level of Some Indıvıdual Fıght Athletes, American Journal of Applied Psychology, 3(2), 22-26.

[21] Çoksevim B., Sarıtaş N., Kaya M., Pepe O. (2008) state of anxiety and continuous anxiety of kick-box athletes at pre-game and post-game, short terms inventory results, Turkey Kick Box Federation Sport Science Journal (1),:1, 23-27.

[22] Martens, R., Burton, D., Vealey, R., Bump, L., and Smith, D. (1990). Development and validation of the Competitive State Anxiety Inventory-2 (CSAI-2. Competitive anxiety in sport IL: Human Kinetics. 1990, 117-213.

[23] Jones, G., Swain, A., and Hardy, L.. (1993). Intensity and direction dimensions of competitive state anxiety and relationships with performance. Journal of Sports Sicences, 1993, (11), 6, 525-532.

[24] Koral J.,Dosseville F. (2009) Combination Of Gradual And Rapid Weight Loss: Effects On Physical Performance And Psychological State Of Elite Judo Athletes, Journal of Sport Science, January 15th, 27(2): 115-120.

[25] Roemmich J. N., Sinning W. E. (1997) Weight Loss AndWrestling Training: Effects On Growth-Related Hormones. JAppl Physiol, June 1, 82 (6): 1760-1764.

The Effect of Swimming Exercise on Motor Development Level in Adolescents with Intellectual Disabilities

Elif Top[*]

Faculty of Sport Sciences, Usak University, Turkey
*Corresponding author: elif.top@usak.edu.tr

Abstract **Objectives:** In this study, it was aimed to analyze the effect of swimming exercise on motor development level in adolescents with intellectual disabilities. **Methods:** A total of 30 mild intellectual disability (MID) individuals between 15-18 age groups participated the study. Bruininks–Oseretsky Test of Motor Proficiency-Second Edition (BOT-2)- Short Form were performed to determine basic motor characteristics of children. BOT-2-Short Form was applied to the participants before and after the ten-month swimming exercise program (60 dk/ 3 days /10 week). **Results:** According to research findings, in terms of body weight, manual dexterity, speed and agility, upper limb coordination, and BOT-2 total point parameters, there was no statistically significant difference found between groups, measurements (pre-test and post-test), groups and their measurements ($p>0.05$). In terms of fine motor precision, and fine motor integration parameters, while there was no statistically significant difference found between groups ($p>0.05$); a significant statistical difference was found between measurements (pre-test and post-test), groups and their measurements ($p<0.05$). In terms of bilateral coordination parameter, while there was no statistically significant difference found between measurements (pre-test and post-test), groups and their measurements ($p>0.05$); a significant statistical difference was found between groups ($p<0.05$). In terms of balance parameter and strength, while there was no statistically significant difference found between groups, groups and measurements ($p>0.05$); statistically significant difference was found between measurements (pre-test and post-test) ($p<0.05$). **Conclusion:** Consequently, regularly applied exercise programmes improve life quality level of individuals with MID by contributing to their motor development level.

Keywords: *motor development, intellectual disabilities, exercise*

1. Introduction

Motor development has been identified as one of the important areas of a child's development [1]. Human motor development is a process of changes continuously. Motor development is seen as a progressive change in movement behaviour and occurs over the human life cycle. However, specialist defined motor development as a study of changes in human behaviour that occur in life, the processes that cause these changes and the factors that influence it [2]. According to data published by schools, the highest population among handicapped students belongs to children with intellectual disabilities (ID) [3]. Intellectual disabilities are characterized by limitations in cognitive functioning and includes severe deficits or limitations in an individual's skills in several areas such as cognitive, motor, psychosocial, language and specific activities of daily living (4). Limitations in motor abilities is a common characteristic in persons with ID, since ID is a condition of deficient brain development, which affects the cognitive as well as the motor functions [4,5]. According to some research, children with MID showed delays in the development of motor skills [6,7,8]. Moreover, results of study showed that the level of motor and cognitive functioning are related in children with ID [8]. Alongside impairments in cognitive and motor function, individuals with ID also account lower levels of physical fitness at all stages of life because of inactive life style, less opportunities for physical exercise, the ID condition itself [9,10]. Individuals with ID have also lower physical fitness levels than general population [11,12,13]. The reason for low level of physical fitness of mentally handicapped children compared to their peers would be that they practice less physical activity models [14]. Since handicapped children survive a sedentary life style, they are exposed to health risk as well [15]. It is reported that physical fitness is necessary for health. Studies reveal that individuals with ID have low level of physical fitness in comparison with their non-handicapped peers [12,16]; and they are statistically in higher risk group in terms of disease, death, and health problem [17]. When individuals with ID participated in planned exercise programs, could improve motor performance parameters, daily activities and quality of life [9,18,19]. Therefore, the present study is conducted to investigate effect of 10-week swimming exercise on motor development levels of individuals with ID aged 15-18.

2. Material and Methods

2.1. Participants

A total of 30 adolescents (age = 17.23 ± 1.43 years) with ID participated in the study. Participants were divided into groups of experimental (6 females, 8 males) and control (5 females, 11 males). Fourteen of the students (mean age = 17.43 ± 1.55 years, height = 156.00 ± 10.60 cm, body weight = 61.85 ± 14.80 kg) comprised the experimental group and attended a 10 week swimming exercise program. Sixteen participants (mean age = 17.06 ± 1.34 years, height = 161.25 ± 10.94 cm, body weight = 60.06 ± 15.73 kg) comprising the control group followed their regular school schedule. Ethical approval was obtained from the University Human Ethics Committee. Parents of all children were informed through form about the study and a written consent was taken from each family about participation in study. It was ensured that all participants received health report for each participant from health institutions before 10-week swimming exercise.

2.2. Level of Intelligence

Before commencement of the study, The intelligence quotients (IQ) of the participants was determined with a Weschler Intelligence Scale test by the Guidance and Research Center of the Uşak City National Education Directorship. Scores obtained through these test were not published since it is not ethical; only educational diagnosis of participants was presented. Based on these diagnosis studies, the participants had intelligence quotients (IQ) that was within a range for individuals with mild intellectual disability (50-70 IQ).

3. Measurements

3.1. Motor Assessment

For motor development evaluation of participants, the BOT-2 Test (Short Form) was utilized. The BOT-2 (Short Form) consists of 14 test items from 8 subtests: (1) Fine motor precision: drawing line through crooked paths and folding paper; (2) Fine motor integration: copying a square and copying a star; (3) Manual dexterity: transferring pennies; (4) Bilateral coordination: jumping in place - same side synchronized and tapping feet and fingers - same sides synchronized; (5) Balance: walking forward on a line and standing on one leg on a balance beam - eyes open; (6) Speed and Agility: jumping on one leg; (7) Upper limb coordination: dropping and catching a ball with both hands, and dribbling a ball with alternating hands; (8) Strength: knee push-ups and sit ups. BOT-2 (Short Form) is a well-known measure of motor proficiency designed to provide clinicians, educators and researchers with useful information to assist them in evaluating the motor skills in students ranging from those who are normally developing to those with moderate motor skill deficits aged 4-21 years [20].

Height: Height measurements of participants were taken while they are standing on a flat surface with bare foot; their body weights were measured as it is distributed equally on both legs while their toes are adjoined and it was contacting with height measurement tool, while their head is on the Frankfort plan, and arms released from shoulders freely on both sides. Two measurements were taken and their averages were calculated and registered [21].

Body Weight: Measurement of body weight was conducted by means of Jawon Make (Model IOI-353) brand body composition analyzer. This device is a system that has a clean steel surface on which bare foot contacts and is capable of making analysis through 5, 50, 250 KHz frequency from one leg to another [22]. Weight was measured with sensitivity of 0.1 while participants were in a light dress and on bare feet.

3.2. Swimming Exercise Program

During 10-week swimming exercises, activities performed by the individuals with ID were prepared based on the Special Olympics Swimming Guide and other resources about swimming [23,24]. Exercises were performed under supervision of 20 helpers and a head coach who are trained about swimming (60 minutes/3 days/10 weeks).

3.3. Statistical Analysis

Windows SPSS IBM 21.0 statistical software is utilized in statistical analysis. For statistical analysis, results were displayed as average values and standard deviation. In comparisons, $\alpha = 0.05$ significance level is taken into consideration. In order to determine whether there is significant difference among groups in terms of age and height values, T-test was conducted for two independent groups. Time-dependent change in all parameters was tested by means of Repeated Measure Anova test in repeated measurements.

4. Results

Results of the study showed that there was no significant difference between average heights of the study group (156,00 ± 10,60 cm) and the control group (161,25 ± 10,94 cm) (t.(28); 1,330). Moreover, there was no significant difference between study group (17,43 ± 1,55 years) and the control group (17,06 ± 1,34 years) in terms of average age (t.(28); ,494) (P>0.05, Table 1).

Table 1. T test Results of Groups Regarding to Height and Age

	Groups	*N*	*Mean*	*Sd*	*MD*	*SE*	*t*	*Sig.*
Height	*Experimental*	14	156.00	10.60	-5.250	2.834	1.330	.194
	Control	16	161.25	10.94		2.736		
Age	*Experimental*	14	17.43	1.55	.366	.416	.693	.494
	Control	16	17.06	1.34		.335		

*p< 0.05.

According to research findings, in terms of body weight parameter, there was no statistically significant difference found between groups, measurements (pre-test and post-test), groups and their measurements (p>0.05). In terms of fine motor precision and fine motor integration parameter, while there was no statistically significant difference found between groups (p>0.05); a significant statistical difference was found between measurements (pre-test and post-test), groups and their measurements (p<0.05) (Table 2).

Table 2. Variance Analysis Results Regarding to Body Weight, Fine motor precision and Fine

			Groups	*N*	*df*	*Mean*	*Sd*	*F*	*Sig.*
Body Weight	*Group*		*Experimental*	14	1	61.84	4.08	.036	.850
			Control	16	28	60.77	3.82		
	Measurements		*Measurement 1*		*1*	*60.96*	*2.80*	*1.970*	*.171*
			Measurement 2		*28*	*61.65*	*2.81*		
	*Group*Measurement*	*Experimental*	*Measurement 1*		*1*	*61.85*	*4.09*	*2.135*	*.155*
			Measurement 2		*28*	*61.82*	*4.11*		
		Control	*Measurement 1*		*1*	*60.06*	*3.82*		
			Measurement 2		*28*	*61.48*	*3.85*		
Fine motor precision	*Group*		*Experimental*	*14*	*1*	*7.42*	*.99*	*.067*	*.798*
			Control	*16*	*28*	*7.78*	*.93*		
	Measurements		*Measurement 1*		*1*	*6.75*	*.68*	*18.155*	*.000**
			Measurement 2		*28*	*8.45*	*.73*		
	*Group*Measurement*	*Experimental*	*Measurement 1*		*1*	*6.14*	*1.00*	*4.905*	*.035**
			Measurement 2		*28*	*8.71*	*1.06*		
		Control	*Measurement 1*		*1*	*7.37*	*.94*		
			Measurement 2		*28*	*8.18*	*.99*		
Fine motor integration	*Group*		*Experimental*	*14*	*1*	*5.71*	*.68*	*.479*	*.494*
			Control	*16*	*28*	*5.06*	*.64*		
	Measurements		*Measurement 1*		*1*	*5.00*	*.52*	*6.895*	*.014**
			Measurement 2		*28*	*5.77*	*.46*		
	*Group*Measurement*	*Experimental*	*Measurement 1*		*1*	*5.00*	*.76*	*4.855*	*.036**
			Measurement 2		*28*	*6.42*	*.67*		
		Control	*Measurement 1*		*1*	*5.00*	*.71*		
			Measurement 2		*28*	*5.12*	*.62*		

*p< 0.05.

According to research findings, in terms of manual dexterity parameter, there was no statistically significant difference found between groups, measurements (pre-test and post-test), groups and their measurements (p>0.05). In terms of bilateral coordination parameter, while there was no statistically significant difference found between measurements (pre-test and post-test), groups and their measurements (p>0.05); a significant statistical difference was found between groups (p<0.05). In terms of balance parameter, while there was no statistically significant difference found between groups, groups and measurements (p>0.05); statistically significant difference was found between measurements (pre-test and post-test) (p<0.05) (Table 3).

Table 3. Variance Analysis Results Regarding to Manual dexterity, Bilateral coordination and Balance

			Groups	*N*	*df*	*Mean*	*Sd*	*F*	*Sig.*
Manual dexterity	*Group*		*Experimental*	14	1	3.53	.50	.000	.995
			Control	16	28	3.53	.47		
	Measurements		*Measurement 1*		*1*	3.66	.36	*1.825*	*.188*
			Measurement 2		*28*	3.40	.35		
	*Group*Measurement*	*Experimental*	*Measurement 1*		*1*	3.64	.53	*.063*	*.803*
			Measurement 2		*28*	3.42	.52		
		Control	*Measurement 1*		*1*	3.68	.49		
			Measurement 2		*28*	3.37	.48		
Bilateral coordination	*Group*		*Experimental*	*14*	*1*	*3.71*	*.63*	*6.077*	*.020**
			Control	*16*	*28*	*1.56*	*.59*		
	Measurements		*Measurement 1*		*1*	*2.48*	*.47*	*.722*	*.403*
			Measurement 2		*28*	*2.79*	*.47*		
	*Group*Measurement*	*Experimental*	*Measurement 1*		*1*	*3.28*	*.68*	*2.401*	*.132*
			Measurement 2		*28*	*4.14*	*.68*		
		Control	*Measurement 1*		*1*	*1.68*	*.64*		
			Measurement 2		*28*	*1.43*	*.64*		
Balance	*Group*		*Experimental*	*14*	*1*	*5.57*	*.56*	*.551*	*.464*
			Control	*16*	*28*	*5.00*	*.52*		
	Measurements		*Measurement 1*		*1*	*4.85*	*.45*	*5.973*	*.021**
			Measurement 2		*28*	*5.71*	*.38*		
	*Group*Measurement*	*Experimental*	*Measurement 1*		*1*	*5.21*	*.66*	*.166*	*.687*
			Measurement 2		*28*	*5.92*	*.56*		
		Control	*Measurement 1*		*1*	*4.50*	*.62*		
			Measurement 2		*28*	*5.50*	*.52*		

*p<0 .05.

Based on the results of the present study, in terms of speed and agility parameter, and upper limb coordination, there was no statistically significant difference found between groups, measurements (pre-test and post-test), groups and their measurements (p>0.05). The results of strength showed that there was a significant difference in measurements (pre-test and post-test) (p<0.05), while it was no found significant difference between groups, and groups and measurements (p>0.05) (Table 4).

According to the results of test parameters of BOT-2 total point, there was no statistically significant difference found between groups, measurements (pre-test and post-test), groups and their measurements (p>0.05) (Table 5).

Table 4. Variance Analysis Results Regarding to Speed and Agility, Upper limb coordination and Strength

			Groups	N	df	Mean	Sd	F	Sig.
Speed and Agility	Group		Experimental	14	1	4.35	.68	.843	.366
			Control	16	28	3.50	.63		
	Measurements		Measurement 1		1	3.80	.46	.396	.534
			Measurement 2		28	4.05	.54		
	Group*Measurement	Experimental	Measurement 1		1	4.35	.67	.396	.534
			Measurement 2		28	4.35	.80		
		Control	Measurement 1		1	3.25	.63		
			Measurement 2		28	3.75	.75		
Upper limb coordination	Group		Experimental	14	1	8.28	.98	4.146	.051
			Control	16	28	5.53	.92		
	Measurements		Measurement 1		1	7.42	.69	3.957	.057
			Measurement 2		28	6.38	.75		
	Group*Measurement	Experimental	Measurement 1		1	8.85	1.01	.039	.846
			Measurement 2		28	7.71	1.10		
		Control	Measurement 1		1	6.00	.94		
			Measurement 2		28	5.06	1.03		
Strength	Group		Experimental	14	1	5.96	.84	1.223	.278
			Control	16	28	4.68	.78		
	Measurements		Measurement 1		1	6.62	.73	15.577	.000*
			Measurement 2		28	4.03	.58		
	Group*Measurement	Experimental	Measurement 1		1	7.92	1.07	4.167	.051
			Measurement 2		28	4.00	.85		
		Control	Measurement 1		1	5.31	1.00		
			Measurement 2		28	4.06	.79		

*p< 0.05.

Table 5. Variance Analysis Results Regarding to Total Point

			Groups	N	df	Mean	Sd	F	Sig.
Total Point	Group		Experimental	14	1	44.57	4.77	1.467	.236
			Control	16	28	36.65	4.46		
	Measurements		Measurement 1		1	40.62	3.33	.000	.991
			Measurement 2		28	40.60	3.30		
	Group*Measurement	Experimental	Measurement 1		1	44.42	4.87	.066	.799
			Measurement 2		28	44.71	4.82		
		Control	Measurement 1		1	36.81	4.55		
			Measurement 2		28	36.50	4.51		

*p< 0.05.

5. Discussion

This study investigated the effect of swimming exercise on motor development level in adolescents with intellectual disabilities. Results of the study showed that there was no statistically significant difference found in terms of body weight, manual dexterity, speed and agility, upper limb coordination, and BOT-2 total point parameters between groups, measurements (pre-test and post-test), groups and their measurements. But, Westendorp et al. [4] found that in the MID group, the object-control subtest scores of the children who participated in sports were significantly higher than the scores for those who did not participate in sports. Moreover, the locomotor skill scores between sports participants and non-participants were not significantly different in the MID group. In a similar study, motor performance on the sub-scale ball skills showed motor problems in 63.6% and 44.3%, in children with mild ID and borderline intellectual functioning, respectively [8]. As stated by Westendorp et al. [4] that even a small problem in intellectual functioning leads to poor object-control skills. Object-control skills are usually practiced in complex play and sport settings that require adaptation to changing environmental circumstances [25].

Muscle strength and balance is essential for many mobility tasks. In terms of fine motor precision, and fine motor integration parameters, while there was no statistically significant difference found between groups; a significant statistical difference was found between measurements (pre-test and post-test), groups and their measurements. In terms of bilateral coordination parameter, while there was no statistically significant difference found between measurements (pre-test and post-test), groups and their measurements; a significant statistical difference was found between groups. In Carmeli et al. [26] study, Group A who received specific muscle and balance exercises, had significantly higher values in balance and muscle strength parameters than the pre training values and Group B who received general exercises. Strength decreases in both group, could be explained lack of motivation of individuals with ID during testing and tendency to stop when uncomfortable in this study [27]. In terms of balance and strength parameter, while there was no statistically significant difference found between groups, groups and measurements; statistically significant difference was found between measurements (pre-test and post-test). Giagazoglou et al. [5] stated that the hippotherapy intervention program resulted in significant improvements in strength parameters, and on the more complex balance task. Blomqvist et al. [28] found that adolescents with ID had significantly lower scores in the balance and muscle performance tests. In a study by Giagazoglou et al. [10], trampoline intervention resulted in significant improvements of participants' performance in all motor and balance tests. Limitations in mobility reported to be common in persons with ID, which suggests that the prevalence of balance problems is also high. There are many reasons which might contribute to limitations in balance and gait capacities with ID. Firstly, ID is a condition of arrest or deficient development of the mind, which does not only affect cognitive functions, but motor functions as well. A second mechanism is premature aging [29].

Low motor performans in children with ID and motor problems could be explained with avoid participation in culturally normative activities like sports [19,30], social and communication problems [30], ID itself, sedentary life style. Therefore, extra training, preferably task-specific is recommended to improve the gross and fine motor skills of children with mild ID. Furthermore, the development of these skills should be an important component of the physical education lessons at schools to promote long-term physical activity and sports participation. In general, it could be said that exercise model which used in this study, had positive effect on the level of individuals' motor development. Consequently, regularly applied exercise programmes improve life quality level of individuals with MID by contributing to their motor development level.

References

[1] Hazel MYL. Assessment of preschoolers' gross motor proficiency: Revisiting Bruininks-Oseretsky Test of Motor Proficiency. Early Child Development and Care (2011); 181(2):189-201.

[2] Borhannudin A, Wan MWJ, Ahmad FMA. The development of gross motor analysis system software: A preliminary concept. Procedia- Social and Behavioral Sciences (2012); 64:501-506.

[3] Faison-Hodge J, Poretta D. Physical activity levels of students with mental retardation and students without disabilities. Adapted Physical Activity Quarterly (2004); 21:139-152.

[4] Westendorp M, Houwen S, Hartman E, Visscher C. Are gross motor skills and sports participation related in children with intellectual disabilities? Research in Developmental Disabilities (2011); 32:1147-1153.

[5] Giagazoglou P, Arabatzi F, Dipla K, Liga M, Kellis E. Effect of a hippotherapy intervention program on static balance and strength in adolescents with intellectual disabilities. Research in Developmental Disabilities (2012); 33:2265-2270.

[6] Rarick GL (ed.). Motor performance of mentally retarded children. In: Physical Activity: Human Growth and Development (ed. G. L. Rarick) (1973); pp. 225-56. Academic Press, NewYork.

[7] Bouffard M. Movement problem solutions by educable mentally handicapped individuals. Adapted Physical Activity Quarterly (1990); 7: 183-97.

[8] Vuijk PJ, Hartman E, Scherder E, Visscher C. Motor performance of children with mild intellectual disability and borderline intellectual functioning. Journal of Intellectual Disability Research (2010); 54(11):955-965.

[9] Frey, G.C., Stanish, H.I., Temple, V.A. (2008). Physical activity of youth with intellectual disability: Review and research agenda. Adapted Physical Activity Quarterly, 25:95-117.

[10] Giagazoglou P, Kokaridas D, Sidiropoulou M, Patsiaouras A, Karra C, Neofotistou K. Effects of a trampoline exercise intervention on motor performance and balance ability of children with intellectual disabilities. Research in Developmental Disabilities (2013); 34:2701-2707.

[11] Temple VA, Frey GC, Stanish HI. Physical activity of adults with mental retardation: Review and research needs. American Journal of Health Promotion (2006); 21(1):2-12.

[12] Pitetti KH, Yarmer DA, Fernhall B. Cardiovascular fitness and body composition of youth with and without mental retardation. Adapted Physical Activity Quarterly (2001); 18:127-141.

[13] Pitetti KH, Yarmer DA. Lower body strength of children and adolescents with and without mental retardation: A comparison. Adapted Physical Activity Quarterly (2002); 19:68-81.

[14] Pitetti KH, Beets MW, Combs C. Physical activity levels of children with intellectual disabilities during school. Medicine and Science in Sports and Exercise (2009); 41(8):1580-1586.

[15] Ayvazoglu NR, Ratliffe T, Kozub FM. Encouraging lifetime physical fitness. Teaching Exceptional Children (2004); 37(2): 16-20.

[16] Gillespie, M. (2003). Cardiovascular fitness of young Canadian children with and without mental retardation. Education and Training in Developmental Disabilities, 38, 296-301.

[17] Phillips AC, Holland AJ. Assessment of objectively measured physical activity levels in individuals with intellectual disabilities with and without Down's Syndrome. PLoS ONE (2011); 6(12).

[18] Chanias AK, Reid G, Hoover ML. Exercise effects on health-related physical fitness of individuals with an intellectual disability: A meta-analysis. Adapted Physical Activity Quarterly (1998); 15:119-140.

[19] Wall AET. The developmental skill-learning gap hypothesis: Implications for children with movement difficulties. Adapted Physical Activity Quarterly (2004); 21:197-218.

[20] Bruininks RH, Bruininks BD. Bruininks-Oseretsky Test of Motor Proficiency (2nd ed.). Windsor: NFER-Nelson (2005).

[21] Lohman TG, Roche AF, Martorell R. Anthropometric Standardization Referance Manual. Illinois: Human Kinetics Books Champaigne (1988).

[22] Chen YC, Tu YK, Huang KC, Chen PC, Chu DC, Lee YL. Pathway from central obesity to childhood asthma. Physical fitness and sedentary time are leading factors. American Journal of Respiratory and Critical Care Medicine (2014); 189(10): 1194-1203.

[23] Special Olympics. Aquatics Coaching Guide. specialolympics.org/soi/files/sports/Aquatics+Coaching+Guide (2004).

[24] Maglischo EW. Swimming Fastest: The essential reference on technique, training, and program design. Champaign, IL: Human Kinetics (2003).

[25] Houwen S, Visscher C, Hartman E, Lemmink KAPM. Gross motor skills and sports participation of children with visual impairments. Research Quarterly for Exercise and Sport (2007); 78:16-23.

[26] Carmeli E, Vaknin TZ, Morad M, Merrick J. Can physical training have an effect on well-being in adults with mild intellectual disability?. Mechanisms of Ageing and Development (2005); 126:299-304.

[27] Graham A, Reid G. Physical fitness of adults with an intellectual disability: A 13-year follow-up study. Research Quarterly for Exercise and Sport (2000); 71: 152-161.

[28] Blomqvist S, Olsson J, Wallin L, Wester A, Rehn B. Adolescents with intellectual disability have reduced postural balance and muscle performance in trunk and lower limbs compared to peers without intellectual disability. Research in Developmental Disabilities (2013); 34:198-206.

[29] Enkelaar L, Smulders E, Valk HSL, Geurts ACH, Weerdesteyn V. A review of balance and gait capacities in relation to falls in persons with intellectual disabilities. Research in Developmental Disabilities (2012); 33: 291-306.

[30] Hartman E, Houwen S, Scherder E, Visscher C. On the relationship between motor performance and executive functioning in children with intellectual disabilities. Journal of Intellectual Disability Research (2010); 54(5):468-477.

Assessing Various Body Composition Measurements as An Appropriate Tool for Estimating Body Fat in National Collegiate Athletic Association Division I Female Collegiate Athletes

Andrew Shim[1,*], Patrick Cross[2], Shannon Norman[1], Patrick Hauer[3]

[1]Division of Kinesiology & Sport Science, The University of South Dakota, Vermillion, SD. USA
[2]Department of Physical Therapy, Briar Cliff University, Sioux City, IA. USA
[3]Department of Physical Therapy, The University of South Dakota, Vermillion, SD. USA
*Corresponding author: andrew.shim@usd.edu

Abstract **Purpose:** The purpose of the study was to determine if various convenient and cost affordable body composition techniques correlate well with more expensive "gold standard" instruments for measuring body composition in female collegiate athletes. **Methods:** Thirty-two Division I track and field and basketball female athletes participated in the study. The host university's Institutional Review Board approved the protocols towards ethical treatment of all subjects before the study commenced. Within one hour, each subject underwent body composition assessments via *air displacement plethysmography* (*ADP*), skinfold (SF) measurements, and bioelectrical impedance analysis (BIA). **Results:** No significant differences were found between basketball and track athletes thus data was normalized. No significant difference in calculated percent body fat was noted between ADP and SF ($p = .002$), but there was a significant difference between ADP and BIA ($p = .478$). Per Pearson correlations, moderate correlations existed between body fat percentages obtained by ADP and SF ($r = .689$) as well as between body fat percentages estimated by ADP and BIA ($r = .447$). **Conclusions:** Results indicate the SF technique had the highest correlation when compared to the BOD POD®. Skinfold measurements obtained with the Harpenden Skinfold Calipers may be used as a quick, affordable, and reliable technique for measuring body fat percentages in female collegiate athletes when performed by an experienced skinfold assessor.

Keywords: *body fat, air displacement plethysmography, skinfold, body composition*

1. Introduction

Obesity is an excess accumulation of body fat and most health complications which arise from being obese are due to excess fat tissue, not from overall body weight [1]. Collegiate athletes need a reliable and cost affordable technique to assess body composition as many coaches are requesting measurements at different times throughout the season [2]. Hydrostatic weighting (HW) is considered to be the gold standard for calculating a person's body composition compared to other popular methods [3,4,5,6]. Other body composition techniques that hold the benchmark for accuracy include deuterium dilution, densitiometry, and dual-energy X-ray absorptiometry, also known as DEXA [7] but are considered costly or inaccessible for the typical college athlete. Air displacement plethysmography (ADP) has also yielded results similar to HW, indicating it may be used as a standard for comparison [4,5,6]. Techniques other than HW and DEXA, such as body mass index (BMI), waist-to-hip ratios (WHR), skinfold (SF) measurements, bioelectrical impedance analysis (BIA), and ADPwere developed because HW and DEXA are not suitable for all patients and can be time consuming [7,8,9,10]. Recently, BMI and WHR are not very popular measurement tools with Division One athletes in the United States. Many collegiate strength coaches and exercise specialists are using either SF through calibrated calipers or BIA to determine body composition. With hundreds of collegiateathletes at each institution, it would be wise to determine if any of these quick and current methods could be correlated to a laboratory tool such as HW or ADP.

2. Literature Review

2.1. Skinfold Technique

The SF technique can be performed at minimal cost, [11,12] provides quick results, does not require a lot of space or expensive equipment, is non-invasive [13], and can be administered to large groups of people. Skinfold measurements vary depending on the SF site, subject's obesity level, and the amount of tension placed on the skin [14]. Errors can also arise if the calipers are not placed in the exact location for consecutive measurements [15]. Inaccurate estimations of percent body fat can arise when equations which were developed for a specific population are applied to another group of people [13,16]. These factors may account for why Williams & Bale [13] noted a significant difference in predicting percent body fat between HW and the SF technique. However, Dixon et al. [5] found no significant differences in percent body fat estimated by ADP, SF, and HW. Additionally, Bentzur et al. [3] noted a high correlation (r = .85) between percent body fat estimated by SF and ADP.

The reliability and validity of the SF technique depends on multiple factors [9,11]. Both of these studies have shown when SF assessors were trained by an expert, more accurate results were obtained. Researchers have also suggested the type of SF caliper used may cause a difference in results [16]. Investigators obtained smaller SF measurements when they used either the Harpenden Caliper or Holtain Caliper when compared to either the Lange Caliper or the Adipometer but inter-rater reliability was greater when the Harpenden and Holtain Calipers were used.

2.2. Bioelectrical Impedance Analysis

Bioelectrical Impedance Analysis (BIA) has been commercially available since the 1980's. It is considered a popular tool to use based on the ease, accessibility, and portability of determining body fat percentage (Prentice & Jebb, 2001). The Body Stat™ is a type of BIA that measures an individual's body composition. The Body Stat™ has been shown to be a quick method that requires little training in determining body composition [8]. The Body Stat™ sends multiple frequency waves throughout the body to determine body composition which includes: fat mass, lean body mass, and total water composition [17]. According to Fornetti et al. [10] there was high reliability in a single trial of the BIA, indicating one trial with the BIA is sufficient. Results have been mixed regarding BIA as Biaggi et al. [4] found no significant differences in estimating percent body fat between ADP and HW or BIA, however, Williams & Bale [13] noted a significant difference did exist in predicting percent body fat between HW and BIA. Also, one previous study did note that leg-to-leg BIA predicted percent body fat significantly lower when compared to HW [5].

2.3. Air Displacement Plethysmography

Research studies have shown no significant differences in estimating percent body fat when comparing HW to ADP [4,5] or DEXA [2]. Dixon et al. [5] observed Division III collegiate wrestlers and found no significant difference between HW, ADP, or SF when estimating body composition. According to Biaggi et al. [4] percent body fat assessed by ADP and by HW was similar to previously reported validation studies. When comparing ADP to DEXA, ADP has been found to be a reliable and valid technique in measuring body composition in female collegiate athletes [2]. In further support, Bentzur et al. [3] discoveredhigh correlational values between body fat percentage measured by ADP and HW incollegiate track and field female athletes. Therefore, ADP could be identified as a valid and reliable method to compare other body fat percentage methods in collegiate female athletes.

2.4. Purpose

The purpose of the study was to determine if various convenient and cost affordable body composition techniques correlate well with more expensive "gold standard" instruments for measuring body composition in female collegiate athletes. It was hypothesized that the Body Stat™ machine is a reliable, valid, convenient, and cost effective tool in which percent body fat will highly correlate with BOD POD® results, in comparison to skinfold calipers used to assess percent body fat.

3. Methods

3.1. Subjects

This study was a quasi-experiemental prospective study design that utilized a sample of convenience. Inclusion criteria included: National Collegiate Athletic Association (NCAA) Division I female collegiate athletes over the age of 18. Exclusion criteria included: student athletes not associated with the research university, non-athletes, club team athletes, males, individuals under the age of 18, or anyone who was pregnant, had a history of cancer, hadelectrical or metal implants, or had a psychosocial fear of electricity. After insuring that the subjects met all inclusion criteria, 19 track athletes and 13 basketball athletes participated in the study. The mean age was 19.53 years with a range of 18-22 years.

3.2. Instruments

A calibrated stadiometer was used to measure height and a standard tape measure was used to measure waist and hip circumference measurements. An electronically calibrated BOD POD® (Life Measurement Inc., Concord, CA) scale was used to measure weight. The BOD POD® Gold Standard Model number BOD POD® 2007A was used to assess percent body fat. The Quads can 4000 Version 4.08 (Body Stat™, British Isles, UK) was used to assess the athletes' hydration status, WHR, BMI, and percent body fat. Harpenden Skinfold Calipers (Baty International, West Sussex, UK) were used to estimate body composition because they have been found to have high inter-rater reliability [16].

3.3. Procedures

The study was approved by the Institutional Review Board at the host university. All protocols and procedures were reviewed by the IRB to ensure ethical treatment of all subjects during the study. The subjects for the study were recruited by the athletic training staff at the university. Informed consent was obtained upon arrival and time was allotted for participants to ask questions. Individuals that desired to participate were given a unique identifier number. Subjects were advised to drink an appropriate amount of water 24-48 hours in advance to ensure proper hydration and to refrain from exercise and food consumption one hour prior to testing. They were also instructed to wear compression shorts and a sports bra or a two piece swimsuit. Testing was performed over a two day period and each athlete had all tests performed within one hour.

Height and weight measurements were taken by the same examiner and recorded to the nearest ¼ inch and thousandth of a pound, respectively. Waist circumference measurements were taken at the top of the iliac crest and hip circumference measurements were taken at the level of the greater trochanters by the same examiner and were recorded to the nearest ¼ inch. The BOD POD® was calibrated according to manufacturer's guidelines. Subjects were asked to remove all jewelry and wear a Lycra swim cap. Subjects also wore either compression shorts and a sports bra or a two-piece bathing suit. The on-screen testing procedures were followed in accordance to the BOD POD® manual. The Siri equation was used to estimate body fat percentage based upon the density obtained by the BOD POD®. The BOD POD® Operator's Manual recommended that this equation be used for the general population, as the subjects included both Caucasian and African American females. Thoracic gas volume was estimated and participants were instructed to remain as still as possible during testing. The temperature, barometric pressure, and relative humidity were maintained within the specified ranges for proper operation of the BOD POD®: 70.5 – 71 degrees F, 29.8 – 29.9 inches, and 51.0 – 51.2% respectively. A printout of the BOD POD® results were given to the athlete and to the athletic trainer or the athlete's coach, based on the signed HIPAA release form.

The Body Stat™ was calibrated prior to testing according to the manufacturer's guidelines [17]. The subject's height, weight, age, gender, activity level, and waist and hip measurements were entered into the Body Stat™ machine. The highest activity level was selected for all subjects. The athlete's skin on the right side of the body was cleaned with an alcohol wipe and electrodes were placed at the following locations: on the dorsum of the hand proximal to the metacarpophalangeal joint, on the dorsum of the hand distal to the wrist joint, on the dorsum of the foot proximal to the metatarsophalangeal joint, and on the dorsum of the foot between the medial and lateral malleoli on the right side of the body. The red lead was placed on the more distal electrode of each limb and the black lead was placed on the more proximal electrode. The subjects were supinein anatomical position for three minutes before testing was performed. All Body Stat™ testing was completed by the same researchers.

The Harpenden Skinfold Calipers were calibrated before testing. Two SF measurements were taken within 15 seconds of each other on the right side of the body at the triceps, suprailiac, and thigh anatomical sites, using the average of the two measurements. The Jackson / Pollock equation was used to estimate body composition. All measurements were completed by an experienced assessor with 25 years of experience and SF certification through the American College of Sports Medicine, Cooper's Institute of Aerobic Research, and National Strength and Conditioning Association.

3.4. Data Analysis

Data was analyzed via Statistical Package for the Social Sciences 19.0. Frequencies and descriptive statistics were used to analyze demographic information including: age, height, weight, waist circumference, hip circumference, BMI, WHR, total body water, total weight, and body fat percentage estimated by BIA, ADP, and SF. No significant differences were found between track and basketball athletes, thus results were combined for the purposes of this study. Paired t-tests were computed to determine if significant differences existed between ADP when compared to BIA and SF. Pearson Correlations were used to analyze the relationships between the body fat percentages obtained by ADP, SF, and BIA.

Table 1. Descriptive Statistics (n = 32)

Variables	Minimum	Maximum	Mean	Standard Deviation
Age (years)	18.00	22.00	19.56	1.16
Height (inches) *	61.00	74.50	67.10	3.17
Height (cm) *	151.90	189.20	170.40	8.10
Weight (kg) *	109.26	191.28	145.45	21.73
Waist (inches)	25.50	36.25	29.37	2.62
Waist (cm)	64.80	92.10	74.60	6.70
Hip (inches)	22.50	43.00	36.13	3.33
Hip (cm)	57.20	109.20	91.80	8.50
BMI	17.50	29.00	22.48	2.52
WHR	0.73	0.88	0.81	0.03
BOD POD (% BF)	13.50	30.80	22.03	4.14
BIA (% BF)	11.30	27.80	19.57	3.68
SF (% BF)	12.30	34.70	21.50	5.69
TBW (kg)	49.80	61.30	55.19	3.38
Total Weight (kg)	109.30	191.30	146.02	21.43

BMI = body mass index; WHR = waist-to-hip ratio; BIA = bioelectrical impedance analysis; SF = skinfold; % BF = percent body fat; TBW = total body water

Table 2. Correlation and P-value between Body Composition Methods to the Bodpod

Bodpod comparison to other body composition methods	Correlation (r)	p-value
ADP to BIA	.447	.010
ADP to SF	.689	.000

ADP = air displacement plethysmography; BIA = bioelectrical impedance analysis; SF = skinfold

4. Results

The study included 32 female subjects between the ages of 18 to 22 years. This study had 100% retention rate and all subjects' data was included in the data analysis. Additional descriptive statistics can be found in Table 1. No significant differences were found between basketball and track athletes, therefore the data was normalized. Paired t-tests yielded a significant difference between percent body fat obtained by ADP and BIA ($p = .002$), however, no significant differences was found between ADP and SF ($p = .478$). Per Pearson correlations, moderate correlations [18] existed between body fat percentages between ADP and SF ($r = .689$). Low correlations (Carter RE, 2011) existed between percent body fat percentages estimated by ADP and BIA ($r = .447$).

5. Discussion

The current study found no significant difference ($p = .478$) in percent body fat estimated by the SF technique, when compared to ADP, but a significant difference ($p = .002$) was noted between body fat percentages estimated by BIA and ADP. Due to the fact that ADP has yielded body composition measurements similar to HW [3,4,5], the current study both contradicts and supports a study conducted with collegiate female athletes by Williams & Bale [13]. In contrast to the findings of the current study, These same authors noted significant differences in predicting percent body fat between HW and the SF technique. In support of the findings of the current study, Williams & Bale [13] also found a significant difference between HW and BIA. The current study contradicts the findings by Biaggi et al. [4] in which no significant differences in estimating percent body fat was found between ADP and HW or BIA.

On the other hand, this current study supports the results by Dixon et al. [5] who found no significant differences in percent body fat estimated by ADP, SF, and HW. Although the current study yielded a moderate correlation [18], between percent body fat estimated by SF and ADP ($r = .689$), the results parallel the trend found by Bentzur et al. [3] who noted a high correlation ($r = .85$) between ADP and SF. The current study revealed a 2.46% mean difference in fat free mass between ADP and BIA, which is similar to the results noted by For netti et al. [10] who found a 2% difference in fat free mass between DEXA and BIA in collegiate female athletes. The current study is also in agreement with the findings of Kispert et al. [15] in that percent body fat estimated in young athletes with the SF technique was more accurate when compared to ADP.

Based on the results of the current study, BIA may not be an appropriate measurement for estimating body composition for female college athletes. For collegiate programs that want a valid, reliable, cost effective, portable, and minimally invasive instrument to assess body composition in female athletes, the current study would support use of Harpenden Skinfold Calipers over other instruments. However, a skilled assessor, or an assessor who has been trained by an expert, would be highly recommended to perform SF measurements. Future studies on a non-athletic population are needed to determine if these results also apply to the general population.

5.1. Limitations

Possible limitations may include errors in height, although these errors were limited by using a standardized protocol and by having the same assessors perform the same measurements each time. Another possible limitation was that all athletes were females from a public Midwestern university and the majority of subjects were Caucasian. Another noted limitation of the study was the Body stat's programming limits with regards to rounding to the nearest standard unit.

6. Conclusion

It was originally hypothesized that the Body Stat™ machine is a reliable, valid, convenient, and cost effective tool in which percent body fat will highly correlate with ADP results, in comparison to other methods used, to assess percent body fat in female collegiate athletes. The results of this study demonstrate that Body Stat™ may not be the most appropriate technique to use on collegiate female athletes when assessing body compositionas they had low correlations in comparison to the BOD POD®. Specifically, the Body Stat™ had significantly different results when compared to the BOD POD®. However, SF measurements, using Harpenden Skinfold Calipers was shown to have the highest percent body fat correlation and revealed no significant difference when compared to the BOD POD® if performed by an expert assessor with years of experience.

References

[1] Prentice AJ, S. Body mass index. *Obesity Reviews*. 2001; 2: 141-147.

[2] Ballard TP, Fafara L, Vukovich MD. Comparison of Bod Pod and DXA in female collegiate athletes. *Med Sci Sports Exerc*. 2004; 36 (4): 731-735.

[3] Bentzur KM, Kravitz L, Lockner DW. Evaluation of the BOD POD for estimating percent body fat in collegiate track and field female athletes: a comparison of four methods. J Strength Cond Res. 2008; 22 (6): 1985-1991.

[4] Biaggi RR, Vollman MW, Nies MA, et al. Comparison of air-displacement plethysmography with hydrostatic weighing

andbioelectrical impedance analysis for the assessment of body composition in healthy adults. *Am J Clin Nutr.* 1999; 69 (5): 898-903.

[5] Dixon CB, Deitrick RW, Pierce JR, Cutrufello PT, Drapeau LL. Evaluation of the BOD POD and leg-to-leg bioelectrical impedance analysis for estimating percent body fat in National Collegiate Athletic Association Division III collegiate wrestlers. *J Strength Cond Res.* 2005; 19 (1): 85-91.

[6] Jensen MD. Research techniques for body composition assessment. J Am Diet Assoc. 1992; 92 (4): 454-460.

[7] Fuller NJ. Comparison of abilities of various interpretations of bio-electrical impedance to predict reference method body composition assessment. *Clin Nutr.* 1993; 12 (4): 236-242.

[8] Jensky-Squires NE, Dieli-Conwright CM, Rossuello A, Erceg DN, McCauley S, Schroeder ET. Validity and reliability of body composition analysers in children and adults. *Br J Nutr.* 2008; 100 (4): 859-865.

[9] Kerr L WS, Bandy WD, Ishee J. Reliability and validity of skinfold measurements of trained versus untrained testers. *Isokinet Exerc Sci.* 1994; 4 (4): 137-140.

[10] Fornetti WC, Pivarnik JM, Foley JM, Fiechtner JJ. Reliability and validity of body composition measures in female athletes. *J Appl Physiol.* 1999; 87 (3): 1114-1122.

[11] Ostojic SM. Estimation of body fat in athletes: skinfolds vs bioelectrical impedance. *J Sports Med Phys Fitness.* 2006; 46 (3): 442-446.

[12] Zando KA RR. The validity and reliability of the Cramer Skyndex Caliper in the estimation of percent body fat. *J Athl Train.* 1987; 22 (1): 23-25.

[13] Williams CA, Bale P. Bias and limits of agreement between hydrodensitometry, bioelectrical impedance and skinfold calipers measures of percentage body fat. *Eur J Appl Physiol Occup Physiol.* 1998; 77 (3): 271-277.

[14] Demura S, Sato S. Suprailiac or abdominal skinfold thickness measured with a skinfold caliper as a predictor of body density in Japanese adults. *Tohoku J Exp Med.* 2007; 213 (1): 51-61.

[15] Kispert CP, Merrifield HH. Interrater reliability of skinfold fat measurements. *Phys Ther.* 1987; 67 (6): 917-920.

[16] Lohman TG, Pollock ML, Slaughter MH, Brandon LJ, Boileau RA. Methodological factors and the prediction of body fat in female athletes. *Med Sci Sports Exerc.* 1984; 16 (1): 92-96.

[17] *BODYSTAT QuadScan 4000 Multi-Frequency BIA Technology Hardware User's Guide* [computer program]. Isle of Man; 2007.

[18] Carter RE LJ, Domholdt E.*Rehabilitation Research Principles and Applications*. 4th ed. St. Louis, MO: ELSEVIER SAUNDERS; 2011: 318.

33

Physical Activity: A Key for the Preclusion of Obesity in Children

Pradeep Singh Chahar*

Assistant Professor Physical Education, Manipal University Jaipur. Jaipur, Rajasthan, India
*Corresponding author: pradeepchahar84@gmail.com

Abstract Childhood obesity is the one of the serious problem globally which keeps on increasing with high rate. Physical activity plays an important role in handling the childhood obesity. Physical activity has long been considered an integral component of weight management, but exercise alone is a reasonably ineffective means for reducing fat percentage. Physical activity along with healthy nutrition boosts the process of fat percentage discount and also helpful in monitoring the hypothalamus part of brain which plays an important role in regulating the food intake. Data suggested that anthropometry is a key component of nutritional status assessment in children especially body mass index, which is quite effective and reliable. Without engaging the children's in physical activity leads to increased chances of obesity, cardiovascular diseases, cancer and diabetes in future and that fastenings the attention of fitness personal and policy makers. Hence, parents and policymakers have to plan accordingly to make their child healthy and fit. This article reviews the available literature regarding the role of physical activity and nutrition in the prevention and handling of childhood obesity along with various anthropometric assessment methods.

Keywords: *childhood obesity, physical activity, nutrition, anthropometry*

1. Introduction

Obesity is emerging as one of the most serious problem discern of the present century especially childhood obesity which is the major public health crunch globally that are on rise. According to WHO, 22 million children (under 5 years of age) are overweight [1]. The prevalence has increased at an alarming rate. Globally, in 2010 the number of overweight children under the age of five is estimated to be over 42 million. Close to 35 million of these are living in developing countries [2]. Obesity is defined as a BMI equal to or greater than 95th percentile for age and sex. It is normally measured in children by plotting body mass index on a standard growth chart using a defined cut-off point [3] and generally caused by imbalance between calories consumption and consumed [4]. Overweight and obese children are likely to stay obese into adulthood and more likely to develop non-communicable diseases like diabetes and cardiovascular diseases at a younger age. Prevention of childhood obesity therefore needs high priority [5,6,7,8]. Children represent the future, and ensuring their healthy growth and development ought to be a prime concern of all societies [9]. Physical inactivity has been identified as the fourth leading risk factor for global mortality causing an estimated 3.2 million deaths globally. Physical activity is defined as any bodily movement produced by skeletal muscles that require energy expenditure [10]. Regular moderate intensity physical activity – such as walking, cycling, or participating in sports – has significant benefits for health. [11,12,13]. Nearly half of American youths 12-21 years of age are not vigorously active on a regular basis. Moreover, physical activity declines dramatically during adolescence [14]. Therefore the purpose of this paper is to highlight the importance of physical activity and nutrition in controlling the childhood obesity along with the assessment techniques.

2. Epidemiology of Childhood Obesity

Obesity was first included in the international classification of diseases in 1948. Since then, an epidemic has developed internationally, affecting all age groups [15]. The combination of our genetic propensity to store fat, the ready availability of calorie dense foods, and sedentary lifestyle promotes overweight. The child's food environment at home and parental obesity are strong determinants [16]. Over the past 40 years, rates of obesity have doubled in 2- to 5-year-olds, quadrupled in 6-to 11-year-olds, and tripled in 12- to 19-year-olds. The causes of childhood obesity are complex and interconnected [17]. Puberty and the following adolescent period are acknowledged as particularly vulnerable times for the development of obesity due to sexual maturation and, in many individuals, a concomitant reduction in physical activity [18]. Childhood obesity and the accompanying health consequences are growing at a fast rate in India [19]. A new study carried out by American researchers suggests that community involvement is important in the fight against childhood obesity [20]. Maternal instinct can be a dicey, since mothers want their child to be well fed, which is not a bad thing. But now-a-days home theatre, play station, unlimited internet has locked up kids at home. Lack of exercise or activity has expanded our children's waste line, making them prone to lifestyle diseases and health problems [21]. Childhood obesity builds a ticking time bomb of sickness in later life - and action to avert ill health should start before the kids attain school going age [22]. A new AIIMS study on 10,000 Delhi schoolchildren has found that 3-4% of them suffered from hypertension, the most common cause of heart-related deaths. Among these were children as young as five year's old [23].

3. Physical Activity and Childhood Obesity

Current research suggests that physical inactivity is inversely correlated with the risk of obesity [24,25,26]. The World Health Organization, the U.S. Dept. of Health and Human Services, and other authorities recommend that for good health, adults should get the equivalent of two and a half hours of moderate-to-vigorous physical activity each week [27,28,29]. Worldwide, people are less active today than they were decades ago. While studies find that sports and leisure activity levels have remained stable or increased slightly [30,31,32,33]. Regular physical activity 45-60 min per day prevents unhealthy weight gain and obesity, whereas sedentary behaviours such as watching television promote them. Regular exercise can markedly reduce body weight and fat mass without dietary caloric restriction in overweight individuals [34]. Local health departments (LHDs) play a crucial role in the identification, management and prevention of obesity [35]. Physical activity and health has been late to emerge as a scientific field and as a target of research, beyond the early impetus provided by medical epidemiologists [36]. The continuum of physical activity behaviour ranges from being inactive to being very physically active. Some individuals can be considered physically active if they are meeting the current recommendations for moderate to vigorous physical activity, yet they may also be very sedentary throughout the rest of their day [37]. The reality is that attaining a healthy weight is difficult if physical activity is not a part of child's lifestyle. One probable cause of childhood overweight and obesity is decreased daily energy expenditure [38]. Evidences clearly showed that regular physical activity helps in reduction of body fat percentage. Children are more active than adults, but their activity levels decline as they move toward adolescence, and significant numbers of young people do not participate in recommended levels of physical activity [39]. Inactivity among children has likely increased because of factors such as dependence on cars for transportation, increased screen time (e.g., television, videogames, internet), and the constraints of the built environment (e.g., urban sprawl, lack of recreational facilities, neighbourhood safety) [40]. Physical activity also has several other aspects that are positive for the obese child's health, such as improving the metabolic profile and psychological wellbeing [41]. In recent years, physical education and recess have been reduced in many schools, resulting in long periods of inactivity during the school day. Without opportunities for physical activity in school, many children will fail to meet minimal activity requirements. Physical education provides youths with meaningful amounts of daily physical activity [42,43,44]. Exercise has long been considered an integral component of weight management, but available evidence suggests that exercise alone is a relatively inefficient means for losing weight. In contrast, regular exercise appears crucial in the prevention of weight gain and successful maintenance of weight loss, and in the fostering of cardiovascular health [45].

4. Endurance Exercise and Obesity

Endurance is the ability to do a single movement under the condition of fatigue. Research suggests that endurance play an important role in preventing the obesity. Endurance exercise helps in reducing skeletal muscle-specific and systemic oxidative damage while improving insulin resistance and cytokine profile associated with obesity, independent of weight loss [46]. Endurance exercise training decreased plasma leptin levels independently of changes in plasma insulin levels and body fat percentage [47]. The relationship between fat mass and leptin, which is also found in humans (48), might be affected by mechanisms acting on fat mass. The insulin hormone is thought to be important in this control mechanism (49). A continuous exercise training protocol can elicit high rates of fat oxidation, increases the contribution of fat to substrate oxidation during exercise [50]. One of the fundamental mechanisms for the positive effects of exercise training in obesity may be related to its effects on fat utilization. Researches proved that an endurance exercise programme is more effective in increasing fat oxidation during exercise [51].

5. Nutrition and Obesity

Good nutrition is just like a good antibiotic or vaccine in preventing illness [52]. Changes in diet and sedentariness are fuelling the obesity epidemic. Good nutrition play an essential parts of a person's overall health and well-being. Insufficient nutrient intake during childhood has been linked to physical and mental health problems as well as emotional and behavioural problems, learning deficiencies, and lower grades [53]. Fundamental causes of the obesity epidemic are sedentary lifestyles and high-fat energy-dense diets, both resulting from the profound changes taking place in society and the behavioural patterns of communities as a consequence of increased urbanization and industrialization and the disappearance of traditional lifestyles [54]. According to the study overweight children, particularly girls, reported eating less bread, cake, and cream, adding less sugar to beverages, and eating sweets and ice cream less frequently than thin and normal-weight children. A higher percentage of the obese group reported skipping one meal and eating no snack at school. Overweight teen-agers appear to be more conscious of their food intake than under- and normal-weight children [55]. As schools have been proposed worldwide as a major setting for tackling childhood obesity it is essential that future policy evaluations measure the long term effectiveness of a range of school food policies in tackling both dietary intake and overweight and obesity [56]. People living in urban areas consume diets distinctly different from those of their rural counterparts. One of the more profound effects is the accelerated change in the structure of diet, only partially explained by economic factors. A second is the emergence of a large proportion of families with both currently malnourished and overweight members [57]. Low birth-weight babies whose families were food insecure in early childhood are almost 28 times more likely than their peers to be overweight or obese at age 4 ½ [52,53]. Gregory et al. [58] reported that the average fat intake of children aged 4-18 years in the UK is close to the government recommendation of 35% energy. On the other hand, some cross-sectional studies have found a positive relationship between fat intake and adiposity in children even after controlling for confounding factors [59,60]. Soft drink intake has been also associated with the prevalence of obesity [61] and type II diabetes [62,63,64,65] among children. While it is possible that drinking soda instead of milk would result in higher intake of total energy, it cannot be concluded definitively that sugar containing soft drinks promote weight gain because they displace dairy products [66]. Fast foods are one of the most advertised products on television and children are often the targeted market. Reducing the huge volume of marketing of energy-dense foods and drinks and fast-food restaurants to young children, particularly through the powerful media of television, is a potential strategy that has been advocated [67].

6. Anthropometric variables for the Assessment of Obesity in Children

Obesity can be assess by a variety of anthropometric variables namely Body mass index, Waist Circumference, hip circumference, Waist to height ratio, waist to hip ratio, different skinfolds of the body, standing height & weight measurement and predictive equations. In addition to this there are some more variables that may also help in assessing the childhood obesity namely upper arm & leg length, head and mid arm circumference. Anthropometry is a key component of nutritional status assessment in children as well as in adults. Comparing anthropometric data from children of different ages is complicated by the fact that children are still growing (We do not expect the height of a 5-year-old to be the same as the height of a 10-year-old!) [68]. But the question is which anthropometric variable is more reliable in comparison to others. One of study suggested that the validity of the anthropometric skinfold thickness in the obese children is low and BMI provides the best estimate of body fat [69]. The childhood obesity working group of the international obesity taskforce recommended the use of body mass index (BMI) cut off points to categorize children as normal weight, overweight, or obese based on age, gender, and BMI [70]. A new function for egen has been developed to allow transformation of child anthropometric data to z-scores using the LMS method. An additional function allows for children to be categorized according to body mass index (weight/height^2) using international cut off points recommended by the Childhood Obesity working group of the international obesity taskforce [68].

7. Molecular Mechanism of Obesity

The command centre for communication between the brain and the body is the hypothalamus. It controls all homeostatic systems, including circadian rhythms, sleep, body temperature, stress regulation, sexual behaviour, and water balance. The hypothalamus also regulates food intake. Hormonal regulators of energy homeostasis can also act on brain reward circuits, most notably on the mesoaccumbens dopamine system [71], to increase or decrease the incentive value of food depending on energy requirements. However, electrical or chemical stimulation of brain areas that regulate food reward can trigger binge-like overeating even in recently fed animals in which homeostatic satiety signals have been engaged [72,73]. Recent research has identified specific molecular mediators of the link between inflammation and insulin resistance in obesity. Study of these mediators and the specific mechanisms underlying inflammation and insulin resistance in obesity holds the promise for novel pharmacotherapy for obesity-related metabolic disease [74]. Leptin, a key appetite-regulating hormone derived from the white adipose tissue, primarily acts on hypothalamic neurons to activate catabolic pathway and inhibit anabolic pathway, which can result in anorexia and weight reduction [75].

8. Conclusion

After gone through the related literature, we may conclude that childhood obesity emerging as an epidemic serious health problem like cardiovascular diseases, cancer, diabetes and many more. Physical inactivity has been identified as the leading risk factor for global mortality. Regular physical activity especially endurance exercise plays an important role in prevention of childhood obesity by enhancing the process of fat oxidation. On the other side research suggested that physical activity, alone is unable to give an effective results towards obesity. Nutrition also have important role to play in reducing the excessive fat percentage along with physical activity. Good nutrition is just like a good antibiotic or vaccine in preventing illness, while high-fat energy-dense diets boost the process of fat formation. Physical activity and diet especially high fat and calorie diet are inversely related in view of reducing extra fat from the body. Parents have to provide such an environment to their child which gives an opportunity for participating in physical activities. We can assess the fat percentage with the help of many anthropometric measures such as body mass index, weight & height of child (growth pattern) and different body parts circumferences. "**Sweat is the Most Effective Medicine for Future Shock**".

References

[1] Obesity retrieved on Nov. 28th, 2013 from http://www.who.int/topics/obesity/en/

[2] Childhood overweight and obesity, retrieved on Nov. 28th, 2013 from http://www.who.int/dietphysicalactivity/childhood/en/index.html

[3] Bhardwaj S, Misra A, Khurana L, Gulati S, Shah P, Vikram NK. Childhood obesity in Asian Indians: A burgeoning cause of insulin resistance, diabetes and sub-clinical inflammation. Asia Pac J Clin Nutr 2008; 17(Suppl 1):172-5.

[4] Sameera Karnik and Amar Kanekar, Childhood obesity: a global public health crisis, International Journal of Preventive Medicine, 2012, 3(1): 1-7.

[5] What is obesity? Retrieved on nov. 25th, 2013 from http://www.medicinenet.com/obesity_weight_loss/page2.htm#what_is_obesity.

[6] Nazeem I. Siddiqui and S. Bose "Prevalence and trends of obesity in Indian school children of different socioeconomic class." Indian Journal of Basic & Applied Medical Research; December 2012: Issue-5, Vol.-2, P. 393-398.

[7] Manu Raj, K. R. Sundaram, Mary Paul, A. S. Deepa, R. Krishna Kumar, Obesity in Indian children: Time trends and relationship with hypertension, The National Medical Journal of India, Vol. 20, No. 6, 2007.

[8] Manu Raj & R. Krishna Kumar, Obesity in children & adolescents, Indian J Med Res 132, November 2010: 598-607.

[9] Childhood overweight and obesity, Retrieved on nov. 25th, 2013 from http://www.who.int/dietphysicalactivity/childhood/en/index.html

[10] Physical activity, Retrieved on nov. 25th, 2013 from http://www.who.int/topics/physical_activity/en/index.html

[11] Child health, Retrieved on nov. 25th, 2013 from http://www.who.int/topics/child_health/en/index.html

[12] Jeon CY, Lokken RP, Hu FB, van Dam RM, Physical activity of moderate intensity and risk of type 2 diabetes: a systematic review, Diabetes Care. 2007 Mar; 30(3):744-52.

[13] Physical Activity for Health, Retrieved on nov. 25th, 2013 from http://www.patient.co.uk/health/Physical-Activity-For-Health.htm

[14] Physical, Activity and Health: A Report of the Surgeon General Executive Summary, U.S. Department of Health and Human Services, Centres for Disease Control and Prevention, National Centre for Chronic Disease Prevention and Health Promotion, The President's Council on Physical Fitness and Sports.

[15] Ruth R Kipping, Russell Jago and Debbie A Lawlor, Obesity in children. Part 1: Epidemiology, measurement, risk factors, and screening, BMJ 2008; 337:a1824.

[16] Moutusi Raychaudhuri and Debmalya Sanyal, Childhood obesity: Determinants, evaluation, and prevention, 16(8), 2012: 192-194.

[17] Nate Whitman, "Physical Activity in Schools is Essential to Reversing Childhood Obesity", Retrieved on nov. 25th, 2013 from http://www.huffingtonpost.com/nate-whitman/physical-activity-in-scho_b_4039563.html.

[18] Andrew P Hills, Lars Bo Andersen and Nuala M Byrne, "Physical activity and obesity in children", *Br J Sports Med* 2011; 45:866-870.

[19] The Times of India (Delhi) Wednesday, November 13, 2013.

[20] The Times of India (Delhi) Friday, March 05, 2010.

[21] The Times of India (Delhi) Saturday, May 4, 2013.

[22] The Times of India (Delhi) Saturday, June 22, 2013.

[23] The Times of India (Delhi) Saturday, October 19, 2013.

[24] Mia Pradinuk, Jean-Pierre Chanoine, Ran D. Goldman, "Obesity and physical activity in children", Canadian Family Physician, 2011 vol. 57 no. 7: 779-782.

[25] Healthy active living for children and youth. Paediatr Child Health 2002; 7(5):339-58.

[26] Spear BA, Barlow SE, Ervin C, Ludwig DS, Saelens BE, Schetzina KE, et al. Recommendations for treatment of child and adolescent overweight and obesity. Pediatrics 2007; 120(Suppl 4):S254-88.

[27] World Health Organization. Global recommendations on physical activity for health; 2011. Accessed January 30, 2012.

[28] Haskell WL, Lee IM, Pate RR, et al. Physical activity and public health: updated recommendation for adults from the American College of Sports Medicine and the American Heart Association. Circulation. 2007; 116:1081-93.

[29] U.S. Dept. of Health and Human Services. 2008 Physical Activity Guidelines for Americans; 2008. Accessed January 30, 2012.

[30] Juneau CE, Potvin L. Trends in leisure-, transport-, and work-related physical activity in Canada 1994-2005. Prev Med. 2010; 51:384-6.

[31] Brownson RC, Boehmer TK, Luke DA. Declining rates of physical activity in the United States: what are the contributors? Annu Rev Public Health. 2005; 26:421-43.

[32] Petersen CB, Thygesen LC, Helge JW, Gronbaek M, Tolstrup JS. Time trends in physical activity in leisure time in the Danish population from 1987 to 2005. Scand J Public Health. 2010; 38:121-8.

[33] Ng SW, Norton EC, Popkin BM. Why have physical activity levels declined among Chinese adults? Findings from the 1991-2006 China Health and Nutrition Surveys. Soc Sci Med. 2009; 68:1305-14.

[34] Lakka TA, Bouchard C., Physical activity, obesity and cardiovascular diseases, Handb Exp Pharmacol. 2005;(170):137-63.

[35] Obesity Prevention/Physical Activity/Nutrition, Retrieved on nov. 25th, 2013 from http://www.naccho.org/topics/HPDP/chronicdisease/oppan.cfm

[36] Morris JN, Heady JA, Raffle PAB, Parks JW, Roberts CG. Coronary heart disease and physical activity of work. Lancet 1953; 1053-1057: 1111-1120.

[37] Claude Bouchard and Peter T. Katzmarzyk, "Physical Activity and Obesity", 2nd Edition, Printed in United States of America, 2010, pp-8-9.

[38] Shephard, R. J. (2005). The obesity epidemic: A challenge to pediatric work physiologists. Pediatric Exercise Science, 17(1), 3-17.

[39] Centers for Disease Control and Prevention. Guidelines for school and community programs to promote lifelong physical activity among young people. MMWR Recomm Rep. 1997; 46: 1-36.

[40] Guy Le Masurier and Charles B. Corbin, "Top 10 Reasons for Quality Physical Education", JOPERD, Volume 77 No. 6, 2006:44-53.

[41] Nowicka P., and Flodmark CE., "Physical activity-key issues in treatment of childhood obesity", Acta Paediatr Suppl. 2007 Apr; 96(454):39-45.

[42] Fairclough, S., & Stratton, G. (2005). 'Physical education makes you fit and healthy': Physical education's contribution to young people's physical activity levels. Health Education Research, 20(1), 14-23.

[43] Flohr, J. A., & Todd, M. K. (2003). Pedometer counts among young adolescents: A comparison between after school activity program participants and non-participants. Medicine & Science in Sports & Exercise, 35(5 Suppl.), S342.

[44] Tudor-Locke, C., Lee, S. M., Morgan, C. F., Beighle, A., & Pangrazi, R. P. (2004). Sex-specifi c activity patterns of the segmented school day. Research Quarterly for Exercise and Sport, 75(1 Suppl.), A-32.

[45] Bensimhon DR, Kraus WE, Donahue MP, "Obesity and physical activity: a review", Am Heart J. 2006 Mar; 151(3):598-603.

[46] I A Samjoo, A Safdar, M J Hamadeh1, S Rahal and M A Tarnopolsky, "The effect of endurance exercise on both skeletal muscle and systemic oxidative stress in previously sedentary obese men", Nutrition & Diabetes, 3, (2013):1-10.

[47] W. J. Pasman, M. S. Westerterp-Plantenga, and W. H. M. Saris, "The effect of exercise training on leptin levels in obese males", Am. J. Physiol. 274 (Endocrinol. Metab. 37), 1998: E280-E286.

[48] Considine, R.V., M.K.Sinha, M.L. Heiman, A. Kriauciunas, T.W.Stephens, M.L. Nyce, J.P. Ohannesian, C.C. Marco, L.J. Mckee, T.L. Bauer and J.F.Caro. Serum immunoreactive-leptin concentrations in normal weight and obese humans, N.Engl. J.Med. 334:292-295,1996.

[49] Cusin, I.,A.Sainsbury, P.Doyle, F.Rohner Jeanrenaud and B. Jeanrenaud, the ob gene and insulin. A relationship leading to clues to the understanding of obesity. Diabetes 44:1467-1470, 1995.

[50] Venables MC, Jeukendrup AE., "Endurance training and obesity: effect on substrate metabolism and insulin sensitivity", Med Sci Sports Exerc. 2008 Mar; 40(3):495-502.

[51] Ellen e. blaak and wim h. m. saris, "substrate oxidation, obesity and exercise training", best practice and research clinical endocrinology and metabolism", vol. 16, no. 4, 2002:667-678.

[52] John Cook and Karen Jeng, "Child Food Insecurity: The Economic Impact on our Nation, A report on research on the impact of food insecurity and hunger on child health, growth and development commissioned by Feeding America and The ConAgra Foods Foundation", Retrieved on dec. 2nd, 2013 from http://feedingamerica.org/sitefiles/child-economy-study.pdf.

[53] Child Nutrition and Obesity, Retrieved on dec. 2nd, 2013 from http://www.childrensdefense.org/policy-priorities/childrens-health/child-nutrition/.

[54] Obesity: preventing and managing the global epidemic, Retrieved on nov. 25th, 2013 from http://www.who.int/nutrition/publications/obesity/WHO_TRS_894/en/.

[55] Kaufmann NA, Poznanski R, Guggenheim K., "Eating habits and opinions of teen-agers on nutrition and obesity", J Am Diet Assoc. 1975 Mar; 66(3):264-8.

[56] Patricia Constante Jaimea and Karen Lockb, "Do school based food and nutrition policies improve diet and reduce obesity?", Preventive Medicine, Volume 48, Issue 1, January 2009: 45-53.

[57] Barry M. Popkin, "The Nutrition Transition and Obesity in the Developing World", J. Nutr. March 1, 2001vol. 131 no. 3: 871S-873S.

[58] Gregory JW, Lowe S: National Diet and Nutrition Survery: Young People Aged 4 to 18 Years: Report of the Diet and Nutrition Survey. London, The Stationery Office: 2000.

[59] Maffeis C, Pinelli L, Schutz Y: Fat intake and adiposity in 8 to 11 year-old obese children, International Journal of Obesity 1996, 20:170-174.

[60] Tucker LA, Seljaas GT, Hager RL: Body fat percentage of children varies according to their diet composition, Journal of the American Dietetic Association 1997, 97:981-986.

[61] Ludwig DS, Peterson KE, Gortmaker SL: Relation between consumption of sugar-sweetened drinks and childhood obesity: a prospective, observational analysis. Lancet 2001, 357:505-508.

[62] Gittelsohn J, Wolever TM, Harris SB, Harris-Giraldo R, Hanley AJ, Zinman B: Specific patterns of food consumption and preparation are associated with diabetes and obesity in a Native Canadian community. J Nutr 1998, 128:541-547.

[63] American Diabetes Association. Type 2 diabetes in children and adolescents. Pediatrics 2000; 105: 671-80.

[64] Pinhas-Hamiel O, Zeitler P. The global spread of type 2 diabetes mellitus in children and adolescents. J. Pediatr 2005; 146: 693-700.

[65] Manu Raj & R. Krishna Kumar, "Obesity in children & adolescents", Indian J Med Res 132, November 2010: 598-607.

[66] Mahshid Dehghan, Noori Akhtar-Danesh and Anwar T Merchant, "Childhood obesity, prevalence and prevention", Nutrition Journal 2005, 4:24.

[67] Swinburn B, Egger G: Preventive strategies against weight gain and obesity. Obes Rev 2002, 3:289-301.

[68] Suzanna Vidmar, John Carlin, and Kylie Hesketh, "Standardizing anthropometric measures in children and adolescents with new functions for egen", The Stata Journal (2004) 4, Number 1, pp. 50-55.

[69] Semiz S, Ozgören E, Sabir N., "Comparison of ultrasonographic and anthropometric methods to assess body fat in childhood obesity. Int J Obes (Lond). 2007 Jan; 31(1):53-8. Epub 2006 Jun 20.

[70] Cole, T. J., M. C. Bellizzi, K. M. Flegal, and W. H. Dietz. 2000. Establishing a standard definition for child overweight and obesity worldwide: international survey. British Medical Journal 320(7244): 1240-1243.

[71] Kenny, P. J. Reward mechanisms in obesity: new insights and future directions. *Neuron* **69**, 664-679 (2011).

[72] Wyrwicka, W., Dobrzecka, C. & Tarnecki, R. On the instrumental conditioned reaction evoked by electrical stimulation of the hypothalamus. *Science* **130**, 336-337 (1959).

[73] Will, M. J., Pratt, W. E. & Kelley, A. E. Pharmacological characterization of high-fat feeding induced by opioid stimulation of the ventral striatum. *Physiol. Behav.* **89**, 226-234 (2006).

[74] O'Rourke RW. Molecular mechanisms of obesity and diabetes: at the intersection of weight regulation, inflammation, and glucose homeostasis. World J Surg. 2009 Oct; 33(10):2007-13.

[75] Chang Hee Jung and Min-Seon Kim, "Molecular mechanisms of central leptin resistance in obesity", Archives of Pharmacal Research, February 2013, Volume 36, Issue 2, pp 201-207.

[76] Emily J. Gallagher and Derek LeRoith, Epidemiology and Molecular Mechanisms Tying Obesity, Diabetes, and the Metabolic Syndrome With Cancer", Diabetes Care August 2013 vol. 36 no. Supplement 2 S233-S239.

[77] Fryar CD, Gu Q, Ogden CL. Anthropometric reference data for children and adults: United States, 2007-2010. National Center for Health Statistics. Vital Health Stat 11(252). 2012.

[78] Russell R. Pate, Thomas N. Robinson and Thomas L. McKenzie, "Promoting Physical Activity in Children and Youth", Circulation, 2006; 114: 1214-1224.

[79] Livingstone B., Epidemiology of childhood obesity in Europe, Eur J. Pediatr. 2000 Sep; 159 Suppl 1:S14-34.

[80] K. R. Fox and M. Hillsdon, "Physical activity and obesity", Volume 8, Issue Supplement s1, pages 115-121, March 2007.

[81] Monica A. F. Lounsbery, Thomas L.McKenzie, James R. Morrow, Shannon M. Monnat, Kathryn A. Holt, "District and School Physical Education Policies: Implications for Physical Education and Recess Time", ann. behav. med. (2013) 45 (Suppl 1):S131-S141.

[82] Wareham NJ, van Sluijs EM, Ekelund U., "Physical activity and obesity prevention: a review of the current evidence", Proc Nutr Soc. 2005 May; 64(2):229-47.

[83] Toni M. Burkhalter and Charles H. Hillman, "A Narrative Review of Physical Activity, Nutrition, and Obesity to Cognition and Scholastic Performance across the Human Lifespan", American Society for Nutrition. Adv. Nutr. 2: 201S-206S, 2011.

34

Prevalence of Obesity among Immigrants Living in Canada

Anup Adhikari*

Anthropometrica, Toronto, Canada
*Corresponding author: dranupadhikari@yahoo.com

Abstract Canadian who were living in Toronto for the past fifteen years after migrating from their own countries and maintaining their own traditional food habits, were studied for their adiposity and body composition. Body composition was analyzed by bio-impedance method using bioelectrical body composition analyzer and BMI was calculated by standard method. Average age, height, weight, fat % and BMI for the males were 34.2 yr (± 12.3), 175.8 cm (± 8.2), 85.5 kg (± 17.5), 23.6 % (± 7.4) and 27.6 kg.m^2 (± 5.2) respectively whereas those for their female counterparts were 30.9 yr (± 11.3), 163.7 cm (± 6.5), 71.1 kg (± 17.1), 31.8 % (± 8.2) and 26.5 kg.m^{-2} (± 5.9) respectively. A wide range of Fat % were observed in both male and female Canadians which were 7.3% - 50.0% for male and 8.5 %-52.6% for female. Similar wide ranges were also observed in BMI where males had a range of 14.6 kg.m^{-2} - 48.5 kg.m^{-2} and female had 15.2 kg.m^{-2} and 50.2 kg.m^{-2}. In males, 66.12 % were in overweight category, out of which 38.74% were in pre-obese and 27.38% were in obese group. Similarly, in females, 52.72% were in overweight category, out of which 30.96% were in pre-obese category and 21.75% were in obese category. High adiposity was also observed both in males and females. The reason might be due to their life style and food habit.

Keywords: *BMI, fat%, over weight, obese, immigrant, Canadian*

1. Introduction

Obesity is a public health challenge throughout the world. The prevalence of obesity has been increased dramatically in past few decades in both developed and developing countries [1,2]. According to the World Health Organization [2] more than 1.4 billion adults aged 20 or older were reported overweight in the year 2008. Of these overweight population, over 200 million men and nearly 300 million women were obese. Once considered to be a high-income country problem, overweight and obesity are now on the rise in low-and –middle-income countries also, particularly in urban settings. In Canada, obesty is a public health challenge and growing concern for the past few years [3,4,5,6]. According to the information reveled from the joint report of Public health Agency of Canada and the Canadian Institute for Health Information [7], the number of obese adults in Canada had been increased tremendously since 1978 and doubled in the 2008 from 13.8% to 25.4 % for adults over 18 years and more. Different studies also revealed that nearly 23% of Canadian population aged 18 or more were suffering from obesity with an additional 36% overweight in the year 2004 [4,8,9].

The aim of the present study was to find out the body fat %, BMI and trend of obesity in the Canadian population those who were settled in Canada for the past 15 years and maintaining their own food habits and culture of eating.

2. Method

2.1. Study Population

Participants were the healthy male and female from Etobicoke (Western part of Toronto), Brampton and Mississauga who came to a local fitness club for enrolling their name for fitness program and first time enrolling themselves in a fitness program. A total of 971 man and women were measured on the very first day prior to their exercise program starts. Out of which, 493 were male and 478 were female. All the subjects were Canadian who immigrated and used to live in Canada for the past fifteen years and migrated mostly from middle Europe, North Africa, Asia and Latin America. Age was calculated in years and was grouped for analysis as 15-20 yr, 21-30 yr, 31-40 yr, 41-50 yr, 51-60 yr, 61-70 yr, 71-80yr. Race, ethnicity and duration of migration period were self reported and those who were in Canada for the past 15 years were chosen for the study. All the participants had participated in the study voluntarily and written concern was taken before the measurements according to club's enrollment rules and regulations.

2.2. Anthropometrical Measurements

For anthropometrical measurements, International Society for the Advancement of Kinanthropometry (ISAK) accredited level 4 criterion Anthropometrist was involved in anthropometrical measurements and training was also given to the other associates who were also involved in the anthropometrical measurements. Anthropometrical measurements were measured according to ISAK manual [10] (2011) for Anthropometrical measurements.

2.2.1. Height and Weight

Height and weight were measured according to the ISAK manual [10] for anthropometrical protocol. The perpendicular distance between the transverse plane of the vertex and the interior aspects of the feet was considered to measure the height and measured with the help of an Anthropometric rod. Similarly, body weight was measured in nearest gram using an electronic digital weighing machine.

2.3 Body Fat %

Body fat percent can be measured by various techniques. Bioelectrical impedance method is one of them to estimate body fat % by applying a small alternating current to the body. Different body tissues have different resistivity and depending on the resistivity body fat % can be estimated with this method [11]. In the present study, whole body fat% was analyzed with Bioelectrical Impedance Analyzer (Quantum II, RJL system, USA). Pre-testing protocols and other specific instructions given by the manufacturer company were followed to avoid error while measuring body fat% with the bio-impedance equipment.

2.4. Body Mass Index (BMI)

BMI was derived by dividing weight (kg) by height (m) squared. BMI categories were based on age specific cut-offs in adolescent. World Health Organization [1] based classification for global database on Body Mass Index (BMI) was used as a cut points for BMI.

Statistical Analysis: For statistical analysis, the software package SPSS 11.0 was used. Mean value and standard deviation were analyzed and presented in the table.

3. Results

Table 1 showed the anthropometrical characteristics, body composition and BMI of men and women studied in the present study. Average 23.6% body fat was observed for the males whereas that of their female counterpart was 31.8% though the ranges were very similar to each other with a wide range. The 95% confidence interval for average 23.6% fat for male was from 22.9 % to 24.3 % and that was for the female was 31.15 to 32.5% with average 31.8 % subcutaneous fat. When body mass index (BMI) was considered, the male groups possessed an average value of 27.6 $kg.m^2$ with a range between 14.6 to 48.5 $kg.m^2$ whereas that of the females was 26.5 $kg.m^2$ with a range between 15.2 $kg.m^2$ to 50.2 $kg.m^2$ which were very similar to each other. The 95 % confidence interval for average BMI of male was from 27.1 to 28.1 $kg.m^2$ whereas that for female counterparts was from 26.0 to 27.0 $kg.m^2$.

The weight category classification based on BMI was presented in Table 3.

Table 2 presented the age group wise information for both male and female. The groups were arranged into 10 years range and 20 years range except for the first group, as the minimum age considered for the study was 15 years for both male and female. The weight category classification based on BMI was presented in Table 3.

95% Confidence Interval level for Fat % and BMI of all age group were shown in Table 4.

The cut points for the classification were based on Body Mass Index (BMI) classified by World Health Organization, which was presented in Table 5.

4. Discussion

Overweight and obesity could be defined as an excessive adiposity that may impair health [2] (WHO 2012). Excess adiposity is a risk factor associated with mature mortality, type 2 diabetes and cardio-vascular diseases [12,13,14,15,16]. In the present study, average body fat% for the men was observed to be 23.6 % (± 7.4) ranging from 7.3 to 50.0 % whereas that of females was 31.8% (± 8.2) ranging from 8.5 to 52.6 % (Table 1).

Table 1. Height, weight, fat% and BMI of Canadian male (n=493) and female (n=478)

	Mean		Standard deviation		Range		95% confidence interval	
	male	female	male	female	male	female	male	female
Age (yr)	34.2	30.9	12.3	11.3	15-74	15-69	-	-
Height (cm)	175.8	163.7	8.2	6.5	150-220	140-182.9	-	-
Weight (kg)	85.5	71.1	17.5	17.1	52.2-156.4	39.1-147.7	-	-
Fat%	23.6	31.8	7.4	8.2	7.3-50	8.5-52.6	22.9-24.3	31.1-32.5
BMI ($kg.m^{-2}$)	27.6	26.5	5.2	5.9	14.6-48.5	15.2-50.2	27.1-28.1	26.0-27.0

When analyzed age wise, fat% increased as age increased both in men and women (Table 2). This might be due to impact of aging on resting metabolic rate as well as on macronutrient oxidation rates besides other factors which supported the study of St-Onge et al [17] with similar findings.

For general population, Body Mass Index (BMI) is as indicator of obesity though it is limited to overall body fat assessment as BMI does not provide complete image on the distribution of body fat. The underlying assumption of using BMI to define obesity was that at a given height, higher weight was associated with increased fatness [15]. As BMI is the result of body weight over height, population with more muscle mass with less height would show more BMI than the population with same height but less muscle mass but excess fat. Thus, BMI may be a good indicator of over weight for general population but limited to athletic population. So, BMI would be a good indicator for obesity and obesity related occurrence of fat for non-athletic population. In the present study, the studied population was non-athletic with regular daily routine activities and out of any exercises for long time prior to their involvement in fitness program. Hence, BMI could be used as appropriate scale for the presently studied population for measuring obesity. Majority of the men and women of the present study were in overweight category (Table 3). 33.06 % men were in normal range whereas a nominal section of 0.81 % were in underweight category. The observed value was very similar to the study reported by Statistics Canada [18] for Canadian adults from 2007 to 2009 where 31.0 % was in normal weight category while only 0.8 % was in underweight category. Out of 66.12 % overweight male of the present study, 38.74 % were in pre-obese category while 27.38 % were in obese category. 17.65 % of obese male population of the present study was in obese class I category whereas a less percent of 6.69 were in obese class II category compared to 3.04 % obese class III category. Very similar value was also reported by Statistics Canada [18] for male Canadians where 24.2 % were in obese category comprising of obese class I, II, and III. Likewise when females of the present study were considered, only 45.39 % were in normal weight range category while 1.88 % was in underweight category. A large percentage of women (52.72 %) of the present study were in overweight category out of which 30.96 % were in pre-obese category and 21.75 % were in obese category. Of these 21.75 % obese female, 3.14 % fell in type III category, 6.69 % in type II category and 11.92 % in type I category. According to The Canada Health Measure survey report of 2007 to 2009, 44.7 % of Canadian women were in normal weight category whereas 29.5 % in overweight category and 23.6 % in obese category comprising of type I, II, III. Thus, the observed value for normal weight category was very similar with the 44.7 % in normal weight category for the Canadian women reported by Canada Health Measure survey which also observed higher incidence of over weight and obesity in Canadian females [18].

Table 2. Age group wise average height, weight, fat% and BMI and weight category of Canadian male (n=493) and female (478), * SD = Standard deviation

Age Group (year)		15-20	21-30	31-40	41-50	51-60	61-70	71-80
Number	M	40	201	115	78	41	16	02
	F	64	215	108	47	37	07	00
Height(cm)	M	176.4	176.5	175.4	175.1	175.8	173.1	174.0
	F	164.7	164.3	162.7	162.8	162.9	163.0	-
SD (height)	M	6.6	7.8	7.9	9.9	9.0	7.3	5.4
	F	6.9	6.3	5.7	7.7	6.0	11.0	-
Weight (kg)	M	80.0	81.6	89.5	88.4	88.9	88.7	96.4
	F	67.4	68.9	74.2	72.7	78.5	76.2	-
SD (weight)	M	16.6	15.4	19.8	17.2	18.7	14.1	14.1
	F	12.9	17.7	16.4	17.7	18.2	12.9	-
Fat%	M	22.8	20.3	25.1	28.3	27.8	30.6	29.1
	F	31.0	29.3	33.9	33.9	37.7	40.1	-
SD (Fat%)	M	7.6	7.1	6.4	8.2	6.3	5.2	7.1
	F	7.4	8.2	7.8	6.9	7.1	4.8	-
BMI ($kg.m^2$)	M	25.6	26.1	29.0	29.2	28.5	29.5	32.0
	F	24.8	25.4	27.9	27.2	29.5	28.7	-
SD (BMI)	M	4.9	4.6	5.8	5.0	4.3	3.7	6.6
	F	4.7	6.1	5.6	5.3	6.1	4.2	-
Under weight	M	2.5 %	1.5 %	0	00.0	00.0	0.00	00.0
	F	3.1 %	3.2 %	-	-	-	14.28%	-
Normal range	M	37.5 %	47.3 %	23.5 %	21.8 %	17.1 %	12.5 %	00.0
	F	54.7 %	55.3 %	33.3 %	40.4 %	18.9 %	-	-
Over weight	M	60 %	51.2 %	76.5 %	78.2 %	83.9 %	-	100 %
	F	42.2 %	41.4 %	66.7 %	59.6 %	81.1 %	57.1 %	-
Pre-obese	M	47.5 %	33.3 %	39.1 %	41.0 %	48.8 %	43.8 %	50 %
	F	26.6 %	25.6 %	35.2 %	34.0 %	48.6 %	28.6 %	-
Obese	M	12.5 %	17.9 %	37.4 %	37.2 %	34.2 %	43.8 %	00.0
	F	15.62%	15.8 %	31.5 %	25.5 %	32.4 %	14.3 %	-
Obese class I	M	7.5 %	10.9 %	23.5 %	21.8 %	26.8 %	43.7 %	0.00
	F	10.9 %	7.9 %	18.5 %	12.8 %	16.2 %	14.3 %	-
Obese class II	M	2.5 %	5.0 %	8.7 %	11.5 %	4.9 %	00.0	50 %
	F	4.7 %	4.2 %	7.41 %	12.8 %	13.5 %	00.0	-
Obese class III	M	2.5 %	2.0 %	5.2 %	3.8 %	2.4 %	00.0	00.0
	F	00.0%	3.7 %	5.6 %	0 %	2.7 %	00.0	-

Age-group wise classification showed that 100 % of men over seventy years were overweight followed by 87.5 % and 83.93 % in the age group of 61-70 and 51-60 yr respectively. The prevalence of overweight in male was further reduced to 78.2 % in 41-50 yr age group followed by 76.52 % in 31 -40 yr group. Surprisingly most of the young male population with age ranged from 15 to 20 years (60 % of total male population studied) were overweight compare to the young girls of same age group (42.2 % of total female population studied) but it was reversed when obesity was considered (Table 2).The reason was not clear but may be due food intake or inactivity. Prevalence of obesity was observed more in the men after 30 year of age than the young population below 30 year and it increased as age went up (Table 3). Similarly, prevalence of obesity was more in women over 30 year than the women below 30 year (Table 2). The observation in the present study was very similar with the findings of Shields et al [19] reported in Statistics Canada [16] where mean BMI rose with age both for males and females.

Table 3. BMI of Canadian male (n=493) and female (n=478)

Categories	BMI	Male number n = 493	Percent in male	Female number n = 478)	Percent in female
Underweight	< 18.5	4	00.81	9	01.88
Severe thinness	< 16.0	2	00.40	3	00.63
Moderate thinners	16 -16.99	1	00.20	1	00.21
Mild thinness	17 -18.49	1	00.20	5	01.04
Normal range	18.5-24.99	163	33.06	217	45.39
Overweight	≥ 25.00	326	66.12	252	52.72
Pre Obese	25 - 29.99	191	38.74	148	30.96
Obese	≥ 30	135	27.38	104	21.75
Obese class I	30 - 34.9	87	17.65	57	11.92
Obese class II	35- 39.9	33	06.69	32	06.69
Obese Class III	≥ 40	15	03.04	15	03.14

It was well known fact that overweight and obesity were the result of energy imbalance between calories consumed and calories expended though the causes and contributors to obesity are a complex phenomenon and depends on various factors like genetic, environment-social and environmental, ethnicity and food habit and some pathological conditions. But in most cases, an increased intake energy rich foods that high in fat and sugars associated with decreased physical activity due to sedentary nature of many forms of work, changing mode of transpiration and increasing urbanization were the some of reasons behind obesity and overweight [2]. The studied population was from different countries migrated to Canada and living in Toronto for the past 15 years but maintaining their own ethnical eating habit and diet. Most of the men and women were with sedentary life style and maintaining there own eating habits, which were basically carbohydrate based ethnical food containing more fats, spices and oils for ethnical way of food preparation which was revealed during the nutritional counselling for the present study.

Table 4. 95% confidence interval for fat % and BMI of male and female at different age groups

Age group		Fat%			BMI		
		mean	95 % confidence interval		mean	95 % confidence interval	
15-20	male	22.8	20.4	25.2	25.6	24.1	27.1
	female	31.0	29.2	32.8	24.8	23.6	26.0
21-30	male	20.3	19.3	21.3	26.1	25.5	26.7
	female	29.3	28.2	30.4	25.4	24.6	26.2
31-40	male	25.1	23.9	26.3	29.0	27.9	30.1
	female	33.9	32.4	35.4	27.9	26.8	29.0
41-50	male	28.3	26.5	30.1	29.2	28.1	30.3
	female	33.9	31.9	35.9	27.2	25.7	28.7
51-60	male	27.8	25.9	29.7	28.5	27.2	29.8
	female	37.7	35.4	40.0	29.5	27.5	31.5
61-70	male	30.6	28.1	33.1	29.5	27.7	31.3
	female	40.1	36.5	43.7	28.7	25.6	31.8
71-80	male	29.1	19.3	38.9	32.0	22.9	41.1
	female	-	-		-	-	

Table 5. The International Classification of adult underweight, overweight and obesity according to BMI (Adapted from WHO 1995,WHO 2000,WHO 2004)

Classification	BMI (kg/m^2)	
Underweight	< 18.50	< 18.50
Severe thinness	< 16.00	< 16.00
Moderate thinness	16.00 - 16.99	16.00 - 16.99
Mild thinness	17.00 - 18.49	17.00 - 18.49
Normal range	18.50 - 24.99	18.50 - 22.99
		23.00 - 24.99
Overweight	≥25.00	≥25.00
Pre-obese	25.00 - 29.99	25.00 - 27.49
		27.50 - 29.99
Obese	≥30.00	≥30.00

5. Conclusion

The prevalence of obesity in the emigrated Canadian population which might be due to less active life style with eating food habits. The study also supported the previous studies indicating prevalence of obesity in Canadian population. It might be concluded that occurrence of overweight increased as age went up which was true for both men and women. The study recommended more active life style for the Canadians with proper balance diet besides other factors.

References

[1] World Health Organization (WHO), Global Database on Body Mass Index. Available from http://apps.who.int/bmi/index.jsp?introPage=in, 2004.

[2] World Health Organization (WHO), Obesity and overweight, Fact sheet No 311, May 2012. Available from www.who.int/mediacentre/factsheets/fs311/en/index.html, 2012.

[3] Gilmore, J., Body mass index and health. Health Reports (Statistics Canada, Catalogue 82-003), 11(1): 31-43, 1999.

[4] Katzmarzyk, P.T., The Canadian obesity epidemic, 1985-1998, *Canadian Medical Association Journal*, 166(8): 1039-1040, 2002.

[5] Tremblay, M.S., Katzmarzyk, P.T., Willms, J.D., Temporal trends in overweight and obesity in Canada, 1981-1996, *International Journal of Obesity*, 26: 538-43,2002.

[6] Tremblay, M.S., Pérez, C.E., Ardern, C.I., Bryan, S.N., Katzmarzyk, P.T., Obesity, overweight and ethnicity, Statistics Canada, Catalogue 82-003. Health Rep 16(4):23-34. 2005.

[7] Public health Agency of Canada and the Canadian Institute for Health Information, Obesity in Canada - A joint report from the Public Health Agency of Canada and The Canadian Institute for Health information. 2011, Available from www.phac-aspc.gc.ca/hp-ps/hl-mvs/oic-oac/index-eng.php.

[8] Shields, M., Tremblay, M.S., Laviolette, M., Craig, C.L., Janssen, I., Gorber, S.C., Fitness of Canadian adults: Results from the 2007-2009 Canadian Health Measures Survey, Statistics Canada, Catalogue no.82-003-X-Health Reports, vol 21, nol, March 2010, available from www.statcan.gc.ca.

[9] Tjepkema, M., Nutrition: Findings from the Canadian Community Health Survey – Adult Obesity in Canada: Measured height and weight, Issue no. 1, Component of Statistics Canada Catalogue no. 82-620-MWE2005001, 2010.

[10] ISAK, International Standards for Anthropometric Assessment. ISAK manual, International Society for the Advancement of Kinanthropometry (ISAK): Lower Hutt, New Zealand, 2011.

[11] Jaffrin, M.Y., Body composition determination by bioimpedance: an update, *Curr. Opin. Clin. Nutr. Metab. Care*, 12(5):482-486, 2009.

[12] Hubert, H.B., Feinleib,M., McNamara, P.M.,Castelli, W.P., Obesity as an independent risk factor for cardiovascular disease: a 26 year follow up of participants in the Framingham Heart Study, *Circulation*, 67(5): 968-977,1983.

[13] Colditz, G.A., Willett, W.C., Stamfer, M.J., Manson, J.E., Hennekens, C.H., Arky, R.A., Speizer, F.E., Weight as a risk factor for clinical diabetes in women, *Am J Epidemiol*, 132(3): 501-513,1990.

[14] Chan, J.M., Rimm, E.B, Colditz, G.A, Stampfer, M.J., Willett, W.C., Obesity, fat distribution and weight gain as a risk factors for clinical diabetes in men, *Diabetes Care*, 17(9):961-969,1994.

[15] Flegal, K.M., Shepherd, J.A., Looker, A.C., Graubard, B.I., Borrud, L.G., Ogden, C.L., Harris, T.B., Everhart, J.E., Schenker, N., Comparisons of percentage body fat, body mass index, waist circumference and waist-stature ratio in adults, *Am J Clin Nutrn*, 89:500-508,2009.

[16] Brenner, D.R., Tepylo, K.,Eny, K.M., Cahill, L.E., Sohemy, A.,Comaprison of body mass index and waist circumference as predictors of cardiometabolic health in a population of young Canadian adults, *Diabetology and Metabolic Syndrome*, 2:28-35,2010.

[17] St-Onge, M.P., Gallagher, D., Body composition changes with aging: The cause or the result of alterations in metabolic rate and macronutrient oxidation?, *Nutrition*, 26(2):152-155, 2010.

[18] Statistics Canada, Catalogue no 82-003-X, Health Reports, January 2010, Available from www.statcan.gc.ca.

[19] Shields, M., Tremblay, M.S., Laviolette, M., Craig, C.L., Janssen, I., Gorber, S.C., Fitness of Canadian adults: Results from the 2007-2009 Canadian Health Measures Survey, Statistics Canada, Catalogue no.82-003-X-Health Reports, vol 21, no 1, March 2010, available from www.statcan.gc.ca.

Hydration Habits of Elite Field Futsal Players during Official Matches: Defenders and Forwards

J. V. García-Jiménez*, J. L. Yuste, J. J. García-Pellicer

Department of Physical Education, University of Murcia, 30100 Murcia, Spain
*Corresponding author: jvgjimenez@um.es

Abstract Futsal is a variant of soccer that is played on a smaller playing surface and mainly indoors. Futsal is played between two teams of five players, and unlimited substitutions per team are permitted. The purpose of this study has been to determine and to compare hydration habits and level of dehydration in elite futsal players during competition in relation to playing position. 4 defenders (DF) and 5 forwards (FW) were studied during 3 official matches (22-26 ºC and relative humidity 32-42.33%) in the Spanish Futsal League (LNFS). Sweat loss was assessed through changes in body mass after correction for fluid intake (*ad libitum*) and urine loss. To analyze this data the statistics used are descriptive and not parametric. Mean sweat lost was higher in FW (2458±670.91 mL) than in DF (1695.56 ± 673.732 mL). Fluid intake was higher in FW (1700.36 ± 857.12 mL) than in DF (1493.33 ± 770.35 mL). FW replaced less total fluid lost (63.64 ± 29.55%) than DF (79.53 ± 38.71%), so FW incurred a mean body mass deficit of 1.23 ± 1.10%, higher than DF (0.59 ± 1.10%). Even FW and DF were aware of the impact that dehydration has on performance. There is a significant correlation between game time and body weight loss (Spearman's Rho = 0.419, $p \leq 0.05$). There is significant difference in sweat lost in relation to playing position ($p = 0.020$; ES = -1.311). We conclude that in these players, during official games, and independently of position, hydration status can be seen to maintain itself through regular substitutions and also the correct level of fluid intake. However, data allow for an individualisation of player hydration strategies, not taking exclusively into account playing position or game time.

Keywords: *dehydration, fluid intake, playing position, competition, futsal*

1. Introduction

Futsal is a variant of soccer that is played on a smaller playing surface (40x20 m.) and mainly played indoors. Futsal is played between two teams of five players, one of whom is the goalkeeper, two defenders and two forwards. Unlimited substitutions per team are permitted. It is an intermittent high intensity sport, where the main energy pathway is the anaerobic metabolism [35,36].

To avoid a reduction in performance during games, players must ingest enough fluid to match their sweat loss [1-6]. Dehydration occurs when fluid loss by sweating is higher than fluid intake [7,8], and it is a limiting factor for mental and physical performance during sport and physical activity [9-17].

A simple way to determine the level of dehydration achieved in futsal players is to weigh the athlete before and after performing the exercise, as the average loss of water through respiration in activity lasting less than 3 hours is barely significant compared to the loss through sweating [18]. The use of pre- to post exercise change in body mass provides a estimation of total fluid loss due to sweating [3,5,16,18]. Therefore, measurement of body weight changes is a simple, non-invasive and valid approach to estimate hydration changes in team sports, by calculating the difference in body weight pre- and post exercise [15,18,19,20,21].

A body water deficit greater than 2% of body weight marks the level of dehydration that can adversely affect physical performance [10,12,13,14,15,16,19,22], and to reduce athlete's cognitive function as perceptual discrimination or reaction time [10,15,22,23,24,25]. This data is particularly relevant to our study because the performance of a futsal player will depend on both their physical condition and cognitive abilities to make right decisions in the shortest time.

Our investigation has studied elite futsal players during official games. The team analyzed is considered one of the best in the world, and the analysis of its players provides valuable information about futsal hydration habits during real competition. In similar articles published by studying first-level players, researchers are required to simulate competitive situations during training sessions [1,4,26,27,28,29].

The aim of this study has been to determine and to compare the water balance and level of dehydration in elite futsal players in relation to playing position during three official matches, through the measurement of weight loss, urine loss and total fluid intake.

2. Materials and Methods

In team sports, individual differences such as body weight, genetic predisposition or heat acclimatization state [15,17,25,29,30], can affect sweat rates of players. It is recommended that players should monitor body weight changes during training/competition to estimate their sweat lost [15]. In addition, hydration level of players can vary considerably depending on their specific position, due to differences in intensity and duration of exercise performed during a match [1,3,31,32]. For this reason, our work has focused on determining and comparing results in variables sweat lost, fluid intake and body weight lost between elite futsal field players (defenders and forwards).

2.1. Participants

9 male futsal players (4 defenders and 5 forwards), from the first team squad of a professional club, were informed and gave their written consent to participate in this study, after the details had been explained to them. All players are professionals, with years of experience. Seven of whom are international with their national teams. The study was approved by the Institutional Review Board of the University of Murcia (Spain). Table 1 shows physical characteristics of players.

Table 1. Physical characteristics of players

Playing position	Defenders (n=4)		Forwards (n=5)	
Variable	Mean±SD	Range	Mean±SD	Range
Age (years)	29.3 ± 5.2	(22 - 33)	26.5 ± 2.46	(24 - 30)
Height (cm.)	176.5 ± 7.3	(169 - 185)	178 ± 9	(169 - 192)
Body mass (kg.)	73.2 ± 5.5	(69 - 85)	78.24 ± 6.99	(67.3 – 84.3)

Due to the difficulty to study other teams in the same level to get a representative sample, the sample selection was done using non-probability sampling, having performed the selection for convenience. Therefore, and because the sample is not representative, we can not infer the results of this research to other futsal teams.

Data were collected during three official matches in the Spanish Futsal League (LNFS), corresponding to gameweeks 25,27 and 29 (Table 2).

Table 2. Timing and climate conditions of matches*

Gameweek	Time	Temperature (ºC)	Relative Humidity (%)
25	18'30h.	22	40
27	13'45h.	26	32
29	18'30h.	24.8	42.33

* All matches were played in Murcia, Spain

2.2. Procedures

A meteorological station OREGON SCIENTIFIC WMR-80 (Oregon®, OR, USA), was used to record temperature and relative humidity, using the average value recorded since the start of warm-up to the final whistle.

To measure body weight we followed the protocol developed by the International Society for the Advancement of Kinanthropometry [33]. We used a scale TANITA BC-350 (Tanita®, Illinois, USA) with 97% reliability, accuracy 0.1 kg. and a measurement range from 0 to 150 kg. Players were weighed without clothing before the warm-up and after the match. Players were asked to micturate and defecate if necessary prior to the pre-warm-up measurement. Before weighing the players at the end of the match, perspiration was wiped of the player's legs, body and face with a towel, as indicated by Barbero et al. [20] in their study.

The percentage of weight loss was calculated using the following formula [34]:

$$\% \text{ Body weight lost}: \left[\begin{pmatrix}\text{Pre}-\text{match weight}\\ -\ \text{Post}-\text{match weight}\end{pmatrix} / \text{Pre}-\text{match weight}\right] \text{x } 100$$

Each player was provided with two individual 500 ml drinks bottles. One of the bottles was filled with water from the brand "Aquadeus", and the other with the sports drink "Gatorade". The players had been consuming these two drinks throughout the season.

The volume of fluid introduced into each bottle was previously measured in a graduated test-tube with capacity of 1000 ml and 1000:10 calibrated. The players were instructed to drink only from their own numbered bottles, just as they were told that in case they need more liquid they should advise the researcher so that he could fill the bottles. Fluid intake was therefore ad libitum. Once the match concluded, by subtracting the amount of liquid remaining in the player's bottle from the amount given to them, the total value for liquid consumed is yielded.

The volume of urine excreted by the players was measured since the warming-up to the end the match. After the first weighing of the players, and there after, each player had to urinate in a sterile and personal container, 1000:10 calibrated and prepared for his urine collection.

Total sweat loss was calculated using the following formula [2]:

$$\text{Sweat loss } = \begin{pmatrix}\text{Pre}-\text{match weight } + \text{ Fluid intake}\\ -\ \text{Post}-\text{match weight}-\text{Urine excreted}\end{pmatrix}$$

Each player's game time was obtained by adding up the minutes played and warm-up time (standardized to 30 minutes). During the game, and because unlimited substitutions per team are permitted, the exact time when the player started and stopped playing was recorded. Finally, the time played was calculated by adding each player's action.

2.3. Statistical Analysis

A 2-way ANOVA was applied to determine reliability (ICCRs), and repeated measures ANOVA for the variables (body weight and fluid volume), obtaining ICC = 1 (95% CI; $p \leq 0{,}001$). In addition, the design of this research is descriptive correlational. Data (game time, weight loss, fluid intake and excreted urine) are presented as mean, ±SD and range, in relation to playing position (defenders or forwards). A non-parametric statistical analysis was applied, using Kruskal-Wallis test to determine differences between playing position of players. Effect size was also calculated using Cohen's d statistics. Spearman's Rho statistic has been applied to establish the correlation between game time and weight lost, with a statistical significance of $p \leq 0.05$. The IBM SPSS 19.0 statistics package was used for the analysis.

3. Results

Table 3 shows that mean sweat lost was higher in forwards (2458 ± 670.91 mL) than in defenders (1695.56 ± 673.732 mL). Also mean fluid intake was higher in forwards (1700.36 ± 857.12 mL) than in defenders (1493.33 ± 770.35 mL). Forwards replaced less total fluid lost (63.64 ± 29.55%) than defenders (79.53 ± 38.71%), so they incurred a body mass deficit of 1.23 ± 1.10%, higher than defenders (0.59 ± 1.10%).

Table 3. Game time and fluid balance summary data in relation to playing position

	Defenders (n=5)		Forwards (n=4)			
Variable	Mean	SD	Mean	SD	p	Effect Size
Total game time (min)	49.78	3.93	50	3.13	0.899	-0.07
Body mass loss (g)	478.89	842.7	968.93	812.5	0.156	0.683
Fluid intake (mL)	1493.33	770.3	1700.36	857.1	0.549	0.293
Excreted urine (mL)	275.55	210.9	210	70.05	0.950	0.538
Sweat loss (mL) *	1695.56	673.7	2458.93	670.9	0.020	-1.31
Percentage of sweat lost replaced (%)	79.53	38.71	63.64	29.55	0.284	0.537
Dehydration (% Body weight lost)	0.59	1.10	1.23	1.10	0.176	0.676

* Significantly different in relation to playing position ($p \leq 0.05$)

There is significant difference in the values of sweat loss in relation to player's position, as indicated by value $p = 0.020$ after applying the Kruskal-Wallis test. Effect size for this variable is -1.311. However there are no significant differences in relation to fluid intake and dehydration of players.

Figure 1 shows that during the three studied matches mean fluid intake was similar in defenders and forwards. However mean sweat loss in forwards was always higher.

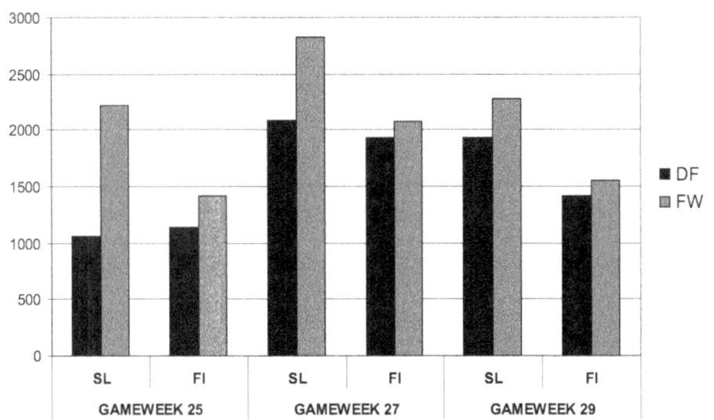

Figure 1. Sweat lost and fluid intake* in relation to playing position**

*** SL: Sweat lost (mL); FI: Fluid intake (mL) **DF = Defenders; FW = Forwards**

Mean game time was similar in defenders (49.78 ± 3.93 min) and forwards (50 ± 3.13 min). In addition, there is a positive relation between game time and level of dehydration (*Spearman's Rho* = 0.419, $p = 0.047$), so dehydration increases if game time increases.

4. Discussion

In this study we have assessed the hydration habits in elite field futsal players during official matches in relation to playing position. The results show that mean sweat lost in forwards is higher than defenders, resulting in higher levels of body weight lost.

Futsal played at highest level demands an excellent physical condition in players due to the physiological demands involved in competition (approximately 90% of maximum heart rate) [35,36]. A high performance player needs an excellent ability to perform high-intensity intermittent exercise, and a rapid recovery during low-intensity activities. In this sense an adequate fluid replacement strategy is essential to avoid reduced performance [2,3,10,15,19,22,23,24]. Unlimited substitutions allow players to increase their chances of ingesting liquids while they are sitting on the bench. Barbero et al. [20] calculated that every field player (defender or forward) had 7.4 opportunities to hydrate per match.

Compared to studies with soccer players, fluid intake in our research (defenders 1493.33 ± 770.35 mL and forwards 1700.36 ± 857.12 mL) was higher than that calculated by Maughan et al. [26] and Shirreffs et al. [27], whose obtained a mean fluid intake of 971 ± 303 mL and 972 ± 335 mL respectively, after having analyzed soccer players during training sessions. In our study, defenders drunk less amount of liquid (1493.33 ± 770.35 mL) than forwards (1700.36 ± 857.12 mL). Mean fluid intake by players in our study exceeds results by Barbero et al. [20] in elite futsal players. Along these lines, another study with elite futsal players [37] obtained an average of 800 mL intake after a training session, less than the total fluid intake by our players. In other team sports, Schröder et al. [38] assessed fluid intake during training and competition in 55 elite basketball players, which mean result was 882 ± 486 mL, less than that obtained in our study.

Despite a similar fluid intake, forwards finished matches with higher levels of dehydration (1.23 ± 1.10) than defenders (0.59 ± 1.10). There is significant difference in sweat lost in relation to playing position ($p = 0.020$; effect size = - 1.31). Mean sweat lost was higher in forwards than in defenders.

This is in accordance with ACSM´s Position Stand [15], which tells of the difficulty in giving a universal recommendation that adequately supplies for the needs of players due to the high variability of results obtained, even among members of the same team. In this context, various publications recommend pay attention to environmental conditions, intensity of effort or fluid intake to explain sweat losses and dehydration [9,10,15,23,29].

The environmental conditions in which the matches were played were similar (22-26°C 32-42,33% RH) because they were played in the same sports hall, which has cooling system.

Game time was similar in defenders and forwards (49.78 ± 3.93 and 50 ± 3.13 min), so to identify physical demands of players in our research, we must study their playing position. Tactics characteristics of each position involving different values of distance or intensity of effort, for instance, between defenders and forwards [30,31,32].

In a study of elite futsal players, defenders covered similar distances to forwards (6185.52 ± 171.35 m versus 6885.06 ± 996.41 m), but duration of high intensity efforts was lower in defenders (13.5 ± 2.5 s versus 55.5 ± 12.5 s), associating this data with lower-intensity efforts [32].

At the end of the games, players incurred a mean body mass deficit of 0.59 ± 1.10% in defenders and 1.23 ± 1.10 in forwards. These values are not associated with a reduction in performance [8,10,15,23]. Due to the characteristics of futsal, it is recommended not to exceed 2% of body weight lost, as dehydration is associated with decreased aerobic performance and increased cardiac work [10,15,16,23], it also affecting motor sensory reactions such as reaction time and perceptual discrimination [23,24].

In similar researches, Barbero et al. [20] Hamouti et al. [37] and Martins et al. [34] studied the level of dehydration in futsal players. The study of Barbero et al. [20] assessed 13 elite futsal players, where mean percentage weight loss after three official matches was 1.1 ± 0.9%, lower than forwards but higher than defenders of our research.

Hamouti et al. [37] obtained 1.2 ± 0.3% body weight lost in elite futsal players after a training session. The mean weight loss rate is similar than that obtained by forwards in our study (1.23 ± 1.10%). Dehydration in defenders was lower (0.59 ± 1.10%).

The study conducted by Martins et al. [34] in futsal players show values of 0.43 ± 0.41% weight loss after assessing 6 players (15-18 years) in training session. These results are lower than those obtained from the players in our study (defenders 0.59 ± 1.10% and forwards 1.23 ± 1.10%).

Regarding other team sports, in an investigation of percentage of weight loss in basketball players, Broad et al. [1] finds mean results were 1%, similar to those obtained in forwards our study (1.23 ± 1.10%). Similar to this, Maughan et al. [26] found a mean 1.59 ± 0.61% weight lost in soccer players during training. Also during a training session with soccer players, Shirreffs et al. [27] results were 1.62%. In both publications [26,27], percentage of weight lost, was higher than in our study (DF 0.59±1.10% and FW 1.23 ± 1.10%).

Even defenders and forwards mean dehydration shows that fluid intake was enough to avoid reduced performance during official games.

5. Conclusions

Independently of playing position, fluid intake in these elite players was enough to offset losses caused by sweat. In a team sport like futsal, hydration status can be well maintained with regular substitutions and correct fluid intake. The results recommend monitoring player's body weight changes to estimate their sweat lost. If necessary, the coach can customize fluid replacement programs for each player, and not exclusively taking into account playing position or game time.

Acknowledgement

We thank players, coaching and managers from *ElPozo Murcia Fútbol Sala* for their participation and collaboration in this study.

References

[1] Broad, E. M., Burke, L.M., Cox, G.R., Heeley, P., Riley, M. (1996). Body weight changes and voluntary fluid intakes during training and competition sessions in team sports. *International Journal of Sport Nutrition and Exercise Metabolism,* 6, 307-320.

[2] Murray, R. (1996). Dehydration, hyperthermia, and athletes: science and practice. *Journal of Athletic Trainning 31(3),* 248-252.

[3] Burke, L.M. (1997). Fluid balance during team sports. *Journal of Sports Science,* 15(3), 287-295.

[4] Cox, G.R., Broad, E.M., Riley, M.D., Burke, L.M. (2002). Body mass changes and voluntary fluid intakes of elite level water polo players and swimmers. *Journal of Science and Medicine in Sport,* 5(3), 183-193.

[5] Maughan, R. J., Gleeson, M. (2004). *The Biochemical Bases of Sports Performance.* Oxford: Oxford University Press.

[6] Roses, J.M., Pujol, P. (2006). Hidratación y Ejercicio Físico. *Apunts de Medicina del Deporte,* 150, 70-77.

[7] Guyton, A.C. (1983). *Fisiología Humana.* México D.F.: Interamericana.

[8] Earle, R.W., Baechle, T.R. (2004). *NSCA's Esentials of Personal Training.* Champaign, IL: Human Kinetics.

[9] López-Román, J., Martínez, A. B., Luque, A., Villegas, J. A. (2008). Estudio comparativo de diferentes procedimentos de hidratación durante un ejercicio de larga duración. *Archivos de Medicina del Deporte,* 25(123), 435-444.

[10] Palacios, N., Franco, L., Manonelles, P., Manuz, B., Villegas, J.A. (2008). Consenso sobre bebidas para el deportista. Composición y pautas de reposición de líquidos. *Archivos de Medicina del Deporte, 126(25),* 245-258.

[11] Sawka M.N., Gonzalez R.R., Young A.J., Muza S.R., Pandolf K.B., Latzka W.A. et al. (1988). Polycythemia and hydration: Effects on thermoregulation and blood volume during exercise-heat stress. *American Journal of Physiology, 255,* 456-463.

[12] González-Alonso, J., Coyle, E.F. (1998) Efectos fisiológicos de la deshidratación. ¿Por qué los deportistas deben ingerir líquidos durante el ejercicio en el calor?. Apunts Educación Física y Deportes, *54,* 46-52.

[13] Cheuvront, S.N., Carter, R., Sawka, M.N. (2003). Fluid balance and endurance exercise performance. *Current Sports Medicine Reports,* 2, 202-208.

[14] Coyle, E.F. (2004). Fluid and fuel intake during exercise. *Journal of Sports Sciences, 22,* 39-55.

[15] Sawka, M.N., Burke, L.M., Eichner, E.R., Maughan, R.J., Montain, S.J., Stachenfeld, N.S. (2007). Exercise and fluid replacement. *Medicine and Science in Sports and Exercise,* 39(2), 377-390.

[16] Wilmore, J.H., Costill, D.L. (2007). *Physiology of Sport and Exercise.* Champaign, IL: Human Kinetics.

[17] Stearns, R.L., Casa, D.J., López, R.M., McDermott, B.P., Ganio, M.S., Decher, N.R. et al. (2009). Influence of hydration status on pacing during trail running in the hear. *Journal of Strength and Condition Research, 23(9),* 2533-2541.

[18] Maughan, R.J., Shirrefs, S.M., Leiper, J.B. (2007). Errors in the estimation of hydration status from changes in body mass. *Journal of Sports Sciences,* 25(7), 797-804.

[19] Murray, R. (2007). Hydration and physical performance. *Journal of the American College of Nutrition, 26(5Suppl),* 542S-548S.

[20] Barbero, J.C., Castagna, C., Granda, J. (2006). Deshidratación y reposición hídrica en fútbol sala. Efectos de un programa de intervención sobre la pérdida de líquidos durante competición. *Motricidad. European Journal of Human Movement,* 17, 97-110.

[21] Harvey, G, Meir, R, Brooks, L, Holloway, K. (2008). The use of body mass changes as a practical measure of dehydration in team sports. *Journal of Sports Science and Medicine,* 11(6): 600-603.

[22] Manore, M.M., Meyer, N.L., Thompson, J. (2008). *Sport Nutrition for Health and Performance.* Champaign, IL: Human Kinetics.

[23] Casa, D. J., Clarkson, P.M., Roberts, W.O. (2005). American College of Sports Medicine roundtable on hydration and physical activity: consensus statements. *Current Sports Medicine Reports,* 4, 115-127.

[24] Montain, S.J. (2008). Hydration recommendations for sport. *Current Sports and Medicine Report,* 7(4), 187-192.

[25] American College of Sports Medicine (2007). ACSM Position Stand on Exercise and Fluid Replacement. *Medicine Science and Sports Exercise,* 39(2), 377-390.

[26] Maughan, R.J., Merson, S.J., Broad, N.P., Shirreffs, S.M. (2004). Fluid and electroyte intake and loss in elite soccer players during training. *International Journal of Sport Nutrition and Exercise Metabolism,* 14(3), 333-346.

[27] Shirreffs, S. M., Aragon-Vargas, L.F., Chamorro, M., Maughan, R.J., Serratosa, L. Zachwieja, J.J. (2005). The sweating response of elite professional soccer players to training in the heat. *International Journal of Sports Medicine,* 26, 90-95.

[28] Martarelli, D., Ugoccioni, F., Stauffacher, F., Spataro, A., Cocchioni, M., Pompei, P. (2009). Assessment of body fluid balance and voluntary drinking in ultimate players during a match. *Journal of Sports Medicine and Physical Fitness, 49(3),* 265-271.

[29] Batchelder, B.C., Krause, B.A., Seegmiller, J.G., Starkey, C.A. (2010= Gastrointestinal temperature increases and hypohydration exists after collegiate men's ice hockey participation. *Journal of Strength and Condition Research, 24(1),* 68-73.

[30] MacLeod, H., Sunderland, C. (2009). Fluid balance and hydration habits of elite male field hockey players during consecutive international matches. *Journal of Strength and Condition Research, 23(4),* 1245-1251.

[31] Aragón-Vargas, L.F., Moncada-Jiménez, J., Hernández-Elizondo, J., Barrenechea, A., Monge-Alvarado, M. (2009). Evaluation of pre-game hydration status, heat stress, and fluid balance during professional soccer competition in the heat. *European Journal of Sport Science,* 9(5), 269-276.

[32] Hernández, J. (2001). Análisis de los parámetros espacio y tiempo en el fútbol sala. La distancia recorrida, el ritmo y dirección del desplazamiento del jugador durante un encuentro de competición. *Apunts: Educación Física y Deportes, 65,* 32-44.

[33] Norton, K., Whittinghan, N., Carter, L., Kerr, D., Gore, C., y Marfell-Jones, M (1996). Measurement techniques in anthropometry. In: K. Norton y T. Olds (Eds.), *Antropométrica.* Sydney: Editorial UNSW.

[34] Martins, M., Aparecida, J., Kleverson, J., Works, R.H., Wagner, R, Bohn, J.H., Coppi, A. (2007). The corporal dehydration of amateur athletes of futsal. *Revista Brasileira de Prescrição e Fisiologia do Exercício,* 1(5), 24-36.

[35] Barbero, J.C., Soto, V.M., Barbero, V., Granda-Vera, J. (2008). Match analysis and heart rate of futsal players during competition. *Journal of Sports Science and Medicine,* 126(1): 63-73.

[36] Castagna, C., D'Ottavio, S., Granda-Vera, J., Barbero, J.C. (2009). Match demands of proffesional futsal: a case study. *Journal of Science and Medicine in Sport,* 12(4): 490-494.

[37] Hamouti, N., Estévez, E., Del Coso, J., Mora, R. (2007). Fluid balance and sweat sodium concentration in elite indoor team sport players during training. Presented at 12th Annual Congress of the ECSS, 11-14 July 2007, Jyvâskylâ, Finland.

[38] Schröder, H., Navarro, E., Mora, H., Seco, J., Torregrosa, J.M., Tramullas, A. (2004). Dietary habits and fluid intake of a group of elite Spanish basketball players: a need for professional advice? *European Journal of Sport Science,* 4(2), 1-15.

Overweight and Physical Activity as a Measure of Age at Menarche in Females

Ajita, Jiwanjot*

Department of Sports Science, Punjabi University, Patiala, Punjab
*Corresponding author: millibrar@gmail.com

Abstract The present study is conducted on 62 girls, out of which 31 girls belong to physically active group with a training age of 8.95 years and 31 girls are from physically inactive group considered as control group. The girls were evaluated for their decimal age, age at menarche, height, weight body fat percentage and BMI. The body mass index and body fat percentages were significantly correlated and an inverse correlation was found. The higher body mass index, the lower was the age at menarche. The physically inactive girls were overweight and also early mature. The age of menarche of physically active girls was significantly delayed as compared to their inactive counterparts.

Keywords: *physical activity, BMI, body fat, menarche*

1. Introduction

With the advancement of technology, there is an increase in the physical inactivity towards every section of society including children also. It has been observed that they have been declining their habitual physical activity even. As a result of which there are certain changes in response to attainment of their growth markers, the very important of which is attainment of puberty. (Mathur and Toriala. 1982; Moisan et al, 1991 and Lalys and Pineau, 2014). In females, age at menarche is very important biological marker to assess the sexual maturation or in other words adolescence. Adolescence growth periods extents for 2.5 to 3 years and it include-Height gain, Weight gain and increase in body fat percentage. (Sidhu and Grewal, 1980; Rokade and Mane, 2009 and Warren,1980). Menarche may be stimulated by attainment of critical weight. According to Frisch(1970) menarche occurs when a girl attain desired body fat a minimum of 17% of body weight is necessary for onset of menarche. It may also occur when enough gonadotropin hormones are released from the pituitary and hypothalamus. Physical activity is also very important parameter to be considered for age at menarche. Research has reported that there is delay in menarche in athletes due to inherent physique, imbalance between energy intake and output and disordered eating habits. (Cavadini et al, 2000, Chang Shu-Hui et al, 2000 and Malina et al, 1973). Body weight, BMI and body composition of a subject are also very important parameters reported in literature to influence the age at menarche (A-Awadhi et al, 2013; Banergee et al, 2007; Deo and Gattorgi, 2004 Lin-Su et al, 2002 and Mohammad et al, 2013). Thus the present study aims to evaluate the age at menarche in physically active and non active girls and to evaluate their relationship with BMI and body composition.

2. Materials and Methods

The study was conducted on 31 physically active and 31 non active girls belonging to Punjabi University Patiala. The data was calculated for age (decimal age), height (cms) and Weight (Kgs). The body mass index was calculated by using formula:

$$\text{Body Mass Index} = \frac{\text{Body Weight (Kg)}}{\text{Height (m)}}$$

Body fat percentage was calculated using four skinfold method. Body density was calculated using biceps, triceps, suprailiac and subscapular skinfold using Durnin and Womersley (1974) method and percent body fat was calculated using Brozek et al (1963) method.

Using the retrospective method, the age of menarche was calculated. It was taken through questionnaire. The entire data were computed statistically using SPSS.

3. Results

In the present study, total 62 girls were studied, out of which 31 girls were physically non active and considered as control group and 31 were physically active belonging to different sportive events with their mean training age of 8.95 years. Table 1 shows the mean and SD values of the decimal age and menarcheal age of the subjects. It has been observed that although there is not statistically significant difference in mean values of their decimal ages of both the groups but the results of the present study shows a difference in the mean ages at menarche in them and it is clear that the non active girls (control group girls) are early maturer as compared to their physically active counterparts and the t-values shows that this difference is statistically significant. The present study although small in number but strongly agree with the previous studies of age at menarche in athletes. (Stager, 1988 and Sidhu and Grewal, 1980).

Table 1. Mean and SD values of decimal age and menarcheal age of the control group and physically active group

Parameters	Control Group (mean ± SD)	Physically Active Girls (mean ± SD)	t-value
Decimal age (yrs)	17.67 ± 1.36	17.53 ± 1.88	0.343
Menarcheal Age (yrs)	13.053 ± 0.44	13.98 ± 0.496	7.78***
Training age (yrs)	--------	8.95 ± 2.99	-----

***significant at 0.05 level

Table 2 & Table 3 shows the mean and SD values of height, weight, body fat percentage, total body fat and lean body mass of the subjects. It is clear from the results that the subjects of both the groups are of same height and the t values shows that the difference their mean height is not statistically significant. The physically inactive girls were overweight and their BMI index is towards higher range and it is also observed that the difference in body weight as well as BMI index is statistically significant with their physically active counterparts. Similar results were observed for mean values of Body fat percentage which also shows a higher range in case of physically inactive girls as compared to their physically active counterparts and the difference is again statistically significant. Table 4 shows the correlation of age at menarche with body mass index and body fat percentage which shows a positive correlation of age at menarche with that of body mass index and body fat percentage.

Table 2. Mean and SD values of Height (cms), Weight (Kg) and BMI (Body Mass Index) of the control group and physically active group

Parameters	Control Group (mean ± SD)	Physically Active Girls (mean ± SD)	t-value
Height (cms)	158.96 ± 4.41	158.72 ± 5.77	0.1844
Weight (Kgs)	58.35 ± 3.70	49.22 ± 6.87	36.52***
BMI	23.12 ± 1.78	19.47 ± 1.92	7.76***

**** significant at 0.05 level.

Table 3. Mean and SD values of Percentage Body Fat, total body fat and lean body mass of the control group and physically active group

Parameters	Control Group (mean ± SD)	Physically Active Girls (mean ± SD)	t-value
Body Fat percentage	21.4 ± 1.68	19.68 ± 2.31	3.38***
Total Body Fat (Kgs)	12.52 ± 1.314	9.75 ± 1.53	7.67***
LBM (kgs)	45.83 ± 3.001	39.977 ± 5.22	5.58***

***significant at 0.05 level

Table 4. Correlation of age at menarche with percentage Body Fat, Body mass Index of the control group and physically active group

Parameters	Control group	Physically active girls
Age at menarche vs BMI	0.25	0.29
Age at menarche vs Body fat %	-0.15	-0.18

4. Discussion

In the present study conducted in Punjabi University Patiala, Punjab it can be concluded that the correlation between BMI and age at menarche is quite high and it is the most important factor to be considered to show its impact on menarche. It can also be concluded that although the timing of puberty is related to the genetic factors, other factors such as geographical location, common health status, nutrition and socioeconomic status but all such factors are also related to the body fat and body weight of the subject thus they can influence the onset of menstruation and its progression. However, the age at menarche reported by the results of the present study for physically inactive girls is (13.05yrs) which is higher than the results available in literature. It may be contributed to the fact that there are other factors also which influence age at menarche and secular trends has also been observed by various studies available in literature (Lalys and Pineau, 2014).

The results of the present study are in agreement with that of a large study (Mandel et al, 2004) in a different population, which found an inverse correlation with BMI. The relationship between BMI and pubertal development in girls appears to be a continuum. However later on and other observations (Bralic et al, 2012; Currie C et al, 2012; Oh CM et al, 2012 & Wronka, 2010) also reported the same findings. As BMI increases through adolescence, it would be an incorrect assumption to extrapolate BMI data in adult life back to the time of menarche. We did not enquire about premature thelarche as a cause of early menarche, although it can be safely assumed that the numbers of such girls were likely to be reassuringly low.

We have used BMI as an index of body fat mass. Although a reasonable tool to estimate adiposity in the community, it is only a ratio and therefore an abstract index. One must therefore exert a degree of caution in its interpretation. Nevertheless, the use of BMI as a surrogate marker of body fat is a more refined method than simple weight measurement, which is liable to be influenced by stature. The influence of body weight on age is contentious. While inadequately balanced diets tend to delay menarche, early and late maturing girls achieved menarche at similar body weights (Frisch and Revelle, 1971), suggesting a critical weight dependency for menarche. Further it has been reported that puberty onset may be related to attainment of a particular height and weight, but that a minimum age requirement must also be met.

5. Conclusion

On the basis of the results of the present study, it can be concluded that Body mass index and Body fat percentage are significantly related to age at menarche. Higher the body mass index lower the age at menarche. The findings add to the evidence that overweight and higher body fat percentage values are contributing factors for early puberty

References

[1] Al-Awadhi N., Al-Kandari N, Al-Hasan T, Almurjan D, Ali S, Al-Taiar A. *Age at menarche and its relationship to body mass index*

among adolescent girls in Kuwait. BMC Public Health, 2013, 12, 13:29.

[2] Bralic I, Tahirovic H, Matanic D, Vrdoljak O, Stojanovic S, Kovacic V, Blazekovic-Milakovic S *Association of early menarche age and overweight/obesity.* J Pediatr Endocrinol Metab. 2012, 25(1-2)57-62.

[3] Banerjee, I., Chakraborty, S., Bhattacharya, N.G., Bandopadhyay, S., Saiyed, H. N., Mukherjee, D. A. *Cohort study of correlation between body mass index and age at menarche in healthy Bengali girls.* J. Ind. Med. Asso. 2007, 105(2): 75-8.

[4] Cavadini, C., Decarli, B., Grim, J., Narring, F., Michand, P.A. *Food habits and sport activity during adolescence: difference between athletic and non-athletic teenagers in Switzerland.* Euro. J. Clin. Nut., 54, Suppl, 2000, 1:516-520.

[5] Chang Shu-Hui, Tzang Shun-Jia, Chang Jung – Yu, chei wei-chu. *Height and weight change across menarche of school girls with early menarche.* Arch Pediatr. Adolescent Med. 2000; 154:880-884.

[6] Curie C, Ahluwalia N, Godeau E, Nic Gabhainn S, Due P and Currie D B. *Is obesity at individual and National level associated with lower age at menarche? Evidence from 34 countries in the Health Behaviour in School-aged children study.* J Adolesc Health, 2012, 50(6): 621-6.

[7] Deo, D.S. and Gattorgi C.H. *Age at Menarche and Associated factors.* Ind. J. Pediatr. 2004:71.

[8] Frisch R, Mc Arthur. *Menstrual cycle: Fatness as determinant of minimum weight for height necessary for the maintenance of onset.* Science. 1974, 185: 949-203.

[9] Lalys L and Pineau JC. *Age at menarche in French population of young school- girls.* Paediatr Int. 2014, 10(1111/ped-12296).

[10] Lin-Su, K., Vogiatzi, M.G., New, M.I. *Body mass index and age at menarche in an adolescent clinic population.*Clin.Pediatr.,2002, 41:501-507.

[11] Malina, R. M., Harper, A. B., Avent, H.H. and Campbell, D. E. *Age of menarche in athletes and non-athletes.* Med. Sc. Sport, 1973,5:11-3.

[12] Mandel D, Zimlichman E, Mimouni FB, Grott O I, Kreiss Y. *Age at menarche and body mass index: a population study.* J. Padiatric Endocrinol Metab; 2004, 17(11):1507-10.

[13] Mathur, N. D., Toriala, L. A.. *Age at Menarche in Nigerian athletes.* Br. J. Sports Med., 1982. 16:250-252.

[14] Mohamad K, Jamshidi L. and Nouri J K. *Is age at menarche related with Body Mass Index.* Iranian J Publ Health. 2013, 42(9):1043-1048.

[15] Moisan, J., Meyer, F., Gingras, S. *Leisure physical activity and age at menarche.* Med. Sci. Sports Exerc., 1991, 23(10): 1170-5(s).

[16] Oh C M, Oh I H, Choi K S, Chol B K, Yoon T Y and Choi J M. *Relationship between body mass index and early menarche of adolescent girls in Seoul.* J Prev Med Public Health. 2012, 45(4): 227-34.

[17] Pehan A, Moghaddam H Y, Najjor L and Akaberi A. *The relationship between menarche age and anthropometric indices of girls in Sabzevar,* Iran. J Pak Med assoc, 2013, 63(1):81-4.

[18] Rajeev A. *Correlation of Body Mass index and total body fat with physical activity patterns in adolescents.* Int J Diabetes Dev Ctries. 2009. 29(3):139-142.

[19] Rokade, A. S., Mane, K. A. *A study of Age at Menarche, The Secular trend and factors associated with it.* The Int. J. Bio. Anthrop. 2009, 1939-459.

[20] Rosenfield RL, Lipton RB and Drum ML. *Thelarche, Pubarche and menarche attainment in children with normal and elevated body mass index.* Pediatrics. 2009, 123(4):1255.

[21] Sidhu, L.S. and Grewal, R. *Age at menarche in various categories of Indian sports women.* Brit. Jour. Sports Med: 1980, 199-203.

[22] Talma H, Schonbeck Y, Van Dommelen P, Bakker B, van Buuren S, Hirasing R A. *Trends in menarcheal age between 1955 and 2009 in Netherlands.* 2013, PLoS One.

[23] Warren, M.P. *The effect of exercise on pubertal progression and reproduction in girls.* Clin.Endocrinol. Metab., 1980, 51:1150-1156.

[24] Wronka I. *Association between BMI and age at menarche in girls from different socio-economic groups.* Anthropol Anz. 2010, 68 (1):43-52.

[25] Zegeye, D. T., Megabam, B., Mulu, A. *Age at menarche and the menstrual pattern of secondary school adolscents in north west Ethiopia.* BMC Women's Health, 2009, 9: 29.

37

Inhibitory Effect of the Kinesio Taping® Method on the Gastrocnemius Muscle

Elizabeth A. Davison[1], Christopher T. Anderson[1], Blake H. Ponist[1], Drew M. Werner[1], Mary E. Jacobs[1], Adam J. Thompson[1,*], Melissa R. Cook[2]

[1]Athletic Training Education, Indiana Wesleyan University, Marion, 46953, USA
[2]Exercise Science, Indiana Wesleyan University, Marion, 46953, USA
*Corresponding author: adam.thompson@indwes.edu

Abstract The Kinesio Taping® method has been studied widely for its claims as a therapeutic taping technique designed to enhance performance and treat a variety of orthopedic, neuromuscular, neurological and other medical conditions. The applications of the Kinesio Taping® method are numerous and this intervention offers a broad range of research inquiry into its effectiveness. This study focuses on the performance benefits of the application of the Kinesio Taping® method. Specific attention was given to the inhibitory effects of the tape application on the gastrocnemius muscle group. Taping for muscle inhibition is indicated when a muscle is overactive as seen in muscular spasm. This study found that the Kinesio Taping® method was effective in inhibiting the muscle activity of the gastrocnemius muscle group without decreasing the performance output of the participants. This is clinically significant for clinicians who are progressing return to activity in patients who are recovering from a lower extremity injury, but still have some functional limitations from their injury. **Purpose:** This research study attempted to determine the effect of Kinesio® Tex Gold™ Tape on muscle inhibition when the tape is externally applied to a muscle group. **Method:** The participating athletes were measured by a Vertec© vertical jump device to determine height jumped as well as the BIOPAC Systems, Inc. (Goleta, CA) MP150 electromyography (EMG) machine to determine the amount of muscular activity. The participants were asked to complete nine single leg jumps on their dominant leg before being taped with Kinesio® Tex Gold™ Tape. The initial three jumps were performed as a warm-up, three more were performed while using the Vertec© to measure jump height, and the final three were performed while attached to the EMG machine to measure electrical activity in the gastrocnemius muscle group. After the initial jumps, each participant's dominant calf was then taped with Kinesio® Tex Gold™ Tape. The tape was applied from insertion to origin to test the inhibitory effects of the Kinesio® Tex Gold™ Tape. After the tape was applied, each participant completed six more maximal vertical jumps on their dominant leg. The first three jumps measured muscular activity, and the last three jumps measured vertical jump height. **Results:** EMG results demonstrated a significant decrease in electrical activity. Electrical activity decreased for 20 participants (74%) while it increased for 7 participants (26%). The decrease in electrical activity found was (t (26) = 2.551, p = .017). The results of the vertical jump test using the Vertec© showed that in the 27 participants, 52% showed an increase in vertical jump height after the Kinesio® Tex Gold™ Tape was applied, 37% showed a decrease in vertical jump height after the application of the tape, and 11% of the participants had no change in vertical jump height. No significant difference was found in the vertical jump height between the without tape and with tape trials (t (26) = -1.120, p = .273). **Conclusion:** Based on this research, it can be concluded there is statistical evidence to show a difference in muscle activity after application of Kinesio® Tex Gold™ Tape. The values obtained from the EMG showed a majority of the participants had a decrease in muscle activity during a single leg vertical jump after being taped. The data found during the study supports the inhibitory basic application technique [2].

Keywords: *Kinesio Taping®, vertical jump, muscle activation, muscle inhibition*

1. Introduction

Created by Dr. Kenzo Kase in the 1970's in Japan, the Kinesio Taping® method eventually made it to the United States in the 1990's. It gained greater worldwide recognition after appearing in the 2008 Olympic Games held in Beijing, China [1]. According to Dr. Kenzo Kase, the Kinesio Taping® method provides multi-day benefits for approximately 3 to 4 days. It can treat orthopedic or neuromuscular conditions, dependent upon the application process [2].

There are many proposed effects which can be gained from using the Kinesio Taping® method. The Kinesio®

Tex Gold™ Tape can be used to normalize muscle function, improve lymphatic and blood flow, reduce pain, correct joint misalignment, and improve proprioception [3]. With the over 1200 recognized applications, there has been proven effects on the following body parts and systems after being applied with Kinesio® Tex Gold™ Tape: skin, fascia, muscles, ligaments, tendons, joints, lymphatic system, and circulatory system [4]. Numerous professional sports such as football, baseball, basketball, cycling, soccer, golf, and tennis use the Kinesio Taping® method [4]. It is designed to be used alongside other treatments such as manual therapy, modalities, and therapeutic exercises [4].

The tape is made of 100% high grade cotton and is latex free. The hypoallergenic tape is heat activated [4]. The thickness of the tape is designed to replicate the thickness of the epidermis. Because of these properties, a single application of tape can remain in place for 3-4 days. It can be worn while bathing, or even swimming. The tape, while still on the paper wrapping, is approximately on a 25% stretch. It is capable of being stretched to 35-40% of its overall resting length. This design allows it to replicate the stretch of muscles and skin. Lastly, a certain amount of stretch/tension must be correctly applied to meet the desired needs. Basic applications require the tape to be applied on a muscle while it is in a stretched position. The stretch of the muscle along with the stretch in the tape may cause convulsions in the skin [2]. It is suggested that these convulsions cause microscopic lifting of the skin which aids in blood and lymphatic flow. These effects help to decrease pain by lifting pressure off the pain receptors [3].

The tape can be applied using various shapes, such as an "I", "Y", "X", "fan", "web", and "donut". The "Y" technique is the most common used when facilitation or inhibition of a muscle is desired. The base of the "Y" is applied approximately 2 inches beyond the origin or insertion of the muscle, depending on the desired effect. The tails of the "Y" are then applied in a fashion that surrounds the muscle. The treatment of muscles typically involves taping from either the origin to the insertion, or the insertion to the origin. When taping from the origin to the insertion, the tape facilitates the muscle. For muscle spasms or over used muscles, the muscle would be taped from insertion to origin to inhibit muscle function. In this approach, the tape is applied at 15-25% tension, or paper-off tension [2].

This study used the "Y" strip application to inhibit the gastrocnemius muscle. With this method, the validity of the inhibitory effect of Kinesio® Tex Gold™ Tape could be measured.

Measurements of single leg countermovement vertical jump height were gathered with the use of the Vertec© (Sports Imports, Hilliard, Ohio) stationary tool used to measure overall vertical height. This assisted in determining if an inhibitory effect would or would not have a direct impact on functional performance. The final component of the study was incorporating the use of the EMG machine, which measures the electrical activity of the muscle. This tool determined the extent to which the Kinesio Taping® method affected the decrease in activity of the target muscle.

2. Methods

2.1. Participants

This research study was conducted with 27 healthy varsity athletes on various athletic teams at an undergraduate institution. The participants' ages ranged from 18 to 23 years. The 21 female and 6 males who participated are approximately 10% of the student athlete population. The following sports were represented: men's and women's track & field, men's and women's basketball, men's and women's soccer, women's cheerleading and volleyball. No subjects had recently participated in high intensity workouts prior to their participation in the study. None of the participants involved in the study had a recent history of lower extremity injury or impairment.

2.2. Procedures

Before participating in the study, the athletes were informed on the process of the experiment and asked to sign an informed consent form approved by the Human Subjects Review Board of the above mentioned undergraduate institution.

All subjects were instructed to perform 3 maximum single leg countermovement jumps on their dominant leg. These jumps were used as a warm-up to familiarize the participants with the testing protocol. Participants then completed three more countermovement maximal vertical jumps on their dominant leg while using the Vertec© to measure the jump height in inches. The height of each jump was recorded individually and then were later averaged. The participants executed 3 additional single leg jumps while connected to the EMG machine to measure muscle activity of the gastrocnemius. Prior to electrode placement, each participant's skin was shaved, abraded and wiped with an alcohol pad to increase conductivity. Bipolar surface electrodes (Model #EL503, BioPac Systems, Inc., Goleta, Ca.) were placed on the skin superficially to the medial and lateral gastrocnemius muscle bellies and the ground lead was attached to the medial malleolus according to the Clinical SEMG Electrode Sites [6] (see Figure 1).

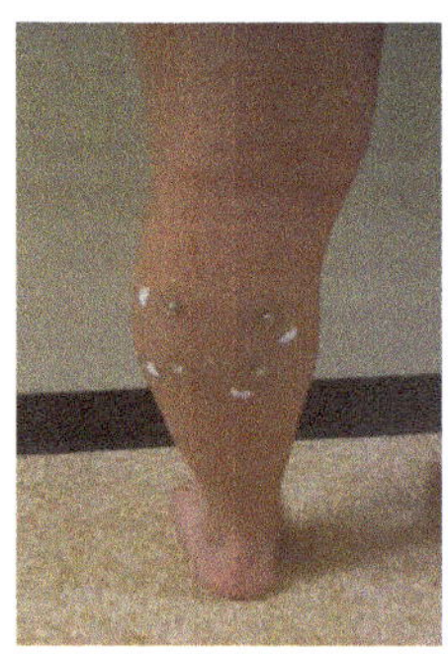

Figure 1. Electrode Placement

The EMG signal was collected on the BioPac MP150 and the gains were set for the TEL 100 transmitter at 2K with a filter of 0.5 Hz. The EMG signal was sampled at 1000 Hz, amplified (analogue differential amplifier, common mode rejection ration >110 dB, total gain 412, noise <0.1μV), analogue –to-digital converted (16-bit) using the AcqKnowledge 4.1 Software (BioPac Systems,

Inc., Goleta, Ca.) [6] and stored in a personal computer for later analysis. No EMG normalization procedures were included in this study's methodology. Participants were then instructed to complete 3 maximal jumps while attached to the EMG machine.

Following those 3 jumps, Kinesio® Tex Gold™ Tape was applied. Kinesio® Tex Gold™ Tape was applied on the dominant leg using a "Y" strip to the gastrocnemius muscle according to the standards of the Kinesio Taping® Lower Extremity Work Book (2) [3]. Participants were instructed to lay prone in a relaxed position on an examination table with the foot hanging off the table. The tape was measured from base of the calcaneus to the middle of the popliteal fossa (Figure 2a). An additional 2 inches was added to the measurement as is standard when using a "Y" strip (Figure 2b).

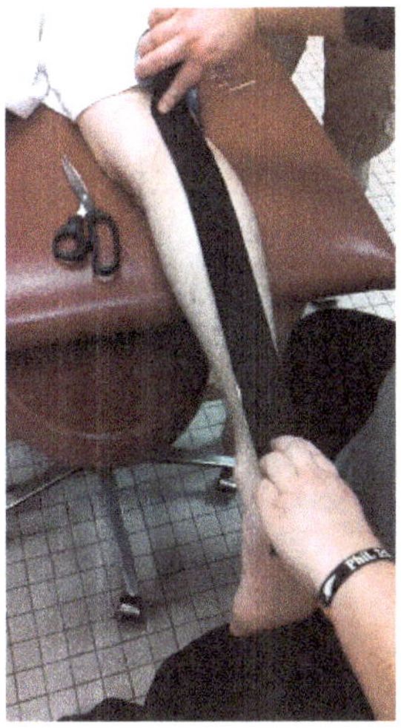

Figure 2a. Step 1: Measure tape length and apply base

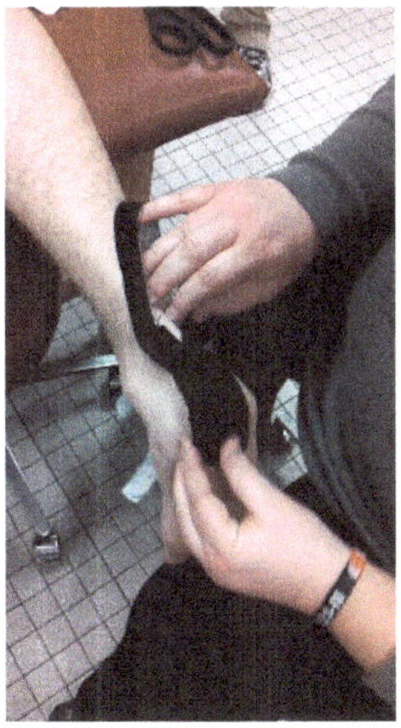

Figure 2b. Step 2: Cut Medial and Lateral Strips

A "Y" strip was cut. The base was applied on the plantar surface of the calcaneus and was rubbed to activate adhesion. The Certified Kinesio Taping Practitioner (CKTPs) then pushed the foot into end range passive dorsiflexion. The tails of the tape were applied with paper off tension to surround the medial and lateral bellies of the gastrocnemius (Figure 3a & Figure 3b). The medial and lateral tails ended approximately at the femoral condyles (Figure 4). The tails were then rubbed to activate the adhesive.

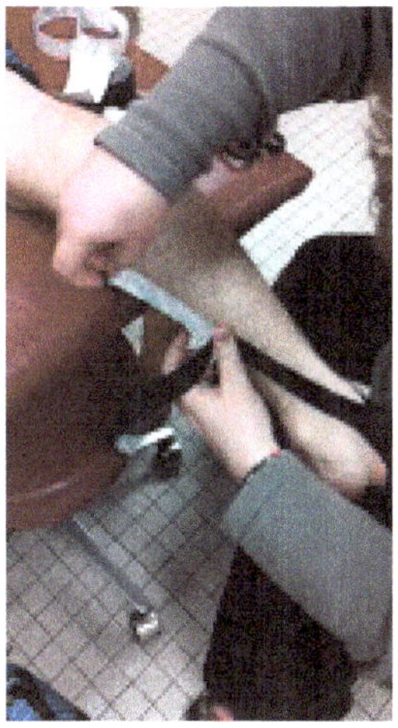

Figure 3a. Step 3: Apply Medial Strip

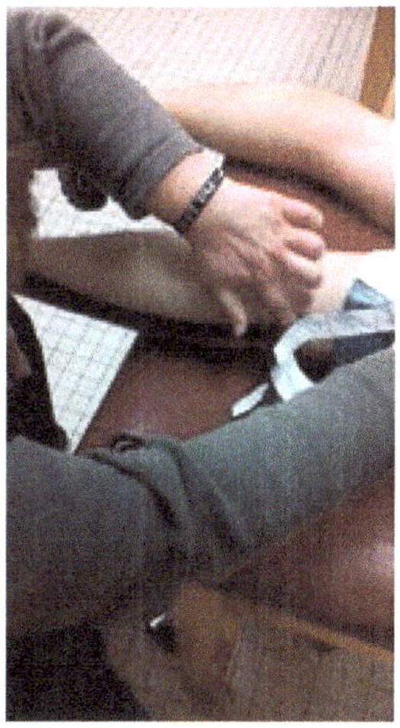

Figure 3b. Step 4: Apply Lateral Strip

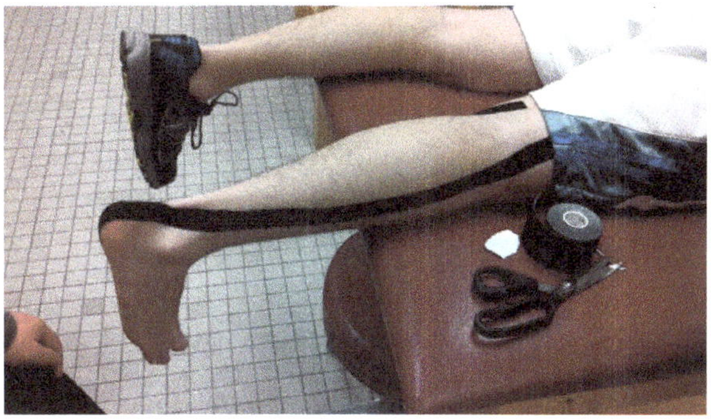

Figure 4. Step 5: Final product/Activate adhesive by rubbing down tape

After 10 minutes, the participants were then reattached to the EMG machine and instructed to perform 3 more jumps under the previous conditions. Participants completed both sets of jumps with electrodes attached consecutively to prevent electrodes from losing conductivity. Finally, the athletes were disconnected from the EMG and performed their final 3 maximal countermovement vertical jumps with the tape applied and using the Vertec© to measure each jump height

2.2. EMG Processing

The raw EMG data from the medial and lateral gastrocnemius were processed by AcqKnowledge

Software[7]. The raw EMG signal was filtered using a band-pass between 10 and 500 Hz, and then the signal was full-wave rectified with a Root Mean Square (RMS) with the time interval set to 30 milliseconds. For this study the time began as the EMG signal exceeded the baseline. The pre-flight phase of jumps 1, 2, and 3 were evaluated separately in order to determine the values of total time length (< 1 sec.) of the pre-flight phase and the total amount of muscle activity or area under the curve (Graph 1). The same process was used to analyze the time of contraction and pre-flight muscle activity of the 3 jumps before and after the Kinesio® Tex Gold™ Tape was applied to the athletes' gastrocnemius (Graph 2) [7]. The EMG activity of the medial and lateral gastrocnemius was only analyzed during the pre-flight phase. The muscle activity for the 3 without tape jumps were averaged, and the same was done for the with tape jumps. The results were recorded in a separate Excel spreadsheet. All data are presented as mean and standard deviations for vertical jump (Graphs 3 and 4) and muscle activity (Graphs 6 and 7). Differences between the means in the vertical jump height and muscle activity for the without tape and with tape jumps were analyzed with a paired samples t-test. The Statistical Package for Social Sciences (SPSS) was used for statistical analysis, with the level for significance being set at 0.05.

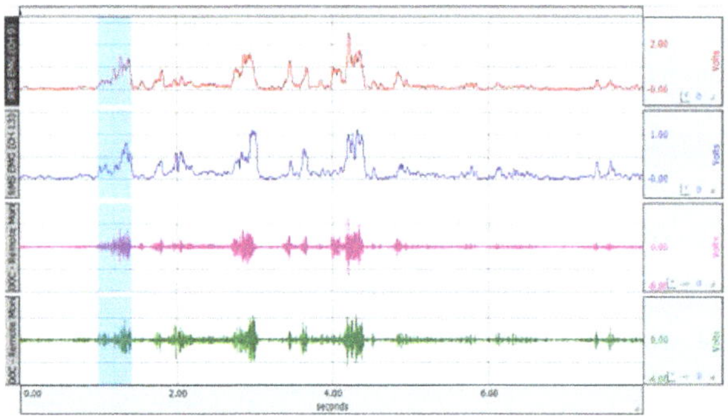

Graph 1. An example of BIOPAC Systems, Inc. MP150 EMG results for athlete without the application of Kinesio® Tex Tape (Jump 1 pre-flight)

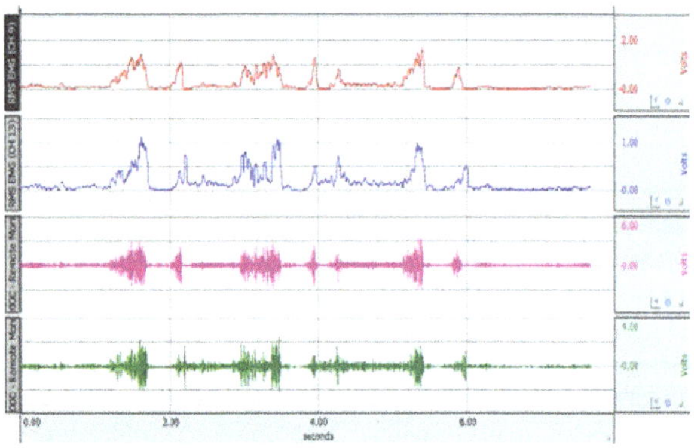

Graph 2. An example of BIOPAC Systems, Inc. MP150 EMG results for athlete with the application of Kinesio® Tex Tape

3. Results

The three vertical jumps with and without tape measured by the Vertec© were averaged. A paired-samples *t* test was calculated to compare the mean vertical jump height without tape to the mean with tape score. The mean vertical jump score without tape was 14.40 in. (sd = 3.14) and the mean on the with tape was 14.62 in. (sd = 3.35) (Graph 3). No significant difference from without tape to with tape was found (t (26) = -1.120, p = .273). The vertical jump test revealed no significant change of height jumped with or without the athlete being taped (Graph 4).

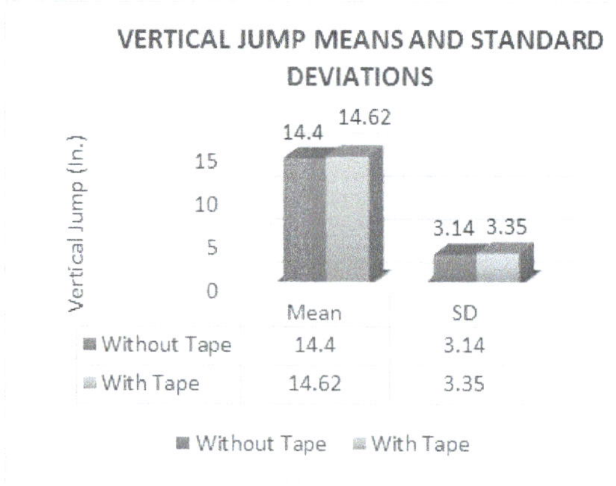

Graph 3. Results of the Vertical Jump Height

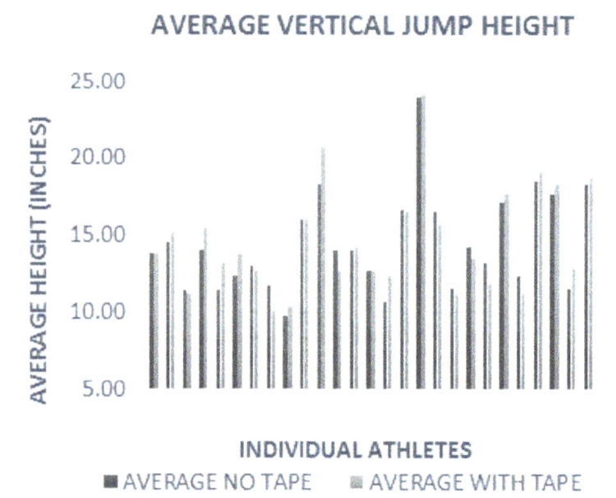

Graph 4. Individual Results of the Vertical Jump Height with/without tape

Individually, 74% (20 participants) showed a decrease in muscle activity with the Kinesio® Tex Gold™ Tape applied; while 26% (7 participants) showed an increase in muscle activity (Graph 5).

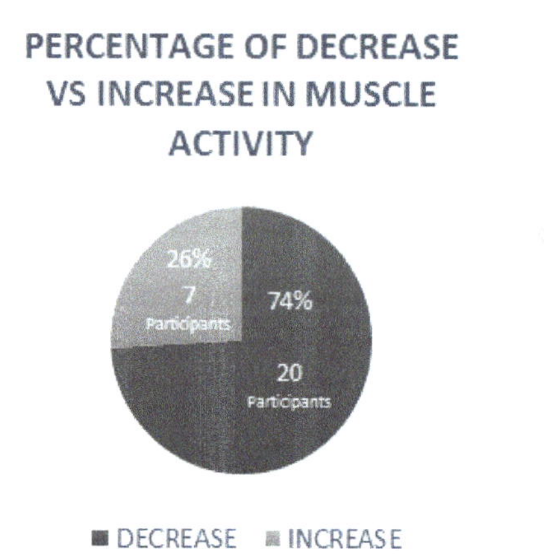

Graph 5. Percentage of Participants who Increased vs. Decreased in Amount of Muscle Activity

The without tape and with tape EMG results were analyzed and compared. The values of the medial and lateral gastrocnemius were combined for each athlete to better understand total gastrocnemius activity. A paired-samples t test was calculated to compare the mean muscle activity without tape to the mean with tape score. The mean muscle activity without tape was 0.8737 mv/s (sd = 0.274) and the mean on the with tape was 0.8044 mv/s (sd = 0.215) (Graphs 6 and 7). A significant decrease from without tape to with tape was found (t (26) = 3.263, p =.017).

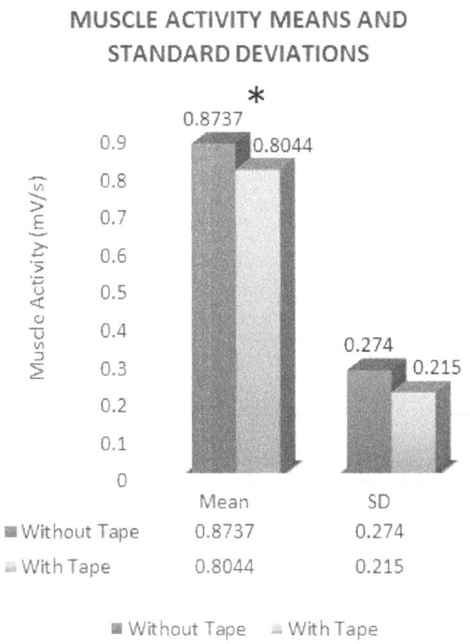

Graph 6. Results of the Muscle Activity; * p< 0.05

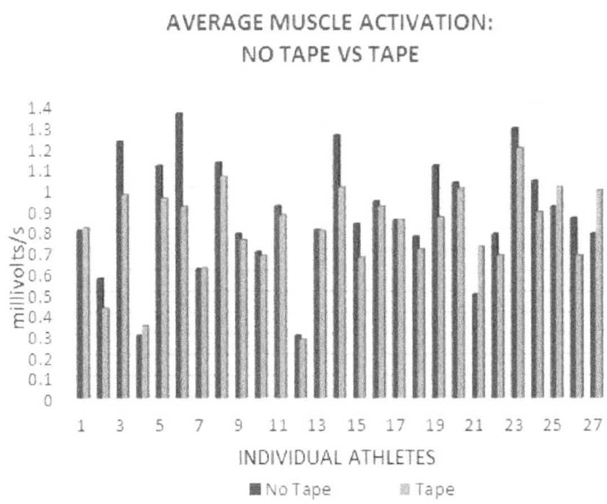

Graph 7. Individual Results of the Muscle Activity with and without tape

4. Discussion

Based on this study, differences were observed between jumps when participants were taped and when they were not taped. The results of the jump height measured by the Vertec© showed half of the participants' jump height increased, but the data collected by the EMG showed muscle activity decreased. When taped, the increased vertical jump heights could have been a result of learned gains and familiarity [8].

This study was designed to investigate the validity of Kinesio® Tex Gold™ Tape to inhibit muscular activity in the gastrocnemius. The data appears to support claims of the Clinical

Therapeutic Applications of the Kinesio Taping® Method (2nd edition), which states the desired outcome for the insertion to origin tape technique is inhibition of a muscle. According to the manual, "For acutely over-used or stretched muscles, the tape is applied from insertion to origin to inhibit muscle function [2]." Many believe that applying an external aid (taping, bracing, etc.) cannot affect an internal pathology. The findings of this study did not wholly agree with existing research on this topic and research methodology. Janwantanakul and Gaogasigam's study showed there were no significant differences in EMG activity of the vastus lateralis and vastus medialus during the application of inhibition and facilitation tapes when compared with no tape condition [9].

The EMG data comparing without tape and with tape jumps contradict other studies which have come to the conclusion of tape not having a significant effect on muscle activity. According to the study by Cools, Witvrouw, Danneels, and Cambier, tape had no major impact on EMG activity in muscles of the shoulder girdle in subjects with good overall health [10]. A study by Lumbroso, Ziv, Vered, and Kalichman looked at the force production in the gastrocnemius and hamstring groups while being taped with the Kinesio Taping® method to inhibit muscle activity. They measured force production 15 minutes after application and again 48 hours after application. They found a significant increase in force production of the muscles 48 hours after the initial tape application [11].

A separate study looked at the effects of facilitating muscle function for vertical jump by using the lateral ankle sprain taping technique by Dr. Kenzo Kase. They had experimental and control groups of participants, the experimental group's tape was applied with 140% of its maximal length and the controls group's tape was applied with paper off tension. Participant's maximal vertical jump was measured for a pre-test, post-test, and 24 hours after tape application. This study found no significant difference in the heights jumped over the three trial periods [12].

The data collected in this study shows that the application of the Kinesio® Tex Gold™ Tape did have a significant effect on electrical activity of the gastrocnemius muscle. As a result, it appears that the insertion to origin taping technique does inhibit the ability for the taped muscle to function fully. It toned down the muscle activity but not enough to have a functional related difference. The vertical height showed no significant different between the without and with tape measurements. Other muscles may have helped to compensate for the "turning down" of the gastrocnemius, resulting in no significant change in the height jumped.

It is important to note the study tested healthy, uninjured college-aged athletes. The Kinesio Taping® manual states that it is designed to inhibit the activity in either an over-used or over stretched muscle, which already have decreased stimulus [2]. It appears the Kinesio® Tex Gold™ Tape may also have the ability to inhibit the activity in a healthy, uninjured muscle.

5. Conclusion

Based on this research, it can be concluded there is statistical evidence to show a difference in muscle activity after application of Kinesio® Tex Gold™ Tape. The values obtained from the EMG show a majority of the participants did have a decrease in muscle activity during a single leg vertical jump after being taped. The data found during the study supports the inhibitory basic application technique [2].

Future studies could focus on the effects facilitation techniques can have on muscle activity for possible performance enhancement. Also, other research can take a more in depth approach of studying the inhibitory taping technique. This can be done by looking at more participants, using a force plate to measure vertical ground reaction force, using intramuscular EMG electrodes, and wearing the tape for a longer period of time before testing. Having a control and a placebo group may help to find a greater change in statistical evidence. A study could divide participants in half, testing the inhibitory effect on half the participants and the effects of facilitating muscle function on the other half.

This study could have been limited by the small percentage of student athletes tested. Athletes from a variety of sports may have distorted data collection in the study. Different performance demands and training methods for each sport could affect the ratio or use of slow twitch and fast twitch muscle fibers. Athletes may have been worn out from doing several maximal vertical jumps within a limited period of time. An alternate warm-up such as biking could have been used to limit the number of jumps being performed. In order to make sure learned effect had no influence on the jump height or muscle activity, the group could have been split in half. Half of the group could have performed the tests with tape first, and then performed the tests without tape and vice versa for the second group.

Additionally, many studies relating to the Kinesio Taping® method are published in other languages. While not insurmountable, this does create a barrier in the investigative process. Many studies are case studies which lack a control group and are performed on healthy patients, similar to this study. Lastly, many studies perform evaluation and collect data immediately after application of the Kinesio Taping® method.

Acknowledgements

The researchers would also like to acknowledge all the participants for being willing to take part in this study.

References

[1] Johannes L. The Wall Street Journal. Aches & claims: Putting on the stripes to ease pain. April 27, 2010. http://www.wsj.com/articles/SB1000142405274. Accessed March 21, 2015

[2] Kase K, Wallis J, Kase T. Clinical therapeutic applications of the kinesio taping method (2nd edition). Tokyo, Japan: Ken Ikai Co. Ltd.; 2003.

[3] Kinesio Taping Association, *Kinesio taping® lower extremity work book (2)*. Tokyo, Japan: Kinesio Taping Association; 2005.

[4] Kase K, (1979). Kinesio. Kinesio Taping Association International Web site. http://www.kinesiotaping.com/about/about-video. Accessed April 15, 2015.

[5] Cram J, Kasman G, *Introduction to surface electromyography*. Gaithersburg, MD: Aspen Publishers, Inc.; 2013.

[6] n. a., Acqknowledge (computer software). Goleta, CA: Biopac Systems, Inc.; 2008.

[7] n. a., MP150 data format acquisition system glp. http://www.biopac.com/. Accessed March 21, 2015.

[8] Taubert M, Bogdan D, Anwander A, Muller K, Horstmann A, Villringer A, Ragert P. Dynamic properties of human brain structure: Learning related changes in cortical areas and associated fiber connections *J Neurosci.* 2010; 30(35): 11670-11677.

[9] Janwantanakul P, Gaogasigam C. Vastus lateralis vastus medialis obliquus muscle activity during the application of inhibition and facilitation taping techniques. *Clin Rehabil.* 2005; 19(1): 12-19.

[10] Cools AM, Witvrouw, EE, Danneels LA, Cambier DC. Does taping influence electromyographic muscle activity in the scapular rotators in healthy shoulders?. *Man Ther.* 2002; 7(3), 154-162.

[11] Lumbroso D, Ziv E, Vered E, Kalichman L, The effect of kinesio tape application on hamstring and gastrocnemius muscles in healthy young adults. *J Bodyw Mov Ther.* 2014; 18(1): 130-138.

[12] Nakajima MA, Baldridge C. The effect of kinesio tape on vertical jump and dynamic postural control. *Int J Sports Phys Ther.* 2013; 8(4): 393-406.

[13] n. a. (2005). *Kinesio Taping® Lower Extremity Work Book (2)*. Kinesio Taping Association. Tokyo, Japan.

[14] n. a. (2013). MP150 data format acquisition system glp. Retrieved from http://www.biopac.com/

[15] Kase, K. (1979). *Kinesio*. Retrieved from http://www.kinesiotaping.com/.

38

Chronic Haematological Profile Study in Brazilian Jiu Jitsu Athletes

Nestor Persio Alvim Agricola[1,*], João Batista Alves de Souza[2], Martha Ribeiro Bonilha[3], Lidia Andreu Guillo[4]

[1]Universidade Federal de Goiás, Regional Jataí, Departamento de Educação Física,
Av. Voluntarios da pátria 1132, Vila Fátima. Jataí, Goiás, Brasil
[2]Universidade Federal de Goiás, Regional Jataí, Departamento de Biomedicina,
R. André Luiz, 42, Vila Fátima. Jataí, Goiás, Brasil
[3]Universidade Federal de Goiás, Regional Jataí, Departamento de Biomedicina,
Av. Petrobras, 91 – bloco 1 apt. 403, Jardim Goiás, Jataí, Goiás, Brasil
[4]Universidade Federal de Goiás, Departamento de Bioquímica e Biologia Molecular, Campus II,
Jardim Samambaia, CP 131. Goiania, Goiás, Brasil
*Corresponding author: nestoralvim@hotmail.com

Abstract This paper will treat about hematological parameters in Brazilian Jiu Jitsu athletes, linking their training with some variations of these parameters. The aim of this study was to evaluate the potentialities of this sport modality in what it has to do with promotion and maintenance of human health. Fourteen athletes have participated in this study that consisted in accompanying them during their training for six months, when monthly blood samples were collected and weekly monitoring of heart rate training were done. Variations in hematological parameters have been compared with the intensity of the training performed all this long. Statistical analyzes performed were Student t test for paired samples when data showed a normal distribution, and Wilcoxon test for paired samples, when data didn't show a normal distribution. Results show that erythrocytes and lymphocytes varied in a very similar way to the intensity of training. Hemoglobin, hematocrit, total leukocytes, neutrophils and platelets varied oppositely to training intensity. RDW, monocytes and eosinophils varied randomly, with no relation to the intensity of training. The training stimulates an increase in the production of red blood cells and hemoglobin, however, the kind of intense training and full contact, with frequent injuries, might cause hemolysis, maintaining low concentrations of these parameters. Jiu Jitsu promotes specific effects both in the red data series as in white ones; and it can be recommended for health maintenance, since, despite the detected variations, all parameters remained under the reference values.

Keywords: *Brazilian Jiu Jitsu, haematological parameters, health*

1. Introduction

Hematological parameters of human health have some factors that can interfere with the interpretation of results, such as altitude, stress, diet, level of physical fitness and exercise. These variables show up as relevant fields of research. In terms of physical training, body adaptations are quite specific to each type or kind of effort. Some authors propose the establishment of reference values of normality for trained people, slightly different from the general parameters [1].

The intensity and duration of training have been indicated as important factors in the variability of several analytes. The nature of the exercise or the sport practice in their volume and intensity can produce various effects demonstrated on several biomarkers, including hematological ones [2]. In this context, test results that come apart from the conventional reference ranges, in athletes, not only can reflect the presence of a particular disease, but can often reveal an adaptation to regular training or changes that occurred during/after the exercise; and it must be clearly recognized to avoid misinterpretation of laboratory data. Thus, the values of some biomarkers in athletes or physically active individuals should be interpreted with some attention.

Brazilian Jiu Jitsu is a fight of intense contact, which takes place predominantly on the ground, in which the fighters try to subdue the opponent using drops, armbars, levers and bottlenecks. The fact of the fight to be developed predominantly on the ground brings some peculiar characteristics to the training itself, marked by intense isometric effort and aerobics [3]. The fight lasts around 8 minutes and requires great endurance in addition to strength, flexibility and motor coordination. During the fight, the athlete is often taken to maximum effort and in order to support five, six or seven fights, as it is common in those kinds of championships, the athlete must hold an excellent cardiorespiratory fitness. The recovery time in a competition between bouts is, mostly, 10 times lower than the total time of the fights added up, revealing the need of a physical condition that's actually ascertained [4].

Although that effort is predominantly of an anaerobic lactic character, the need for recovery and discarding of lactate requires the athlete a great aerobic capacity [4]. Throughout the year of training, athletes alternate periods of high intensity of training when the competitions are near, with periods of low intensity and even a period of rest at the end of the scheduled competitions. The energy expenditure is high and this maximum or submaximal effort often leads to muscle, joint and bone injuries. A Jiu Jitsu athlete rarely practices with any pain from injuries or microlesions acquired in previous training sessions.

There are several studies on hematological parameters in athletes or people who work out regularly. These are divided primarily on studies of chronic effects, checked by monitoring the changes in parameters during training practice time, and the severe effects, checked by comparison, in the values of the parameters, before and after the section or sections of training. Studies of chronic effects in general seek modifications of a long-lasting character and that can point direct correlations with human health.

Among most of standard results found in chronic effects studies, the decrease stands out in hemoglobin concentration during the training period [5,6,8,9]. Apparently, the continuing training enhances the gas transport capacity of erythrocytes and consequently reduces the need for hemoglobin, which in its turn, reduces its concentration. However, this effect is obtained in elite athletes that undergo systematic training that aims competitions, and not in moderately trained people. The isolated training, done sporadically, does not change the hemoglobin parameters in people who work out in various practices, compared to baseline [7]. The decreases in concentration of erythrocytes, in hematocrit values and in the concentration of mean corpuscular hemoglobin (MCHC) are also mentioned as a result of intense and regular training [6,8,9]. However, these observed changes do not refer to a morphological change in the cells, but an improvement in the entire system of capitation and transport of gases as one effect of *endurance* training. On the other side, some studies have not observed any decrease in the concentration of any red blood parameter, and there are also studies that observed the opposite effect, an increase in hemoglobin concentration after the training period [10,11].

Concerning the white series parameters, the most common result found in similar studies is leukocytosis [11,12,13]. Authors attribute this increase of leukocytes to a white blood cell demargination which, due the increase in blood flow, falls into the bloodstream, enlisted as a possible inflammatory response caused by microlesions in the tissues. In addition to the increased leukocyte, there are reports of an increase in neutrophils and monocytes concentration, and a decrease in the concentration of eosinophils [11,12,13] and lymphocytes [14]. Neutrophilia is also attributed to the mobilization of bone marrow cells, and lymphopenia is associated with high concentrations of cortisol, typically originated from an intense effort. Reports of decrease in concentrations of lymphocytes and eosinophils are also associated with the migration of these cells to those inflammatory sites caused by microlesions due muscular effort.

Thus, this paper aims to discuss the results of hematological parameters in Brazilian Jiu Jitsu athletes checked over six months compared with heart rate training data, characteristic in intense physical effort, in order to recognize this modality in its particularities related to intensity and physical effort and its effects on the body; and also to consider its potential in relation to human health.

2. Materials and Methods

This study involved 14 volunteers with a mean age of 27 (± 4.56) years, Jiu Jitsu athletes with at least 2 years of practice in this modality and competitors in regional and national tournaments. The athletes were monitored for six months in their training routine (2014), when monthly blood samples collection were done before each training session.

4 ml of whole blood was collected using BD Vacutainer™ tubes containing EDTA K2, in vacuum puncture needle BD Eclipse™ about 10 minutes before starting each training session. CBCs were performed on the KX-21N Sysmex™ device and included erythrocytes, hemoglobin, hematocrit, MCV (Mean Corpuscular Volume), MCH (Mean Corpuscular Hemoglobin), MCHC (Mean Corpuscular Hemoglobin Concentration), RDW (Red Cell Distribution Width), platelets count, total leukocytes, neutrophils, lymphocytes, and the sum of monocytes, eosinophils and basophils. Smears were also made, which were stained by quick panoptic method for obtaining differential counting of monocytes, basophils and eosinophils. The blood counts were performed at the Laboratory of Biomedical Sciences II of the course of Biomedicine in UFG Regional Jataí.

Heart rate was weekly monitored, during the trainings, by a frequency counter. The heart rate monitoring meant to compare the variations in blood counts with the intensity of training, and for this, the mean heart rate was calculated for each month of training. All statistical analysis was performed using the software R i386 version 3.1.1. Tables and graphs were constructed using the software Office Excel 2007. Statistical tests performed in this study were Test t-student for paired samples, when data showed a normal distribution, and the Wilcoxon test for paired samples, when data did not show a normal distribution.

That study was submitted to the Ethics Committees in Research of the Federal University of Goiás and was approved by the opinion 692.581 on 05/16/2014. Volunteers signed a Free and Clarified Consent Term before the start of the study, ensuring the confidentiality, according to the ethical standards in research with human beings. This study was conducted in accordance with Resolution 466/2012 of the National Health Council and with Resolution 196/1996 from the same council and the Declaration of Helsinki.

3. Results

3.1. Evaluation of Cardiac Frequency

During these six months follow-up of Brazilian Jiu Jitsu athletes, results of the mean heart rate (Figure 1) reflected the variation of the intensity used in trainings [15].

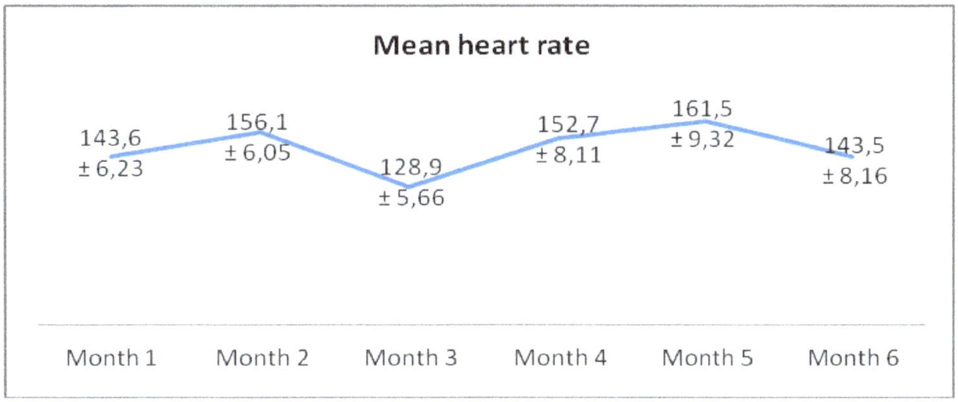

Figure 1. Monthly mean heart rate

As shown in Figure 1, the monitored training period had two peaks of greater intensity over 6 months: the first peak happened circa the second month and the other near the fifth month of training. This occurred due competitions in which the athletes have participated, thus the training sessions were carried out with more intensity. Periods of lower mean heart rate were periods of preparation and recovery, characterized by lower intensity.

3.2. Red Series

Erythrocytes data (million/mm³), hematocrit (%) hemoglobin (g/dl), MCV (ft), MCH (pg), MCHC (g/dl), RDW (%) and platelets (mil/mm³), are expressed in Table 1 as mean ± standard deviation.

Table 1. Data of red series

	Month 1	Month 2	Month 3	Month 4	Month 5	Month 6
Red blood cells (million/mm³)	5,25 ± 0,424	5,27 ± 0,463	4,93 ± 0,402*	5,14 ± 0,342*	5,17 ± 0,422	5,38 ± 0,446
Hematocrit (%)	44,00 ± 3,24	43,85 ± 2,32	44,60 ± 3,06	43,90 ± 2,83	44,74 ± 3,17	47,75 ± 3,73*
Hemoglobin (g/dl)	14,16 ± 1,21	14,34 ± 1,19	15,32 ± 1,14**	14,36 ± 1,17	14,99 ± 1,39	15,37 ± 1,49*
MCV (ft)	84,35 ± 9,71	83,83 ± 8,37	91,04 ±10,45**	85,77 ± 8,44	87,02 ± 9,39	89,20 ± 9,09**
MCH (pg)	27,28 ± 3,63	27,49 ± 3,71	31,28 ± 3,96**	28,06 ± 3,24	29,16 ± 3,84**	28,73 ± 3,78
MCHC (g/dl)	32,27 ± 0,74	32,69 ± 1,73	33,96 ± 0,83*	32,65 ± 0,83	33,42 ± 1,04**	32,10 ± 1,10
RDW (%)	13,74 ± 0,72	12,97 ± 1,54	13,07 ± 0,95**	14,02 ± 0,96**	13,12 ± 1,03	13,02 ± 0,81**
Platelets (mil/mm³)	225,0 ± 50,31	240,3 ± 55,18*	264,6 ± 67,64*	213,6 ± 56,35	182,1 ± 60,29	248,5 ± 61,59*

* significant difference from month # 1, with p<0,05 (Student t-test for paired samples).
** significant difference from month # 1, with p<0,05 (Wilcoxon test for paired samples)

The behavior of the red series parameters can be compared with data from heart rate or from intensity of training. For red blood cell values (Figure 2) it was showed a significant decrease between the first month and the third month, with P-value = 0.0004 and also between the first and the fourth month, with P-value = 0.025. The measurement of erythrocytes concentration showed a normal distribution by the Shapiro-wilk test over the 6 months of follow-up. Red blood cells ranged from a very similar way to the heart rate itself; markedly differing only in the sixth month of follow-up.

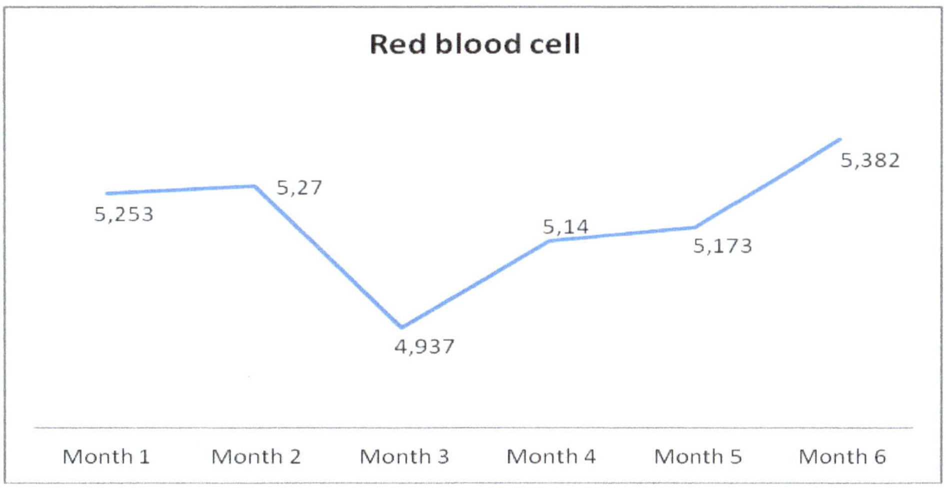

Figure 2. Variation of red blood cells

In hematocrit data a significant difference was only detected in the sixth month of study (P-value = 0.002), compared to the values of the first month. The distribution of hematocrit presented normality in five out of the six months of tests and it may vary in a less intense way.

Hemoglobin (Figure 3) presented significant increase in the third month (P-value = 0.014) and in the six month (P-value = 0.01). As for the distribution of hemoglobin levels it didn't show normal distribution to four of the six months tested. The hemoglobin values varied differently from the intensity of training, by having higher peaks in the values during the months that came after higher intense training. Months of higher mean hemoglobin are the months of lower intensity of training (Figure 3).

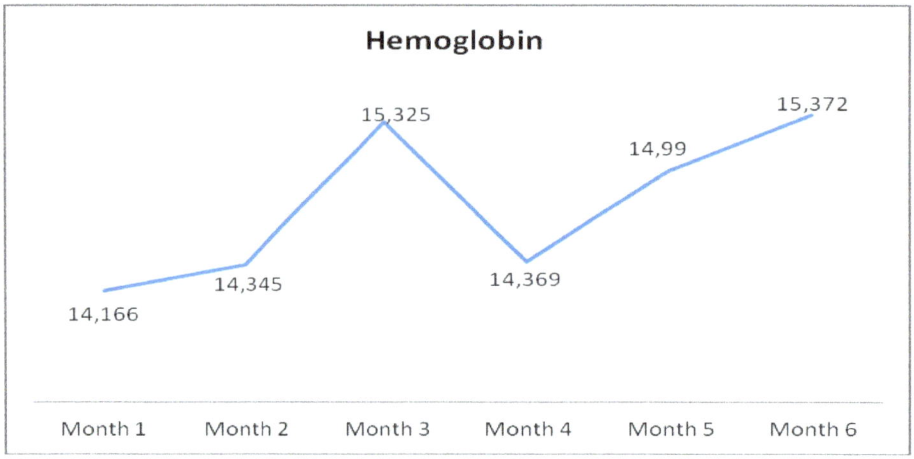

Figure 3. Hemoglobin variation

RDW values varied randomly with no reference to the intensity of those training data. However, there was significant statistical difference between the first and third month (P-value = 0.023), between the first and the fourth month (P-value = 0.024) and between the first and sixth month (P-value = 0.021).

MCV, MCH and MCHC data rarely presented normal distribution, thus they were tested by paired Wilcoxon test. MCV showed significant difference in third month (P-value = 0.015) and sixth month (P-value = 0.015) compared to the first month. As for MCH and MCHC values, there was a significant difference in the third and fifth month, if compared to the first month.

3.3. White Series

Total leukocytes, neutrophils, lymphocytes, monocytes and eosinophils data (all measured in cells/mm³ of blood) are shown in Table 2 as mean ± standard deviation:

Table 2. White series data

	Month 1	Month 2	Month 3	Month 4	Month 5	Month 6
Total leukocytes	6966,6 ± 1305,7	7218,1 ± 1373,9	7966,6 ± 1527,5*	7292,3 ± 1694,3	7340,0 ± 1119,7	7518,1 ± 2059,5
Netrophils	3792,3 ± 1028,0	3842,7 ± 1410,1	4576,6 ± 1348,2*	4047,2 ± 1756,9	4117,5 ± 947,7*	4478,4 ± 1810,0
Linphocytes	2852,5 ± 716,5	2839,0 ± 519,1	2760,0 ± 441,7	2767,3 ± 730,9	2777,6 ± 507,3	2597,1 ± 515,4
Monocytes	234,8 ± 58,5	323,0 ± 135,3	401,5 ± 120,2*	314,8 ± 81,7*	304,4 ± 110,3	279,7 ± 78,4
Eosinophils	86,8 ± 41,7	194,0 ± 85,3*	177,0 ± 71,7*	162,8 ± 67,6*	139,7 ± 60,8*	162,8 ± 66,3*

* significant difference from month # 1, with $p<0,05$ (Student t-test for paired samples).

All white series parameters showed normal distribution (Shapiro-Wilk test), except for eosinophils in months 1 and 4. Basophils statistically could not be tested because they are cells that were rarely observed throughout the study period.

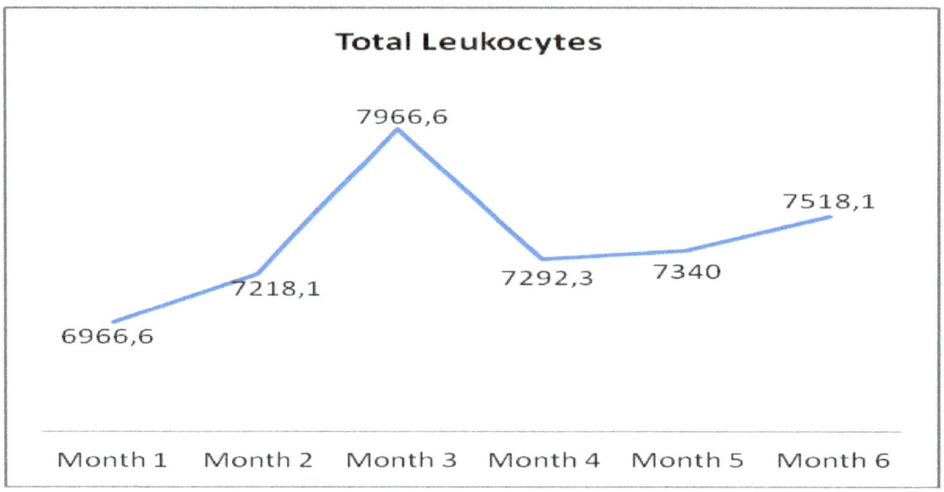

Figure 4. Variation of total leukocytes

Among the total leukocytes values, there is a significant difference only in month # 3 when compared to month # 1, with P-value = 0.004 (Figure 4). Month # 6, compared with # 1, did not show significant difference due to a high standard deviation. The mean values of total leukocytes presented subsequent peaks to those two of training intensity ones, indicating an increase in months 3 and 6 when compared to month # 1, coinciding with those peaks of high hemoglobin values. Neutrophils values follow the same increasing tendency in months succeeding months of higher intensity in the training (months 3 and 6), following also the hemoglobin peaks (Figure 5).

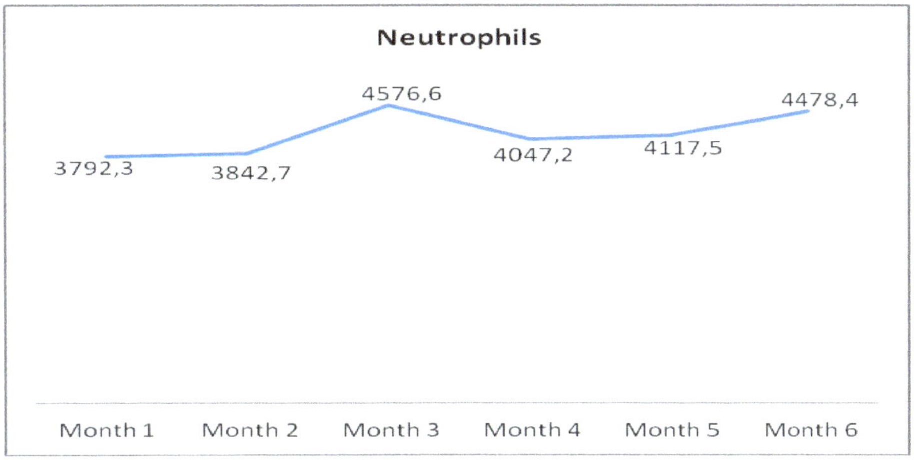

Figure 5. Variation of neutrophils

For neutrophils values, month # 3 shows significant difference from month # 1 (P-value = 0.002). Although the sixth month shows an increase compared to the first month, this increase was not statistically significant. However, month # 5 shows significant difference from month # 1 (P-value = 0.032).

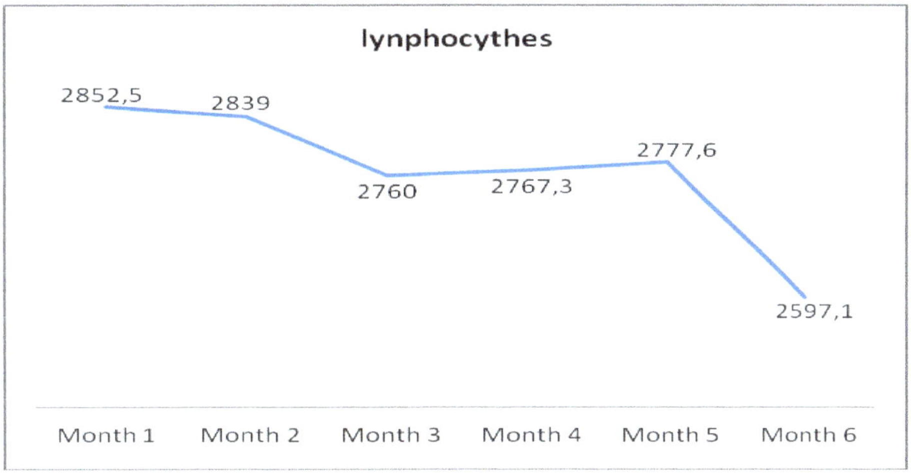

Figure 6. Variation of lymphocytes

Lymphocytes have a continuous decline over the study period, but there was no statistically significant variation in any month when compared to month # 1. Lymphocyte values may vary subtly, but inversely to the values of total leukocytes and neutrophils, with the lowest values found exactly in months # 3 and # 6. This variation, however, was not significant from a statistical point of view. Lymphocytes behave in an inverse way to red blood cells, hematocrit, hemoglobin, total leukocytes and neutrophils, revealing an almost steady decline over the 6 months (Figure 6).

Monocytes vary randomly and do not appear to follow the patterns of the other cell types. A significant variation was observed in third month (P-value = 0.003) and in fourth month (P-value = 0.033), relative to the first month. Eosinophils also vary out of the established patterns checked in neutrophils and lymphocytes, with significant variation over all months compared to month # 1.

Platelet parameters showed statistically significant changes in months 2 (P-value = 0.044), 3 (P-value = 0.002) and 6 (P-value = 0.006) compared to month 1. The variation in mean platelet in athletes draws a graph similar to neutrophils one, signifying a possible relationship between these two variables. The striking difference between the two graphs is observed only in the fifth month, which in neutrophil graph shows an increase if compared to the fourth month, and in the platelet graph shows a decrease when compared to the fourth month.

4. Discussion

Hematologic parameters seem to show no variation according to a well-defined pattern associated with body exercise. What can be perceived in most of those cited studies is that physical exercise influences these parameters, but it seems to vary according to the intensity and exercise's duration, and especially according to the type of training. The findings are not unanimous much less conclusive and require new and deeper studies. There is no single concept that can discourse and explain the variability between different sports practices or how they may be compared to each other. The level of physical effort or the volume/intensity of work can't characterize the difference between the different categories. Data from blood counts collected in this study and in other similar ones demonstrate this. Athletic modalities with similarities in training intensity present hematological parameters that vary differently, which requires, therefore, other classifications or concepts that can find justification for the phenomenon.

Erythrocytes values may vary similarly to the values obtained for heart rate. Hemoglobin values vary in a reverse way from the heart rate, showing higher values in months of lower intensity. This tends to confirm the explanation in which the most intense training enhances the gas transport system, reducing the need for hemoglobin [6,16]. Thus, in months of lower intensity, the body starts producing hemoglobin again in greater quantity, as seen in months 3 and 6, because the improvement is only checked in really intense training periods.

However, this result may have another explanation. In months of higher intensity of training, low concentrations of hemoglobin has been observed. This might suggest that the stress due intense training after the preparation for competitions has led to a loss of erythrocytes. Oxidative stress, cause of cellular damages in muscle tissue, leads to micro lesions originated from high tension and effort, causing hemolysis and maintaining low concentrations of erythrocytes, even before an intense stimulus of production of those cells [2,17]. Thus, in months of post competition characterized by a lower intensity of effort, the micro lesions would be less frequent, and the hemolysis in decrease, revealing higher concentration of erythrocytes. Reports of decrease in hemoglobin concentrations, including values below the international standard of normality, due to the high physical effort, are related to the stress in muscle and joint structures underwent to high stress [18,19]. Combat sports, and specifically the Brazilian jiu jitsu, are propitious to these lesions [19,20,21].

Regarding the white series, the leukocyte count varied very similarly to hemoglobin one, i.e., in months after a stronger intensity there is an increase in leukocyte concentration. This graph says much more in what relates to neutrophils, as long as the lymphocytes vary inversely. The specialized literature reports an increase in the concentration of neutrophils and a decreased in lymphocytes induced by exercise [23,24]. However, this reaction occurs only under maximum or submaximal effort [25,26]. In this study the same effect can be observed mainly in months of lower intensity of training.

5. Conclusion

Brazilian Jiu Jitsu fight has as characteristic a very intense contact between athletes, which may facilitate the dissemination of viral or bacterial infections within the group, like in school environments, and it may affect the average values of some of these parameters, mainly in white series. In addition, the Jiu Jitsu exposes the athlete to high physical effort, demanding a lot from joints and tendons, which ends up turning to a very common inflammation in these structures, changing parameters of blood cells associated with the immune system.

However, it can't be stated that the training has no influence in those parameters, and therefore the hypothesis that the blood count parameters are affected by physical effort is sustained. The maintenance of lower hemoglobin concentrations in high-intensity training periods is evidence that the athlete suffers frequent injuries, which would be responsible for hemolysis of those cells. The body would have stimulated an increase in the production of red blood cells in intense training; however, the oxidative stress generated by that same intense training would lead to a decrease in concentrations of red blood cells and especially hemoglobin. Notwithstanding, this reaction doesn't confirm itself in white series, demonstrating an immune response mobilization, with an increase of neutrophils and lower lymphocyte, precisely in the subsequent months to the greater intensity.

This type of fight shows to be indicated for the maintenance of human health parameters, since all parameters verified during the study were within the reference standards accepted worldwide. It should be highlighted, however, the fact that several studies have come to affirm that parameters of normality must be reviewed when it's about trained athletes, with consequences that can reach issues related to doping in sports [2,6,16,18,22]. Further studies, with different designs, are necessary to confirm some of the hypotheses raised here for more accurate conclusions.

Statement of Competing Interests

The authors have no competing interests

References

[1] Nunes L A S. Estudo dos parâmetros hematológicos em pessoas fisicamente ativas. Campinas (SP): Dissertação (mestrado) – Universidade Estadual de Campinas, Instituto de Biologia, 2006.

[2] Sanchis-Gomar F, Lippi G. Physical activity - an important preanalytical variable. Biochemia Medica 2014; 24(1):68-79.

[3] Bradão F, Fernandes H M, Alves J V, Fonseca S, Reis V M. Hematological and biochemical markers after a Brazilian Jiu-Jitsu tournament in world-class athletes. Revista Brasileira de Cineantromopetria e Desempenho Humano.

[4] Del Vecchio F B, Bianchi S, Hirata S M, Chacon-Mikahil M P T. Análise Morfo-funcional de praticantes de Brazilian Jiu Jitsu e estudo da temporalidade e da quantificação das ações motoras na modalidade. Movimento & Percepção, Espirito Santo do Pinhal, SP, v.7, n.10, jan./jun. 2007.

[5] Boyadjiev N, Taralov Z. Red blood cell variables in highly trained pubescent athletes: a comparative analysis. Br J Sports Med 2000;34:200-4.

[6] Banfi G, Del Fabbro M. Behaviour of reticulocyte counts and immature reticulocyte fraction during a competitive season in elite athletes of four different sports. Int J Lab Hematol 2007;29:127-31.

[7] Schumacher Y O, Schmid A, Grathwohl D, Bultermann D, Berg A. Hematological indices and iron status in athletes of various sports and performances. Med Sci Sports Exerc 2002;34:869-75.

[8] Wirnitzer K C, Faulhaber M. Hemoglobin and hematocrit during an 8 day mountainbike race: A field study. Journal of Sports Science and Medicine 2007;6:265-66.

[9] Hu M, Finni T, Sedliak M, Zhou W, Alen M, Cheng, S. Seasonal variation of red blood cell variables in physically inactive men: effects of strength training. Int J Sports Med 2008;29:564-8.

[10] Diaz V, Lombardi G, Ricci C, Jacobs R A, Montalvo Z, Lundby C. Reticulocyte and haemoglobin profiles in elite triathletes over four consecutive seasons. Int J Lab Hematol 2011;33:638-44.

[11] Lombardi G, Ricci C, Banfi G. Effect of winter swimming on haematological parameters. Biochem Med 2011;21:71-8.

[12] Hammouda O, Chtourou H, Chahed H, Ferchichi S, Chaouachi A, Kallel C. High intensity exercise affects diurnal variation of some biological markers in trained subjects. Int J Sports Med 2012;33:886-91.

[13] Oliveira C A M, Rogatto G P, Luciano E. Efeitos do treinamento físico de alta intensidade sobre os leucócitos de ratos diabéticos. Rev Bras Med Esporte _ Vol. 8, Nº 6 – Nov/Dez, 2002.

[14] Bachur J A, Quemelo Q R, Bachur C A K, Domenciano J C, Martins C H G, Stoppa M A, Neto T L B, Garcia S B. Evaluation of the effect of hypothermia by cold water immersion on blood neutrophils and lymphocytes of rats submitted to acute exercise. Rev. Bras. Hematol. Hemoter. 2008;30(6):470-474.

[15] Henríquez O C, Báez S M E, Von Oetinger A, Cañas J R, Ramírez C R. Autonomic control of heart rate after exercise in trained wrestlers. Biology of Sport, Vol. 30 No2, 2013.

[16] Lippi G, Salvagno G L, Danese E, Tarperi C, Guidi G C, Schena F. Variation of Red Blood Cell Distribution Width and Mean Platelet Volume after Moderate Endurance Exercise. Advances in Hematology, Volume 2014, Article ID 192173, 4 pages.

[17] Latunde-Dada G O. Iron metabolism in athletes – achieving a gold standard. European Journal of Haematology 90 (10-15), 2012.

[18] Rietjens G J, Kuipers H, Hartgens F, Keizer H A. Red blood cell profile of elite olympic distance triathletes. A three-year follow-up. Int J Sports Med. 2002 Aug;23(6):391-6.

[19] Bledsoe G H, Hsu E B, Grabowski J G, Brill J D, Li G. Incidence of injury in professional Mixed Martial Arts competitions. Journal of Sports Science and Medicine (2006) CSSI, 136-142. http://www.jssm.org.

[20] Scarpi M J, Conte M, Rossin R A, Skubs R, Lenk R E, Brant R. Association between two different types of strangling and intraocular pressure variation in jiu-jitsu athletes. Arq Bras Oftalmol. 2009;72(3):341-5.

[21] Ide B N, Padilha D A. Possíveis lesões decorrentes da aplicação das técnicas do jiu-jitsu desportivo. Efdeportes, Buenos Aires - Año 10 - N° 83 - Abril de 2005. http://www.efdeportes.com.

[22] Schumacher Y O, Jankovits R, Bültermann D, Schmid A, Berg A. Hematological indices in elite cyclists. Scand J Med Sci Sports.

[23] Costa Rosa L F P B, Vaisberg M W. Influências do exercício na resposta imune. Rev Bras Med Esporte 2002; 8(4):167-72.

[24] Oliveira C A M, Rogatto G P, Luciano E. Effects of high intensity physical training on the leukocytes of diabetic rats. Rev Bras Med Esporte _ Vol. 8, Nº 6 – Nov/Dez, 2002.

[25] Bradão F, Fernandes H M, Alves J V, Fonseca S, Reis V M. Hematological and biochemical markers after a Brazilian Jiu-Jitsu tournament in world-class athletes. Revista Brasileira de Cineantromopetria e Desempenho Humano.

[26] Gonçalves L C, Bessa A, Freitas-Dias R, Werneck-de-Castro J P S, Bassini A, Cameron L C A. sportomics strategy to analyze the ability of arginine to modulate both ammonia and lymphocyte levels in blood after high-intensity exercise. Journal of the International Society of Sports Nutrition 2012, 9:30. http://www.jissn.com/content/9/1/30.

Permissions

All chapters in this book were first published in AJSSM, by Science and Education Publishing; hereby published with permission under the Creative Commons Attribution License or equivalent. Every chapter published in this book has been scrutinized by our experts. Their significance has been extensively debated. The topics covered herein carry significant findings which will fuel the growth of the discipline. They may even be implemented as practical applications or may be referred to as a beginning point for another development.

The contributors of this book come from diverse backgrounds, making this book a truly international effort. This book will bring forth new frontiers with its revolutionizing research information and detailed analysis of the nascent developments around the world.

We would like to thank all the contributing authors for lending their expertise to make the book truly unique. They have played a crucial role in the development of this book. Without their invaluable contributions this book wouldn't have been possible. They have made vital efforts to compile up to date information on the varied aspects of this subject to make this book a valuable addition to the collection of many professionals and students.

This book was conceptualized with the vision of imparting up-to-date information and advanced data in this field. To ensure the same, a matchless editorial board was set up. Every individual on the board went through rigorous rounds of assessment to prove their worth. After which they invested a large part of their time researching and compiling the most relevant data for our readers.

The editorial board has been involved in producing this book since its inception. They have spent rigorous hours researching and exploring the diverse topics which have resulted in the successful publishing of this book. They have passed on their knowledge of decades through this book. To expedite this challenging task, the publisher supported the team at every step. A small team of assistant editors was also appointed to further simplify the editing procedure and attain best results for the readers.

Apart from the editorial board, the designing team has also invested a significant amount of their time in understanding the subject and creating the most relevant covers. They scrutinized every image to scout for the most suitable representation of the subject and create an appropriate cover for the book.

The publishing team has been an ardent support to the editorial, designing and production team. Their endless efforts to recruit the best for this project, has resulted in the accomplishment of this book. They are a veteran in the field of academics and their pool of knowledge is as vast as their experience in printing. Their expertise and guidance has proved useful at every step. Their uncompromising quality standards have made this book an exceptional effort. Their encouragement from time to time has been an inspiration for everyone.

The publisher and the editorial board hope that this book will prove to be a valuable piece of knowledge for researchers, students, practitioners and scholars across the globe.

List of Contributors

Masakatsu Nakada
National Defense Academy of Japan, 1-10-20 Hashirimizu, Yokosuka, Kanagawa, Japan

Shinichi Demura
Graduate School of Natural Science & Technology, Kanazawa University, Kakuma, Kanazawa, Ishikawa, Japan

Mostafa Dehghani
Department of Physiology, Physical Education and Sports Science Faculty, Shahid Chamran University, Ahvaz, Iran

Saeid Shakerian and Massood Nikbakht
Department of Physiology, Physical Education Faculty, Shahid Chamran University, Ahvaz, Iran

Mohammad Kazem Gharib Nasseri
Physiology Research Center, Jondishapoor Medical Sciences University, Ahvaz, Iran

Sedigheh Heidari Nejad
Department of Sports Management, Physical Education Faculty, Shahid Chamran University, Ahvaz, Iran

Roan Mukherjee
Department of Human Physiology, Hazaribag College of Dental Sciences and Hospital, Demotand, Hazaribag, Jharkhand, India

Prakash C. Dhara
Ergonomics and Sports Physiology Division, Department of Human Physiology with CommunityHealth, Vidyasagar University, Medinipore, West Bengal, India

Gholam A. Ghasemi, Vahid Zolaktaf and Minasian V
Department of Exercise science , University of Isfahan, Isfahan, Iran

Khosravi Ibrahim
Department of Exercise Rehab, Faculty of Exercise Sciences, University of Isfahan, Isfahan, Iran

D. Dixon
Applied Sport and Exercise Sciences, School of Health Sport and Bioscience, University of East London. London, UK

Nikolaidis P.T.
Department of Physical and Cultural Education, Hellenic Army Academy, Athens, Greece Exercise Physiology Laboratory, Nikaia, Greece

Shankarashis Mukherjee, Neepa Banerjee, Surjani Chatterjee, Sandipan Chatterjee, Ayan Chatterjee, Tanaya Santra and Bijan Saha
Human Performance Analytics and Facilitation Unit, Department of Physiology, University of Calcutta, Kolkata, India

R. Moore and J. Radford
Sport Industry Research Centre, Sheffield Hallam University, Sheffield, England

J. Álvarez-Medina, V. Murillo-Lorente and L. Giménez-Salillas
Faculty of Health Sciences, Department of Physical Medicine and Nursing, University of Zaragoza, Zaragoza, Spain

P. Manonelles-Marqueta
Spanish Federation of Sports Medicine (FEMEDE), Pamplona, Spain

Fabian Vasquez, Erik Diaz, Lydia Lera, Loretta Vasquez, Alyerina Anziani and Raquel Burrows
Institute of Nutrition and Food Technology (INTA), University of Chile

D. Berdejo-del-Fresno
England Futsal National Squad, The Football Association and The International Futsal Academy (United Kingdom)

R. Moore
Research Fellow, Sport Industry Research Centre, Sheffield Hallam University (United Kingdom)

M. W. Laupheimer
England Futsal National Squad, The Football Association and The International Futsal Academy (United Kingdom)
Senior Clinical Lecturer in Sports and Exercise Medicine, Queen Mary University of London (United Kingdom)

Ranjit Biswas
Department of Computer Science, Jamia Hamdard University, Hamdard Nagar, New Delhi, INDIA

Kenji Takahashi
Faculty of Community Health Care, Department of Judo Physical Therapy, Teikyo Heisei University, Uruidominami 4-1 Ichihara, chiba, Japan

Shin-ichi Demura
Graduate School of Natural Science & Technology, Kanazawa University, Kakuma, Kanazawa, Ishikawa, Japan

Mansi Chopra and Anupa Siddhu
Department of Food and Nutrition, Lady Irwin College, Sikandra Road, New Delhi- 110001, University of Delhi, India

Ünsal Tazegül
Dumlupinar, Turkey

Aytekin Soykan
School of Physical Education and Sports, Marmara University, Stanbul, Turkey

Hein F.M. Lodewijkx
Department of Psychology, Open University, Heerlen, The Netherlands

Borut Kirn and Vito Starc
Medical Faculty, University of Ljubljana, Ljubljana, Slovenia

A. Paz-Franco
Physical Coach, Al Wahda Futsal, Abu Dhabi, UAE

A. Bores-Cerezal
Physical Coach, Spain National Team, Spain

R. Barcala-Furelos
Special Didactics, University of Vigo, Spain

M. Mecias-Calvo
Physical Coach, Santiago Futsal, Spain

C Aouichaoui, Y Trabelsi, Z Tabka and E Bouhlel
Laboratory of Physiology and Lung Function Testing, Faculty of Medicine Ibn-El-Jazzar, University of Sousse, Sousse, Tunisia

M Dogui
Laboratory of Physiology, Faculty of Medicine, Monastir, Tunisia

JP Richalet
Laboratory of Cellular and Functional Responses to Hypoxia, University of Paris 13, Bobigny, France

H. Kubota
Faculty of Education, Gifu University, Gifu, Japan

S. Demura
Graduate School of Natural Science & Technology, Kanazawa University, Ishikawa, Japan

M. Uchiyama
Research and Education Center for Comprehensive Science, Akita Prefectural University, Akita, Japan

K. Takahashi
Faculty of Community Health Care, Department of Judo Physical Therapy, Teikyo Heisei University, Chiba, Japan

Adhikari Anup
Anthropmetrica, Toronto, Canada

Pervin Nahida and Rumy Nazrul Islam
Bangladesh Institute of Sports (BKSP), Dhaka, Bangladesh

Ali Kitab
Bangladesh Athletic Federation, Dhaka, Bangladesh

J. Cachón-Zagalaz, A. Lara-Sánchez and M. L. Zagalaz-Sánchez
University of Jaén, Jaén, Spain

P. Valdivia-Moral
University of Huelva, Huelva, Spain

D. Berdejo-del-Fresno
The Football Association, London, England

Sheffield FC Futsal, D. Berdejo-del-Fresno
The Football Association, London, England
Sheffield FC Futsal, England

M. W. Laupheimer
The Football Association, London, England
Queen Mary, University of London, England
Sports & MSK Physician BUPA, London, England

Tabka Z
Université de Sousse, Laboratoire de Physiologie et des Explorations Fonctionnelles, Faculté de Médecine de Sousse, Sousse, Tunisie

Trabelsi Y
Université de Sousse, Laboratoire de Physiologie et des Explorations Fonctionnelles, Faculté de Médecine de Sousse, Sousse, Tunisie
Université de Sfax, Institut Supérieur du Sport et de l'Education Physique de Sfax, Sfax, Tunisie

Aouichaoui C
Université de Sousse, Laboratoire de Physiologie et des Explorations Fonctionnelles, Faculté de Médecine de Sousse, Sousse, Tunisie
Université de Sfax, Institut Supérieur du Sport et de l'Education Physique de Sfax, Sfax, Tunisie
Université de Gafsa, Institut Supérieur du Sport et de l'Education Physique de Gafsa, Gafsa, Tunisie

Richalet JP
Université Paris 13, Laboratoire "Réponses Cellulaires et Fonctionnelles à l'hypoxie" EA 2363, Bobigny, France

Rafael Reimann Baptista, Luis Felipe Silveira, Fábio Rodrigo Suñé, Fernanda Martins Marquesan, Gustavo Sandri Heidner, Mariana Kloeckner Pires Dias and Luciano Castro
School of Physical Education, Pontifical Catholic University of Rio Grande do Sul, Porto Alegre, Brazil

Ramon Cruz
Faculdade de Educação Física e Desporto, Universidade Federal de Juiz de Fora, Juiz de Fora, Brazil

Francisco de Assis Manoel and Bruno Pereira Melo
Departamento de Educação Física, Universidade Estadual de Maringá, Maringá, Brazil

Sandro Fernandes da Silva
Departamento de Educação Física, Universidade Federal de Lavras, Lavras, Brazil

Rita R. Culross
Louisiana State University, School of Education, 301 Peabody Hall, Baton Rouge, LA

Saeed Rahmaty, Keivan Khoramipour and Mostafa Saboory
Department of Sports and Physical Education, Tehran University

Pooneh Dehghan
Imaging Department, Taleghani Hospital Research Development Unit, Shahid Beheshti University of Medical Sciences

Veysel Küçük and Hamdi Sancaklı
Marmara University, School of Physical Education and Sports, İstanbul, Turkey

Ünsal Tazegül
GaziUniversity, School of Physical Education and Sports, Ankara, Turkey

Mehmet Haşim Akgül
Mehmet Akif Ersoy, University, School of Physical Educationand Sports, Burdur, Turkey

A. Serdar Yücel
Fırat University, Faculty of Sports Sciences, Elazig, Turkey

Elif Top
Faculty of Sport Sciences, Usak University, Turkey

Andrew Shim and Shannon Norman
Division of Kinesiology & Sport Science, The University of South Dakota, Vermillion, SD. USA

Patrick Cross
Department of Physical Therapy, Briar Cliff University, Sioux City, IA. USA

Patrick Hauer
Department of Physical Therapy, The University of South Dakota, Vermillion, SD. USA

Pradeep Singh Chahar
Assistant Professor Physical Education, Manipal University Jaipur. Jaipur, Rajasthan, India

Anup Adhikari
Anthropometrica, Toronto, Canada

J. V. García-Jiménez, J. L. Yuste and J. J. García-Pellicer
Department of Physical Education, University of Murcia, 30100 Murcia, Spain

Ajita, Jiwanjot
Department of Sports Science, Punjabi University, Patiala, Punjab

Elizabeth A. Davison, Christopher T. Anderson, Blake H. Ponist, Drew M. Werner, Mary E. Jacobs and Adam J. Thompson
Athletic Training Education, Indiana Wesleyan University, Marion, 46953, USA

Melissa R. Cook
Exercise Science, Indiana Wesleyan University, Marion, 46953, USA

Nestor Persio Alvim Agricola
Universidade Federal de Goiás, Regional Jataí, Departamento de Educação Física, Av. Voluntarios da pátria 1132, Vila Fátima. Jataí, Goiás, Brasil

João Batista Alves de Souza
Universidade Federal de Goiás, Regional Jataí, Departamento de Biomedicina, R. André Luiz, 42, Vila Fátima. Jataí, Goiás, Brasil

Martha Ribeiro Bonilha
Universidade Federal de Goiás, Regional Jataí, Departamento de Biomedicina, Av. Petrobras, 91 - bloco 1 apt. 403, Jardim Goiás, Jataí, Goiás, Brasil

Lidia Andreu Guillo
Universidade Federal de Goiás, Departamento de Bioquímica e Biologia Molecular, Campus II, Jardim Samambaia, CP 131. Goiania, Goiás, Brasil

Index

Electromagnetism: Theory, Concepts and Applications

Editor: Ewen Murray

NY RESEARCH PRESS
New York

Published by NY Research Press
118-35 Queens Blvd., Suite 400,
Forest Hills, NY 11375, USA
www.nyresearchpress.com

Electromagnetism: Theory, Concepts and Applications
Edited by Ewen Murray

International Standard Book Number: 978-1-63238-603-8 (Hardback)

Cataloging-in-Publication Data

Electromagnetism : theory, concepts and applications / edited by Ewen Murray.
p. cm.
Includes bibliographical references and index.
ISBN 978-1-63238-603-8
1. Electromagnetism. 2. Metamaterials. I. Murray, Ewen.
QC760 .E44 2018
537--dc23

Printed in China.

Contents

Preface

The study of the electromagnetic force and the relation between electrically charged particles is known as electromagnetism. It is a sub-branch of physics and includes the study of magnetic field, light, electric field, etc. Other topics covered under this field are gravitation, strong interaction, and weak interaction. It also focuses on the properties of electrons. The book studies, analyses and upholds the pillars of the subject and its utmost significance in modern times. The various sub-fields of electromagnetism along with technological progress that have future implications are glanced at in it. For someone with an interest and eye for detail, this textbook covers the most significant topics in this field. It will provide comprehensive knowledge to the readers.

To facilitate a deeper understanding of the contents of this book a short introduction of every chapter is written below:

Chapter 1- The branch of physics which studies electromagnetic force is known as electromagnetism. It plays a crucial rule in forming the internal properties of any objects. This chapter is an overview of the subject matter incorporating all the major aspects of electromagnetism.

Chapter 2- The interaction that takes place between electric charges and currents is studied under the subject of classical electromagnetism. Electric charge, charge conservation and Liénard-Wiechert potential are some topics discussed in regard to classical electromagnetism. This chapter will provide an integrated understanding of classical electromagnetism.

Chapter 3- Ampere, coulomb, charge number, tesla, Siemens, farad, ohm, watt, volt and weber are some measurement units in electromagnetism. The base unit of electric current is known as ampere whereas the unit used for electric charge is known as coulomb. The measurement units in electromagnetism are discussed in this chapter.

Chapter 4- The ability of some materials to conduct electricity with no resistance is known as superconductivity. There are a number of criteria used in classifying superconductors. Some of these are response to a magnetic field, by critical temperature, by material and by theory of operation. The chapter on superconductivity offers an insightful focus, keeping in mind the complex subject matter.

I owe the completion of this book to the never-ending support of my family, who supported me throughout the project.

Editor

1

An Introduction to Electromagnetism

The branch of physics which studies electromagnetic force is known as electromagnetism. It plays a crucial rule in forming the internal properties of any objects. This chapter is an overview of the subject matter incorporating all the major aspects of electromagnetism.

Electromagnetism

Electromagnetism is a branch of physics involving the study of the electromagnetic force, a type of physical interaction that occurs between electrically charged particles. The electromagnetic force usually exhibits electromagnetic fields such as electric fields, magnetic fields, and light and is one of the four fundamental interactions (commonly called forces) in nature. The other three fundamental interactions are the strong interaction, the weak interaction, and gravitation.

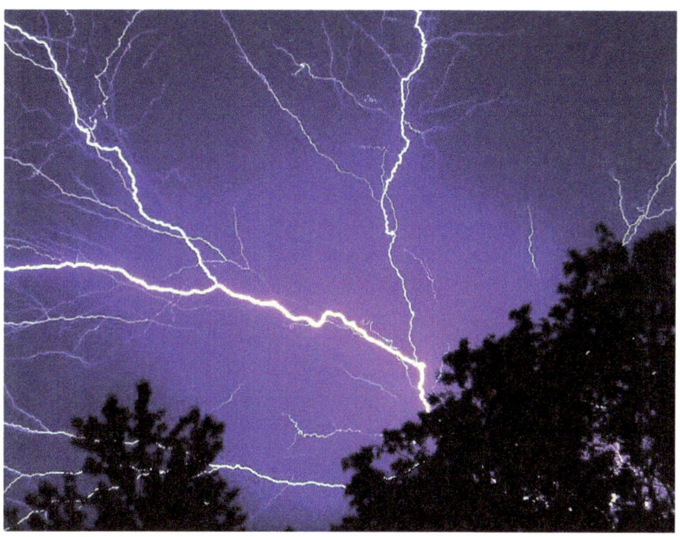

Lightning is an electrostatic discharge that travels between two charged regions.

The word *electromagnetism* is a compound form of two Greek terms, which means “magnesian stone”, a type of iron ore. Electromagnetic phenomena are defined in terms of the electromagnetic force, sometimes called the Lorentz force, which includes both electricity and magnetism as different manifestations of the same phenomenon.

The electromagnetic force plays a major role in determining the internal properties of most objects encountered in daily life. Ordinary matter takes its form as a result of intermolecular forces between individual atoms and molecules in matter, and is a manifestation of the electromagnetic force. Electrons are bound by the electromagnetic force to atomic nuclei, and their orbital shapes and their influence on nearby atoms with their electrons is described by quantum mechanics. The electromagnetic force governs the processes involved in chemistry, which arise from interactions between the electrons of neighboring atoms.

There are numerous mathematical descriptions of the electromagnetic field. In classical electrodynamics, electric fields are described as electric potential and electric current. In Faraday's law, magnetic fields are associated with electromagnetic induction and magnetism, and Maxwell's equations describe how electric and magnetic fields are generated and altered by each other and by charges and currents.

The theoretical implications of electromagnetism, particularly the establishment of the speed of light based on properties of the "medium" of propagation (permeability and permittivity), led to the development of special relativity by Albert Einstein in 1905.

Although electromagnetism is considered one of the four fundamental forces, at high energy the weak force and electromagnetic force are unified as a single electroweak force. In the history of the universe, during the quark epoch the unified force broke into the two separate forces as the universe cooled.

History of the Theory

Originally, electricity and magnetism were considered to be two separate forces. This view changed, however, with the publication of James Clerk Maxwell's 1873 *A Treatise on Electricity and Magnetism* in which the interactions of positive and negative charges were shown to be mediated by one force. There are four main effects resulting from these interactions, all of which have been clearly demonstrated by experiments:

1. Electric charges *attract* or *repel* one another with a force inversely proportional to the square of the distance between them: unlike charges attract, like ones repel.

2. Magnetic poles (or states of polarization at individual points) attract or repel one another in a manner similar to positive and negative charges and always exist as pairs: every north pole is yoked to a south pole.

3. An electric current inside a wire creates a corresponding circumferential magnetic field outside the wire. Its direction (clockwise or counter-clockwise) depends on the direction of the current in the wire.

4. A current is induced in a loop of wire when it is moved toward or away from a magnetic field, or a magnet is moved towards or away from it; the direction of current depends on that of the movement.

While preparing for an evening lecture on 21 April 1820, Hans Christian Ørsted made a surprising observation. As he was setting up his materials, he noticed a compass needle deflected away from magnetic north when the electric current from the battery he was using was switched on and off. This deflection convinced him that magnetic fields radiate from all sides of a wire carrying an electric current, just as light and heat do, and that it confirmed a direct relationship between electricity and magnetism.

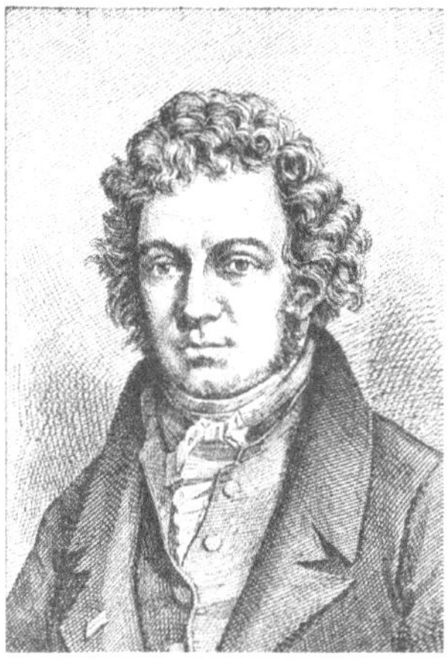

André-Marie Ampère

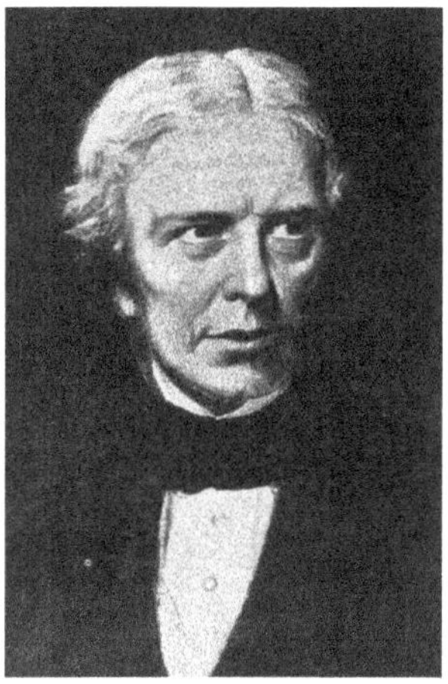

Michael Faraday

At the time of discovery, Ørsted did not suggest any satisfactory explanation of the phenomenon, nor did he try to represent the phenomenon in a mathematical framework. However, three months later he began more intensive investigations. Soon thereafter he published his findings, proving that an electric current produces a magnetic field as it flows through a wire. The CGS unit of magnetic induction (oersted) is named in honor of his contributions to the field of electromagnetism.

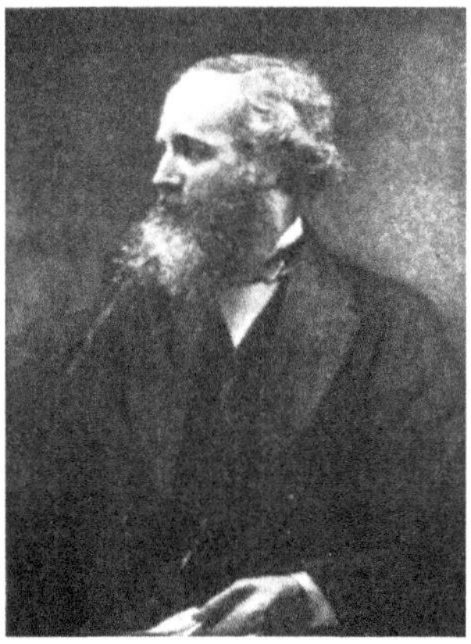

James Clerk Maxwell

His findings resulted in intensive research throughout the scientific community in electrodynamics. They influenced French physicist André-Marie Ampère's developments of a single mathematical form to represent the magnetic forces between current-carrying conductors. Ørsted's discovery also represented a major step toward a unified concept of energy.

This unification, which was observed by Michael Faraday, extended by James Clerk Maxwell, and partially reformulated by Oliver Heaviside and Heinrich Hertz, is one of the key accomplishments of 19th century mathematical physics. It has had far-reaching consequences, one of which was the understanding of the nature of light. Unlike what was proposed by electromagnetic theory of that time, light and other electromagnetic waves are at present seen as taking the form of quantized, self-propagating oscillatory electromagnetic field disturbances called photons. Different frequencies of oscillation give rise to the different forms of electromagnetic radiation, from radio waves at the lowest frequencies, to visible light at intermediate frequencies, to gamma rays at the highest frequencies.

Ørsted was not the only person to examine the relationship between electricity and magnetism. In 1802, Gian Domenico Romagnosi, an Italian legal scholar, deflected a magnetic needle using a Voltaic pile. The factual setup of the experiment is not completely clear, so if current flew across the needle or not. An account of the discovery was published in 1802 in an Italian newspaper, but it was largely overlooked by the contemporary scientific community, because Romagnosi seemingly did not belong to this community.

Fundamental Forces

The electromagnetic force is one of the four known fundamental forces. The other fundamental forces are:

- the weak nuclear force, which binds to all known particles in the Standard Model, and causes certain forms of radioactive decay. (In particle physics though, the electroweak interaction is the unified description of two of the four known fundamental interactions of nature: electromagnetism and the weak interaction);
- the strong nuclear force, which binds quarks to form nucleons, and binds nucleons to form nuclei;
- the gravitational force.

All other forces (e.g., friction, contact forces) are derived from these four fundamental forces (including momentum which is carried by the movement of particles).

The electromagnetic force is the one responsible for practically all the phenomena one encounters in daily life above the nuclear scale, with the exception of gravity. Roughly speaking, all the forces involved in interactions between atoms can be explained by the electromagnetic force acting between the electrically charged atomic nuclei and electrons of the atoms. Electromagnetic forces also explain how these particles carry momentum by their movement. This includes the forces we experience in "pushing" or "pulling" ordinary material objects, which result from the intermolecular forces that act between the individual molecules in our bodies and those in the objects. The electromagnetic force is also involved in all forms of chemical phenomena.

A necessary part of understanding the intra-atomic and intermolecular forces is the effective force generated by the momentum of the electrons' movement, such that as electrons move between interacting atoms they carry momentum with them. As a collection of electrons becomes more confined, their minimum momentum necessarily increases due to the Pauli exclusion principle. The behaviour of matter at the molecular scale including its density is determined by the balance between the electromagnetic force and the force generated by the exchange of momentum carried by the electrons themselves.

Classical Electrodynamics

In 1600, William Gilbert proposed, in his *De Magnete*, that electricity and magnetism, while both capable of causing attraction and repulsion of objects, were distinct effects. Mariners had noticed that lightning strikes had the ability to disturb a compass needle, but the link between lightning and electricity was not confirmed until Benjamin Franklin's proposed experiments in 1752. One of the first to discover and publish a link between man-made electric current and magnetism was Romagnosi, who in 1802 noticed that connecting a wire across a voltaic pile deflected a nearby compass needle. However, the effect did not become widely known until 1820, when Ørsted performed a similar experiment. Ørsted's work influenced Ampère to produce a theory of electromagnetism that set the subject on a mathematical foundation.

A theory of electromagnetism, known as classical electromagnetism, was developed by various physicists the period between 1820 and 1873 when it culminated in the publication of a treatise by James Clerk Maxwell, which unified the preceding developments into a single theory and discovered the electromagnetic nature of light. In classical electromagnetism, the behavior of the electromagnetic field is described by a set of equations known as Maxwell's equations, and the electromagnetic force is given by the Lorentz force law.

One of the peculiarities of classical electromagnetism is that it is difficult to reconcile with classical mechanics, but it is compatible with special relativity. According to Maxwell's equations, the speed of light in a vacuum is a universal constant that is dependent only on the electrical permittivity and magnetic permeability of free space. This violates Galilean invariance, a long-standing cornerstone of classical mechanics. One way to reconcile the two theories (electromagnetism and classical mechanics) is to assume the existence of a luminiferous aether through which the light propagates. However, subsequent experimental efforts failed to detect the presence of the aether. After important contributions of Hendrik Lorentz and Henri Poincaré, in 1905, Albert Einstein solved the problem with the introduction of special relativity, which replaced classical kinematics with a new theory of kinematics compatible with classical electromagnetism.

In addition, relativity theory implies that in moving frames of reference a magnetic field transforms to a field with a nonzero electric component and conversely, a moving electric field transforms to a nonzero magnetic component, thus firmly showing that the phenomena are two sides of the same coin. Hence the term "electromagnetism".

Quantum Mechanics

Early Quantum Theory

In a second paper published in 1905, Albert Einstein undermined the very foundations of classical electromagnetism. In his theory of the photoelectric effect, for which he won the Nobel prize in physics, he posited that light could exist in discrete particle-like quantities, which later came to be called photons. Einstein's theory of the photoelectric effect extended the insights that appeared in the solution of the ultraviolet catastrophe presented by Max Planck in 1900 and who coined the term "quanta" . In his work, Planck showed that hot objects emit electromagnetic radiation in discrete packets ("quanta"), which leads to a finite total energy emitted as black body radiation. Both of these results were in direct contradiction with the classical view of light as a continuous wave. Planck's and Einstein's theories were progenitors of quantum mechanics, which, when formulated in 1925, necessitated the invention of a quantum theory of electromagnetism.

Quantum Electrodynamics

Maxwell's equations have been superseded by quantum electrodynamics (QED). Richard Feynman called it "the jewel of physics" for its extremely accurate predictions of quantities like the Lamb shift, and measurement of the magnetic moment of the electron. The electromagnetic field is quantized by imagining that at every point in space and time is a quantum harmonic oscillator. The empty field (vacuum state) fluctuates randomly as a consequence of the uncertainty principle. This theory, completed in the 1940s–1950s, is one of the most accurate theories known to physics in situations where perturbation theory can be applied. Like classical electromagnetism, QED is a linear U(1) gauge group.

Electroweak Interaction

The electroweak interaction is a unified field theory description of two of the four known fundamental interactions of nature: electromagnetism and the weak interaction. It is a SU(2) × U(1) gauge group. Although these two forces appear very different at everyday low energies, the theory models them as two different aspects of the same force. At energies greater than 100 GeV, called the unification energy, the two forces merge into a single electroweak force. Thus when the universe was hot enough (approximately 10^{15} K, a temperature that was exceeded until shortly after the Big Bang) the electromagnetic force and weak force were merged into the electroweak force. With the cooling of the universe, at the end of the electroweak epoch, the electroweak force separated into the electromagnetic force and the weak force. During the following quark epoch, it was still too hot for quarks to combine into hadrons and they moved about freely.

Chaotic and Emergent Phenomena

The mathematical models used in classical electromagnetism, quantum electrodynamics (QED) and the standard model all view the electromagnetic force as a linear set of equations. In these theories electromagnetism is a U(1) gauge theory, whose topological properties do not allow any complex nonlinear interaction of a field with and on itself. For example, in the QED vacuum the field fluctuates randomly as a consequence of the uncertainty principle but these fluctuations cancel each other out with no overall observable effect. However, there are many observed nonlinear physical electromagnetic phenomena such as Aharonov–Bohm (AB) and Altshuler–Aronov– Spivak (AAS) effects, Berry, Aharonov– Anandan, Pancharatnam and Chiao–Wu phase rotation effects, Josephson effect, Quantum Hall effect, the de Haas–van Alphen effect, the Sagnac effect and many other physically observable phenomena which would indicate that the electromagnetic potential field has real physical meaning rather than being a mathematical artifact and therefore an all encompassing theory would not confine electromagnetism as a local force as is currently done, but as a SU(2) gauge theory or higher geometry. Higher symmetries allow for nonlinear, aperiodic behaviour which manifest as a variety of complex non-equilibrium phenomena that do not arise in the linearised U(1) theory, such as multiple stable states, symmetry breaking, chaos and emergence. In higher symmetry groups, the electromagnetic field is not a calm, randomly fluctuating, passive substance, but can at times can be viewed as a turbulent virtual plasma that can have complex vortices, entangled states and a rich nonlinear structure.

What are called Maxwell's equation's today are in fact a simplified version of the original equations reformulated by Heaviside, FitzGerald, Lodge and Hertz. The original equations used Hamilton's more expressive quaternion notation, a kind of Clifford algebra, which fully subsumes the standard Maxwell vectorial equations largely used today. In the late 1880s there was a debate over the relative merits of vector analysis and quaternions. According to Heaviside the electromagnetic potential field was purely metaphysical, an arbitrary mathematical fiction, that needed to be *"murdered"*. It was concluded that there was no need for the greater physical insights provided by the quaternions if the theory was purely local in nature. Local vector analysis has become the dominant way of using Maxwell's equations ever since. However, this strictly vectorial approach as led to a restrictive topological understanding in some areas of electromagnetism, for example, a full understanding of the energy transfer dynamics in Tesla's oscillator-shuttle-circuit can be achieved only in quaternionic algebra or higher SU(2) symmetries. It has often been argued that quaternions are not compatible with special relativity, but multiple papers have shown ways of incorporating relativity.

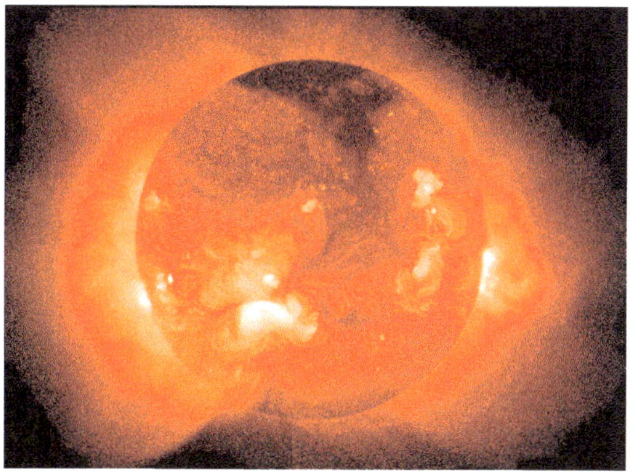

Plasma vortices give rise to solar flares on the sun

A good example of nonlinear electromagnetics is in high energy dense plasmas, where vortical phenomena occur which seemingly violate the second law of thermodynamics by increasing the energy gradient within the electromagnetic field and violate Maxwell's laws by creating ion currents which capture and concentrate their own and surrounding magnetic fields. In particular Lorentz force law, which elaborates Maxwell's equations is violated by these force free vortices. These apparent violations are due to the fact that the traditional conservation laws in classical and quantum electrodynamics (QED) only display linear U(1) symmetry (in particular, by the extended Noether theorem, conservation laws such as the laws of thermodynamics need not always apply to dissipative systems, which are expressed in gauges of higher symmetry). The second law of thermodynamics states that in a closed linear system entropy flow can be only be positive (or exactly zero at the end of a cycle). However, negative entropy (i.e. increased order, structure or self-organisation) can spontaneously appear in an open nonlinear thermodynamic system that is far from equilibrium, so long as this emergent order accelerates the overall flow of entropy in the total system.

Given the complex and adaptive behaviour that arises from nonlinear systems considerable attention in recent years has gone into studying a new class of phase transitions which occur at absolute zero temperature. These are quantum phase transitions which are driven by electomagnetic field fluctuations as a consequence of zero-point energy A good example of a spontaneous phase transition that are attributed to zero-point fluctuations can be found in superconductors. Superconductivity is one of the best known empirically quantified macroscopic electromagnetic phenomena whose basis is recognised to be quantum mechanical in origin. The behaviour of the electric and magnetic fields under superconductivity is governed by the London equations. However, it has been questioned in a series of journal articles whether the quantum mechanically canonised London equations can be given a purely classical derivation. Bostick for instance, has claimed to show that the London equations do indeed have a classical origin that applies to superconductors and to some collisionless plasmas as well. In particular it has been asserted that the Beltrami vortices in the plasma focus display the same paired flux-tube morphology as Type II superconductors. Others have also pointed out this connection, Fröhlich has shown that the hydrodynamic equations of compressible fluids, together with the London equations, lead to a macroscopic parameter (μ = electric charge density / mass density), without involving either quantum phase factors or Planck's constant. In essence, it has been asserted that Beltrami plasma vortex structures are able to at least simulate the morphology of Type I and Type II superconductors. This occurs because the *"organised"* dissipative energy of the vortex configuration comprising the ions and electrons far exceeds the *"disorganised"* dissipative random thermal energy. The transition from disorganised fluctuations to organised helical structures is a phase transition involving a change in the condensate's energy (i.e. the ground state or zero-point energy) but *without any associated rise in temperature*. This is an example of zero-point energy having multiple stable states and where the overall system structure is independent of a reductionist or deterministic view, that *"classical"* macroscopic order can also causally affect quantum phenomena.

Quantities and Units

Electromagnetic units are part of a system of electrical units based primarily upon the magnetic properties of electric currents, the fundamental SI unit being the ampere. The units are:

- ampere (electric current)
- coulomb (electric charge)
- farad (capacitance)
- henry (inductance)
- ohm (resistance)
- siemens (conductance)
- tesla (magnetic flux density)
- volt (electric potential)

- watt (power)
- weber (magnetic flux)

In the electromagnetic cgs system, electric current is a fundamental quantity defined via Ampère's law and takes the permeability as a dimensionless quantity (relative permeability) whose value in a vacuum is unity. As a consequence, the square of the speed of light appears explicitly in some of the equations interrelating quantities in this system.

SI electromagnetism units				
Symbol	**Name of Quantity**	**Derived Units**	**Unit**	**Base Units**
I	electric current	ampere (SI base unit)	A	A (= W/V = C/s)
Q	electric charge	coulomb	C	A·s
$U, \Delta V, \Delta\varphi; E$	potential difference; electromotive force	volt	V	$kg \cdot m^2 \cdot s^{-3} \cdot A^{-1}$ (= J/C)
$R; Z; X$	electric resistance; impedance; reactance	ohm	Ω	$kg \cdot m^2 \cdot s^{-3} \cdot A^{-2}$ (= V/A)
ρ	resistivity	ohm metre	Ω·m	$kg \cdot m^3 \cdot s^{-3} \cdot A^{-2}$
P	electric power	watt	W	$kg \cdot m^2 \cdot s^{-3}$ (= V·A)
C	capacitance	farad	F	$kg^{-1} \cdot m^{-2} \cdot s^4 \cdot A^2$ (= C/V)
E	electric field strength	volt per metre	V/m	$kg \cdot m \cdot s^{-3} \cdot A^{-1}$ (= N/C)
D	electric displacement field	coulomb per square metre	C/m²	$A \cdot s \cdot m^{-2}$
ε	permittivity	farad per metre	F/m	$kg^{-1} \cdot m^{-3} \cdot s^4 \cdot A^2$
χ_e	electric susceptibility	(dimensionless)	–	–
$G; Y; B$	conductance; admittance; susceptance	siemens	S	$kg^{-1} \cdot m^{-2} \cdot s^3 \cdot A^2$ (= Ω^{-1})
κ, γ, σ	conductivity	siemens per metre	S/m	$kg^{-1} \cdot m^{-3} \cdot s^3 \cdot A^2$
B	magnetic flux density, magnetic induction	tesla	T	$kg \cdot s^{-2} \cdot A^{-1}$ (= Wb/m² = $N \cdot A^{-1} \cdot m^{-1}$)
	magnetic flux	weber	Wb	$kg \cdot m^2 \cdot s^{-2} \cdot A^{-1}$ (= V·s)
H	magnetic field strength	ampere per metre	A/m	$A \cdot m^{-1}$
L, M	inductance	henry	H	$kg \cdot m^2 \cdot s^{-2} \cdot A^{-2}$ (= Wb/A = V·s/A)
μ	permeability	henry per metre	H/m	$kg \cdot m \cdot s^{-2} \cdot A^{-2}$
χ	magnetic susceptibility	(dimensionless)	–	–
J	current density	ampere per square metre	A/m²	$C \cdot m^{-2} \cdot s^{-1}$

Formulas for physical laws of electromagnetism (such as Maxwell's equations) need to be adjusted depending on what system of units one uses. This is because there is no one-to-one correspondence between electromagnetic units in SI and those in CGS, as is the case for mechanical units. Furthermore, within CGS, there are several plausible choices of electromagnetic units, leading to different unit "sub-systems", including Gaussian, "ESU", "EMU", and Heaviside–Lorentz. Among these choices, Gaussian units are the most common today, and in fact the phrase "CGS units" is often used to refer specifically to CGS-Gaussian units.

History of Electromagnetic Theory

The history of electromagnetic theory begins with ancient measures to understand atmospheric electricity, in particular lightning. People then had little understanding of electricity, and were unable to explain the phenomena. Scientific understanding into the nature of electricity grew throughout the eighteenth and nineteenth centuries through the work of researchers such as Ampère, Coulomb, Faraday and Maxwell.

In the 19th century it had become clear that electricity and magnetism were related, and their theories were unified: wherever charges are in motion electric current results, and magnetism is due to electric current. The source for electric field is electric charge, whereas that for magnetic field is electric current (charges in motion).

Ancient and Classical History

The knowledge of static electricity dates back to the earliest civilizations, but for millennia it remained merely an interesting and mystifying phenomenon, without a theory to explain its behavior and often confused with magnetism. The ancients were acquainted with rather curious properties possessed by two minerals, amber and magnetic iron ore. Amber, when rubbed, attracts lightweight objects, such as feathers; magnetic iron ore has the power of attracting iron.

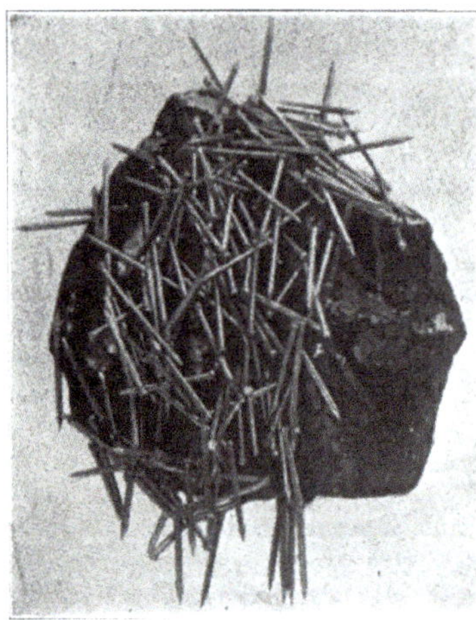

The discovery of the *property of magnets*

Magnets were first found in a natural state; certain iron oxides were discovered in various parts of the world, notably in Magnesia in Asia Minor, that had the property of attracting small pieces of iron, which is shown here.

Based on his find of an Olmec hematite artifact in Central America, the American astronomer John Carlson has suggested that "the Olmec may have discovered and used the geomagnetic lodestone compass earlier than 1000 BC". If true, this "predates the Chinese discovery of the geomagnetic lodestone compass by more than a millennium". Carlson speculates that the Olmecs may have used similar artifacts as a directional device for astrological or geomantic purposes, or to orient their temples, the dwellings of the living or the interments of the dead. The earliest Chinese literature reference to *magnetism* lies in a 4th-century BC book called *Book of the Devil Valley Master*. "The lodestone makes iron come or it attracts it."

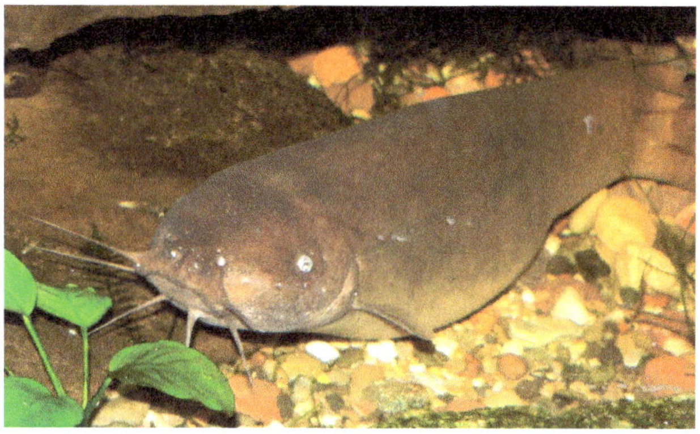

Electric catfish are found in tropical Africa and the Nile River

Long before any knowledge of electromagnetism existed, people were aware of the effects of electricity. Lightning and other manifestations of electricity such as St. Elmo's fire were known in ancient times, but it was not understood that these phenomena had a common origin. Ancient Egyptians were aware of shocks when interacting with electric fish (such as the electric catfish) or other animals (such as electric eels). The shocks from animals were apparent to observers since pre-history by a variety of peoples that came into contact with them. Texts from 2750 BCE by the ancient Egyptians referred to these fish as "thunderer of the Nile" and saw them as the "protectors" of all the other fish. Another possible approach to the discovery of the identity of lightning and electricity from any other source, is to be attributed to the Arabs, who before the 15th century used the same Arabic word for lightning (*barq*) and the electric ray.

Thales of Miletus, writing at around 600 BC, noted that rubbing fur on various substances such as amber would cause them to attract specks of dust and other light objects. Thales wrote on the effect now known as static electricity. The Greeks noted that if they rubbed the amber for long enough they could even get an electric spark to jump.

The electrostatic phenomena was again reported millennia later by Roman and Arabic naturalists and physicians. Several ancient writers, such as Pliny the Elder and Scribonius Largus, attested to the numbing effect of electric shocks delivered by catfish and torpedo rays. Pliny in his books writes: "The ancient Tuscans by their learning hold that there are nine gods that send forth lightning and those of eleven sorts." This was in general the early pagan idea of lightning. The ancients held some concept that shocks could travel along conducting objects. Patients suffering from ailments such as gout or headache were directed to touch electric fish in the hope that the powerful jolt might cure them.

A number of objects found in Iraq in 1938 dated to the early centuries AD (Sassanid Mesopotamia), called the Baghdad Battery, resembles a galvanic cell and is believed by some to have been used for electroplating. The claims are controversial because of supporting evidence and theories for the uses of the artifacts, physical evidence on the objects conducive for electrical functions, and if they were electrical in nature. As a result, the nature of these objects is based on speculation, and the function of these artifacts remains in doubt.

Middle Ages and the Renaissance

Magnetic attraction was once accounted for by Aristotle and Thales as the working of a soul in the stone.

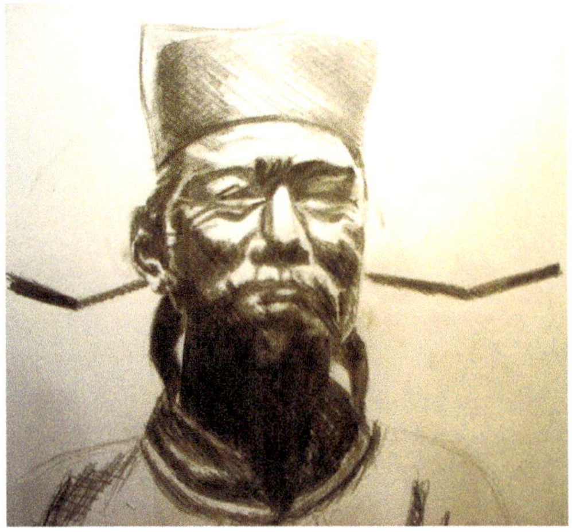

Shen Kuo wrote *Dream Pool Essays*; Shen also first described the magnetic needle.

In the 11th century, the Chinese scientist Shen Kuo (1031–1095) was the first person to write of the magnetic needle compass and that it improved the accuracy of navigation by employing the astronomical concept of true north *(Dream Pool Essays*, AD 1088), and by the 12th century the Chinese were known to use the lodestone compass for navigation. In 1187, Alexander Neckam was the first in Europe to describe the compass and its use for navigation.

Magnetism was one of the few sciences which progressed in medieval Europe; for in the thirteenth century Peter Peregrinus, a native of Maricourt in Picardy, made a discovery of fundamental importance. The French 13th century scholar conducted experiments on magnetism and wrote the first extant treatise describing the properties of magnets and pivoting compass needles. The dry compass was invented around 1300 by Italian inventor Flavio Gioja.

Archbishop Eustathius of Thessalonica, Greek scholar and writer of the 12th century, records that *Woliver*, king of the Goths, was able to draw sparks from his body. The same writer states that a certain philosopher was able while dressing to draw sparks from his clothes, a result seemingly akin to that obtained by Robert Symmer in his silk stocking experiments, a careful account of which may be found in the 'Philosophical Transactions,' 1759.

Italian physician Gerolamo Cardano wrote about electricity in *De Subtilitate* (1550) distinguishing, perhaps for the first time, between electrical and magnetic forces.

Toward the late 16th century, a physician of Queen Elizabeth's time, Dr. William Gilbert, in *De Magnete*, expanded on Cardano's work and invented the New Latin word *electricus* from (*elektron*), the Greek word for "amber". Gilbert, a native of Colchester, Fellow of St John's College, Cambridge, and sometime President of the College of Physicians, was one of the earliest and most distinguished English men of science — a man whose work Galileo thought enviably great. He was appointed Court physician, and a pension was settled on him to set him free to continue his researches in Physics and Chemistry.

Gilbert undertook a number of careful electrical experiments, in the course of which he discovered that many substances other than amber, such as sulphur, wax, glass, etc., were capable of manifesting electrical properties. Gilbert also discovered that a heated body lost its electricity and that moisture prevented the electrification of all bodies, due to the now well-known fact that moisture impaired the insulation of such bodies. He also noticed that electrified substances attracted all other substances indiscriminately, whereas a magnet only attracted iron. The many discoveries of this nature earned for Gilbert the title of *founder of the electrical science*. By investigating the forces on a light metallic needle, balanced on a point, he extended the list of electric bodies, and found also that many substances, including metals and natural magnets, showed no attractive forces when rubbed. He noticed that dry weather with north or east wind was the most favourable atmospheric condition for exhibiting electric phenomena—an observation liable to misconception until the difference between conductor and insulator was understood.

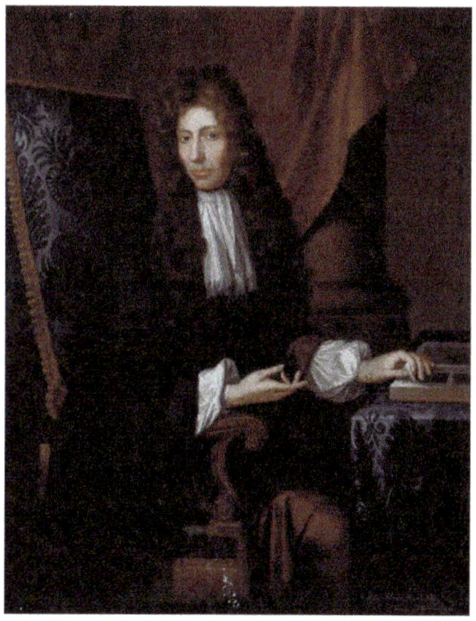

Robert Boyle

Gilbert's work was followed up by Robert Boyle (1627–1691), the famous natural philosopher who was once described as "father of Chemistry, and uncle of the Earl of Cork." Boyle was one of the founders of the Royal Society when it met privately in Oxford, and became a member of the Council after the Society was incorporated by Charles II. in 1663. He worked frequently at the new science of electricity, and added several substances to Gilbert's list of electrics. He left a detailed account of his researches under the title of *Experiments on the Origin of Electricity*. Boyle, in 1675, stated that electric attraction and repulsion can act across a vacuum. One of his important discoveries was that electrified bodies in a vacuum would attract light substances, thus indicating that the electrical effect did not depend upon the air as a medium. He also added resin to the then known list of electrics.

This was followed in 1660 by Otto von Guericke, who invented an early electrostatic generator. By the end of the 17th Century, researchers had developed practical means of generating electricity by friction with an electrostatic generator, but the development of electrostatic machines did not begin in earnest until the 18th century, when they became fundamental instruments in the studies about the new science of electricity.

The first usage of the word *electricity* is ascribed to Sir Thomas Browne in his 1646 work, *Pseudodoxia Epidemica*.

The first appearance of the term *electromagnetism* on the other hand comes from an earlier date: 1641. *Magnes*, by the Jesuit luminary Athanasius Kircher, carries on page 640 the provocative chapter-heading: "*Elektro-magnetismos* i.e. On the Magnetism of amber, or electrical attractions and their causes"

18th Century

Improving the Electric Machine

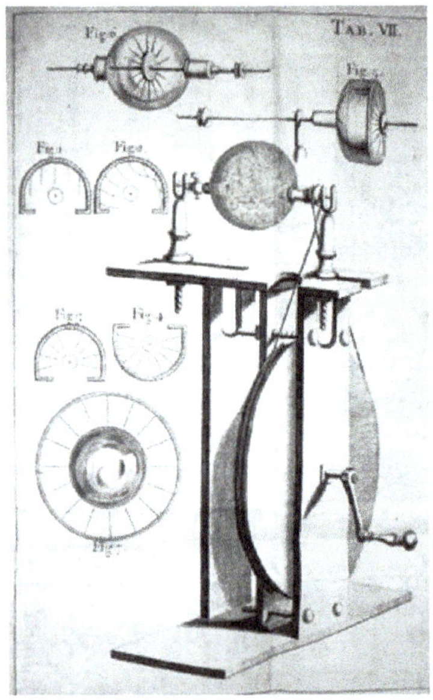

Generator built by Francis Hauksbee

The electric machine was subsequently improved by Francis Hauksbee, Litzendorf, and by Prof. Georg Matthias Bose, about 1750. Litzendorf, researching for Christian August Hausen, substituted a glass ball for the sulphur ball of Guericke. Bose was the first to employ the "prime conductor" in such machines, this consisting of an iron rod held in the hand of a person whose body was insulated by standing on a block of resin. Ingenhousz, during 1746, invented electric machines made of plate glass. Experiments with the electric machine were largely aided by the discovery of the property of a glass plate, when coated on both sides with tinfoil, of accumulating a charge of electricity when connected with a source of electromotive force. The electric machine was soon further improved by Andrew Gordon, a Scotsman, Professor at Erfurt, who substituted a glass cylinder in place of a glass globe; and by Giessing of Leipzig who added a "rubber" consisting of a cushion of woollen material. The collector, consisting of a series of metal points, was added to the machine by Benjamin Wilson about 1746, and in 1762, John Canton of England (also the inventor of the first pith-ball electroscope) improved the efficiency of electric machines by sprinkling an amalgam of tin over the surface of the rubber.

Electrics and Non-electrics

In 1729, Stephen Gray conducted a series of experiments that demonstrated the difference between conductors and non-conductors (insulators), showing amongst other things that a metal wire and even pack thread conducted electricity, whereas silk did not. In one of his experiments he sent an electric current through 800 feet of hempen thread which was suspended at intervals by loops of silk thread. When he tried to conduct the same experiment substituting the silk for finely spun brass wire, he found that the electric current was no longer carried throughout the hemp cord, but instead seemed to vanish into the brass wire. From this experiment he classified substances into two categories: "electrics" like glass, resin and silk and "non-electrics" like metal and water. "Non-electrics" conducted charges while "electrics" held the charge.

Vitreous and Resinous

Intrigued by Gray's results, in 1732, C. F. du Fay began to conduct several experiments. In his first experiment, Du Fay concluded that all objects except metals, animals, and liquids could be electrified by rubbing and that metals, animals and liquids could be electrified by means of an electric machine, thus discrediting Gray's "electrics" and "non-electrics" classification of substances.

In 1737 Du Fay and Hauksbee independently discovered what they believed to be two kinds of frictional electricity; one generated from rubbing glass, the other from rubbing resin. From this, Du Fay theorized that electricity consists of two electrical fluids, "vitreous" and "resinous", that are separated by friction and that neutralize each other when combined. This two-fluid theory would later give rise to the concept of *positive* and *negative* electrical charges devised by Benjamin Franklin.

Leyden Jar

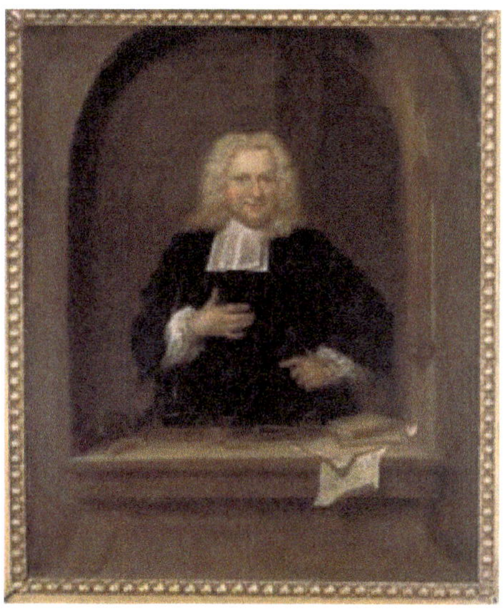

Pieter van Musschenbroek

The Leyden jar, a type of capacitor for electrical energy in large quantities, was invented independently by Ewald Georg von Kleist on 11 October 1744 and by Pieter van Musschenbroek in 1745—1746 at Leiden University (the latter location giving the device its name). William Watson, when experimenting with the Leyden jar, discovered in 1747 that a discharge of static electricity was equivalent to an electric current. Capacitance was first observed by Von Kleist of Leyden in 1754. Von Kleist happened to hold, near his electric machine, a small bottle, in the neck of which there was an iron nail. Touching the iron nail accidentally with his other hand he received a severe electric shock. In much the same way Musschenbroeck assisted by Cunaens received a more severe shock from a somewhat similar glass bottle. Sir William Watson of England greatly improved this device, by covering the bottle, or jar, outside and in with tinfoil. This piece of electrical apparatus will be easily recognized as the well-known Leyden jar, so called by the Abbot Nollet of Paris, after the place of its discovery.

In 1741, John Ellicott "proposed to measure the strength of electrification by its power to raise a weight in one scale of a balance while the other was held over the electrified body and pulled to it by its attractive power". As early as 1746, Jean-Antoine Nollet (1700–1770) had performed experiments on the propagation speed of electricity. By involving 200 monks connected from hand to hand by a 7-m iron wire so as to form a circle of about 1.6 km, he was able to prove that this speed is finite, even though very high. In 1749, Sir William Watson conducted numerous experiments to ascertain the velocity of electricity in a wire. These experiments, although perhaps not so intended, also demonstrated the possibility of transmitting signals to a distance by electricity. In these experiments, the signal appeared to travel the 12,276-foot length of the insulated wire instantaneously. Le Monnier in France had previously made somewhat similar experiments, sending shocks through an iron wire 1,319 feet long.

About 1750, first experiments in electrotherapeutics were made. Various experimenters made tests to ascertain the physiological and therapeutical effects of electricity. Demainbray in Edinburgh examined the effects of electricity upon plants and concluded that the growth of two myrtle trees was quickened by electrification. These myrtles were electrified "during the whole month of October, 1746, and they put forth branches and blossoms sooner than other shrubs of the same kind not electrified.". Abbé Ménon in France tried the effects of a continued application of electricity upon men and birds and found that the subjects experimented on lost weight, thus apparently showing that electricity quickened the excretions. The efficacy of electric shocks in cases of paralysis was tested in the county hospital at Shrewsbury, England, with rather poor success.

Late 18th Century

Benjamin Franklin promoted his investigations of electricity and theories through the famous, though extremely dangerous, experiment of having his son fly a kite through a storm-threatened sky. A key attached to the kite string sparked and charged a Leyden jar, thus establishing the link between lightning and electricity. Following these experiments, he invented a lightning rod. It is either Franklin (more frequently) or Ebenezer Kinnersley of Philadelphia (less frequently) who is considered to have established the convention of positive and negative electricity.

Theories regarding the nature of electricity were quite vague at this period, and those prevalent were more or less conflicting. Franklin considered that electricity was an imponderable fluid pervading everything, and which, in its normal condition, was uniformly distributed in all substances. He assumed that the electrical manifestations obtained by rubbing glass were due to the production of an excess of the electric fluid in that substance and that the manifestations produced by rubbing wax were due to a deficit of the fluid. This theory was opposed by Robert Symmer's "Two-fluid" theory in 1759. By Symmer's theory, the vitreous and resinous electricities were regarded as imponderable fluids, each fluid being composed of mutually repellent particles while the particles of the opposite electricities are mutually attractive. When the two fluids unite as a result of their attraction for one another, their effect upon external objects is neutralized. The act of rubbing a body decomposes the fluids, one of which remains in excess on the body and manifests itself as vitreous or resinous electricity.

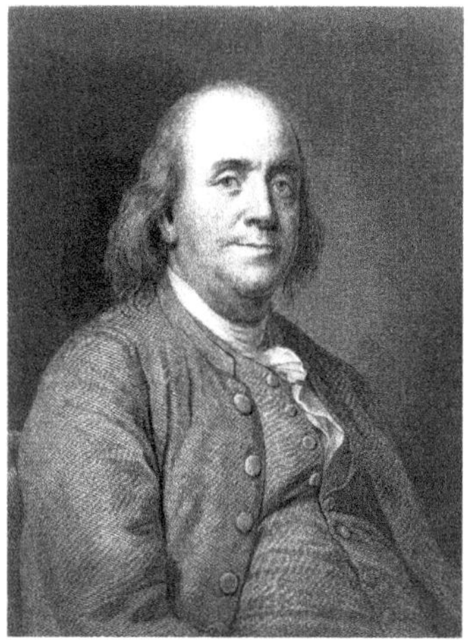

Benjamin Franklin

Up to the time of Franklin's historic kite experiment, the identity of the electricity developed by rubbing and by electrostatic machines (frictional electricity) with lightning had not been generally established. Dr. Wall, Abbot Nollet, Hauksbee, Stephen Gray and John Henry Winkler had indeed suggested the resemblance between the phenomena of "electricity" and "lightning", Gray having intimated that they only differed in degree. It was doubtless Franklin, however, who first proposed tests to determine the sameness of the phenomena. In a letter to Peter Comlinson of London, on 19 October 1752, Franklin, referring to his kite experiment, wrote,

"At this key the phial (Leyden jar) may be charged; and from the electric fire thus obtained spirits may be kindled, and all the other electric experiments be formed which are usually done by the help of a rubbed glass globe or tube, and thereby the sameness of the electric matter with that of lightning be completely demonstrated."

On 10 May 1742 Thomas-François Dalibard, at Marley (near Paris), using a vertical iron rod 40 feet long, obtained results corresponding to those recorded by Franklin and somewhat prior to the date of Franklin's experiment. Franklin's important demonstration of the sameness of frictional electricity and lightning doubtless added zest to the efforts of the many experimenters in this field in the last half of the 18th century, to advance the progress of the science.

Franklin's observations aided later scientists such as Michael Faraday, Luigi Galvani, Alessandro Volta, André-Marie Ampère and Georg Simon Ohm, whose collective work provided the basis for modern electrical technology and for whom fundamental units of electrical measurement are named. Others who would advance the field of knowledge included William Watson, Georg Matthias Bose, Smeaton, Louis-Guillaume Le Monnier, Jacques de Romas, Jean Jallabert, Giovanni Battista Beccaria, Tiberius Cavallo, John Canton, Robert Symmer, Abbot Nollet, John Henry Winkler, Richman, Dr. Wilson, Kinnersley, Joseph Priestley, Franz Aepinus, Edward Hussey Délavai, Henry Cavendish, and Charles-Augustin de Coulomb. Descriptions of many of the experiments and discoveries of these early electrical scientists may be found in the scientific publications of the time, notably the *Philosophical Transactions*, *Philosophical Magazine*, *Cambridge Mathematical Journal*, *Young's Natural Philosophy*, Priestley's *History of Electricity*, Franklin's *Experiments and Observations on Electricity*, Cavalli's *Treatise on Electricity* and De la Rive's *Treatise on Electricity*.

Henry Elles was one of the first people to suggest links between electricity and magnetism. In 1757 he claimed that he had written to the Royal Society in 1755 about the links between electricity and magnetism, asserting that "there are some things in the power of magnetism very similar to those of electricity" but he did "not by any means think them the same". In 1760 he similarly claimed that in 1750 he had been the first "to think how the electric fire may be the cause of thunder". Among the more important of the electrical research and experiments during this period were those of Franz Aepinus, a noted German scholar (1724–1802) and Henry Cavendish of London, England.

Franz Aepinus is credited as the first to conceive of the view of the reciprocal relationship of electricity and magnetism. In his work *Tentamen Theoria Electricitatis et Magnetism*, published in Saint Petersburg in 1759, he gives the following amplification of Franklin's theory, which in some of its features is measurably in accord with present-day views: "The particles of the electric fluid repel each other, attract and are attracted by the particles of all bodies with a force that decreases in proportion as the distance increases; the electric fluid exists in the pores of bodies; it moves unobstructedly through non-electric (conductors), but moves with difficulty in insulators; the manifestations of electricity are due to the unequal distribution of the fluid in a body, or to the approach of bodies unequally charged with the fluid." Aepinus formulated a corresponding theory of magnetism excepting that, in the case of magnetic phenomena, the fluids only acted on the particles of iron. He also made numerous electrical experiments apparently showing that, in order to manifest electrical effects, tourmaline must be heated to between 37.5°C and 100 °C. In fact, tourmaline remains unelectrified when its temperature is uniform, but manifests electrical properties when its temperature is rising or falling. Crystals that manifest electrical properties in this way are termed pyroelectric; along with tourmaline, these include sulphate of quinine and quartz.

Henry Cavendish independently conceived a theory of electricity nearly akin to that of Aepinus. In 1784, he was perhaps the first to utilize an electric spark to produce an explosion of hydrogen and oxygen in the proper proportions that would create pure water. Cavendish also discovered the inductive capacity of dielectrics (insulators), and, as early as 1778, measured the specific inductive capacity for beeswax and other substances by comparison with an air condenser.

Around 1784 C. A. Coulomb devised the torsion balance, discovering what is now known as Coulomb's law: the force exerted between two small electrified bodies varies inversely as the square of the distance, not as Aepinus in his theory of electricity had assumed, merely inversely as the distance. According to the theory advanced by Cavendish, "the particles attract and are attracted inversely as some less power of the distance than the cube." *A large part of the domain of electricity became virtually annexed by Coulomb's discovery of the law of inverse squares.*

Through the experiments of William Watson and others proving that electricity could be transmitted to a distance, the idea of making practical use of this phenomenon began, around 1753, to engross the minds of inquisitive people. To this end, suggestions as to the employment of electricity in the transmission of intelligence were made. The first of the methods devised for this purpose was probably that of Georges Lesage in 1774. This method consisted of 24 wires, insulated from one another and each having had a pith ball connected to its distant end. Each wire represented a letter of the alphabet. To send a message, a desired wire was charged momentarily with electricity from an electric machine, whereupon the pith ball connected to that wire would fly out. Other methods of telegraphing in which frictional electricity was employed were also tried, some of which are described in the history on the telegraph.

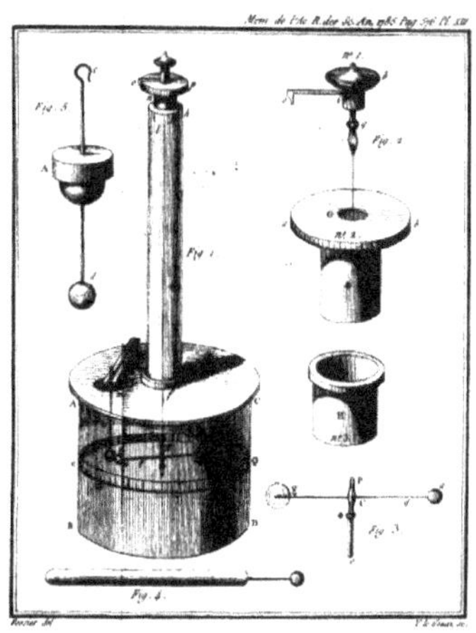

Drawing of Coulomb's torsion balance. From Plate 13 of his 1785 memoir

The era of galvanic or voltaic electricity represented a revolutionary break from the historical focus on frictional electricity. Alessandro Volta discovered that chemical reactions could be used to create positively charged anodes and negatively charged cathodes. When a conductor was attached between these, the difference in the electrical potential (also known as voltage) drove a current between them through the conductor. The potential difference between two points is measured in units of volts in recognition of Volta's work.

The first mention of voltaic electricity, although not recognized as such at the time, was probably made by Johann Georg Sulzer in 1767, who, upon placing a small disc of zinc under his tongue and a small disc of copper over it, observed a peculiar taste when the respective metals touched at their edges. Sulzer assumed that when the metals came together they were set into vibration, acting upon the nerves of the tongue to produce the effects noticed. In 1790, Prof. Luigi Alyisio Galvani of Bologna, while conducting experiments on "animal electricity", noticed the twitching of a frog's legs in the presence of an electric machine. He observed that a frog's muscle, suspended on an iron balustrade by a copper hook passing through its dorsal column, underwent lively convulsions without any extraneous cause, the electric machine being at this time absent.

To account for this phenomenon, Galvani assumed that electricity of opposite kinds existed in the nerves and muscles of the frog, the muscles and nerves constituting the charged coatings of a Leyden jar. Galvani published the results of his discoveries, together with his hypothesis, which engrossed the attention of the physicists of that time. The most prominent of these was Volta, professor of physics at Pavia, who contended that the results observed by Galvani were the result of the two metals, copper and iron, acting as electromotors, and that the muscles of the frog played the part of a conductor, completing the circuit. This precipitated a long discussion between the adherents of the conflicting views. One group agreed with Volta that the electric current was the result of an electromotive force of contact at the two metals; the other adopted a modification of Galvani's view and asserted that the current was the result of a chemical affinity between the metals and the acids in the pile. Michael Faraday wrote in the preface to his *Experimental Researches*, relative to the question of whether metallic contact is productive of a part of the electricity of the voltaic pile: "I see no reason as yet to alter the opinion I have given; ... but the point itself is of such great importance that I intend at the first opportunity renewing the inquiry, and, if I can, rendering the proofs either on the one side or the other, undeniable to all."

Even Faraday himself, however, did not settle the controversy, and while the views of the advocates on both sides of the question have undergone modifications, as subsequent investigations and discoveries demanded, up to 1918 diversity of opinion on these points continued to crop out. Volta made numerous experiments in support of his theory and ultimately developed the pile or battery, which was the precursor of all subsequent chemical batteries, and possessed the distinguishing merit of being the first means by which a prolonged continuous current of electricity was obtainable. Volta communicated a description of his pile to the Royal Society of London and shortly thereafter Nicholson and Cavendish (1780) produced the decomposition of water by means of the electric current, using Volta's pile as the source of electromotive force.

19th Century

Early 19th Century

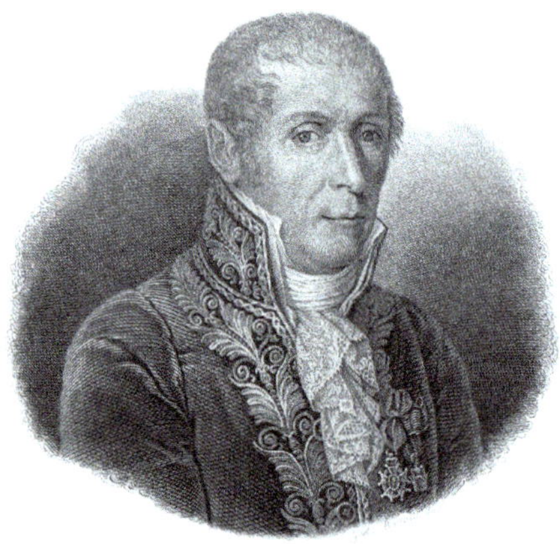

Alessandro Volta

In 1800 Alessandro Volta constructed the first device to produce a large electric current, later known as the electric battery. Napoleon, informed of his works, summoned him in 1801 for a command performance of his experiments. He received many medals and decorations, including the Légion d'honneur.

Davy in 1806, employing a voltaic pile of approximately 250 cells, or couples, decomposed potash and soda, showing that these substances were respectively the oxides of potassium and sodium, metals which previously had been unknown. These experiments were the beginning of electrochemistry, the investigation of which Faraday took up, and concerning which in 1833 he announced his important law of electrochemical equivalents, viz.: "*The same quantity of electricity — that is, the same electric current — decomposes chemically equivalent quantities of all the bodies which it traverses; hence the weights of elements separated in these electrolytes are to each other as their chemical equivalents.*" Employing a battery of 2,000 elements of a voltaic pile Humphry Davy in 1809 gave the first public demonstration of the electric arc light, using for the purpose charcoal enclosed in a vacuum.

Somewhat important to note, it was not until many years after the discovery of the voltaic pile that the sameness of annual and frictional electricity with voltaic electricity was clearly recognized and demonstrated. Thus as late as January 1833 we find Faraday writing in a paper on the electricity of the electric ray. "*After an examination of the experiments of Walsh, Ingenhousz, Henry Cavendish, Sir*

H. Davy, and Dr. Davy, no doubt remains on my mind as to the identity of the electricity of the torpedo with common (frictional) *and voltaic electricity; and I presume that so little will remain on the mind of others as to justify my refraining from entering at length into the philosophical proof of that identity. The doubts raised by Sir Humphry Davy have been removed by his brother, Dr. Davy; the results of the latter being the reverse of those of the former. ... The general conclusion which must, I think, be drawn from this collection of facts* (a table showing the similarity, of properties of the diversely named electricities) *is, that electricity, whatever may be its source, is identical in its nature."*

It is proper to state, however, that prior to Faraday's time the similarity of electricity derived from different sources was more than suspected. Thus, William Hyde Wollaston, wrote in 1801: "*This similarity in the means by which both electricity and galvanism (voltaic electricity) appear to be excited in addition to the resemblance that has been traced between their effects shows that they are both essentially the same and confirm an opinion that has already been advanced by others, that all the differences discoverable in the effects of the latter may be owing to its being less intense, but produced in much larger quantity.*" In the same paper Wollaston describes certain experiments in which he uses very fine wire in a solution of sulphate of copper through which he passed electric currents from an electric machine. This is interesting in connection with the later day use of almost similarly arranged fine wires in electrolytic receivers in wireless, or radio-telegraphy.

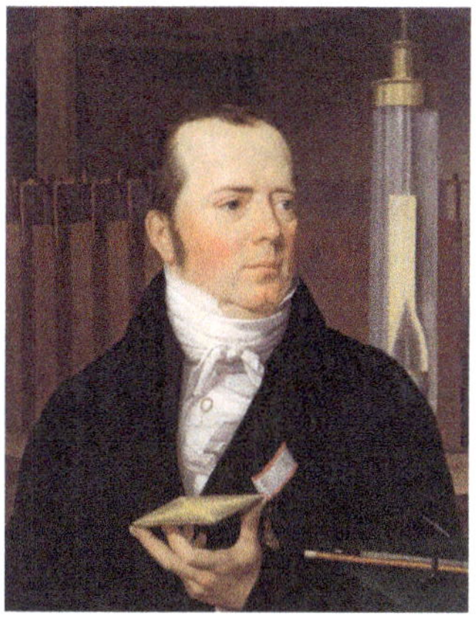

Hans Christian Ørsted

In the first half of the 19th century many very important additions were made to the world's knowledge concerning electricity and magnetism. For example, in 1819 Hans Christian Ørsted of Copenhagen discovered the deflecting effect of an electric current traversing a wire upon- a suspended magnetic needle.

This discovery gave a clue to the subsequently proved intimate relationship between electricity and magnetism which was promptly followed up by Ampère who shortly thereafter (1821) announced his celebrated theory of electrodynamics, relating to the force that one current exerts upon another, by its electro-magnetic effects, namely:

1. Two parallel portions of a circuit attract one another if the currents in them are flowing in the same direction, and repel one another if the currents flow in the opposite direction.
2. Two portions of circuits crossing one another obliquely attract one another if both the cur-

rents flow either towards or from the point of crossing, and repel one another if one flows to and the other from that point.

3. When an element of a circuit exerts a force on another element of a circuit, that force always tends to urge the second one in a direction at right angles to its own direction.

Ampere brought a multitude of phenomena into theory by his investigations of the mechanical forces between conductors supporting currents and magnets.

The German physicist Seebeck discovered in 1821 that when heat is applied to the junction of two metals that had been soldered together an electric current is set up. This is termed thermoelectricity. Seebeck's device consists of a strip of copper bent at each end and soldered to a plate of bismuth. A magnetic needle is placed parallel with the copper strip. When the heat of a lamp is applied to the junction of the copper and bismuth an electric current is set up which deflects the needle.

Around this time, Siméon Denis Poisson attacked the difficult problem of induced magnetization, and his results, though differently expressed, are still the theory, as a most important first approximation. It was in the application of mathematics to physics that his services to science were performed. Perhaps the most original, and certainly the most permanent in their influence, were his memoirs on the theory of electricity and magnetism, which virtually created a new branch of mathematical physics.

George Green wrote *An Essay on the Application of Mathematical Analysis to the Theories of Electricity and Magnetism* in 1828. The essay introduced several important concepts, among them a theorem similar to the modern Green's theorem, the idea of potential functions as currently used in physics, and the concept of what are now called Green's functions. George Green was the first person to create a mathematical theory of electricity and magnetism and his theory formed the foundation for the work of other scientists such as James Clerk Maxwell, William Thomson, and others.

Peltier in 1834 discovered an effect opposite to thermoelectricity, namely, that when a current is passed through a couple of dissimilar metals the temperature is lowered or raised at the junction of the metals, depending on the direction of the current. This is termed the Peltier effect. The variations of temperature are found to be proportional to the strength of the current and not to the square of the strength of the current as in the case of heat due to the ordinary resistance of a conductor. This second law is the C^2R law, discovered experimentally in 1841 by the English physicist Joule. In other words, this important law is that the heat generated in any part of an electric circuit is directly proportional to the product of the resistance of this part of the circuit and to the square of the strength of current flowing in the circuit.

In 1822 Johann Schweigger devised the first galvanometer. This instrument was subsequently much improved by Wilhelm Weber (1833). In 1825 William Sturgeon of Woolwich, England, invented the horseshoe and straight bar electromagnet, receiving therefor the silver medal of the Society of Arts. In 1837 Carl Friedrich Gauss and Weber (both noted workers of this period) jointly invented a reflecting galvanometer for telegraph purposes. This was the forerunner of the Thomson reflecting and other exceedingly sensitive galvanometers once used in submarine signaling and still widely employed in electrical measurements. Arago in 1824 made the important discovery that when a copper disc is rotated in its own plane, and if a magnetic needle be freely suspended on a pivot over the disc, the needle will rotate with the disc. If on the other hand the needle is fixed it will tend to retard the motion of the disc. This effect was termed Arago's rotations.

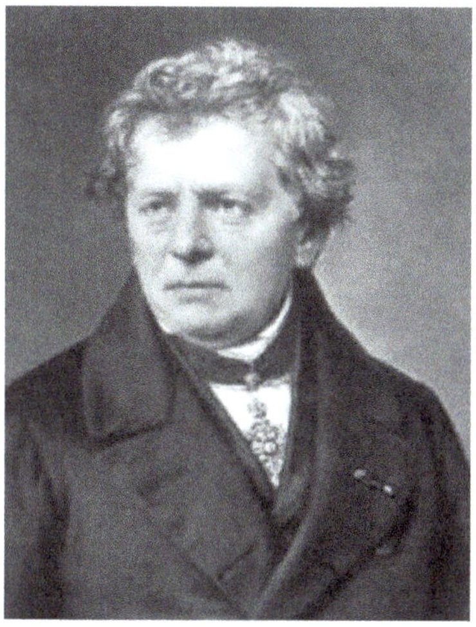

Georg Simon Ohm

Futile attempts were made by Charles Babbage, Peter Barlow, John Herschel and others to explain this phenomenon. The true explanation was reserved for Faraday, namely, that electric currents are induced in the copper disc by the cutting of the magnetic lines of force of the needle, which currents in turn react on the needle. Georg Simon Ohm did his work on resistance in the years 1825 and 1826, and published his results in 1827 as the book *Die galvanische Kette, mathematisch bearbeitet*. He drew considerable inspiration from Fourier's work on heat conduction in the theoretical explanation of his work. For experiments, he initially used voltaic piles, but later used a thermocouple as this provided a more stable voltage source in terms of internal resistance and constant potential difference. He used a galvanometer to measure current, and knew that the voltage between the thermocouple terminals was proportional to the junction temperature. He then added test wires of varying length, diameter, and material to complete the circuit. He found that his data could be modeled through a simple equation with variable composed of the reading from a galvanometer, the length of the test conductor, thermocouple junction temperature, and a constant of the entire setup. From this, Ohm determined his law of proportionality and published his results. In 1827, he announced the now famous law that bears his name, that is:

Electromotive force = Current × Resistance

Ohm brought into order a host of puzzling facts connecting electromotive force and electric current in conductors, which all previous electricians had only succeeded in loosely binding together qualitatively under some rather vague statements. Ohm found that the results could be summed up in such a simple law and by Ohm's discovery a large part of the domain of electricity became annexed to theory.

Faraday and Henry

The discovery of electromagnetic induction was made almost simultaneously, although independently, by Michael Faraday, who was first to make the discovery in 1831, and Joseph Henry in 1832. Henry's discovery of self-induction and his work on spiral conductors using a copper coil were made public in 1835, just before those of Faraday.

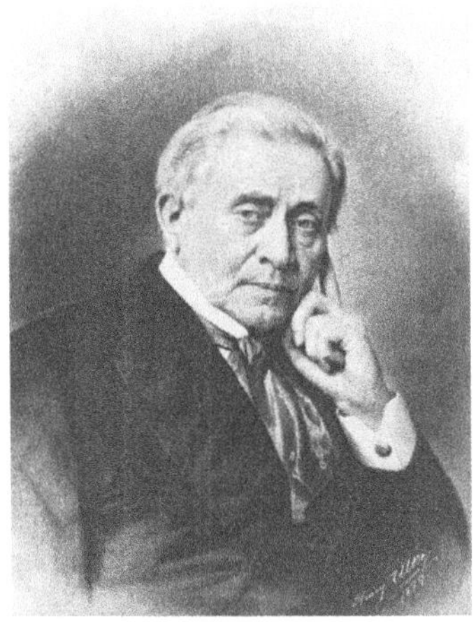

Joseph Henry

In 1831 began the epoch-making researches of Michael Faraday, the famous pupil and successor of Humphry Davy at the head of the Royal Institution, London, relating to electric and electromagnetic induction. The remarkable researches of Faraday, the *prince of experimentalists*, on electrostatics and electrodynamics and the induction of currents. These were rather long in being brought from the crude experimental state to a compact system, expressing the real essence. Faraday was not a competent mathematician, but had he been one, he would have been greatly assisted in his researches, have saved himself much useless speculation, and would have anticipated much later work. He would, for instance, knowing Ampere's theory, by his own results have readily been led to Neumann's theory, and the connected work of Helmholtz and Thomson. Faraday's studies and researches extended from 1831 to 1855 and a detailed description of his experiments, deductions and speculations are to be found in his compiled papers, entitled Experimental Researches in Electricity.' Faraday was by profession a chemist. He was not in the remotest degree a mathematician in the ordinary sense — indeed it is a question if in all his writings there is a single mathematical formula.

The experiment which led Faraday to the discovery of electromagnetic induction was made as follows: He constructed what is now and was then termed an induction coil, the primary and secondary wires of which were wound on a wooden bobbin, side by side, and insulated from one another. In the circuit of the primary wire he placed a battery of approximately 100 cells. In the secondary wire he inserted a galvanometer. On making his first test he observed no results, the galvanometer remaining quiescent, but on increasing the length of the wires he noticed a deflection of the galvanometer in the secondary wire when the circuit of the primary wire was made and broken. This was the first observed instance of the development of electromotive force by electromagnetic induction.

He also discovered that induced currents are established in a second closed circuit when the current strength is varied in the first wire, and that the direction of the current in the secondary circuit is opposite to that in the first circuit. Also that a current is induced in a secondary circuit when another circuit carrying a current is moved to and from the first circuit, and that the approach or withdrawal of a magnet to or from a closed circuit induces momentary currents in the latter. In short, within the space of a few months Faraday discovered by experiment virtually all the laws and facts now known concerning electro-magnetic induction and magneto-electric induction.

Upon these discoveries, with scarcely an exception, depends the operation of the telephone, the dynamo machine, and incidental to the dynamo electric machine practically all the gigantic electrical industries of the world, including electric lighting, electric traction, the operation of electric motors for power purposes, and electro-plating, electrotyping, etc.

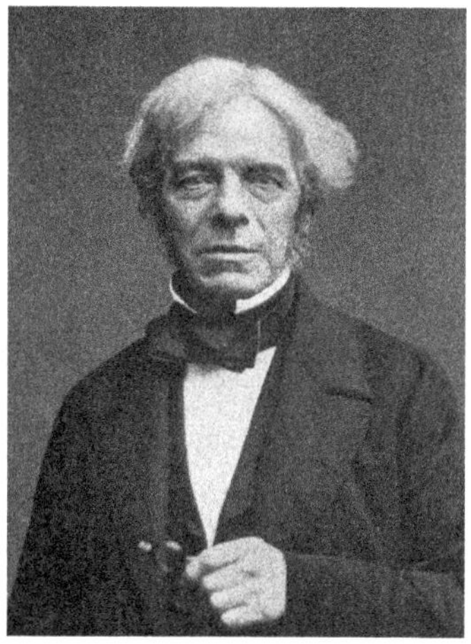

Michael Faraday

In his investigations of the peculiar manner in which iron filings arrange themselves on a cardboard or glass in proximity to the poles of a magnet, Faraday conceived the idea of magnetic "lines of force" extending from pole to pole of the magnet and along which the filings tend to place themselves. On the discovery being made that magnetic effects accompany the passage of an electric current in a wire, it was also assumed that similar magnetic lines of force whirled around the wire. For convenience and to account for induced electricity it was then assumed that when these lines of force are "*cut*" by a wire in passing across them or when the lines of force in rising and falling cut the wire, a current of electricity is developed, or to be more exact, an electromotive force is developed in the wire that sets up a current in a closed circuit. Faraday advanced what has been termed the *molecular theory of electricity* which assumes that electricity is the manifestation of a peculiar condition of the molecule of the body rubbed or the ether surrounding the body. Faraday also, by experiment, discovered paramagnetism and diamagnetism, namely, that all solids and liquids are either attracted or repelled by a magnet. For example, iron, nickel, cobalt, manganese, chromium, etc., are paramagnetic (attracted by magnetism), whilst other substances, such as bismuth, phosphorus, antimony, zinc, etc., are repelled by magnetism or are diamagnetic.

Brugans of Leyden in 1778 and Le Baillif and Becquerel in 1827 had previously discovered diamagnetism in the case of bismuth and antimony. Faraday also rediscovered specific inductive capacity in 1837, the results of the experiments by Cavendish not having been published at that time. He also predicted the retardation of signals on long submarine cables due to the inductive effect of the insulation of the cable, in other words, the static capacity of the cable. In 1816 telegraph pioneer Francis Ronalds had also observed signal retardation on his buried telegraph lines, attributing it to induction.

The 25 years immediately following Faraday's discoveries of electromagnetic induction were fruitful in the promulgation of laws and facts relating to induced currents and to magnetism. In 1834 Heinrich Lenz and Moritz von Jacobi independently demonstrated the now familiar fact that the currents induced in a coil are proportional to the number of turns in the coil. Lenz also announced at that time his important law that, in all cases of electromagnetic induction the induced currents have such a direction that their reaction tends to stop the motion that produces them, a law that was perhaps deducible from Faraday's explanation of Arago's rotations.

The induction coil was first designed by Nicholas Callan in 1836. In 1845 Joseph Henry, the American physicist, published an account of his valuable and interesting experiments with induced currents of a high order, showing that currents could be induced from the secondary of an induction coil to the primary of a second coil, thence to its secondary wire, and so on to the primary of a third coil, etc. Heinrich Daniel Ruhmkorff further developed the induction coil, the Ruhmkorff coil was patented in 1851, and he utilized long windings of copper wire to achieve a spark of approximately 2 inches (50 mm) in length. In 1857, after examining a greatly improved version made by an American inventor, Edward Samuel Ritchie, Ruhmkorff improved his design (as did other engineers), using glass insulation and other innovations to allow the production of sparks more than 300 millimetres (12 in) long.

Middle 19th Century

Up to the middle of the 19th century, indeed up to about 1870, electrical science was, it may be said, a sealed book to the majority of electrical workers. Prior to this time a number of handbooks had been published on electricity and magnetism, notably Auguste de La Rive's exhaustive ' *Treatise on Electricity,*' in 1851 (French) and 1853 (English); August Beer's *Einleitung in die Elektrostatik, die Lehre vom Magnetismus und die Elektrodynamik*, Wiedemann's ' *Galvanismus,*' and Reiss' '*Reibungsal-elektricitat.*' But these works consisted in the main in details of experiments with electricity and magnetism, and but little with the laws and facts of those phenomena. Henry d'Abria published the results of some researches into the laws of induced currents, but owing to their complexity of the investigation it was not productive of very notable results. Around the mid-19th century, Fleeming Jenkin's work on ' *Electricity and Magnetism* ' and Clerk Maxwell's ' *Treatise on Electricity and Magnetism* ' were published.

These books were departures from the beaten path. As Jenkin states in the preface to his work the science of the schools was so dissimilar from that of the practical electrician that it was quite impossible to give students sufficient, or even approximately sufficient, textbooks. A student he said might have mastered de la Rive's large and valuable treatise and yet feel as if in an unknown country and listening to an unknown tongue in the company of practical men. As another writer has said, with the coming of Jenkin's and Maxwell's books all impediments in the way of electrical students were removed, *"the full meaning of Ohm's law becomes clear; electromotive force, difference of potential, resistance, current, capacity, lines of force, magnetization and chemical affinity were measurable, and could be reasoned about, and calculations could be made about them with as much certainty as calculations in dynamics"*.

About 1850, Kirchhoff published his laws relating to branched or divided circuits. He also showed mathematically that according to the then prevailing electrodynamic theory, electricity would be propagated along a perfectly conducting wire with the velocity of light. Helmholtz investigated mathematically the effects of induction upon the strength of a current and deduced therefrom equations, which experiment confirmed, showing amongst other important points the retarding effect of self-induction under certain conditions of the circuit.

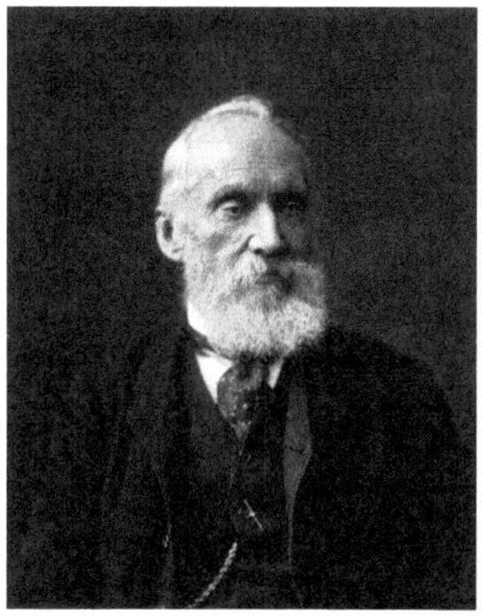

Sir William Thomson

In 1853, Sir William Thomson (later Lord Kelvin) predicted as a result of mathematical calculations the oscillatory nature of the electric discharge of a condenser circuit. To Henry, however, belongs the credit of discerning as a result of his experiments in 1842 the oscillatory nature of the Leyden jar discharge. He wrote: *The phenomena require us to admit the existence of a principal discharge in one direction, and then several reflex actions backward and forward, each more feeble than the preceding, until the equilibrium is obtained.* These oscillations were subsequently observed by B. W. Feddersen (1857) who using a rotating concave mirror projected an image of the electric spark upon a sensitive plate, thereby obtaining a photograph of the spark which plainly indicated the alternating nature of the discharge. Sir William Thomson was also the discoverer of the electric convection of heat (the "Thomson" effect). He designed for electrical measurements of precision his quadrant and absolute electrometers. The reflecting galvanometer and siphon recorder, as applied to submarine cable signaling, are also due to him.

About 1876 the American physicist Henry Augustus Rowland of Baltimore demonstrated the important fact that a static charge carried around produces the same magnetic effects as an electric current. The Importance of this discovery consists in that it may afford a plausible theory of magnetism, namely, that magnetism may be the result of directed motion of rows of molecules carrying static charges.

After Faraday's discovery that electric currents could be developed in a wire by causing it to cut across the lines of force of a magnet, it was to be expected that attempts would be made to construct machines to avail of this fact in the development of voltaic currents. The first machine of this kind was due to Hippolyte Pixii, 1832. It consisted of two bobbins of iron wire, opposite which the poles of a horseshoe magnet were caused to rotate. As this produced in the coils of the wire an alternating current, Pixii arranged a commutating device (commutator) that converted the alternating current of the coils or armature into a direct current in the external circuit. This machine was followed by improved forms of magneto-electric machines due to Ritchie, Saxton, Clarke 1834, Stohrer 1843, Nollet 1849, Shepperd 1856, Van Maldern, Siemens, Wilde and others.

A notable advance in the art of dynamo construction was made by Mr. S. A. Varley in 1866 and by Dr. Charles William Siemens and Mr. Charles Wheatstone, who independently discovered that when a coil of wire, or armature, of the dynamo machine is rotated between the poles (or in the "field") of an electromagnet, a weak current is set up in the coil due to residual magnetism in the iron of the electromagnet, and that if the circuit of the armature be connected with the circuit of the electromagnet, the weak current developed in the armature increases the magnetism in the field. This further increases the magnetic lines of force in which the armature rotates, which still further increases the current in the electromagnet, thereby producing a corresponding increase in the field magnetism, and so on, until the maximum electromotive force which the machine is capable of developing is reached. By means of this principle the dynamo machine develops its own magnetic field, thereby much increasing its efficiency and economical operation. Not by any means, however, was the dynamo electric machine perfected at the time mentioned.

In 1860 an important improvement had been made by Dr. Antonio Pacinotti of Pisa who devised the first electric machine with a ring armature. This machine was first used as an electric motor, but afterward as a generator of electricity. The discovery of the principle of the reversibility of the dynamo electric machine (variously attributed to Walenn 1860; Pacinotti 1864 ; Fontaine, Gramme 1873; Deprez 1881, and others) whereby it may be used as an electric motor or as a generator of electricity has been termed one of the greatest discoveries of the 19th century.

In 1872 the drum armature was devised by Hefner-Alteneck. This machine in a modified form was subsequently known as the Siemens dynamo. These machines were presently followed by the Schuckert, Gulcher, Fein, Brush, Hochhausen, Edison and the dynamo machines of numerous other inventors. In the early days of dynamo machine construction the machines were mainly arranged as direct current generators, and perhaps the most important application of such machines at that time was in electro-plating, for which purpose machines of low voltage and large current strength were employed.

Beginning about 1887 alternating current generators came into extensive operation and the commercial development of the transformer, by means of which currents of low voltage and high current strength are transformed to currents of high voltage and low current strength, and vice versa, in time revolutionized the transmission of electric power to long distances. Likewise the introduction of the rotary converter (in connection with the "step-down" transformer) which converts alternating currents into direct currents (and vice versa) has effected large economies in the operation of electric power systems.

Before the introduction of dynamo electric machines, voltaic, or primary, batteries were extensively used for electro-plating and in telegraphy. There are two distinct types of voltaic cells, namely, the "open" and the "closed", or "constant", type. The open type in brief is that type which operated on closed circuit becomes, after a short time, polarized; that is, gases are liberated in the cell which settle on the negative plate and establish a resistance that reduces the current strength. After a brief interval of open circuit these gases are eliminated or absorbed and the cell is again ready for operation. Closed circuit cells are those in which the gases in the cells are absorbed as quickly as liberated and hence the output of the cell is practically uniform. The Leclanché and Daniell cells, respectively, are familiar examples of the "open" and "closed" type of voltaic cell. The "open" cells are used very extensively at present, especially in the dry cell form, and in annunciator and other open circuit signal systems. Batteries of the Daniell or "gravity" type were employed almost generally in the United States and Canada as the source of electromotive force in telegraphy before the dynamo machine became available, and still are largely used for this service or as "local" cells. Batteries of the "gravity" and the Edison-Lalande types are still much used in "closed circuit" systems.

In the late 19th century, the term luminiferous aether, meaning light-bearing aether, was a conjectured medium for the propagation of light. The word *aether* stems via Latin from the Greek, from a root meaning to kindle, burn, or shine. It signifies the substance which was thought in ancient times to fill the upper regions of space, beyond the clouds.

Maxwell

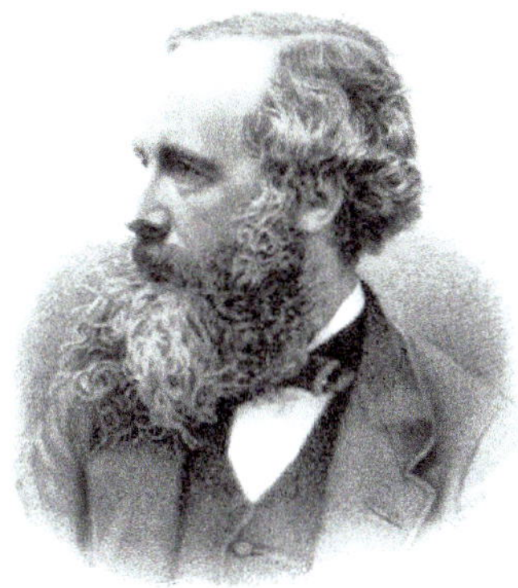

James Clerk Maxwell

In 1864 James Clerk Maxwell of Edinburgh announced his electromagnetic theory of light, which was perhaps the greatest single step in the world's knowledge of electricity. Maxwell had studied and commented on the field of electricity and magnetism as early as 1855/6 when *On Faraday's lines of force* was read to the Cambridge Philosophical Society. The paper presented a simplified model of Faraday's work, and how the two phenomena were related. He reduced all of the current knowledge into a linked set of differential equations with 20 equations in 20 variables. This work was later published as *On Physical Lines of Force* in March 1861. In order to determine the force which is acting on any part of the machine we must find its momentum, and then calculate the rate at which this momentum is being changed. This rate of change will give us the force. The method of calculation which it is necessary to employ was first given by Lagrange, and afterwards developed, with some modifications, by Hamilton's equations. It is usually referred to as Hamilton's principle; when the equations in the original form are used they are known as Lagrange's equations. Now Maxwell logically showed how these methods of calculation could be applied to the electro-magnetic field. The energy of a dynamical system is partly kinetic, partly potential. Maxwell supposes that the magnetic energy of the field is kinetic energy, the electric energy potential.

Around 1862, while lecturing at King's College, Maxwell calculated that the speed of propagation of an electromagnetic field is approximately that of the speed of light. He considered this to be more than just a coincidence, and commented "*We can scarcely avoid the conclusion that light consists in the transverse undulations of the same medium which is the cause of electric and magnetic phenomena.*"

Working on the problem further, Maxwell showed that the equations predict the existence of waves of oscillating electric and magnetic fields that travel through empty space at a speed that could be predicted from simple electrical experiments; using the data available at the time, Maxwell obtained a velocity of 310,740,000 m/s. In his 1864 paper *A Dynamical Theory of the Electromagnetic Field,* Maxwell wrote, *The agreement of the results seems to show that light and magnetism are affections of the same substance, and that light is an electromagnetic disturbance propagated through the field according to electromagnetic laws.*

As already noted herein Faraday, and before him, Ampère and others, had inklings that the luminiferous ether of space was also the medium for electric action. It was known by calculation and experiment that the velocity of electricity was approximately 186,000 miles per second; that is, equal to the velocity of light, which in itself suggests the idea of a relationship between -electricity and "light." A number of the earlier philosophers or mathematicians, as Maxwell terms them, of the 19th century, held the view that electromagnetic phenomena were explainable by action at a distance. Maxwell, following Faraday, contended that the seat of the phenomena was in the medium. The methods of the mathematicians in arriving at their results were synthetical while Faraday's methods were analytical. Faraday in his mind's eye saw lines of force traversing all space where the mathematicians saw centres of force attracting at a distance. Faraday sought the seat of the phenomena in real actions going on in the medium; they were satisfied that they had found it in a power of action at a distance on the electric fluids.

Both of these methods, as Maxwell points out, had succeeded in explaining the propagation of light as an electromagnetic phenomenon while at the same time the fundamental conceptions of what the quantities concerned are, radically differed. The mathematicians assumed that insulators were barriers to electric currents; that, for instance, in a Leyden jar or electric condenser the electricity was accumulated at one plate and that by some occult action at a distance electricity of an opposite kind was attracted to the other plate.

Maxwell, looking further than Faraday, reasoned that if light is an electromagnetic phenomenon and is transmissible through dielectrics such as glass, the phenomenon must be in the nature of electromagnetic currents in the dielectrics. He therefore contended that in the charging of a condenser, for instance, the action did not stop at the insulator, but that some "displacement" currents are set up in the insulating medium, which currents continue until the resisting force of the medium equals that of the charging force. In a closed conductor circuit, an electric current is also a displacement of electricity.

The conductor offers a certain resistance, akin to friction, to the displacement of electricity, and heat is developed in the conductor, proportional to the square of the current(as already stated herein), which current flows as long as the impelling electric force continues. This resistance may be likened to that met with by a ship as it displaces in the water in its progress. The resistance of the dielectric is of a different nature and has been compared to the compression of multitudes of springs, which, under compression, yield with an increasing back pressure, up to a point where the total back pressure equals the initial pressure. When the initial pressure is withdrawn the energy expended in compressing the "springs" is returned to the circuit, concurrently with the return of the springs to their original condition, this producing a reaction in the opposite direction. Consequently, the current due to the displacement of electricity in a conductor may be continuous, while the displacement currents in a dielectric are momentary and, in a circuit or medium which contains but little resistance compared with capacity or inductance reaction, the currents of discharge are of an oscillatory or alternating nature.

Maxwell extended this view of displacement currents in dielectrics to the ether of free space. Assuming light to be the manifestation of alterations of electric currents in the ether, and vibrating at the rate of light vibrations, these vibrations by induction set up corresponding vibrations in adjoining portions of the ether, and in this way the undulations corresponding to those of light are propagated as an electromagnetic effect in the ether. Maxwell's electromagnetic theory of light obviously involved the existence of electric waves in free space, and his followers set themselves the task of experimentally demonstrating the truth of the theory. By 1871, he presented the *Remarks on the mathematical classification of physical quantities.*

End of the 19th Century

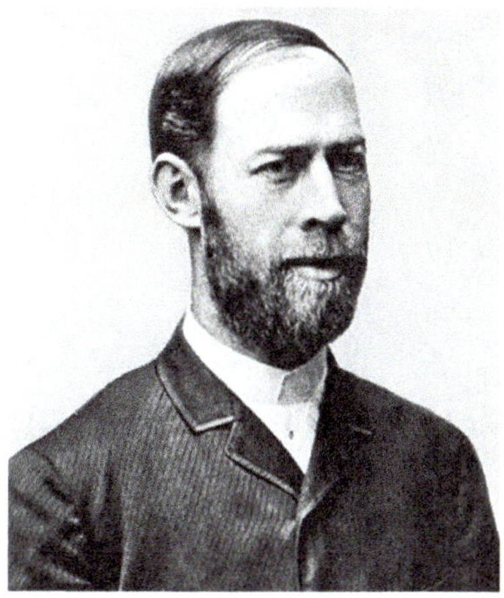

Heinrich Hertz

In 1887, the German physicist Heinrich Hertz in a series of experiments proved the actual existence electromagnetic waves, showing that transverse free space electromagnetic waves can travel over some distance as predicted by Maxwell and Faraday. Hertz published his work in a book titled: *Electric waves: being researches on the propagation of electric action with finite velocity through space.* The discovery of electromagnetic waves in space led to the development in the closing years of the 19th century of radio.

The electron as a unit of charge in electrochemistry was posited by G. Johnstone Stoney in 1874, who also coined the term *electron* in 1894. Plasma was first identified in a Crookes tube, and so described by Sir William Crookes in 1879 (he called it "radiant matter"). The place of electricity in leading up to the discovery of those beautiful phenomena of the Crookes Tube (due to Sir William Crookes), viz., Cathode rays, and later to the discovery of Roentgen or X-rays, must not be overlooked, since without electricity as the excitant of the tube the discovery of the rays might have been postponed indefinitely. It has been noted herein that Dr. William Gilbert was termed the founder of electrical science. This must, however, be regarded as a comparative statement.

Oliver Heaviside was a self-taught scholar who reformulated Maxwell's field equations in terms of electric and magnetic forces and energy flux, and independently co-formulated vector analysis. His series of articles continued the work entitled "*Electromagnetic Induction and its Propagation*", commenced in *The Electrician* in 1885 to nearly 1887 (ed., the latter part of the work dealing with the propagation of electromagnetic waves along wires through the dielectric surrounding them), when the great pressure on space and the want of readers appeared to necessitate its abrupt discontinuance. (A straggler piece appeared December 31, 1887.) He wrote an interpretation of the transcendental formulae of electromagnetism. Following the real object of true naturalists when they employ mathematics to assist them, he wrote to find out the connections of known phenomena, and by deductive reasoning, to obtain a knowledge of electromagnetic phenomena. Although at odds with the scientific establishment for most of his life, Heaviside changed the face of mathematics and science for years to come.

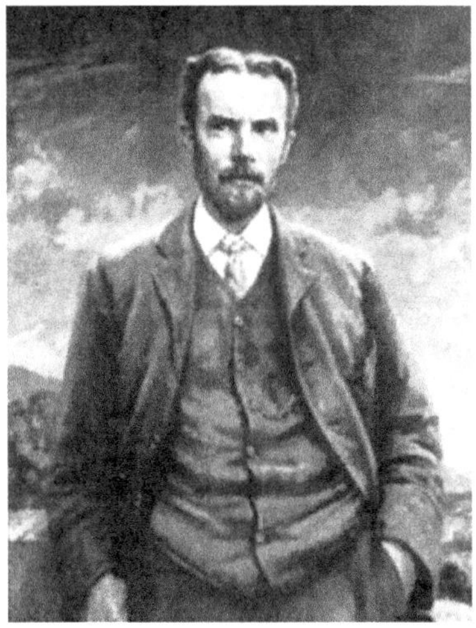

Oliver Heaviside

Of the changes in the field of electromagnetic theory, certain conclusions from *Electro-Magnetic Theory* by Heaviside are, if not drawn, at least indicated in this book. Two of them may be stated as follows:

1. That magnetism is a phenomenon of motion and not a statical phenomenon; also that this motion is more likely to be translational than vortical.

2. That all electric currents are phenomena consequent upon the emission of electro-magnetic wave disturbances in the aether, and that the proper treatment of all the phenomena of currents and magnetic flux should be considered as the consequence, and not as the cause, of electro-magnetic waves.

The ultimate results of his work are twofold. (1) The first ultimate result is purely mathematical, which is important only to those who study mathematical physics. The system of *vectorial algebra* as developed by Mr. Heaviside was used because of ease for physical investigations to the methods of quaternions. (2) The second ultimate result is physical. It consists in more closely uniting the more recondite problems of telegraphy, telephony, *Teslaic phenomena* and *Hertzian phenomena* with the fundamental properties of the aether. In elucidating this connection, the merit of the book appears most prominently as a stepping-stone to the goal in the full view of all physical analysis, namely, the resolution of all physical phenomena to the activities of the aether, and of matter in the aether, under the laws of dynamics.

During the late 1890s a number of physicists proposed that electricity, as observed in studies of electrical conduction in conductors, electrolytes, and cathode ray tubes, consisted of discrete units, which were given a variety of names, but the reality of these units had not been confirmed in a compelling way. However, there were also indications that the cathode rays had wavelike properties.

Faraday, Weber, Helmholtz, Clifford and others had glimpses of this view; and the experimental works of Zeeman, Goldstein, Crookes, J. J. Thomson and others had greatly strengthened this view. Weber predicted that electrical phenomena were due to the existence of electrical atoms, the influence of which on one another depended on their position and relative accelerations and velocities. Helmholtz and others also contended that the existence of electrical atoms followed from Faraday's laws of electrolysis, and Johnstone Stoney, to whom is due the term "electron", showed that each chemical ion of the decomposed electrolyte carries a definite and constant quantity of electricity, and inasmuch as these charged ions are separated on the electrodes as neutral substances there must be an instant, however brief, when the charges must be capable of existing separately as electrical atoms; while in 1887, Clifford wrote: "There is great reason to believe that every material atom carries upon it a small electric current, if it does not wholly consist of this current."

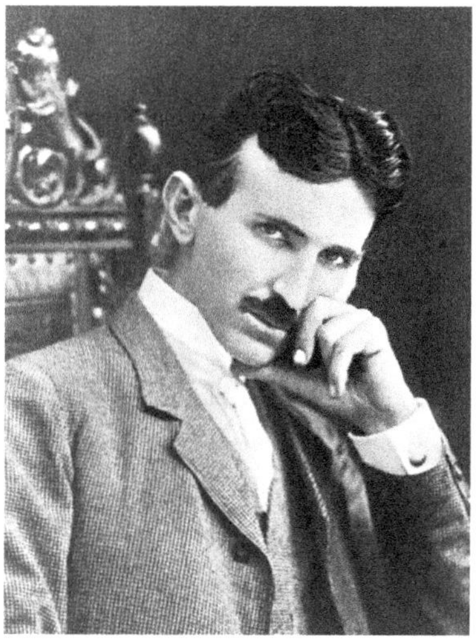

Nikola Tesla, c. 1896

The Serbian American engineer Nikola Tesla learned of Hertz' experiments at the Exposition Universelle in 1889 and launched into his own experiments in high frequency and high potential current developing "high-frequency" alternators (which operated around 15,000 hertz).. He concluded from his observations that Maxwell and Hertz were wrong about the existence of airborne electromagnetic waves (which he attributed it to what he called "electrostatic thrusts") but saw great potential in Maxwell's idea that electricity and light were part of the same phenomena, seeing it as a way to create a new type of wireless electric lighting. By 1893 he was giving lectures on "On Light and Other High Frequency Phenomena", including a demonstration where he would light a Geissler tubes wirelessly. Tesla worked for many years after that trying to develop a wireless power distribution system.

In 1896, J. J. Thomson performed experiments indicating that cathode rays really were particles, found an accurate value for their charge-to-mass ratio e/m, and found that e/m was independent of cathode material. He made good estimates of both the charge e and the mass m, finding that cathode ray particles, which he called "corpuscles", had perhaps one thousandth of the mass of the least massive ion known (hydrogen). He further showed that the negatively charged particles produced by radioactive materials, by heated materials, and by illuminated materials, were universal. The nature of the Crookes tube "cathode ray" matter was identified by Thomson in 1897.

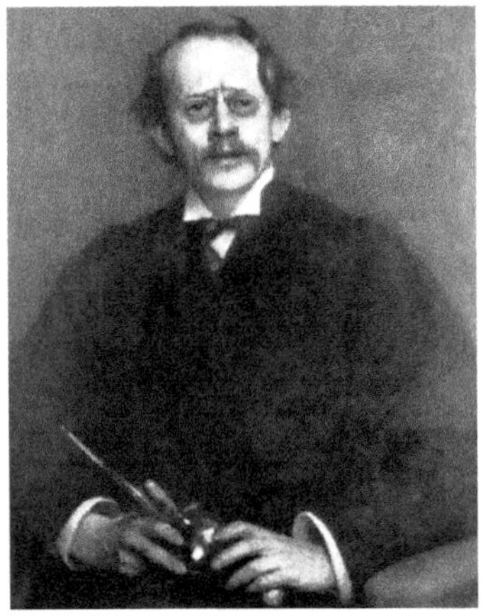

J. J. Thomson

In the late 19th century, the Michelson–Morley experiment was performed by Albert A. Michelson and Edward W. Morley at what is now Case Western Reserve University. It is generally considered to be the evidence against the theory of a luminiferous aether. The experiment has also been referred to as "the kicking-off point for the theoretical aspects of the Second Scientific Revolution." Primarily for this work, Michelson was awarded the Nobel Prize in 1907. Dayton Miller continued with experiments, conducting thousands of measurements and eventually developing the most accurate interferometer in the world at that time. Miller and others, such as Morley, continue observations and experiments dealing with the concepts. A range of proposed aether-dragging theories could explain the null result but these were more complex, and tended to use arbitrary-looking coefficients and physical assumptions.

By the end of the 19th century electrical engineers had become a distinct profession, separate from physicists and inventors. They created companies that investigated, developed and perfected the techniques of electricity transmission, and gained support from governments all over the world for starting the first worldwide electrical telecommunication network, the telegraph network. Pioneers in this field included Werner von Siemens, founder of Siemens AG in 1847, and John Pender, founder of Cable & Wireless.

The first public demonstration of a "alternator system" took place in 1886. Large two-phase alternating current generators were built by a British electrician, J. E. H. Gordon, in 1882. Lord Kelvin and Sebastian Ferranti also developed early alternators, producing frequencies between 100 and 300 hertz. After 1891, polyphase alternators were introduced to supply currents of multiple differing phases. Later alternators were designed for varying alternating-current frequencies between sixteen and about one hundred hertz, for use with arc lighting, incandescent lighting and electric motors.

The possibility of obtaining the electric current in large quantities, and economically, by means of dynamo electric machines gave impetus to the development of incandescent and arc lighting. Until these machines had attained a commercial basis voltaic batteries were the only available source of current for electric lighting and power. The cost of these batteries, however, and the difficulties of maintaining them in reliable operation were prohibitory of their use for practical lighting purposes. The date of the employment of arc and incandescent lamps may be set at about 1877.

Even in 1880, however, but little headway had been made toward the general use of these illuminants; the rapid subsequent growth of this industry is a matter of general knowledge. The employment of storage batteries, which were originally termed secondary batteries or accumulators, began about 1879. Such batteries are now utilized on a large scale as auxiliaries to the dynamo machine in electric power-houses and substations, in electric automobiles and in immense numbers in automobile ignition and starting systems, also in fire alarm telegraphy and other signal systems.

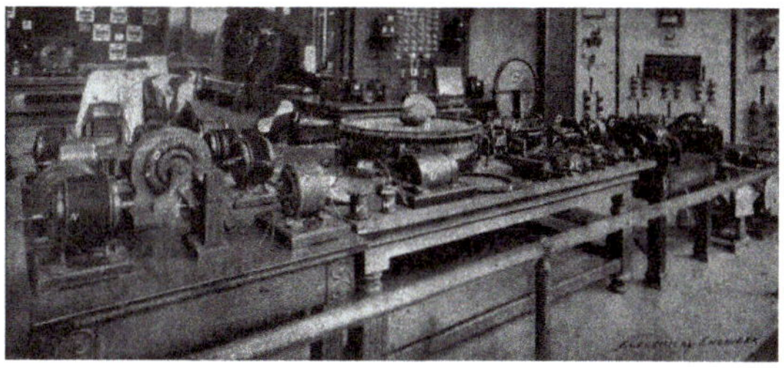

World's Fair Tesla presentation

In 1893, the World's Columbian International Exposition was held in a building which was devoted to electrical exhibits. General Electric Company (backed by Edison and J. P. Morgan) had proposed to power the electric exhibits with direct current at the cost of one million dollars. However, Westinghouse proposed to illuminate the Columbian Exposition in Chicago with alternating current for half that price, and Westinghouse won the bid. It was an historical moment and the beginning of a revolution, as George Westinghouse introduced the public to electrical power by illuminating the Exposition.

Second Industrial Revolution

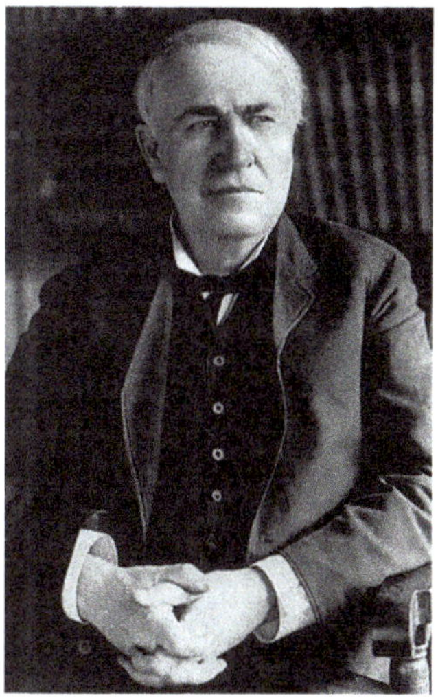

Thomas Edison

Between 1885 and 1890 Galileo Ferraris in Italy, Nikola Tesla in the United States, and Mikhail Dolivo-Dobrovolsky in Germany explored poly-phase currents combined with electromagnetic induction leading to the development of practical AC induction motors. The AC induction motor helped usher in the Second Industrial Revolution. The rapid advance of electrical technology in the latter 19th and early 20th centuries led to commercial rivalries. In the War of Currents in the late 1880s, George Westinghouse and Thomas Edison became adversaries due to Edison's promotion of direct current (DC) for electric power distribution over alternating current (AC) advocated by Westinghouse.

Several inventors helped develop commercial systems. Samuel Morse, inventor of a long-range telegraph; Thomas Edison, inventor of the first commercial electrical energy distribution network; George Westinghouse, inventor of the electric locomotive; Alexander Graham Bell, the inventor of the telephone and founder of a successful telephone business.

In 1871 the electric telegraph had grown to large proportions and was in use in every civilized country in the world, its lines forming a network in all directions over the surface of the land. The system most generally in use was the electromagnetic telegraph due to S. F. B. Morse of New York, or modifications of his system. Submarine cables connecting the Eastern and Western hemispheres were also in successful operation at that time.

When, however, in 1918 one views the vast applications of electricity to electric light, electric railways, electric power and other purposes (all it may be repeated made possible and practicable by the perfection of the dynamo machine), it is difficult to believe that no longer ago than 1871 the author of a book published in that year, in referring to the state of the art of applied electricity at that time, could have truthfully written: "The most important and remarkable of the uses which have been made of electricity consists in its application to telegraph purposes". The statement was, however, quite accurate and perhaps the time could have been carried forward to the year 1876 without material modification of the remarks. In that year the telephone, due to Alexander Graham Bell, was invented, but it was not until several years thereafter that its commercial employment began in earnest. Since that time also the sister branches of electricity just mentioned have advanced and are advancing with such gigantic strides in every direction that it is difficult to place a limit upon their progress. Electrical devices account of the use of electricity in the arts and industries.

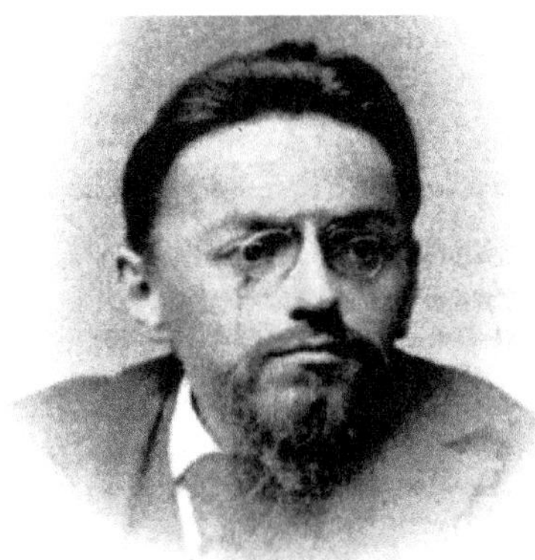

Charles Proteus Steinmetz, theoretician of alternating current.

The 1880s saw the spread of large scale commercial electric power systems, first used for lighting and eventually for electro-motive power and heating. Systems early on used alternating current and direct current. Large centralized power generation became possible when it was recognized that alternating current electric power lines could use transformers to take advantage of the fact that each doubling of the voltage would allow the same size cable to transmit the same amount of power four times the distance. Transformer were used to raise voltage at the point of generation (a representative number is a generator voltage in the low kilovolt range) to a much higher voltage (tens of thousands to several hundred thousand volts) for primary transmission, followed to several downward transformations, for commercial and residential domestic use.

The International Electro-Technical Exhibition of 1891 featuring the long distance transmission of high-power, three-phase electric current. It was held between 16 May and 19 October on the disused site of the three former "Westbahnhöfe" (Western Railway Stations) in Frankfurt am Main. The exhibition featured the first long distance transmission of high-power, three-phase electric current, which was generated 175 km away at Lauffen am Neckar. As a result of this successful field trial, three-phase current became established for electrical transmission networks throughout the world.

Much was done in the direction in the improvement of railroad terminal facilities, and it is difficult to find one steam railroad engineer who would have denied that all the important steam railroads of this country were not to be operated electrically. In other directions the progress of events as to the utilization of electric power was expected to be equally rapid. In every part of the world the power of falling water, nature's perpetual motion machine, which has been going to waste since the world began, is now being converted into electricity and transmitted by wire hundreds of miles to points where it is usefully and economically employed.

The first windmill for electricity production was built in Scotland in July 1887 by the Scottish electrical engineer James Blyth. Across the Atlantic, in Cleveland, Ohio a larger and heavily engineered machine was designed and constructed in 1887–88 by Charles F. Brush, this was built by his engineering company at his home and operated from 1886 until 1900. The Brush wind turbine had a rotor 56 feet (17 m) in diameter and was mounted on a 60-foot (18 m) tower. Although large by today's standards, the machine was only rated at 12 kW; it turned relatively slowly since it had 144 blades. The connected dynamo was used either to charge a bank of batteries or to operate up to 100 incandescent light bulbs, three arc lamps, and various motors in Brush's laboratory. The machine fell into disuse after 1900 when electricity became available from Cleveland's central stations, and was abandoned in 1908.

20th Century

Various units of electricity and magnetism have been adopted and named by representatives of the electrical engineering institutes of the world, which units and names have been confirmed and legalized by the governments of the United States and other countries. Thus the volt, from the Italian Volta, has been adopted as the practical unit of electromotive force, the ohm, from the enunciator of Ohm's law, as the practical unit of resistance; the ampere, after the eminent French scientist of that name, as the practical unit of current strength, the henry as the practical unit of inductance, after Joseph Henry and in recognition of his early and important experimental work in mutual induction.

Dewar and John Ambrose Fleming predicted that at absolute zero, pure metals would become perfect electromagnetic conductors (though, later, Dewar altered his opinion on the disappearance of resistance believing that there would always be some resistance). Walther Hermann Nernst developed the third law of thermodynamics and stated that absolute zero was unattainable. Carl von Linde and William Hampson, both commercial researchers, nearly at the same time filed for patents on the Joule–Thomson effect. Linde's patent was the climax of 20 years of systematic investigation of established facts, using a regenerative counterflow method. Hampson's design was also of a regenerative method. The combined process became known as the Linde–Hampson liquefaction process. Heike Kamerlingh Onnes purchased a Linde machine for his research. Zygmunt Florenty Wróblewski conducted research into electrical properties at low temperatures, though his research ended early due to his accidental death. Around 1864, Karol Olszewski and Wroblewski predicted the electrical phenomena of dropping resistance levels at ultra-cold temperatures. Olszewski and Wroblewski documented evidence of this in the 1880s. A milestone was achieved on 10 July 1908 when Onnes at the Leiden University in Leiden produced, for the first time, liquified helium and achieved superconductivity.

In 1900, William Du Bois Duddell develops the Singing Arc and produced melodic sounds, from a low to a high-tone, from this arc lamp.

Lorentz and Poincaré

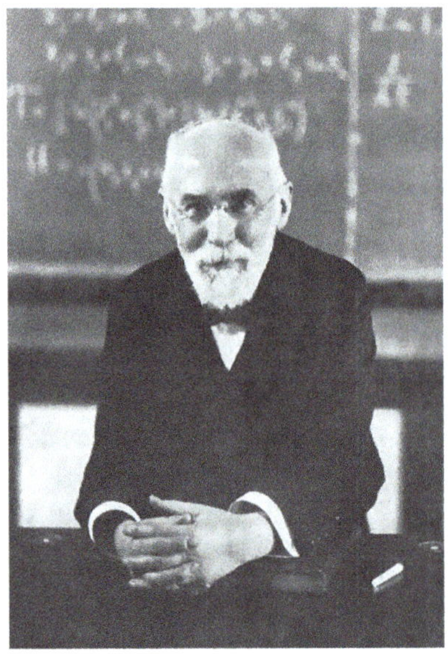

Hendrik Lorentz

Between 1900 and 1910, many scientists like Wilhelm Wien, Max Abraham, Hermann Minkowski, or Gustav Mie believed that all forces of nature are of electromagnetic origin (the so-called "electromagnetic world view"). This was connected with the electron theory developed between 1892 and 1904 by Hendrik Lorentz. Lorentz introduced a strict separation between matter (electrons) and the aether, whereby in his model the ether is completely motionless, and it won't be set in motion in the neighborhood of ponderable matter. Contrary to other electron models before, the electromagnetic field of the ether appears as a mediator between the electrons, and changes in this field can propagate not faster than the speed of light.

In 1896, three years after submitting his thesis on the Kerr effect, Pieter Zeeman disobeyed the direct orders of his supervisor and used laboratory equipment to measure the splitting of spectral lines by a strong magnetic field. Lorentz theoretically explained the Zeeman effect on the basis of his theory, for which both received the Nobel Prize in Physics in 1902. A fundamental concept of Lorentz's theory in 1895 was the "theorem of corresponding states" for terms of order v/c. This theorem states that a moving observer (relative to the ether) makes the same observations as a resting observer. This theorem was extended for terms of all orders by Lorentz in 1904. Lorentz noticed, that it was necessary to change the space-time variables when changing frames and introduced concepts like physical length contraction (1892) to explain the Michelson–Morley experiment, and the mathematical concept of local time (1895) to explain the aberration of light and the Fizeau experiment. That resulted in the formulation of the so-called Lorentz transformation by Joseph Larmor (1897, 1900) and Lorentz (1899, 1904). As Lorentz later noted (1921, 1928), he considered the time indicated by clocks resting in the aether as "true" time, while local time was seen by him as a heuristic working hypothesis and a mathematical artifice. Therefore, Lorentz's theorem is seen by modern historians as being a mathematical transformation from a "real" system resting in the aether into a "fictitious" system in motion.

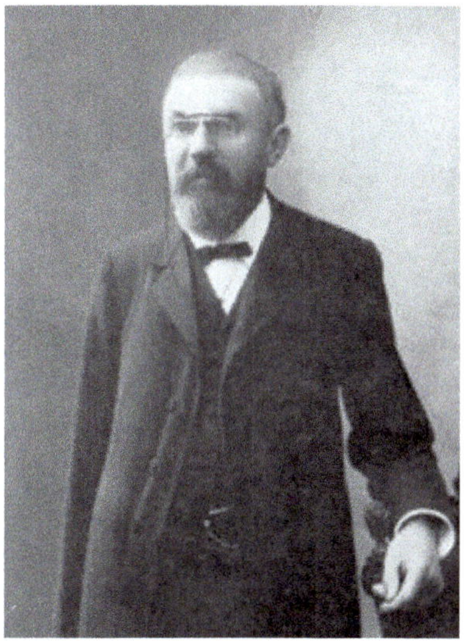

Henri Poincaré

Continuing the work of Lorentz, Henri Poincaré between 1895 and 1905 formulated on many occasions the principle of relativity and tried to harmonize it with electrodynamics. He declared simultaneity only a convenient convention which depends on the speed of light, whereby the constancy of the speed of light would be a useful postulate for making the laws of nature as simple as possible. In 1900 he interpreted Lorentz's local time as the result of clock synchronization by light signals, and introduced the electromagnetic momentum by comparing electromagnetic energy to what he called a "fictitious fluid" of mass $m = E/c^2$. And finally in June and July 1905 he declared the relativity principle a general law of nature, including gravitation. He corrected some mistakes of Lorentz and proved the Lorentz covariance of the electromagnetic equations. Poincaré also suggested that there exist non-electrical forces to stabilize the electron configuration and asserted that gravitation is a non-electrical force as well, contrary to the electromagnetic world view. However, historians pointed out that he still used the notion of an ether and distinguished between "apparent" and "real" time and therefore didn't invent special relativity in its modern understanding.

Einstein's *Annus Mirabilis*

In 1905, while he was working in the patent office, Albert Einstein had four papers published in the *Annalen der Physik*, the leading German physics journal. These are the papers that history has come to call the *Annus Mirabilis papers*:

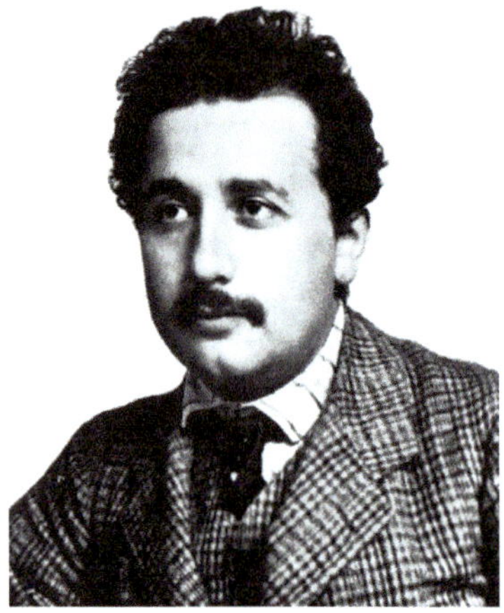

Albert Einstein, 1905

- His paper on the particulate nature of light put forward the idea that certain experimental results, notably the photoelectric effect, could be simply understood from the postulate that light interacts with matter as discrete "packets" (quanta) of energy, an idea that had been introduced by Max Planck in 1900 as a purely mathematical manipulation, and which seemed to contradict contemporary wave theories of light (Einstein 1905a). This was the only work of Einstein's that he himself called "revolutionary."
- His paper on Brownian motion explained the random movement of very small objects as direct evidence of molecular action, thus supporting the atomic theory. (Einstein 1905b)
- His paper on the electrodynamics of moving bodies introduced the radical theory of special relativity, which showed that the observed independence of the speed of light on the observer's state of motion required fundamental changes to the notion of simultaneity. Consequences of this include the time-space frame of a moving body slowing down and contracting (in the direction of motion) relative to the frame of the observer. This paper also argued that the idea of a luminiferous aether—one of the leading theoretical entities in physics at the time—was superfluous. (Einstein 1905c)
- In his paper on mass–energy equivalence (previously considered to be distinct concepts), Einstein deduced from his equations of special relativity what later became the well-known expression: $E = mc^2$, suggesting that tiny amounts of mass could be converted into huge amounts of energy. (Einstein 1905d)

All four papers are today recognized as tremendous achievements—and hence 1905 is known as Einstein's "Wonderful Year". At the time, however, they were not noticed by most physicists as being important, and many of those who did notice them rejected them outright. Some of this work—such as the theory of light quanta—remained controversial for years.

Mid-20th Century

The first formulation of a quantum theory describing radiation and matter interaction is due to Paul Dirac, who, during 1920, was first able to compute the coefficient of spontaneous emission of an atom. Paul Dirac described the quantization of the electromagnetic field as an ensemble of harmonic oscillators with the introduction of the concept of creation and annihilation operators of particles. In the following years, with contributions from Wolfgang Pauli, Eugene Wigner, Pascual Jordan, Werner Heisenberg and an elegant formulation of quantum electrodynamics due to Enrico Fermi, physicists came to believe that, in principle, it would be possible to perform any computation for any physical process involving photons and charged particles. However, further studies by Felix Bloch with Arnold Nordsieck, and Victor Weisskopf, in 1937 and 1939, revealed that such computations were reliable only at a first order of perturbation theory, a problem already pointed out by Robert Oppenheimer. At higher orders in the series infinities emerged, making such computations meaningless and casting serious doubts on the internal consistency of the theory itself. With no solution for this problem known at the time, it appeared that a fundamental incompatibility existed between special relativity and quantum mechanics.

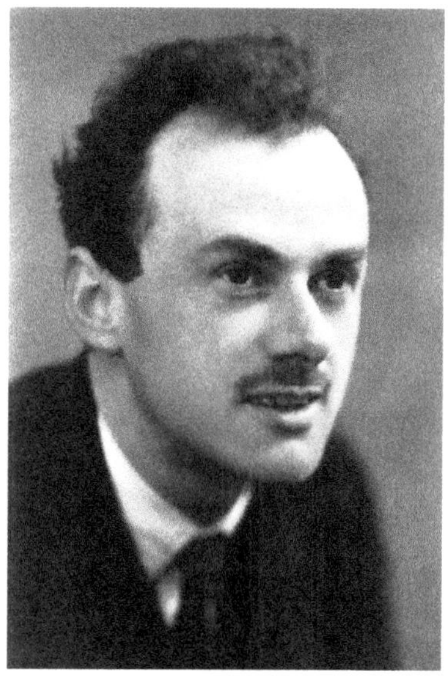

Paul Dirac

In December 1938, the German chemists Otto Hahn and Fritz Strassmann sent a manuscript to *Naturwissenschaften* reporting they had detected the element barium after bombarding uranium with neutrons; simultaneously, they communicated these results to Lise Meitner. Meitner, and her nephew Otto Robert Frisch, correctly interpreted these results as being nuclear fission. Frisch confirmed this experimentally on 13 January 1939. In 1944, Hahn received the Nobel Prize in Chemistry for the discovery of nuclear fission. Some historians who have documented the history of the discovery of nuclear fission believe Meitner should have been awarded the Nobel Prize with Hahn.

Difficulties with the Quantum theory increased through the end of 1940. Improvements in microwave technology made it possible to take more precise measurements of the shift of the levels of a hydrogen atom, now known as the Lamb shift and magnetic moment of the electron. These experiments unequivocally exposed discrepancies which the theory was unable to explain. With the invention of bubble chambers and spark chambers in the 1950s, experimental particle physics discovered a large and ever-growing number of particles called hadrons. It seemed that such a large number of particles could not all be fundamental.

Shortly after the end of the war in 1945, Bell Labs formed a Solid State Physics Group, led by William Shockley and chemist Stanley Morgan; other personnel including John Bardeen and Walter Brattain, physicist Gerald Pearson, chemist Robert Gibney, electronics expert Hilbert Moore and several technicians. Their assignment was to seek a solid-state alternative to fragile glass vacuum tube amplifiers. Their first attempts were based on Shockley's ideas about using an external electrical field on a semiconductor to affect its conductivity. These experiments failed every time in all sorts of configurations and materials. The group was at a standstill until Bardeen suggested a theory that invoked surface states that prevented the field from penetrating the semiconductor. The group changed its focus to study these surface states and they met almost daily to discuss the work. The rapport of the group was excellent, and ideas were freely exchanged.

As to the problems in the electron experiments, a path to a solution was given by Hans Bethe. In 1947, while he was traveling by train to reach Schenectady from New York, after giving a talk at the conference at Shelter Island on the subject, Bethe completed the first non-relativistic computation of the shift of the lines of the hydrogen atom as measured by Lamb and Retherford. Despite the limitations of the computation, agreement was excellent. The idea was simply to attach infinities to corrections at mass and charge that were actually fixed to a finite value by experiments. In this way, the infinities get absorbed in those constants and yield a finite result in good agreement with experiments. This procedure was named renormalization.

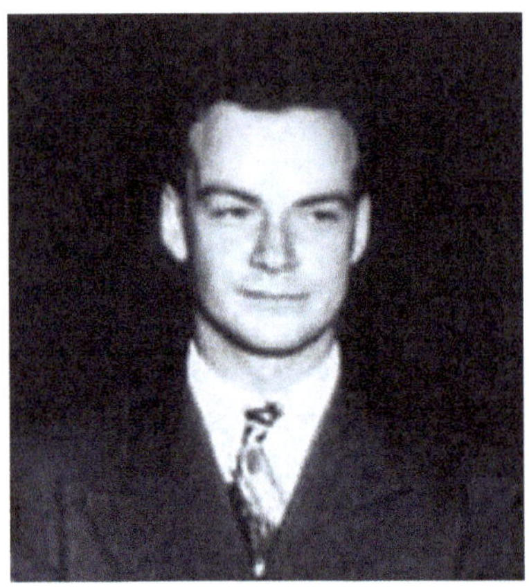

Richard Feynman

Based on Bethe's intuition and fundamental papers on the subject by Shin'ichirō Tomonaga, Julian Schwinger, Richard Feynman and Freeman Dyson, it was finally possible to get fully covariant formulations that were finite at any order in a perturbation series of quantum electrodynamics. Shin'ichirō Tomonaga, Julian Schwinger and Richard Feynman were jointly awarded with a Nobel Prize in Physics in 1965 for their work in this area. Their contributions, and those of Freeman Dyson, were about covariant and gauge-invariant formulations of quantum electrodynamics that allow computations of observables at any order of perturbation theory. Feynman's mathematical technique, based on his diagrams, initially seemed very different from the field-theoretic, operator-based approach of Schwinger and Tomonaga, but Freeman Dyson later showed that the two approaches were equivalent. Renormalization, the need to attach a physical meaning at certain divergences appearing in the theory through integrals, has subsequently become one of the fundamental aspects of quantum field theory and has come to be seen as a criterion for a theory's general acceptability. Even though renormalization works very well in practice, Feynman was never entirely comfortable with its mathematical validity, even referring to renormalization as a "shell game" and "hocus pocus". QED has served as the model and template for all subsequent quantum field theories. Peter Higgs, Jeffrey Goldstone, and others, Sheldon Glashow, Steven Weinberg and Abdus Salam independently showed how the weak nuclear force and quantum electrodynamics could be merged into a single electroweak force.

Robert Noyce credited Kurt Lehovec for the *principle of p–n junction isolation* caused by the action of a biased p-n junction (the diode) as a key concept behind the integrated circuit. Jack Kilby recorded his initial ideas concerning the integrated circuit in July 1958 and successfully demonstrated the first working integrated circuit on September 12, 1958. In his patent application of February 6, 1959, Kilby described his new device as "a body of semiconductor material ... wherein all the components of the electronic circuit are completely integrated." Kilby won the 2000 Nobel Prize in Physics for his part of the invention of the integrated circuit. Robert Noyce also came up with his own idea of an integrated circuit half a year later than Kilby. Noyce's chip solved many practical problems that Kilby's had not. Noyce's chip, made at Fairchild Semiconductor, was made of silicon, whereas Kilby's chip was made of germanium.

Philo Farnsworth developed the Farnsworth–Hirsch Fusor, or simply fusor, an apparatus designed by Farnsworth to create nuclear fusion. Unlike most controlled fusion systems, which slowly heat a magnetically confined plasma, the fusor injects high temperature ions directly into a reaction chamber, thereby avoiding a considerable amount of complexity. When the Farnsworth-Hirsch Fusor was first introduced to the fusion research world in the late 1960s, the Fusor was the first device that could clearly demonstrate it was producing fusion reactions at all. Hopes at the time were high that it could be quickly developed into a practical power source. However, as with other fusion experiments, development into a power source has proven difficult. Nevertheless, the fusor has since become a practical neutron source and is produced commercially for this role.

Parity Violation

The mirror image of an electromagnet produces a field with the opposite polarity. Thus the north and south poles of a magnet have the same symmetry as left and right. Prior to 1956, it was believed that this symmetry was perfect, and that a technician would be unable to distinguish the north and south poles of a magnet except by reference to left and right. In that year, T. D. Lee and C. N. Yang predicted the nonconservation of parity in the weak interaction. To the surprise of many physicists, in 1957 C. S. Wu and collaborators at the U.S. National Bureau of Standards demonstrated that under suitable conditions for polarization of nuclei, the beta decay of cobalt-60 preferentially releases electrons toward the south pole of an external magnetic field, and a somewhat higher number of gamma rays toward the north pole. As a result, the experimental apparatus does not behave comparably with its mirror image.

Electroweak Theory

The first step towards the Standard Model was Sheldon Glashow's discovery, in 1960, of a way to combine the electromagnetic and weak interactions. In 1967, Steven Weinberg and Abdus Salam incorporated the Higgs mechanism into Glashow's electroweak theory, giving it its modern form. The Higgs mechanism is believed to give rise to the masses of all the elementary particles in the Standard Model. This includes the masses of the W and Z bosons, and the masses of the fermions - i.e. the quarks and leptons. After the neutral weak currents caused by Zboson exchange were discovered at CERN in 1973, the electroweak theory became widely accepted and Glashow, Salam, and Weinberg shared the 1979 Nobel Prize in Physics for discovering it. The W and Z bosons were discovered experimentally in 1981, and their masses were found to be as the Standard Model predicted. The theory of the strong interaction, to which many contributed, acquired its modern form around 1973–74, when experiments confirmed that the hadrons were composed of fractionally charged quarks. With the establishment of quantum chromodynamics in the 1970s finalized a set of fundamental and exchange particles, which allowed for the establishment of a "standard model" based on the mathematics of gauge invariance, which successfully described all forces except for gravity, and which remains generally accepted within the domain to which it is designed to be applied.

The 'standard model' groups the electroweak interaction theory and quantum chromodynamics into a structure denoted by the gauge group $SU(3)\times SU(2)\times U(1)$. The formulation of the unification of the electromagnetic and weak interactions in the standard model is due to Abdus Salam, Steven Weinberg and, subsequently, Sheldon Glashow. After the discovery, made at CERN, of the existence of neutral weak currents, mediated by the Z boson foreseen in the standard model, the physicists Salam, Glashow and Weinberg received the 1979 Nobel Prize in Physics for their electroweak theory. Since then, discoveries of the bottom quark (1977), the top quark (1995) and the tau neutrino (2000) have given credence to the standard model. Because of its success in explaining a wide variety of experimental results.

Electrodynamic Tethers

Before the start of the 21st century, the electrodynamic tether being oriented at an angle to the local vertical between the object and a planet with a magnetic field cut the Earth's magnetic field and generated a current; thereby it converted some of the orbiting body's kinetic energy to electrical energy. The tether's far end can be left bare, making electrical contact with the ionosphere, creating a generator. As part of a *tether propulsion* system, crafts can use long, strong conductors to change the orbits of spacecraft. It has the potential to make space travel significantly cheaper. It is a simplified, very low-budget magnetic sail. It can be used either to accelerate or brake an orbiting spacecraft. When direct current is pumped through the tether, it exerts a force against the magnetic field, and the tether accelerates the spacecraft.

21st Century

Electromagnetic Technologies

There are a range of emerging energy technologies. By 2007, solid state micrometer-scale electric double-layer capacitors based on advanced superionic conductors had been for low-voltage electronics such as deep-sub-voltage nanoelectronics and related technologies (the 22 nm technological node of CMOS and beyond). Also, the nanowire battery, a lithium-ion battery, was invented by a team led by Dr. Yi Cui in 2007.

Magnetic Resonance

Reflecting the fundamental importance and applicability of Magnetic resonance imaging in medicine, Paul Lauterbur of the University of Illinois at Urbana-Champaign and Sir Peter Mansfield of the University of Nottingham were awarded the 2003 Nobel Prize in Physiology or Medicine for their "*discoveries concerning magnetic resonance imaging*". The Nobel citation acknowledged Lauterbur's insight of using magnetic field gradients to determine spatial localization, a discovery that allowed rapid acquisition of 2D images.

Wireless Electricity

Wireless electricity is a form of wireless energy transfer, the ability to provide electrical energy to remote objects without wires. The term WiTricity was coined in 2005 by Dave Gerding and later used for a project led by Prof. Marin Soljačić in 2007. The MIT researchers successfully demonstrated the ability to power a 60 watt light bulb wirelessly, using two 5-turn copper coils of 60 cm (24 in) diameter, that were 2 m (7 ft) away, at roughly 45% efficiency. This technology can potentially be used in a large variety of applications, including consumer, industrial, medical and military. Its aim is to reduce the dependence on batteries. Further applications for this technology include transmission of information—it would not interfere with radio waves and thus could be used as a cheap and efficient communication device without requiring a license or a government permit.

Unified Theories

As of 2010, there is still no hard evidence that nature is described by a Grand Unified Theory (GUT). The Higgs particle has been tentatively verified,. The discovery of neutrino oscillations indicates that the Standard Model is incomplete and has led to renewed interest toward certain GUT such as $SO(10)$. One of the few possible experimental tests of certain GUT is proton decay and also fermion masses. There are a few more special tests for supersymmetric GUT. The gauge coupling strengths of QCD, the weak interaction and hypercharge seem to meet at a common length scale called the GUT scale and equal approximately to 10^{16} GeV, which is slightly suggestive. This interesting numerical observation is called the gauge coupling unification, and it works particularly well if one assumes the existence of superpartners of the Standard Model particles. Still it is possible to achieve the same by postulating, for instance, that ordinary (non supersymmetric) $SO(10)$ models break with an intermediate gauge scale, such as the one of Pati–Salam group.

The Theory of Everything (TOE) is a putative theory of theoretical physics that fully explains and links together all known physical phenomena, and, ideally, has predictive power for the outcome of any experiment that could be carried out in principle. M-Theory is not yet complete, but the underlying structure of the mathematics has been established and is in agreement with not only all the string theories, but with all of our scientific observations of the universe. Furthermore, it has passed many tests of internal mathematical consistency that many other attempts to combine quantum mechanics and gravity had failed. Unfortunately, until we can find some way to observe higher dimensions (impossible with our current level of technology) M-Theory has a very difficult time making predictions which can be tested in a laboratory. Technologically, it may never be possible for it to be "proven". Physicist and author Michio Kaku has remarked that M-Theory may present us with a "Theory of Everything" which is so concise that its underlying formula would fit on a T-shirt. Stephen Hawking originally believed that M-Theory may be the ultimate theory but later suggested that the search for understanding of mathematics and physics will never be complete.

Open Problems

The magnetic monopole in the *quantum* theory of magnetic charge started with a paper by the physicist Paul A.M. Dirac in 1931. The detection of magnetic monopoles is an open problem in experimental physics. In some theoretical models, magnetic monopoles are unlikely to be observed, because they are too massive to be created in particle accelerators, and also too rare in the Universe to enter a particle detector with much probability.

After more than twenty years of intensive research, the origin of high-temperature superconductivity is still not clear, but it seems that instead of *electron-phonon* attraction mechanisms, as in conventional superconductivity, one is dealing with genuine *electronic* mechanisms (e.g. by antiferromagnetic correlations), and instead of s-wave pairing, d-wave pairings are substantial. One goal of all this research is room-temperature superconductivity.

Electromagnetic Field

An electromagnetic field (also EMF or EM field) is a physical field produced by electrically charged objects. It affects the behavior of charged objects in the vicinity of the field. The electromagnetic field extends indefinitely throughout space and describes the electromagnetic interaction. It is one of the four fundamental forces of nature (the others are gravitation, weak interaction and strong interaction).

The field can be viewed as the combination of an electric field and a magnetic field. The electric field is produced by stationary charges, and the magnetic field by moving charges (currents); these two are often described as the sources of the field. The way in which charges and currents interact with the electromagnetic field is described by Maxwell's equations and the Lorentz force law.

From a classical perspective in the history of electromagnetism, the electromagnetic field can be regarded as a smooth, continuous field, propagated in a wavelike manner; whereas from the perspective of quantum field theory, the field is seen as quantized, being composed of individual particles.

Structure

The electromagnetic field may be viewed in two distinct ways: a continuous structure or a discrete structure.

Continuous Structure

Classically, electric and magnetic fields are thought of as being produced by smooth motions of charged objects. For example, oscillating charges produce electric and magnetic fields that may be viewed in a 'smooth', continuous, wavelike fashion. In this case, energy is viewed as being transferred continuously through the electromagnetic field between any two locations. For instance, the metal atoms in a radio transmitter appear to transfer energy continuously. This view is useful to a certain extent (radiation of low frequency), but problems are found at high frequencies.

Discrete Structure

The electromagnetic field may be thought of in a more 'coarse' way. Experiments reveal that in some circumstances electromagnetic energy transfer is better described as being carried in the form of packets called quanta (in this case, photons) with a fixed frequency. Planck's relation links the photon energy E of a photon to its frequency ν through the equation:

$$E = h\nu$$

where h is Planck's constant, and ν is the frequency of the photon . Although modern quantum optics tells us that there also is a semi-classical explanation of the photoelectric effect—the emission of electrons from metallic surfaces subjected to electromagnetic radiation—the photon was historically (although not strictly necessarily) used to explain certain observations. It is found that increasing the intensity of the incident radiation (so long as one remains in the linear regime) increases only the number of electrons ejected, and has almost no effect on the energy distribution of their ejection. Only the frequency of the radiation is relevant to the energy of the ejected electrons.

This quantum picture of the electromagnetic field (which treats it as analogous to harmonic oscillators) has proved very successful, giving rise to quantum electrodynamics, a quantum field theory describing the interaction of electromagnetic radiation with charged matter. It also gives rise to quantum optics, which is different from quantum electrodynamics in that the matter itself is modelled using quantum mechanics rather than quantum field theory.

Dynamics

In the past, electrically charged objects were thought to produce two different, unrelated types of field associated with their charge property. An electric field is produced when the charge is stationary with respect to an observer measuring the properties of the charge, and a magnetic field as well as an electric field is produced when the charge moves, creating an electric current with respect to this observer. Over time, it was realized that the electric and magnetic fields are better thought of as two parts of a greater whole — the electromagnetic field. Until 1820, when the Danish physicist H. C. Ørsted discovered the effect of electricity through a wire on a compass needle, electricity and magnetism had been viewed as unrelated phenomena. In 1831, Michael Faraday, one of the great thinkers of his time, made the seminal observation that time-varying magnetic fields could induce electric currents and then, in 1864, James Clerk Maxwell published his famous paper *A Dynamical Theory of the Electromagnetic Field.*

Once this electromagnetic field has been produced from a given charge distribution, other charged objects in this field will experience a force in a similar way that planets experience a force in the gravitational field of the sun. If these other charges and currents are comparable in size to the sources producing the above electromagnetic field, then a new net electromagnetic field will be produced. Thus, the electromagnetic field may be viewed as a dynamic entity that causes other charges and currents to move, and which is also affected by them. These interactions are described by Maxwell's equations and the Lorentz force law. This discussion ignores the radiation reaction force.

Feedback Loop

The behavior of the electromagnetic field can be divided into four different parts of a loop:

- the electric and magnetic fields are generated by electric charges,
- the electric and magnetic fields interact with each other,
- the electric and magnetic fields produce forces on electric charges,
- the electric charges move in space.

A common misunderstanding is that (a) the quanta of the fields act in the same manner as (b) the charged particles that generate the fields. In our everyday world, charged particles, such as electrons, move slowly through matter with a drift velocity of a fraction of a centimeter (or inch) per second, but fields propagate at the speed of light - approximately 300 thousand kilometers (or 186 thousand miles) a second. The mundane speed difference between charged particles and field quanta is on the order of one to a million, more or less. Maxwell's equations relate (a) the presence and movement of charged particles with (b) the generation of fields. Those fields can then affect the force on, and can then move other slowly moving charged particles. Charged particles can move at relativistic speeds nearing field propagation speeds, but, as Einstein showed, this requires enormous field energies, which are not present in our everyday experiences with electricity, magnetism, matter, and time and space.

The feedback loop can be summarized in a list, including phenomena belonging to each part of the loop:

- charged particles generate electric and magnetic fields
- the fields interact with each other
    - changing electric field acts like a current, generating 'vortex' of magnetic field
    - Faraday induction: changing magnetic field induces (negative) vortex of electric field
    - Lenz's law: negative feedback loop between electric and magnetic fields
- fields act upon particles
    - Lorentz force: force due to electromagnetic field
        - electric force: same direction as electric field
        - magnetic force: perpendicular both to magnetic field and to velocity of charge
- particles move
    - current is movement of particles
- particles generate more electric and magnetic fields; cycle repeats

Mathematical Description

There are different mathematical ways of representing the electromagnetic field. The first one views the electric and magnetic fields as three-dimensional vector fields. These vector fields each have a value defined at every point of space and time and are thus often regarded as functions of the space and time coordinates. As such, they are often written as $E(x, y, z, t)$ (electric field) and $B(x, y, z, t)$ (magnetic field).

If only the electric field (E) is non-zero, and is constant in time, the field is said to be an electrostatic field. Similarly, if only the magnetic field (B) is non-zero and is constant in time, the field is said to be a magnetostatic field. However, if either the electric or magnetic field has a time-dependence, then both fields must be considered together as a coupled electromagnetic field using Maxwell's equations.

With the advent of special relativity, physical laws became susceptible to the formalism of tensors. Maxwell's equations can be written in tensor form, generally viewed by physicists as a more elegant means of expressing physical laws.

The behaviour of electric and magnetic fields, whether in cases of electrostatics, magnetostatics, or electrodynamics (electromagnetic fields), is governed by Maxwell's equations. In the vector field formalism, these are:

$$\nabla \cdot \boldsymbol{E} = \frac{\rho}{\varepsilon_0} \text{ (Gauss's law)}$$

$$\nabla \cdot \boldsymbol{B} = 0 \text{ (Gauss's law for magnetism)}$$

$$\nabla \times \boldsymbol{E} = -\frac{\partial \boldsymbol{B}}{\partial t} \text{ (Faraday's law)}$$

$$\nabla \times \boldsymbol{B} = \mu_0 \boldsymbol{J} + \mu_0 \varepsilon_0 \frac{\partial \boldsymbol{E}}{\partial t} \text{ (Maxwell–Ampère law)}$$

where ρ is the charge density, which can (and often does) depend on time and position, is the permittivity of free space, ϵ_0 is the permeability of free space, and J is the current density vector, also a function of time and position. The units used above are the standard SI units. Inside a linear material, Maxwell's equations change by switching the permeability and permittivity of free space with the permeability and permittivity of the linear material in question. Inside other materials which possess more complex responses to electromagnetic fields, these terms are often represented by complex numbers, or tensors.

The Lorentz force law governs the interaction of the electromagnetic field with charged matter.

When a field travels across to different media, the properties of the field change according to the various boundary conditions. These equations are derived from Maxwell's equations. The tangential components of the electric and magnetic fields as they relate on the boundary of two media are as follows:

$$\mathbf{E}_1 = \mathbf{E}_2$$

$$\boldsymbol{H}_1 = \boldsymbol{H}_2 \text{ (current-free)}$$

$$\boldsymbol{D}_1 = \boldsymbol{D}_2 \text{ (charge-free)}$$

$$\mathbf{B}_1 = \mathbf{B}_2$$

The angle of refraction of an electric field between media is related to the permittivity (ε) of each medium:

$$\frac{\tan\theta_1}{\tan\theta_2} = \frac{\varepsilon_{r2}}{\varepsilon_{r1}}$$

The angle of refraction of a magnetic field between media is related to the permeability (μ) of each medium:

$$\frac{\tan\theta_1}{\tan\theta_2} = \frac{\mu_{r2}}{\mu_{r1}}$$

Properties of the Field

Reciprocal Behavior of Electric and Magnetic Fields

The two Maxwell equations, Faraday's Law and the Ampère-Maxwell Law, illustrate a very practical feature of the electromagnetic field. Faraday's Law may be stated roughly as 'a changing magnetic field creates an electric field'. This is the principle behind the electric generator.

Ampere's Law roughly states that 'a changing electric field creates a magnetic field'. Thus, this law can be applied to generate a magnetic field and run an electric motor.

Behavior of the Fields in the Absence of Charges or Currents

Maxwell's equations take the form of an electromagnetic wave in a volume of space not containing charges or currents (free space) – that is, where ρ and J are zero. Under these conditions, the electric and magnetic fields satisfy the electromagnetic wave equation:

$$\left(\nabla^2 - \frac{1}{c^2}\frac{\partial^2}{\partial t^2}\right)\boldsymbol{E} = 0$$

$$\left(\nabla^2 - \frac{1}{c^2}\frac{\partial^2}{\partial t^2}\right)\mathbf{B} = 0$$

James Clerk Maxwell was the first to obtain this relationship by his completion of Maxwell's equations with the addition of a displacement current term to Ampere's Circuital law.

Relation to and Comparison with other Physical Fields

Being one of the four fundamental forces of nature, it is useful to compare the electromagnetic field with the gravitational, strong and weak fields. The word 'force' is sometimes replaced by 'interaction' because modern particle physics models electromagnetism as an exchange of particles known as gauge bosons.

Electromagnetic and Gravitational Fields

Sources of electromagnetic fields consist of two types of charge – positive and negative. This contrasts with the sources of the gravitational field, which are masses. Masses are sometimes described as *gravitational charges*, the important feature of them being that there are only positive masses and no negative masses. Further, gravity differs from electromagnetism in that positive masses attract other positive masses whereas same charges in electromagnetism repel each other.

The relative strengths and ranges of the four interactions and other information are tabulated below:

Theory	Interaction	mediator	Relative Magnitude	Behavior	Range
Chromodynamics	Strong interaction	gluon	10^{38}	1	10^{-15} m
Electrodynamics	Electromagnetic interaction	photon	10^{36}	$1/r^2$	infinite
Flavordynamics	Weak interaction	W and Z bosons	10^{25}	$1/r^5$ to $1/r^7$	10^{-16} m
Geometrodynamics	Gravitation	graviton	10^0	$1/r^2$	infinite

Applications

Static E and M fields and static EM Fields

When an EM field is not varying in time, it may be seen as a purely electrical field or a purely magnetic field, or a mixture of both. However the general case of a static EM field with both electric and magnetic components present, is the case that appears to most observers. Observers who see only an electric or magnetic field component of a static EM field, have the other (electric or magnetic) component suppressed, due to the special case of the immobile state of the charges that produce the EM field in that case. In such cases the other component becomes manifest in other observer frames.

A consequence of this, is that any case that seems to consist of a "pure" static electric or magnetic field, can be converted to an EM field, with both E and M components present, by simply moving the observer into a frame of reference which is moving with regard to the frame in which only the "pure" electric or magnetic field appears. That is, a pure static electric field will show the familiar magnetic field associated with a current, in any frame of reference where the charge moves. Likewise, any new motion of a charge in a region that seemed previously to contain only a magnetic field, will show that the space now contains an electric field as well, which will be found to produces an additional Lorentz force upon the moving charge.

Thus, electrostatics, as well as magnetism and magnetostatics, are now seen as studies of the static EM field when a particular frame has been selected to suppress the other type of field, and since an EM field with both electric and magnetic will appear in any other frame, these "simpler" effects are merely the observer's.

Time-varying EM fields in Maxwell's Equations

An EM field that varies in time has two "causes" in Maxwell's equations. One is charges and currents (so-called "sources"), and the other cause for an E or M field is a change in the other type of field (this last cause also appears in "free space" very far from currents and charges).

An electromagnetic field very far from currents and charges (sources) is called electromagnetic radiation (EMR) since it radiates from the charges and currents in the source, and has no "feedback" effect on them, and is also not affected directly by them in the present time (rather, it is indirectly produced by a sequences of changes in fields radiating out from them in the past). EMR consists of the radiations in the electromagnetic spectrum, including radio waves, microwave, infrared, visible light, ultraviolet light, X-rays, and gamma rays.

A notable application of visible light is that this type of energy from the Sun powers all life on Earth that either makes or uses oxygen.

A changing electromagnetic field which is physically close to currents and charges will have a dipole characteristic that is dominated by either a changing electric dipole, or a changing magnetic dipole. This type of dipole field near sources is called an electromagnetic *near-field*.

Changing *electric* dipole fields, as such, are used commercially as near-fields mainly as a source of dielectric heating. Otherwise, they appear parasitically around conductors which absorb EMR, and around antennas which have the purpose of generating EMR at greater distances.

Changing *magnetic* dipole fields (i.e., magnetic near-fields) are used commercially for many types of magnetic induction devices. These include motors and electrical transformers at low frequencies, and devices such as metal detectors and MRI scanner coils at higher frequencies. Sometimes these high-frequency magnetic fields change at radio frequencies without being far-field waves and thus radio waves. Far-field effects (EMR) in the quantum picture of radiation, are represented by ordinary photons.

Health and Safety

The potential health effects of the very low frequency EMFs surrounding power lines and electrical devices are the subject of on-going research and a significant amount of public debate. The US National Institute for Occupational Safety and Health (NIOSH) and other US government agencies do not consider EMFs a proven health hazard. NIOSH has issued some cautionary advisories but stresses that the data are currently too limited to draw good conclusions.

The potential effects of electromagnetic fields on human health vary widely depending on the frequency and intensity of the fields.

Electric Potential

An electric potential (also called the *electric field potential* or the *electrostatic potential*) is the amount of work needed to move a unit positive charge from a reference point to a specific point inside the field without producing any acceleration. Typically, the reference point is *Earth* or a point at *Infinity*, although any point beyond the influence of the electric field charge can be used.

According to theoretical electromagnetics, electric potential is a scalar quantity denoted by V, equal to the electric potential energy of any charged particle at any location (measured in joules) divided by the charge of that particle (measured in coulombs). By dividing out the charge on the particle a remainder is obtained that is a property of the electric field itself.

This value can be calculated in either a static (time-invariant) or a dynamic (varying with time) electric field at a specific time in units of joules per coulomb ($J\ C^{-1}$), or volts (V). The electric potential at infinity is assumed to be zero.

A generalized electric scalar potential is also used in electrodynamics when time-varying electromagnetic fields are present, but this can not be so simply calculated. The electric potential and the magnetic vector potential together form a four vector, so that the two kinds of potential are mixed under Lorentz transformations.

Introduction

Classical mechanics explores concepts such as force, energy, potential etc. Force and potential energy are directly related. A net force acting on any object will cause it to accelerate. As an object moves in the direction in which the force accelerates it, its potential energy decreases: the gravitational potential energy of a cannonball at the top of a hill is greater than at the base of the hill. As it rolls downhill its potential energy decreases, being translated to motion, inertial (kinetic) energy.

It is possible to define the potential of certain force fields so that the potential energy of an object in that field depends only on the position of the object with respect to the field. Two such force fields are the gravitational field and an electric field (in the absence of time-varying magnetic fields). Such fields must affect objects due to the intrinsic properties of the object (e.g., mass or charge) and the position of the object.

Objects may possess a property known as electric charge and an electric field exerts a force on charged objects. If the charged object has a positive charge the force will be in the direction of the electric field vector at that point while if the charge is negative the force will be in the opposite direction. The magnitude of the force is given by the quantity of the charge multiplied by the magnitude of the electric field vector.

Electrostatics

The electric potential at a point r in a static electric field E is given by the line integral

$$V_E = -\int_C \boldsymbol{E} \cdot \mathrm{d}\ell$$

where C is an arbitrary path connecting the point with zero potential to r. When the curl $\nabla \times$ E is zero, the line integral above does not depend on the specific path C chosen but only on its endpoints. In this case, the electric field is conservative and determined by the gradient of the potential:

$$\boldsymbol{E} = -\nabla V_E .$$

Then, by Gauss's law, the potential satisfies Poisson's equation:

$$\nabla \cdot \quad = \nabla \cdot \left(-\nabla V_E\right) = -\nabla \ V_E = \rho / \varepsilon \ ,$$

where ρ is the total charge density (including bound charge) and $\nabla\cdot$ denotes the divergence.

The concept of electric potential is closely linked with potential energy. A test charge q has an electric potential energy U_E given by

$$U_E = qV .$$

The potential energy and hence also the electric potential is only defined up to an additive constant: one must arbitrarily choose a position where the potential energy and the electric potential are zero.

These equations cannot be used if the curl $\nabla \times E \neq 0$, i.e., in the case of a *nonconservative electric field*. The generalization of electric potential to this case is described below.

Electric Potential Due to a Point Charge

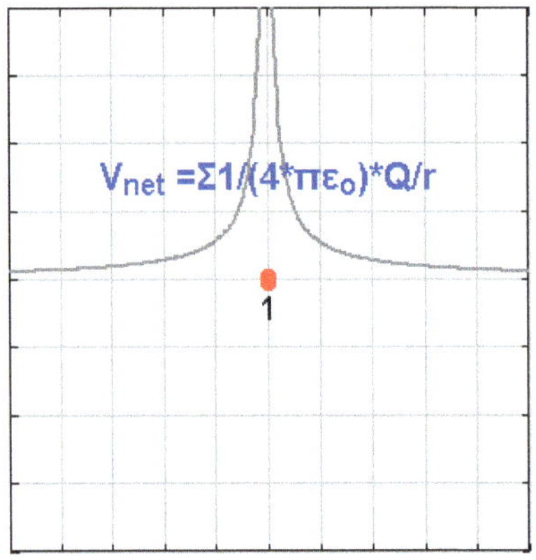

The electric potential created by a charge Q is $V=Q/(4\pi\varepsilon_0 r)$. Different values of Q will make different values of electric potential V (shown in the image).

The electric potential created by a point charge Q, at a distance r from the charge (relative to the potential at infinity), can be shown to be:

$$V_{\mathbf{E}} = \frac{1}{4\pi\varepsilon_0}\frac{Q}{r},$$

where ε_0 is the dielectric constant (permittivity of vacuum). This is known as the Coulomb potential.

The electric potential due to a system of point charges is equal to the sum of the point charges' individual potentials. This fact simplifies calculations significantly, since addition of potential (scalar) fields is much easier than addition of the electric (vector) fields.

The equation given above for the electric potential (and all the equations used here) are in the forms required by SI units. In some other (less common) systems of units, such as CGS-Gaussian, many of these equations would be altered.

Generalization to Electrodynamics

When time-varying magnetic fields are present (which is true whenever there are time-varying electric fields and vice versa), it is not possible to describe the electric field simply in terms of a scalar potential V because the electric field is no longer conservative: $\int_C \boldsymbol{E}\cdot d\ell$ is path-dependent because $\nabla \times \boldsymbol{E} \neq \boldsymbol{0}$ (Faraday's law of induction).

Instead, one can still define a scalar potential by also including the magnetic vector potential A. In particular, A is defined to satisfy:

$$\mathbf{B} = \nabla \times \mathbf{A},$$

where B is the magnetic field. Because the divergence of the magnetic field is always zero due to the absence of magnetic monopoles, such an A can always be found. Given this, the quantity,

$$\mathbf{F} = \mathbf{E} + \frac{\partial \mathbf{A}}{\partial t}$$

is a conservative field by Faraday's law and one can therefore write,

$$\boldsymbol{E} = -\nabla V - \frac{\partial \boldsymbol{A}}{\partial t},$$

where V is the scalar potential defined by the conservative field F.

The electrostatic potential is simply the special case of this definition where A is time-invariant. On the other hand, for time-varying fields,

$$-\int_a^b \boldsymbol{E} \cdot \mathrm{d}\ell \neq V_{(b)} - V_{(a)},$$

unlike electrostatics.

Units

The SI unit of electric potential is the volt (in honor of Alessandro Volta), which is why a difference in electric potential between two points is known as voltage. Older units are rarely used today. Variants of the centimeter gram second system of units included a number of different units for electric potential, including the abvolt and the statvolt.

Galvani Potential Versus Electrochemical Potential

Inside metals (and other solids and liquids), the energy of an electron is affected not only by the electric potential, but also by the specific atomic environment that it is in. When a voltmeter is connected between two different types of metal, it measures not the electric potential difference, but instead the potential difference corrected for the different atomic environments. The quantity measured by a voltmeter is called electrochemical potential or fermi level, while the pure unadjusted electric potential is sometimes called Galvani potential. The terms "voltage" and "electric potential" are a bit ambiguous in that, in practice, they can refer to *either* of these in different contexts.

Electric Current

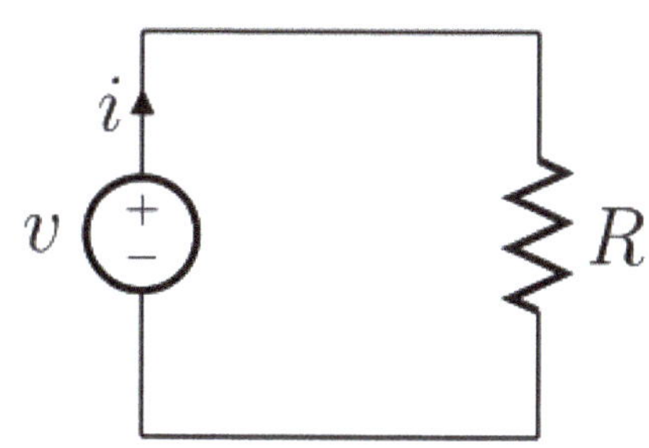

A simple electric circuit, where current is represented by the letter *i*. The relationship between the voltage (V), resistance (R), and current (I) is V=IR; this is known as Ohm's law.

An electric current is a flow of electric charge. In electric circuits this charge is often carried by moving electrons in a wire. It can also be carried by ions in an electrolyte, or by both ions and electrons such as in an ionised gas (plasma).

The SI unit for measuring an electric current is the ampere, which is the flow of electric charge across a surface at the rate of one coulomb per second. Electric current is measured using a device called an ammeter.

Electric currents cause Joule heating, which creates light in incandescent light bulbs. They also create magnetic fields, which are used in motors, inductors and generators.

The moving charged particles in an electric current are called charge carriers. In metals, one or more electrons from each atom are loosely bound to the atom, and can move freely about within the metal. These conduction electrons are the charge carriers in metal conductors.

Symbol

The conventional symbol for current is I, which originates from the French phrase *intensité de courant*, (current intensity). Current intensity is often referred to simply as *current*. The I symbol was used by André-Marie Ampère, after whom the unit of electric current is named, in formulating Ampère's force law (1820). The notation travelled from France to Great Britain, where it became standard, although at least one journal did not change from using C to I until 1896.

Conventions

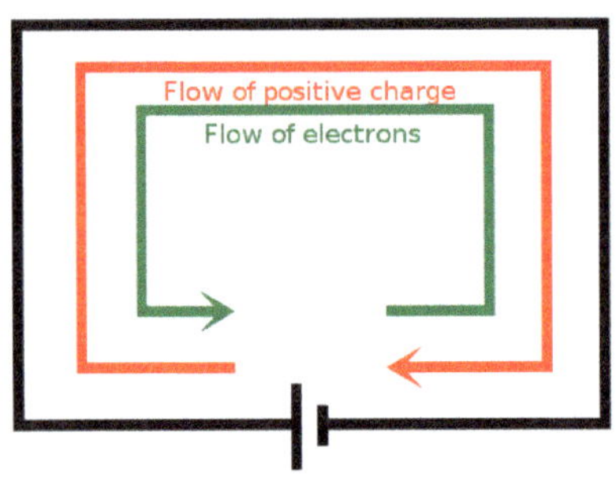

The electrons, the charge carriers in an electrical circuit, flow in the opposite direction of the conventional electric current.

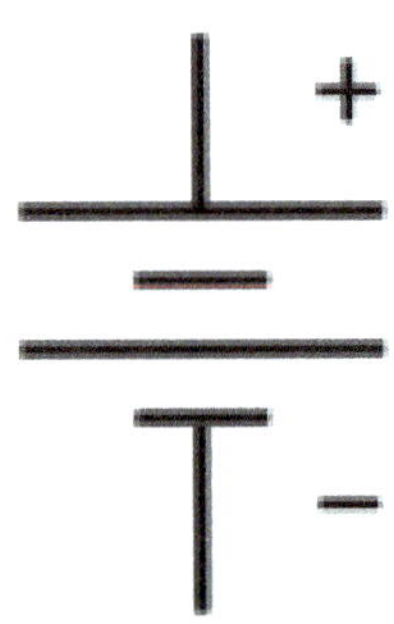

The symbol for a battery in a circuit diagram.

In a conductive material, the moving charged particles which constitute the electric current are called charge carriers. In metals, which make up the wires and other conductors in most electrical circuits, the positively charged atomic nuclei are held in a fixed position, and the negatively charged electrons are free to move, carrying their charge from one place to another. In other materials, notably the semiconductors, the charge carriers can be positive *or* negative, depending on the dopant used. Positive and negative charge carriers may even be present at the same time, as happens in an electrochemical cell.

A flow of positive charges gives the same electric current, and has the same effect in a circuit, as an equal flow of negative charges in the opposite direction. Since current can be the flow of either positive or negative charges, or both, a convention is needed for the direction of current that is independent of the type of charge carriers. The direction of *conventional current* is arbitrarily defined as the same direction as positive charges flow.

The consequence of this convention is that electrons, the charge carriers in metal wires and most other parts of electric circuits, flow in the opposite direction of conventional current flow in an electrical circuit.

Reference Direction

Since the current in a wire or component can flow in either direction, when a variable I is defined to represent that current, the direction representing positive current must be specified, usually by an arrow on the circuit schematic diagram. This is called the *reference direction* of current I. If the current flows in the opposite direction, the variable I has a negative value.

When analyzing electrical circuits, the actual direction of current through a specific circuit element is usually unknown. Consequently, the reference directions of currents are often assigned arbitrarily. When the circuit is solved, a negative value for the variable means that the actual direction of current through that circuit element is opposite that of the chosen reference direction. In electronic circuits, the reference current directions are often chosen so that all currents are toward ground. This often corresponds to the actual current direction, because in many circuits the power supply voltage is positive with respect to ground.

Ohm's Law

Ohm's law states that the current through a conductor between two points is directly proportional to the potential difference across the two points. Introducing the constant of proportionality, the resistance, one arrives at the usual mathematical equation that describes this relationship:

$$I = \frac{V}{R}$$

where I is the current through the conductor in units of amperes, V is the potential difference measured *across* the conductor in units of volts, and R is the resistance of the conductor in units of ohms. More specifically, Ohm's law states that the R in this relation is constant, independent of the current.

Alternating and Direct Current

In alternating current (AC) systems, the movement of electric charge periodically reverses direction. AC is the form of electric power most commonly delivered to businesses and residences. The usual waveform of an AC power circuit is a sine wave. Certain applications use different waveforms, such as triangular or square waves. Audio and radio signals carried on electrical wires are also examples of alternating current. An important goal in these applications is recovery of information encoded (or *modulated*) onto the AC signal.

In contrast, direct current (DC) is the unidirectional flow of electric charge, or a system in which the movement of electric charge is in one direction only. Direct current is produced by sources such as batteries, thermocouples, solar cells, and commutator-type electric machines of the dynamo type. Direct current may flow in a conductor such as a wire, but can also flow through semiconductors, insulators, or even through a vacuum as in electron or ion beams. An old name for direct current was *galvanic current.*

Occurrences

Natural observable examples of electrical current include lightning, static electric discharge, and the solar wind, the source of the polar auroras.

Man-made occurrences of electric current include the flow of conduction electrons in metal wires such as the overhead power lines that deliver electrical energy across long distances and the smaller wires within electrical and electronic equipment. Eddy currents are electric currents that occur in conductors exposed to changing magnetic fields. Similarly, electric currents occur, particularly in the surface, of conductors exposed to electromagnetic waves. When oscillating electric currents flow at the correct voltages within radio antennas, radio waves are generated.

In electronics, other forms of electric current include the flow of electrons through resistors or through the vacuum in a vacuum tube, the flow of ions inside a battery or a neuron, and the flow of holes within a semiconductor.

Current Measurement

Current can be measured using an ammeter.

At the circuit level, there are various techniques that can be used to measure current:

- Shunt resistors
- Hall effect current sensor transducers
- Transformers (however DC cannot be measured)
- Magnetoresistive field sensors

Resistive Heating

Joule heating, also known as *ohmic heating* and *resistive heating*, is the process by which the passage of an electric current through a conductor releases heat. It was first studied by James Prescott Joule in 1841. Joule immersed a length of wire in a fixed mass of water and measured the temperature rise due to a known current through the wire for a 30 minute period. By varying the current and the length of the wire he deduced that the heat produced was proportional to the square of the current multiplied by the electrical resistance of the wire.

$$Q \propto I^2 R$$

This relationship is known as Joule's First Law. The SI unit of energy was subsequently named the joule and given the symbol J. The commonly known unit of power, the watt, is equivalent to one joule per second.

Electromagnetism

Electromagnet

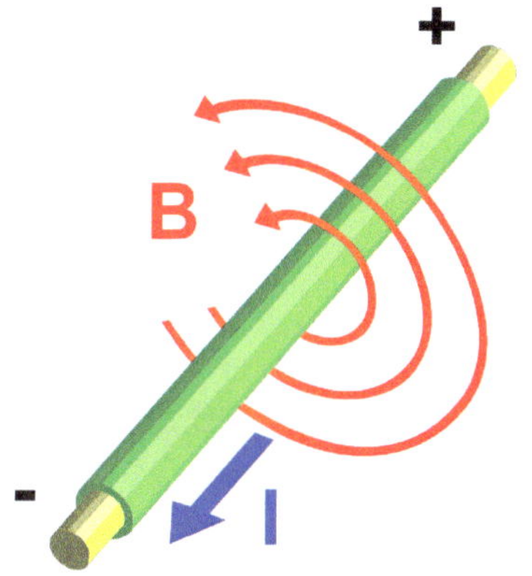

According to Ampère's law, an electric current produces a magnetic field.

In an electromagnet a coil, of a large number of circular turns of insulated wire, wrapped on a cylindrical core, behaves like a magnet when an electric current flows through it. When the current is switched off, the coil loses its magnetism immediately. We call such a device as an electromagnet.

Electric current produces a magnetic field. The magnetic field can be visualized as a pattern of circular field lines surrounding the wire that persists as long as there is current.

Magnetism can also produce electric currents. When a changing magnetic field is applied to a conductor, an Electromotive force (EMF) is produced, and when there is a suitable path, this causes current.

Electric current can be directly measured with a galvanometer, but this method involves breaking the electrical circuit, which is sometimes inconvenient. Current can also be measured without breaking the circuit by detecting the magnetic field associated with the current. Devices used for this include Hall effect sensors, current clamps, current transformers, and Rogowski coils.

Radio Waves

When an electric current flows in a suitably shaped conductor at radio frequencies radio waves can be generated. These travel at the speed of light and can cause electric currents in distant conductors.

Conduction Mechanisms in Various Media

In metallic solids, electric charge flows by means of electrons, from lower to higher electrical potential. In other media, any stream of charged objects (ions, for example) may constitute an electric current. To provide a definition of current independent of the type of charge carriers, *conventional current* is defined as moving in the same direction as the positive charge flow. So, in metals where the charge carriers (electrons) are negative, conventional current is in the opposite direction as the electrons. In conductors where the charge carriers are positive, conventional current is in the same direction as the charge carriers.

In a vacuum, a beam of ions or electrons may be formed. In other conductive materials, the electric current is due to the flow of both positively and negatively charged particles at the same time. In still others, the current is entirely due to positive charge flow. For example, the electric currents in electrolytes are flows of positively and negatively charged ions. In a common lead-acid electrochemical cell, electric currents are composed of positive hydrogen ions (protons) flowing in one direction, and negative sulfate ions flowing in the other. Electric currents in sparks or plasma are flows of electrons as well as positive and negative ions. In ice and in certain solid electrolytes, the electric current is entirely composed of flowing ions.

Metals

In a metal, some of the outer electrons in each atom are not bound to the individual atom as they are in insulating materials, but are free to move within the metal lattice. These conduction electrons can serve as charge carriers, carrying a current. Metals are particularly conductive because there are a large number of these free electrons, typically one per atom in the lattice. With no external electric field applied, these electrons move about randomly due to thermal energy but, on average, there is zero net current within the metal. At room temperature, the average speed of these random motions is 10^6 metres per second. Given a surface through which a metal wire passes, electrons move in both directions across the surface at an equal rate. As George Gamow wrote in his popular science book, *One, Two, Three...Infinity* (1947), "The metallic substances differ from all other materials by the fact that the outer shells of their atoms are bound rather loosely, and often let one of their electrons go free. Thus the interior of a metal is filled up with a large number of unattached electrons that travel aimlessly around like a crowd of displaced persons. When a metal wire is subjected to electric force applied on its opposite ends, these free electrons rush in the direction of the force, thus forming what we call an electric current."

When a metal wire is connected across the two terminals of a DC voltage source such as a battery, the source places an electric field across the conductor. The moment contact is made, the free electrons of the conductor are forced to drift toward the positive terminal under the influence of this field. The free electrons are therefore the charge carrier in a typical solid conductor.

For a steady flow of charge through a surface, the current I (in amperes) can be calculated with the following equation:

$$I = \frac{Q}{t},$$

where Q is the electric charge transferred through the surface over a time t. If Q and t are measured in coulombs and seconds respectively, I is in amperes.

More generally, electric current can be represented as the rate at which charge flows through a given surface as:

$$I = \frac{dQ}{dt}.$$

Electrolytes

Electric currents in electrolytes are flows of electrically charged particles (ions). For example, if an electric field is placed across a solution of Na^+ and Cl^- (and conditions are right) the sodium ions move towards the negative electrode (cathode), while the chloride ions move towards the positive electrode (anode). Reactions take place at both electrode surfaces, absorbing each ion.

Water-ice and certain solid electrolytes called proton conductors contain positive hydrogen ions ("protons") that are mobile. In these materials, electric currents are composed of moving protons, as opposed to the moving electrons in metals.

In certain electrolyte mixtures, brightly coloured ions are the moving electric charges. The slow progress of the colour makes the current visible.

Gases and Plasmas

In air and other ordinary gases below the breakdown field, the dominant source of electrical conduction is via relatively few mobile ions produced by radioactive gases, ultraviolet light, or cosmic rays. Since the electrical conductivity is low, gases are dielectrics or insulators. However, once the applied electric field approaches the breakdown value, free electrons become sufficiently accelerated by the electric field to create additional free electrons by colliding, and ionizing, neutral gas atoms or molecules in a process called avalanche breakdown. The breakdown process forms a plasma that contains enough mobile electrons and positive ions to make it an electrical conductor. In the process, it forms a light emitting conductive path, such as a spark, arc or lightning.

Plasma is the state of matter where some of the electrons in a gas are stripped or "ionized" from their molecules or atoms. A plasma can be formed by high temperature, or by application of a high electric or alternating magnetic field as noted above. Due to their lower mass, the electrons in a plasma accelerate more quickly in response to an electric field than the heavier positive ions, and hence carry the bulk of the current. The free ions recombine to create new chemical compounds (for example, breaking atmospheric oxygen into single oxygen [$O_2 \rightarrow 2O$], which then recombine creating ozone [O_3]).

Vacuum

Since a "perfect vacuum" contains no charged particles, it normally behaves as a perfect insulator. However, metal electrode surfaces can cause a region of the vacuum to become conductive by injecting free electrons or ions through either field electron emission or thermionic emission. Thermionic emission occurs when the thermal energy exceeds the metal's work function, while field electron emission occurs when the electric field at the surface of the metal is high enough to cause tunneling, which results in the ejection of free electrons from the metal into the vacuum. Externally heated electrodes are often used to generate an electron cloud as in the filament or indirectly heated cathode of vacuum tubes. Cold electrodes can also spontaneously produce electron clouds via thermionic emission when small incandescent regions (called cathode spots or anode spots) are formed. These are incandescent regions of the electrode surface that are created by a localized high current. These regions may be initiated by field electron emission, but are then sustained by localized thermionic emission once a vacuum arc forms. These small electron-emitting regions can form quite rapidly, even explosively, on a metal surface subjected to a high electrical field. Vacuum tubes and sprytrons are some of the electronic switching and amplifying devices based on vacuum conductivity.

Superconductivity

Superconductivity is a phenomenon of exactly zero electrical resistance and expulsion of magnetic fields occurring in certain materials when cooled below a characteristic critical temperature. It was discovered by Heike Kamerlingh Onnes on April 8, 1911 in Leiden. Like ferromagnetism and atomic spectral lines, superconductivity is a quantum mechanical phenomenon. It is characterized by the Meissner effect, the complete ejection of magnetic field lines from the interior of the superconductor as it transitions into the superconducting state. The occurrence of the Meissner effect indicates that superconductivity cannot be understood simply as the idealization of *perfect conductivity* in classical physics.

Semiconductor

In a semiconductor it is sometimes useful to think of the current as due to the flow of positive "holes" (the mobile positive charge carriers that are places where the semiconductor crystal is missing a valence electron). This is the case in a p-type semiconductor. A semiconductor has electrical conductivity intermediate in magnitude between that of a conductor and an insulator. This means a conductivity roughly in the range of 10^{-2} to 10^{4} siemens per centimeter ($S{\cdot}cm^{-1}$).

In the classic crystalline semiconductors, electrons can have energies only within certain bands (i.e. ranges of levels of energy). Energetically, these bands are located between the energy of the ground state, the state in which electrons are tightly bound to the atomic nuclei of the material, and the free electron energy, the latter describing the energy required for an electron to escape entirely from the material. The energy bands each correspond to a large number of discrete quantum states of the electrons, and most of the states with low energy (closer to the nucleus) are occupied, up to a particular band called the *valence band*. Semiconductors and insulators are distinguished from metals because the valence band in any given metal is nearly filled with electrons under usual operating conditions, while very few (semiconductor) or virtually none (insulator) of them are available in the *conduction band*, the band immediately above the valence band.

The ease of exciting electrons in the semiconductor from the valence band to the conduction band depends on the band gap between the bands. The size of this energy band gap serves as an arbitrary dividing line (roughly 4 eV) between semiconductors and insulators.

With covalent bonds, an electron moves by hopping to a neighboring bond. The Pauli exclusion principle requires that the electron be lifted into the higher anti-bonding state of that bond. For delocalized states, for example in one dimension – that is in a nanowire, for every energy there is a state with electrons flowing in one direction and another state with the electrons flowing in the other. For a net current to flow, more states for one direction than for the other direction must be occupied. For this to occur, energy is required, as in the semiconductor the next higher states lie above the band gap. Often this is stated as: full bands do not contribute to the electrical conductivity. However, as a semiconductor's temperature rises above absolute zero, there is more energy in the semiconductor to spend on lattice vibration and on exciting electrons into the conduction band. The current-carrying electrons in the conduction band are known as *free electrons*, though they are often simply called *electrons* if that is clear in context.

Current Density and Ohm's Law

Current density is a measure of the density of an electric current. It is defined as a vector whose magnitude is the electric current per cross-sectional area. In SI units, the current density is measured in amperes per square metre.

$$I = \int \vec{J} \cdot d\vec{A}$$

where I is current in the conductor, $\vec{J}$ is the current density, and $d\vec{A}$ is the differential cross-sectional area vector.

The current density (current per unit area) $\vec{J}$ in materials with finite resistance is directly proportional to the electric field $\vec{E}$ in the medium. The proportionality constant is called the conductivity σ of the material, whose value depends on the material concerned and, in general, is dependent on the temperature of the material:

$$\vec{J} = \sigma \vec{E}$$

The reciprocal of the conductivity σ of the material is called the resistivity ρ of the material and the above equation, when written in terms of resistivity becomes:

$$\vec{J} = \frac{\vec{E}}{\rho} \text{ or}$$

$$\vec{E} = \rho \vec{J}$$

Conduction in semiconductor devices may occur by a combination of drift and diffusion, which is proportional to diffusion constant D and charge density α_q . The current density is then:

$$J = \sigma E + Dq\nabla n,$$

with q being the elementary charge and n the electron density. The carriers move in the direction of decreasing concentration, so for electrons a positive current results for a positive density gradient. If the carriers are holes, replace electron density n by the negative of the hole density p .

In linear anisotropic materials, σ, ρ and D are tensors.

In linear materials such as metals, and under low frequencies, the current density across the conductor surface is uniform. In such conditions, Ohm's law states that the current is directly proportional to the potential difference between two ends (across) of that metal (ideal) resistor (or other ohmic device):

$$I = \frac{V}{R},$$

where I is the current, measured in amperes; V is the potential difference, measured in volts; and R is the resistance, measured in ohms. For alternating currents, especially at higher frequencies, skin effect causes the current to spread unevenly across the conductor cross-section, with higher density near the surface, thus increasing the apparent resistance.

Drift Speed

The mobile charged particles within a conductor move constantly in random directions, like the particles of a gas. (More accurately, a Fermi gas.) To create a net flow of charge, the particles must also move together with an average drift rate. Electrons are the charge carriers in metals and they follow an erratic path, bouncing from atom to atom, but generally drifting in the opposite direction of the electric field. The speed they drift at can be calculated from the equation:

$$I = nAvQ,$$

where

I is the electric current

n is number of charged particles per unit volume (or charge carrier density)

A is the cross-sectional area of the conductor

v is the drift velocity, and

Q is the charge on each particle.

Typically, electric charges in solids flow slowly. For example, in a copper wire of cross-section 0.5 mm^2, carrying a current of 5 A, the drift velocity of the electrons is on the order of a millimetre per second. To take a different example, in the near-vacuum inside a cathode ray tube, the electrons travel in near-straight lines at about a tenth of the speed of light.

Any accelerating electric charge, and therefore any changing electric current, gives rise to an electromagnetic wave that propagates at very high speed outside the surface of the conductor. This speed is usually a significant fraction of the speed of light, as can be deduced from Maxwell's Equations, and is therefore many times faster than the drift velocity of the electrons. For example, in AC power lines, the waves of electromagnetic energy propagate through the space between the wires, moving from a source to a distant load, even though the electrons in the wires only move back and forth over a tiny distance.

The ratio of the speed of the electromagnetic wave to the speed of light in free space is called the velocity factor, and depends on the electromagnetic properties of the conductor and the insulating materials surrounding it, and on their shape and size.

The magnitudes (not the natures) of these three velocities can be illustrated by an analogy with the three similar velocities associated with gases.

- The low drift velocity of charge carriers is analogous to air motion; in other words, winds.
- The high speed of electromagnetic waves is roughly analogous to the speed of sound in a

gas (these waves move through the medium much faster than any individual particles do)

- The random motion of charges is analogous to heat – the thermal velocity of randomly vibrating gas particles.

Lorentz Force

In physics (particularly in electromagnetism) the Lorentz force is the combination of electric and magnetic force on a point charge due to electromagnetic fields. A particle of charge q moving with velocity v in the presence of an electric field E and a magnetic field B experiences a force:

$$\boldsymbol{F} = q\boldsymbol{E} + q\boldsymbol{v} \times \boldsymbol{B}$$

(in SI units). Variations on this basic formula describe the magnetic force on a current-carrying wire (sometimes called Laplace force), the electromotive force in a wire loop moving through a magnetic field (an aspect of Faraday's law of induction), and the force on a charged particle which might be travelling near the speed of light (relativistic form of the Lorentz force).

The first derivation of the Lorentz force is commonly attributed to Oliver Heaviside in 1889, although other historians suggest an earlier origin in an 1865 paper by James Clerk Maxwell. Hendrik Lorentz derived it a few years after Heaviside.

Equation

Charged Particle

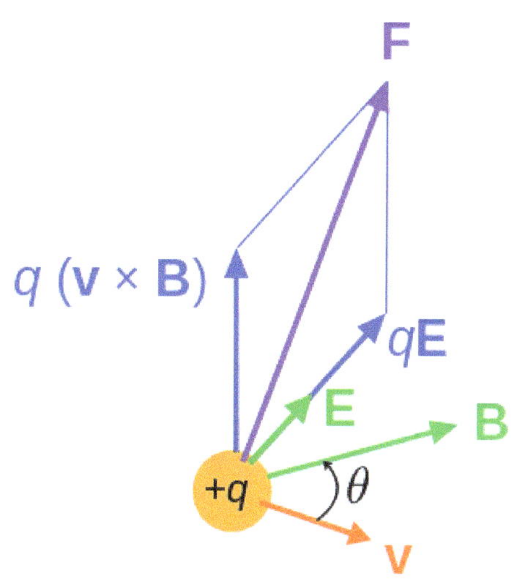

Lorentz force **F** on a charged particle (of charge q) in motion (instantaneous velocity **v**). The **E** field and **B** field vary in space and time.

The force F acting on a particle of electric charge q with instantaneous velocity v, due to an external electric field E and magnetic field B, is given by (in SI units):

$$\boldsymbol{F} = q(\boldsymbol{E} + \boldsymbol{v} \times \boldsymbol{B})$$

where × is the vector cross product. All boldface quantities are vectors. More explicitly stated:

$$\boldsymbol{F}(\boldsymbol{r}, \dot{\boldsymbol{r}}, t, q) = q[\boldsymbol{E}(\boldsymbol{r}, t) + \dot{\boldsymbol{r}} \times \boldsymbol{B}(\boldsymbol{r}, t)]$$

in which r is the position vector of the charged particle, t is time, and the overdot is a time derivative.

A positively charged particle will be accelerated in the *same* linear orientation as the E field, but will curve perpendicularly to both the instantaneous velocity vector v and the B field according to the right-hand rule (in detail, if the fingers of the right hand are extended to point in the direction of v and are then curled to point in the direction of B, then the extended thumb will point in the direction of F).

The term qE is called the electric force, while the term qv × B is called the magnetic force. According to some definitions, the term "Lorentz force" refers specifically to the formula for the magnetic force, with the *total* electromagnetic force (including the electric force) given some other (nonstandard) name.The term "Lorentz force" will refer only to the expression for the total force.

The magnetic force component of the Lorentz force manifests itself as the force that acts on a current-carrying wire in a magnetic field. In that context, it is also called the Laplace force.

Continuous Charge Distribution

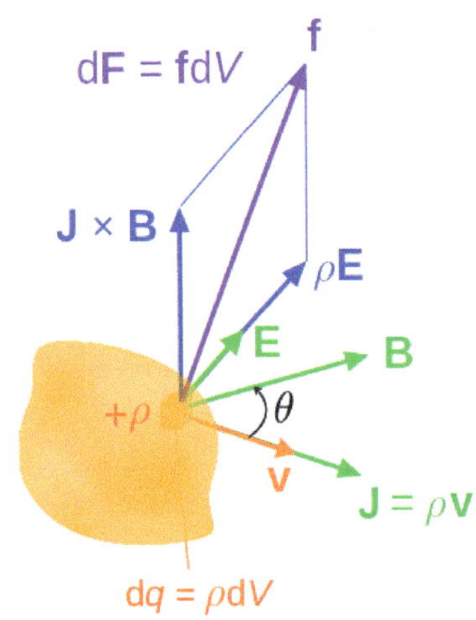

Lorentz force (per unit 3-volume) **f** on a continuous charge distribution (charge density ρ) in motion. The 3-current density **J** corresponds to the motion of the charge element dq in volume element dV and varies throughout the continuum.

For a continuous charge distribution in motion, the Lorentz force equation becomes:

$$\mathrm{d}\boldsymbol{F} = \mathrm{d}q\left(\boldsymbol{E} + \boldsymbol{v} \times \boldsymbol{B}\right)$$

where dF is the force on a small piece of the charge distribution with charge dq. If both sides of this equation are divided by the volume of this small piece of the charge distribution dV, the result is:

$$\mathbf{f} = \rho(\mathbf{E} + \mathbf{v} \times \mathbf{B})$$

where f is the *force density* (force per unit volume) and ρ is the charge density (charge per unit volume). Next, the current density corresponding to the motion of the charge continuum is

$$\mathbf{J} = \rho\mathbf{v}$$

so the continuous analogue to the equation is

$$\boldsymbol{f} = \rho\boldsymbol{E} + \boldsymbol{J} \times \boldsymbol{B}$$

The total force is the volume integral over the charge distribution:

$$\mathbf{F} = \iiint(\rho\mathbf{E} + \mathbf{J} \times \mathbf{B})\mathrm{d}V.$$

By eliminating ρ and J, using Maxwell's equations, and manipulating using the theorems of vector calculus, this form of the equation can be used to derive the Maxwell stress tensor σ, in turn this can be combined with the Poynting vector S to obtain the electromagnetic stress–energy tensor T used in general relativity.

In terms of σ and S, another way to write the Lorentz force (per unit volume) is

$$\mathbf{f} = \nabla \cdot \sigma - \frac{1}{c^2}\frac{\partial \mathbf{S}}{\partial t}$$

where c is the speed of light and ∇· denotes the divergence of a tensor field. Rather than the amount of charge and its velocity in electric and magnetic fields, this equation relates the energy flux (flow of *energy* per unit time per unit distance) in the fields to the force exerted on a charge distribution.

Equation in cgs Units

The above-mentioned formulae use SI units which are the most common among experimentalists, technicians, and engineers. In cgs-Gaussian units, which are somewhat more common among theoretical physicists, one has instead

$$\boldsymbol{F} = q_{\mathrm{cgs}}\left(\boldsymbol{E}_{\mathrm{cgs}} + \frac{\boldsymbol{v}}{c} \times \boldsymbol{B}_{\mathrm{cgs}}\right).$$

where c is the speed of light. Although this equation looks slightly different, it is completely equivalent, since one has the following relations:

$$q_{\mathrm{cgs}} = \frac{q_{\mathrm{SI}}}{\sqrt{4\pi\epsilon_0}}, \quad \boldsymbol{E}_{\mathrm{cgs}} = \sqrt{4\pi\epsilon_0}\,\boldsymbol{E}_{\mathrm{SI}}, \quad \boldsymbol{B}_{\mathrm{cgs}} = \sqrt{4\pi/\mu_0}\,\boldsymbol{B}_{\mathrm{SI}}, \quad c = \frac{1}{\sqrt{\epsilon_0\mu_0}}.$$

where ε_0 is the vacuum permittivity and μ_0 the vacuum permeability. In practice, the subscripts "cgs" and "SI" are always omitted, and the unit system has to be assessed from context.

History

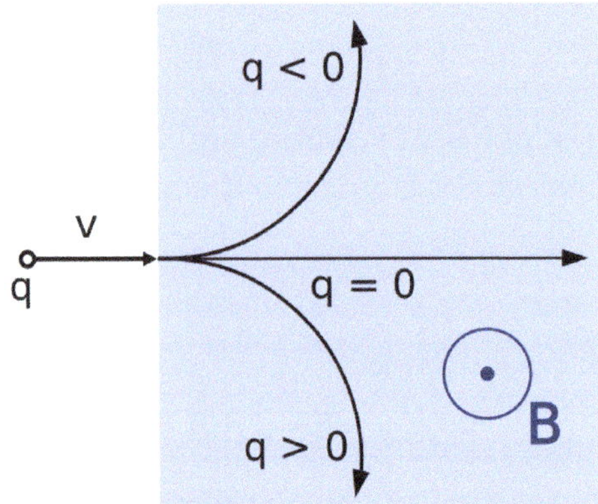

Trajectory of a particle with a positive or negative charge *q* under the influence of a magnetic field *B*, which is directed perpendicularly out of the screen.

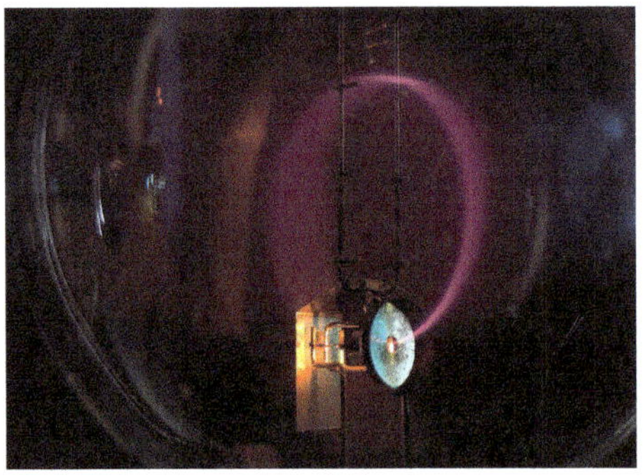

Beam of electrons moving in a circle, due to the presence of a magnetic field. Purple light is emitted along the electron path, due to the electrons colliding with gas molecules in the bulb. A Teltron tube is used in this example.

Early attempts to quantitatively describe the electromagnetic force were made in the mid-18th century. It was proposed that the force on magnetic poles, by Johann Tobias Mayer and others in 1760,and electrically charged objects, by Henry Cavendish in 1762, obeyed an inverse-square law. However, in both cases the experimental proof was neither complete nor conclusive. It was not until 1784 when Charles-Augustin de Coulomb, using a torsion balance, was able to definitively show through experiment that this was true. Soon after the discovery in 1820 by H. C. Ørsted that a magnetic needle is acted on by a voltaic current, André-Marie Ampère that same year was able to devise through experimentation the formula for the angular dependence of the force between two current elements. In all these descriptions, the force was always given in terms of the properties of the objects involved and the distances between them rather than in terms of electric and magnetic fields.

The modern concept of electric and magnetic fields first arose in the theories of Michael Faraday, particularly his idea of lines of force, later to be given full mathematical description by Lord Kelvin and James Clerk Maxwell. From a modern perspective it is possible to identify in Maxwell's 1865 formulation of his field equations a form of the Lorentz force equation in relation to electric currents, however, in the time of Maxwell it was not evident how his equations related to the forces on moving charged objects. J. J. Thomson was the first to attempt to derive from Maxwell's field equations the electromagnetic forces on a moving charged object in terms of the object's properties and external fields. Interested in determining the electromagnetic behavior of the charged particles in cathode rays, Thomson published a paper in 1881 wherein he gave the force on the particles due to an external magnetic field as

$$\mathbf{F} = \frac{q}{2}\mathbf{v} \times \mathbf{B}.$$

Thomson derived the correct basic form of the formula, but, because of some miscalculations and an incomplete description of the displacement current, included an incorrect scale-factor of a half in front of the formula. Oliver Heaviside invented the modern vector notation and applied it to Maxwell's field equations; he also (in 1885 and 1889) had fixed the mistakes of Thomson's derivation and arrived at the correct form of the magnetic force on a moving charged object. Finally, in 1892, Hendrik Lorentz derived the modern form of the formula for the electromagnetic force which includes the contributions to the total force from both the electric and the magnetic fields. Lorentz began by abandoning the Maxwellian descriptions of the ether and conduction. Instead, Lorentz made a distinction between matter and the luminiferous aether and sought to apply the Maxwell equations at a microscopic scale. Using Heaviside's version of the Maxwell equations for a stationary ether and applying Lagrangian mechanics, Lorentz arrived at the correct and complete form of the force law that now bears his name.

Trajectories of Particles Due to The Lorentz Force

In many cases of practical interest, the motion in a magnetic field of an electrically charged particle (such as an electron or ion in a plasma) can be treated as the superposition of a relatively fast circular motion around a point called the guiding center and a relatively slow drift of this point. The drift speeds may differ for various species depending on their charge states, masses, or temperatures, possibly resulting in electric currents or chemical separation.

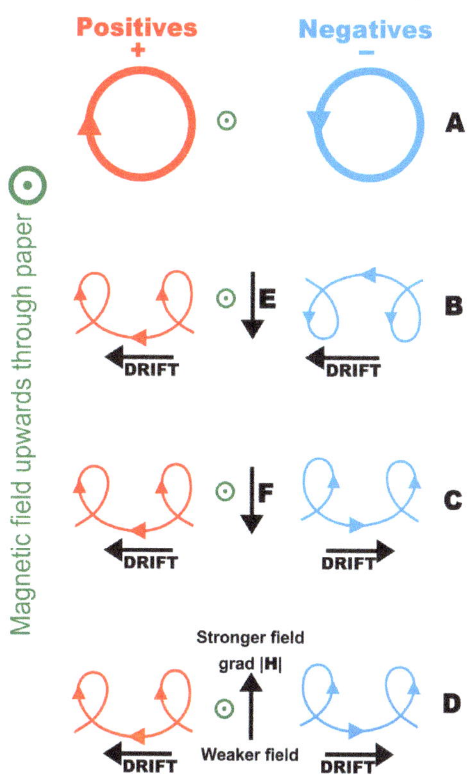

Charged particle drifts in a homogeneous magnetic field. (A) No disturbing force (B) With an electric field, E (C) With an independent force, F (e.g. gravity) (D) In an inhomogeneous magnetic field, grad H.

Significance of The Lorentz Force

While the modern Maxwell's equations describe how electrically charged particles and currents or moving charged particles give rise to electric and magnetic fields, the Lorentz force law completes that picture by describing the force acting on a moving point charge q in the presence of electromagnetic fields. The Lorentz force law describes the effect of E and B upon a point charge, but such electromagnetic forces are not the entire picture. Charged particles are possibly coupled to other forces, notably gravity and nuclear forces. Thus, Maxwell's equations do not stand separate from other physical laws, but are coupled to them via the charge and current densities. The response of a point charge to the Lorentz law is one aspect; the generation of E and B by currents and charges is another.

In real materials the Lorentz force is inadequate to describe the collective behavior of charged particles, both in principle and as a matter of computation. The charged particles in a material medium not only respond to the E and B fields but also generate these fields. Complex transport equations must be solved to determine the time and spatial response of charges, for example, the Boltzmann equation or the Fokker–Planck equation or the Navier–Stokes equations. For example, magnetohydrodynamics, fluid dynamics, electrohydrodynamics, superconductivity, stellar evolution. An entire physical apparatus for dealing with these matters has developed. For example, Green–Kubo relations and Green's function (many-body theory).

Lorentz Force Law as the Definition of E and B

In many textbook treatments of classical electromagnetism, the Lorentz force Law is used as the *definition* of the electric and magnetic fields E and B. To be specific, the Lorentz force is understood to be the following empirical statement:

> *The electromagnetic force **F** on a test charge at a given point and time is a certain function of its charge* q *and velocity **v**, which can be parameterized by exactly two vectors **E** and **B**, in the functional form:*

$$\boldsymbol{F} = q(\boldsymbol{E} + \boldsymbol{v} \times \boldsymbol{B})$$

This is valid, even for particles approaching the speed of light (that is, magnitude of $v = |v| = c$). So the two vector fields E and B are thereby defined throughout space and time, and these are called the "electric field" and "magnetic field". The fields are defined everywhere in space and time with respect to what force a test charge would receive regardless of whether a charge is present to experience the force.

As a definition of E and B, the Lorentz force is only a definition in principle because a real particle (as opposed to the hypothetical "test charge" of infinitesimally-small mass and charge) would generate its own finite E and B fields, which would alter the electromagnetic force that it experiences. In addition, if the charge experiences acceleration, as if forced into a curved trajectory by some external agency, it emits radiation that causes braking of its motion. For example Bremsstrahlung and synchrotron light. These effects occur through both a direct effect (called the radiation reaction force) and indirectly (by affecting the motion of nearby charges and currents). Moreover, net force must include gravity, electroweak, and any other forces aside from electromagnetic force.

Force on a Current-carrying Wire

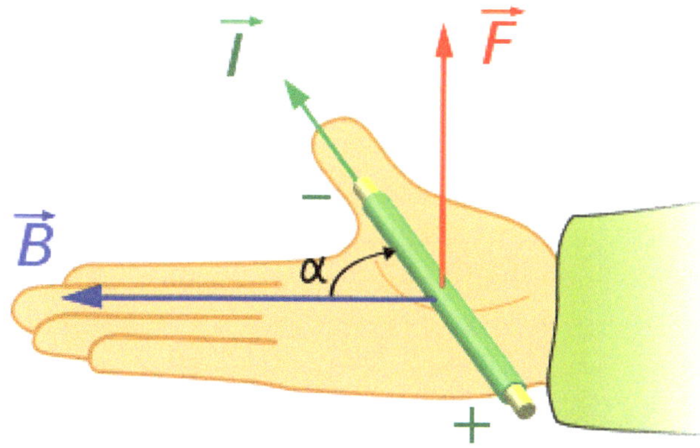

Right-hand rule for a current-carrying wire in a magnetic field *B*

When a wire carrying an electric current is placed in a magnetic field, each of the moving charges, which comprise the current, experiences the Lorentz force, and together they can create a macroscopic force on the wire (sometimes called the Laplace force). By combining the Lorentz force law above with the definition of electric current, the following equation results, in the case of a straight, stationary wire:

$$\boldsymbol{F} = I\boldsymbol{\ell} \times \boldsymbol{B}$$

where ℓ is a vector whose magnitude is the length of wire, and whose direction is along the wire, aligned with the direction of conventional current flow *I*.

If the wire is not straight but curved, the force on it can be computed by applying this formula to each infinitesimal segment of wire *d*ℓ, then adding up all these forces by integration. Formally, the net force on a stationary, rigid wire carrying a steady current *I* is

$$\mathbf{F} = I\int \mathrm{d}\boldsymbol{\ell} \times \mathbf{B}$$

This is the net force. In addition, there will usually be torque, plus other effects if the wire is not perfectly rigid.

One application of this is Ampère's force law, which describes how two current-carrying wires can attract or repel each other, since each experiences a Lorentz force from the other's magnetic field.

EMF

The magnetic force ($q\mathrm{v} \times \mathrm{B}$) component of the Lorentz force is responsible for *motional* electromotive force (or *motional EMF*), the phenomenon underlying many electrical generators. When a conductor is moved through a magnetic field, the magnetic field exerts opposite forces on electrons and nuclei in the wire, and this creates the EMF. The term "motional EMF" is applied to this phenomenon, since the EMF is due to the *motion* of the wire.

In other electrical generators, the magnets move, while the conductors do not. In this case, the EMF is due to the electric force ($q\mathrm{E}$) term in the Lorentz Force equation. The electric field in question is created by the changing magnetic field, resulting in an *induced* EMF, as described by the Maxwell–Faraday equation (one of the four modern Maxwell's equations).

Both of these EMFs, despite their apparently distinct origins, are described by the same equation, namely, the EMF is the rate of change of magnetic flux through the wire. (This is Faraday's law of induction). Einstein's special theory of relativity was partially motivated by the desire to better understand this link between the two effects. In fact, the electric and magnetic fields are different facets of the same electromagnetic field, and in moving from one inertial frame to another, the solenoidal vector field portion of the E-field can change in whole or in part to a B-field or *vice versa*.

Lorentz Force and Faraday's Law of Induction

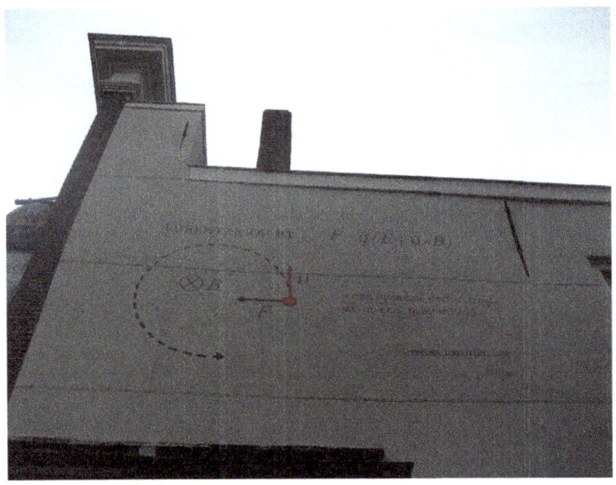

Lorentz force -image on a wall in Leiden

Given a loop of wire in a magnetic field, Faraday's law of induction states the induced electromotive force (EMF) in the wire is:

$$\mathcal{E} = -\frac{\mathrm{d}\Phi_B}{\mathrm{d}t}$$

where

$$\Phi_B = \iint_{\Sigma(t)} \mathrm{d}\boldsymbol{A} \cdot \boldsymbol{B}(\boldsymbol{r}, t)$$

is the magnetic flux through the loop, B is the magnetic field, $\Sigma(t)$ is a surface bounded by the closed contour $\partial\Sigma(t)$, at all at time t, dA is an infinitesimal vector area element of $\Sigma(t)$ (magnitude is the area of an infinitesimal patch of surface, direction is orthogonal to that surface patch).

The *sign* of the EMF is determined by Lenz's law. Note that this is valid for not only a *stationary* wire – but also for a *moving* wire.

From Faraday's law of induction (that is valid for a moving wire, for instance in a motor) and the Maxwell Equations, the Lorentz Force can be deduced. The reverse is also true, the Lorentz force and the Maxwell Equations can be used to derive the Faraday Law.

Let $\Sigma(t)$ be the moving wire, moving together without rotation and with constant velocity v and $\Sigma(t)$ be the internal surface of the wire. The EMF around the closed path $\partial\Sigma(t)$ is given by:

$$=\oint_{\partial\Sigma(\ )} \mathrm{d}\ \cdot\ \ /$$

where

$$\boldsymbol{E} = \boldsymbol{F} / q$$

is the electric field and $\mathrm{d}\ell$ is an infinitesimal vector element of the contour $\partial\Sigma(t)$.

Both $\mathrm{d}\ell$ and dA have a sign ambiguity; to get the correct sign, the right-hand rule is used, as in the Kelvin–Stokes theorem.

The above result can be compared with the version of Faraday's law of induction that appears in the modern Maxwell's equations, called here the *Maxwell–Faraday equation*:

$$\nabla \times \mathbf{E} = -\frac{\partial \mathbf{B}}{\partial t}.$$

The Maxwell–Faraday equation also can be written in an *integral form* using the Kelvin–Stokes theorem.

So we have, the Maxwell Faraday equation:

$$\oint_{\partial \acute{O}(t)} \mathrm{d}\ell \cdot \mathbf{E}(\mathbf{r},\ t) = -\iint_{\acute{O}(t)} \mathrm{d}\mathbf{A} \cdot \frac{\mathrm{d}\mathbf{B}(\mathbf{r},\ t)}{\mathrm{d}t}$$

and the Faraday Law,

$$\oint_{\partial\Sigma(t)} \mathrm{d}\ell \cdot \boldsymbol{F} / q(\boldsymbol{r}, t) = -\frac{\mathrm{d}}{\mathrm{d}t} \iint_{\Sigma(t)} \mathrm{d}\boldsymbol{A} \cdot \boldsymbol{B}(\boldsymbol{r}, t).$$

The two are equivalent if the wire is not moving. Using the Leibniz integral rule and that *div* B = 0, results in,

$$\oint_{\partial \acute{O}(t)} \mathrm{d}\ell \cdot \mathbf{F} / q(\mathbf{r},t) = -\iint_{\acute{O}(t)} \mathrm{d}\mathbf{A} \cdot \frac{\partial}{\partial t}\mathbf{B}(\mathbf{r},t) + \oint_{\partial \acute{O}(t)} \mathbf{v} \times \mathbf{B}\mathrm{d}\ell$$

and using the Maxwell Faraday equation,

$$\oint_{\partial\Sigma(t)} \mathrm{d}\ell \cdot \boldsymbol{F} / q(\boldsymbol{r}, t) = \oint_{\partial\Sigma(t)} \mathrm{d}\ell \cdot \boldsymbol{E}(\boldsymbol{r}, t) + \oint_{\partial\Sigma(t)} \boldsymbol{v} \times \boldsymbol{B}(\boldsymbol{r}, t)\mathrm{d}\ell$$

since this is valid for any wire position it implies that,

$$\boldsymbol{F} = q\boldsymbol{E}(\boldsymbol{r}, t) + q\boldsymbol{v} \times \boldsymbol{B}(\boldsymbol{r}, t).$$

Faraday's law of induction holds whether the loop of wire is rigid and stationary, or in motion or in process of deformation, and it holds whether the magnetic field is constant in time or changing. However, there are cases where Faraday's law is either inadequate or difficult to use, and application of the underlying Lorentz force law is necessary.

If the magnetic field is fixed in time and the conducting loop moves through the field, the magnetic flux Φ_B linking the loop can change in several ways. For example, if the B-field varies with position, and the loop moves to a location with different B-field, Φ_B will change. Alternatively, if the loop changes orientation with respect to the B-field, the B · dA differential element will change because of the different angle between B and dA, also changing Φ_B. As a third example, if a portion of the circuit is swept through a uniform, time-independent B-field, and another portion of the circuit is held stationary, the flux linking the entire closed circuit can change due to the shift in relative position of the circuit's component parts with time (surface $\partial\Sigma(t)$ time-dependent). In all three cases, Faraday's law of induction then predicts the EMF generated by the change in Φ_B.

Note that the Maxwell Faraday's equation implies that the Electric Field E is non conservative when the Magnetic Field B varies in time, and is not expressible as the gradient of a scalar field, and not subject to the gradient theorem since its rotational is not zero.

Lorentz Force in Terms of Potentials

The E and B fields can be replaced by the magnetic vector potential A and (scalar) electrostatic potential ϕ by

$$\mathbf{E} = -\nabla\phi - \frac{\partial \mathbf{A}}{\partial t}$$

$$\boldsymbol{B} = \nabla \times \boldsymbol{A}$$

where ∇ is the gradient, ∇· is the divergence, ∇× is the curl.

The force becomes

$$\boldsymbol{F} = q\left[-\nabla\phi - \frac{\partial \boldsymbol{A}}{\partial t} + \boldsymbol{v} \times (\nabla \times \boldsymbol{A})\right]$$

and using an identity for the triple product simplifies to

$$\boldsymbol{F} = q\left[-\nabla\phi - \frac{\partial \boldsymbol{A}}{\partial t} + \nabla(\boldsymbol{v} \cdot \boldsymbol{A}) - (\boldsymbol{v} \cdot \nabla)\boldsymbol{A}\right]$$

using the chain rule, the total derivative of A is:

$$\frac{\mathrm{d}\boldsymbol{A}}{\mathrm{d}t} = \frac{\partial \boldsymbol{A}}{\partial t} + (\boldsymbol{v} \cdot \nabla)\boldsymbol{A}$$

so the above expression can be rewritten as;

$$F = q\left[-\nabla(\phi - \mathbf{v}\cdot\mathbf{A}) - \frac{d\mathbf{A}}{\mathrm{d}t} \right]$$

which can take the convenient Euler–Lagrange form

$$\boldsymbol{F} = q\left[-\nabla_x(\phi - \dot{\boldsymbol{x}}\cdot \boldsymbol{A}) + \frac{\mathrm{d}}{\mathrm{d}t}\nabla_{\dot{x}}(\phi - \dot{\boldsymbol{x}}\cdot \boldsymbol{A}) \right]$$

Lorentz Force and Analytical Mechanics

The Lagrangian for a charged particle of mass m and charge q in an electromagnetic field equivalently describes the dynamics of the particle in terms of its *energy*, rather than the force exerted on it. The classical expression is given by:

$$L = \frac{m}{2}\dot{\boldsymbol{r}}\cdot\dot{\boldsymbol{r}} + q\boldsymbol{A}\cdot\dot{\boldsymbol{r}} - q\phi$$

where A and ϕ are the potential fields as above. Using Lagrange's equations, the equation for the Lorentz force can be obtained.

Derivation of Lorentz force from classical Lagrangian (SI units)

For an A field, a particle moving with velocity $\mathrm{v} = \dot{r}$ has potential momentum $q\mathbf{A}(\mathbf{r},t)$, so its potential energy is $q\boldsymbol{A}(\boldsymbol{r},t)\cdot\dot{\boldsymbol{r}}$. For a ϕ field, the particle's potential energy is $q\phi(\boldsymbol{r},t)$.

The total potential energy is then:

$$V = q\phi - q\boldsymbol{A}\cdot\dot{\boldsymbol{r}}$$

and the kinetic energy is:

$$T = \frac{m}{2}\dot{\mathbf{r}}\cdot\dot{\mathbf{r}}$$

hence the Lagrangian:

$$L = T - V = \frac{m}{2}\dot{\mathbf{r}}\cdot\dot{\mathbf{r}} + q\mathbf{A}\cdot\dot{\mathbf{r}} - q\phi$$

$$L = \frac{m}{2}(\dot{x}^2 + \dot{y}^2 + \dot{z}^2) + q(\dot{x}A_x + \dot{y}A_y + \dot{z}A_z) - q\phi$$

Lagrange's equations are

$$\frac{\mathrm{d}}{\mathrm{d}t}\frac{\partial L}{\partial \dot{x}} = \frac{\partial L}{\partial x}$$

(same for y and z). So calculating the partial derivatives:

$$\begin{aligned}\frac{\mathrm{d}}{\mathrm{d}t}\frac{\partial L}{\partial \dot{x}} &= m\ddot{x} + q\frac{\mathrm{d}A_x}{\mathrm{d}t} \\ &= m\ddot{x} + \frac{q}{\mathrm{d}t}\left(\frac{\partial A_x}{\partial t}dt + \frac{\partial A_x}{\partial x}dx + \frac{\partial A_x}{\partial y}dy + \frac{\partial A_x}{\partial z}dz\right) \\ &= m\ddot{x} + q\left(\frac{\partial A_x}{\partial t} + \frac{\partial A_x}{\partial x}\dot{x} + \frac{\partial A_x}{\partial y}\dot{y} + \frac{\partial A_x}{\partial z}\dot{z}\right)\end{aligned}$$

$$\frac{\partial L}{\partial x} = -q\frac{\partial \phi}{\partial x} + q\left(\frac{\partial A_x}{\partial x}\dot{x} + \frac{\partial A_y}{\partial x}\dot{y} + \frac{\partial A_z}{\partial x}\dot{z}\right)$$

equating and simplifying:

$$m\ddot{x} + q\left(\frac{\partial A_x}{\partial t} + \frac{\partial A_x}{\partial x}\dot{x} + \frac{\partial A_x}{\partial y}\dot{y} + \frac{\partial A_x}{\partial z}\dot{z}\right) = -q\frac{\partial \phi}{\partial x} + q\left(\frac{\partial A_x}{\partial x}\dot{x} + \frac{\partial A_y}{\partial x}\dot{y} + \frac{\partial A_z}{\partial x}\dot{z}\right)$$

$$\begin{aligned}F_x &= -q\left(\frac{\partial \phi}{\partial x} + \frac{\partial A_x}{\partial t}\right) + q\left[\dot{y}\left(\frac{\partial A_y}{\partial x} - \frac{\partial A_x}{\partial y}\right) + \dot{z}\left(\frac{\partial A_z}{\partial x} - \frac{\partial A_x}{\partial z}\right)\right] \\ &= qE_x + q[\dot{y}(\nabla \times \boldsymbol{A})_z - \dot{z}(\nabla \times \boldsymbol{A})_y] \\ &= qE_x + q[\dot{\boldsymbol{r}} \times (\nabla \times \boldsymbol{A})]_x \\ &= qE_x + q(\dot{\boldsymbol{r}} \times \boldsymbol{B})_x\end{aligned}$$

and similarly for the y and z directions. Hence the force equation is:

$$\boldsymbol{F} = q(\boldsymbol{E} + \dot{\boldsymbol{r}} \times \boldsymbol{B})$$

The potential energy depends on the velocity of the particle, so the force is velocity dependent, so it is not conservative.

The relativistic Lagrangian is

$$L = -mc^2\sqrt{1 - \left(\frac{\dot{\mathbf{r}}}{c}\right)^2} + e\mathbf{A}(\mathbf{r}) \cdot \dot{\mathbf{r}} - e\phi(\mathbf{r})$$

The action is the relativistic arclength of the path of the particle in space time, minus the potential energy contribution, plus an extra contribution which quantum mechanically is an extra phase a charged particle gets when it is moving along a vector potential.

Derivation of Lorentz Force from Relativistic Lagrangian (SI units)

The equations of motion derived by extremizing the action.

$$\frac{\mathrm{d}\boldsymbol{P}}{\mathrm{d}t} = \frac{\partial L}{\partial \boldsymbol{r}} = e\frac{\partial \boldsymbol{A}}{\partial \boldsymbol{r}} \cdot \dot{\boldsymbol{r}} - e\frac{\partial \phi}{\partial \boldsymbol{r}}$$

$$\boldsymbol{P} - e\boldsymbol{A} = \frac{m\dot{\boldsymbol{r}}}{\sqrt{1 - \left(\frac{\dot{\boldsymbol{r}}}{c}\right)^2}}$$

are the same as Hamilton's equations of motion:

$$\frac{\mathrm{d}\boldsymbol{r}}{\mathrm{d}t} = \frac{\partial}{\partial \boldsymbol{p}}\left(\sqrt{(\boldsymbol{P} - e\boldsymbol{A})^2 + (mc^2)^2} + e\phi\right)$$

$$\frac{\mathrm{d}\boldsymbol{p}}{\mathrm{d}t} = -\frac{\partial}{\partial \boldsymbol{r}}\left(\sqrt{(\boldsymbol{P} - e\boldsymbol{A})^2 + (mc^2)^2} + e\phi\right)$$

both are equivalent to the noncanonical form:

$$\frac{\mathrm{d}}{\mathrm{d}t}\left(\frac{m\dot{\boldsymbol{r}}}{\sqrt{1 - \left(\frac{\dot{\boldsymbol{r}}}{c}\right)^2}}\right) = e\left(\boldsymbol{E} + \dot{\boldsymbol{r}} \times \boldsymbol{B}\right).$$

This formula is the Lorentz force, representing the rate at which the EM field adds relativistic momentum to the particle.

Relativistic form of The Lorentz force

Field Tensor

Using the metric signature (1, −1, −1, −1), the Lorentz force for a charge q can be written in covariant form:

$$\frac{\mathrm{d}p^\alpha}{\mathrm{d}\tau} = qF^{\alpha\beta}U_\beta$$

where p^α is the four-momentum, defined as

$$p^\alpha = \left(p_0, p_1, p_2, p_3\right) = \left(\gamma mc, p_x, p_y, p_z\right),$$

τ the proper time of the particle, $F^{\alpha\beta}$ the contravariant electromagnetic tensor

$$F^{\alpha\beta} = \begin{pmatrix} 0 & -E_x/c & -E_y/c & -E_z/c \\ E_x/c & 0 & -B_z & B_y \\ E_y/c & B_z & 0 & -B_x \\ E_z/c & -B_y & B_x & 0 \end{pmatrix}$$

and U is the covariant 4-velocity of the particle, defined as:

$$U_\beta = (U_0, U_1, U_2, U_3) = \gamma(c, -v_x, -v_y, -v_z),$$

in which

$$\gamma(v) = \frac{1}{\sqrt{1-\frac{v^2}{c^2}}} = \frac{1}{\sqrt{1-\frac{v_x^2+v_y^2+v_z^2}{c^2}}}$$

is the Lorentz factor.

The fields are transformed to a frame moving with constant relative velocity by:

$$F'^{\mu\nu} = \Lambda^\mu{}_\alpha \Lambda^\nu{}_\beta F^{\alpha\beta},$$

where $\Lambda^\mu{}_\alpha$ is the Lorentz transformation tensor.

Translation to Vector Notation

The $\alpha = 1$ component (x-component) of the force is

$$\frac{\mathrm{d}p^1}{\mathrm{d}\tau} = qU_\beta F^{1\beta} = q\left(U_0F^{10} + U_1F^{11} + U_2F^{12} + U_3F^{13}\right).$$

Substituting the components of the covariant electromagnetic tensor F yields

$$\frac{\mathrm{d}p^1}{\mathrm{d}\tau} = q\left[U_0\left(\frac{E_x}{c}\right) + U_2(-B_z) + U_3(B_y)\right].$$

Using the components of covariant four-velocity yields

$$\begin{aligned}\frac{\mathrm{d}p^1}{\mathrm{d}\tau} &= q\gamma\left[c\left(\frac{E_x}{c}\right) + (-v_y)(-B_z) + (-v_z)(B_y)\right] \\ &= q\gamma\left(E_x + v_yB_z - v_zB_y\right) \\ &= q\gamma\left[E_x + (\boldsymbol{v}\times\boldsymbol{B})_x\right].\end{aligned}$$

The calculation for $\alpha = 2, 3$ (force components in the y and z directions) yields similar results, so collecting the 3 equations into one:

$$\frac{\mathrm{d}\boldsymbol{p}}{\mathrm{d}\tau} = q\gamma\left(\boldsymbol{E} + \boldsymbol{v} \times \boldsymbol{B}\right),$$

and since differentials in coordinate time dt and proper time $d\tau$ are related by the Lorentz factor,

$$dt = \gamma(v)d\tau,$$

so we arrive at

$$\frac{\mathrm{d}\boldsymbol{p}}{\mathrm{d}t} = q\left(\boldsymbol{E} + \boldsymbol{v} \times \boldsymbol{B}\right).$$

This is precisely the Lorentz force law, however, it is important to note that p is the relativistic expression,

$$\boldsymbol{p} = \gamma(v)m_0\boldsymbol{v}.$$

Lorentz force in Spacetime Algebra (STA)

The electric and magnetic fields are dependent on the velocity of an observer, so the relativistic form of the Lorentz force law can best be exhibited starting from a coordinate-independent expression for the electromagnetic and magnetic fields $\mathcal{F}$, and an arbitrary time-direction, γ_0. This can be settled through Space-Time Algebra (or the geometric algebra of space-time), a type of Clifford's Algebra defined on a pseudo-euclidian space, as

$$\boldsymbol{E} = (\mathcal{F} \cdot \gamma_0)\gamma_0$$

and

$$i\boldsymbol{B} = (\mathcal{F} \wedge \gamma_0)\gamma_0$$

$\mathcal{F}$ is a space-time bivector (an oriented plane segment, just like a vector is an oriented line segment), which has six degrees of freedom corresponding to boosts (rotations in space-time planes) and rotations (rotations in space-space planes). The dot product with the vector γ_0 pulls a vector (in the space algebra) from the translational part, while the wedge-product creates a trivector (in the space algebra) who is dual to a vector which is the usual magnetic field vector. The relativistic velocity is given by the (time-like) changes in a time-position vector $v = \dot{x}$, where

$$v^2 = 1,$$

(which shows our choice for the metric) and the velocity is

$$\boldsymbol{v} = cv \wedge \gamma_0 / (v \cdot \gamma_0).$$

The proper (invariant is an inadequate term because no transformation has been defined) form of the Lorentz force law is simply

$$F = q\mathcal{F} \cdot v$$

Note that the order is important because between a bivector and a vector the dot product is anti-symmetric. Upon a space time split like one can obtain the velocity, and fields as above yielding the usual expression.

Applications

The Lorentz force occurs in many devices, including:

- Cyclotrons and other circular path particle accelerators
- Mass spectrometers
- Velocity Filters
- Magnetrons
- Lorentz force velocimetry

In its manifestation as the Laplace force on an electric current in a conductor, this force occurs in many devices including:

- Electric motors
- Railguns
- Linear motors
- Loudspeakers
- Magnetoplasmadynamic thrusters
- Electrical generators
- Homopolar generators
- Linear alternators

Fundamental Interaction

In physics, the fundamental interactions, also known as fundamental forces, are the interactions that do not appear to be reducible to more basic interactions. There are four conventionally accepted fundamental interactions—gravitational, electromagnetic, strong, and weak. Each one is described mathematically as a *field*. The gravitational force is modelled as a continuous classical field. The other three, part of the Standard Model of particle physics, are described as discrete quantum fields, and their interactions are each carried by a *quantum*, an *elementary particle*.

The strong and weak interactions have short ranges, producing forces at minuscule, subatomic distances; these forces govern nuclear interactions. The strong interaction, which is carried by the gluon particle, is responsible for the binding of quarks together to form hadrons, such as protons and neutrons. As a residual effect, it creates the nuclear force that binds the latter particles to form atomic nuclei. The weak interaction, which is carried by the W and Z particles, also acts on the nucleus, mediating radioactive decay. The other two, electromagnetism and gravity, produce significant forces at macroscopic scales where the effects can be seen directly in everyday life. The electromagnetic force, carried by the photon, creates electric and magnetic fields, which are responsible for chemical bonding and are used in electrical technology. Electromagnetic forces tend to cancel each other out when large collections of objects are considered, so over the largest distances (on the scale of planets and galaxies), gravity tends to be the dominant force.

All four fundamental forces are believed to be related, and to unite into a single force at high energies on a minuscule scale, the Planck scale, but particle accelerators cannot produce the enormous energies required to experimentally probe this. A goal of theoretical physicists working beyond the Standard Model is to quantize the gravitational field, yielding a theory of quantum gravity (QG) which would unite gravity in a common theoretical framework with the other three forces. Other theorists seek to unite the electroweak and strong fields within a Grand Unified Theory (GUT). Some theories, notably string theory, seek both QG and GUT within one framework, unifying all four fundamental interactions along with mass generation within a theory of everything (ToE). A few researchers have interpreted various anomalous observations in physics as evidence for a fifth force, but this is not widely accepted.

The four fundamental interactions of nature						
Property/Interaction	**Gravitation**	**Weak**	**Electromagnetic**	**Strong**	
		(Electroweak)		**Fundamental**	**Residual**
Acts on:	Mass - Energy	Flavor	Electric charge	Color charge	Atomic nuclei
Particles experiencing:	All	Quarks, leptons	Electrically charged	Quarks, Gluons	Hadrons
Particles mediating:	Not yet observed (Graviton hypothesised)	W^+, W^- and Z^0	γ (photon)	Gluons	π, ρ and ω mesons
Strength at the scale of quarks:	10^{-41}	10^{-4}	1	60	Not applicable to quarks
Strength at the scale of protons/neutrons:	10^{-36}	10^{-7}	1	Not applicable to hadrons	20

History

Classical Theory

In his 1687 theory, Isaac Newton postulated space as an infinite and unalterable physical structure existing before, within, and around all objects while their states and relations unfold at a constant pace everywhere, thus absolute space and time. Inferring that all objects bearing mass approach at a constant rate, but collide by impact proportional to their masses, Newton inferred that matter exhibits an attractive force. His law of universal gravitation mathematically stated it to span the entire universe instantly (despite absolute time), or, if not actually a force, to be instant interaction among all objects (despite absolute space.) As conventionally interpreted, Newton's theory of motion modelled a *central force* without a communicating medium. Thus Newton's theory violated the first principle of mechanical philosophy, as stated by Descartes, *No action at a distance*. Conversely, during the 1820s, when explaining magnetism, Michael Faraday inferred a *field* filling space and transmitting that force. Faraday conjectured that ultimately, all forces unified into one.

In the early 1870s, James Clerk Maxwell unified electricity and magnetism as effects of an electromagnetic field whose third consequence was light, travelling at constant speed in a vacuum. The electromagnetic field theory contradicted predictions of Newton's theory of motion, unless physical states of the luminiferous aether—presumed to fill all space whether within matter or in a vacuum and to manifest the electromagnetic field—aligned all phenomena and thereby held valid the Newtonian principle relativity or invariance.

The Standard Model

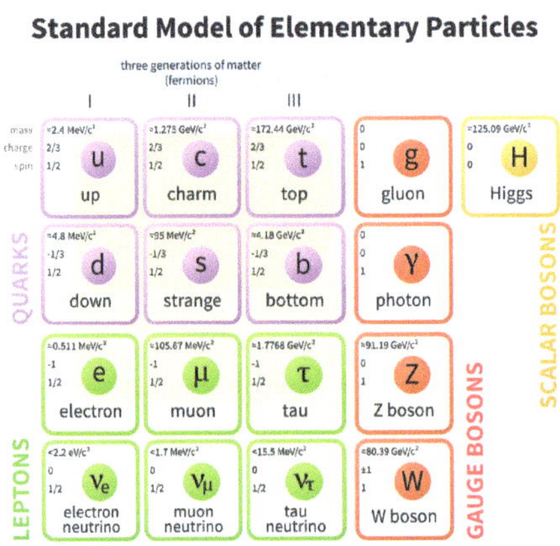

The Standard Model of elementary particles, with the fermions in the first three columns, the gauge bosons in the fourth column, and the Higgs boson in the fifth column.

The Standard Model of particle physics was developed throughout the latter half of the 20th century. In the Standard Model, the electromagnetic, strong, and weak interactions associate with elementary particles, whose behaviours are modelled in quantum mechanics (QM). For predictive success with QM's probabilistic outcomes, particle physics conventionally models QM events across a field set to special relativity, altogether relativistic quantum field theory (QFT). Force particles, called gauge bosons—*force carriers* or *messenger particles* of underlying fields—interact with matter particles, called fermions. Everyday matter is atoms, composed of three fermion types: up-quarks and down-quarks constituting, as well as electrons orbiting, the atom's nucleus. Atoms interact, form molecules, and manifest further properties through electromagnetic interactions among their electrons absorbing and emitting photons, the electromagnetic field's force carrier, which if unimpeded traverse potentially infinite distance. Electromagnetism's QFT is quantum electrodynamics (QED).

The electromagnetic interaction was modelled with the weak interaction, whose force carriers are W and Z bosons, traversing the minuscule distance, in electroweak theory (EWT). Electroweak interaction would operate at such high temperatures as soon after the presumed Big Bang, but, as the early universe cooled, split into electromagnetic and weak interactions. The strong interaction, whose force carrier is the gluon, traversing minuscule distance among quarks, is modeled in quantum chromodynamics (QCD). EWT, QCD, and the Higgs mechanism, whereby the Higgs field manifests Higgs bosons that interact with some quantum particles and thereby endow those particles with mass comprise particle physics' Standard Model (SM). Predictions are usually made using calculational approximation methods, although such perturbation theory is inadequate to model some experimental observations (for instance bound states and solitons.) Still, physicists widely accept the Standard Model as science's most experimentally confirmed theory.

Beyond the Standard Model, some theorists work to unite the electroweak and strong interactions within a Grand Unified Theory (GUT). Some attempts at GUTs hypothesize "shadow" particles, such that every known matter particle associates with an undiscovered force particle, and vice versa, altogether supersymmetry (SUSY). Other theorists seek to quantize the gravitational field by the modelling behaviour of its hypothetical force carrier, the graviton and achieve quantum gravity (QG). One approach to QG is loop quantum gravity (LQG). Still other theorists seek both QG and GUT within one framework, reducing all four fundamental interactions to a Theory of Everything (ToE). The most prevalent aim at a ToE is string theory, although to model matter particles, it added SUSY to force particles—and so, strictly speaking, became superstring theory. Multiple, seemingly disparate superstring theories were unified on a backbone, M-theory. Theories beyond the Standard Model remain highly speculative, lacking great experimental support.

Overview of The Fundamental Interactions

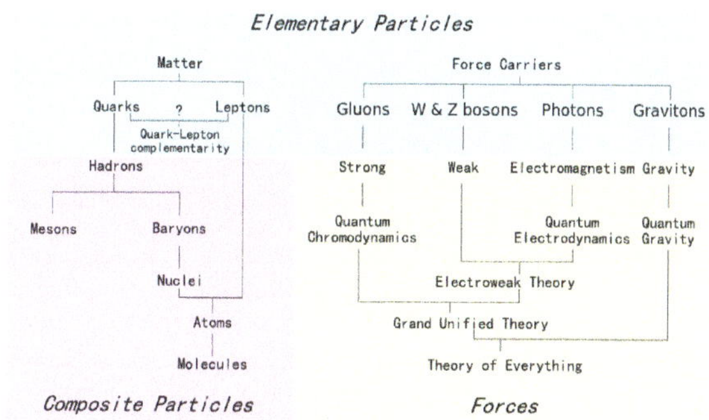

An overview of the various families of elementary and composite particles, and the theories describing their interactions. Fermions are on the left, and Bosons are on the right.

In the conceptual model of fundamental interactions, matter consists of fermions, which carry properties called charges and spin $\pm\frac{1}{2}$ (intrinsic angular momentum $\pm\frac{\hbar}{2}$, where ħ is the reduced Planck constant). They attract or repel each other by exchanging bosons.

The interaction of any pair of fermions in perturbation theory can then be modelled thus:

Two fermions go in → *interaction* by boson exchange → Two changed fermions go out.

The exchange of bosons always carries energy and momentum between the fermions, thereby changing their speed and direction. The exchange may also transport a charge between the fermions, changing the charges of the fermions in the process (e.g., turn them from one type of fermion to another). Since bosons carry one unit of angular momentum, the fermion's spin direction will flip from $+\frac{1}{2}$ to $-\frac{1}{2}$ (or vice versa) during such an exchange (in units of the reduced Planck's constant).

Because an interaction results in fermions attracting and repelling each other, an older term for "interaction" is force.

According to the present understanding, there are four fundamental interactions or forces: gravitation, electromagnetism, the weak interaction, and the strong interaction. Their magnitude and behaviour vary greatly, as described in the table below. Modern physics attempts to explain every observed physical phenomenon by these fundamental interactions. Moreover, reducing the number of different interaction types is seen as desirable. Two cases in point are the unification of:

- Electric and magnetic force into electromagnetism;
- The electromagnetic interaction and the weak interaction into the electroweak interaction.

Both magnitude ("relative strength") and "range", as given in the table, are meaningful only within a rather complex theoretical framework. It should also be noted that the table below lists properties of a conceptual scheme that is still the subject of ongoing research.

Interaction	Current theory	Mediators	Relative strength	Long-distance behavior	Range (m)
Strong	Quantum chromodynamics (QCD)	gluons	10^{38}	1	10^{-15}
Electromagnetic	Quantum electrodynamics (QED)	photons	10^{36}	$\frac{1}{r^2}$	∞
Weak	Electroweak Theory (EWT)	W and Z bosons	10^{25}	$\frac{1}{r}e^{-m_{W,Z}\,r}$	10^{-18}
Gravitation	General relativity (GR)	gravitons (hypothetical)	1	$\frac{1}{r^2}$	∞

The modern (perturbative) quantum mechanical view of the fundamental forces other than gravity is that particles of matter (fermions) do not directly interact with each other, but rather carry a charge, and exchange virtual particles (gauge bosons), which are the interaction carriers or force mediators. For example, photons mediate the interaction of electric charges, and gluons mediate the interaction of color charges.

The Interactions

Gravity

Gravitation is by far the weakest of the four interactions. The weakness of gravity can easily be demonstrated by suspending a pin using a simple magnet (such as a refrigerator magnet). The magnet is able to hold the pin against the gravitational pull of the entire Earth.

Yet gravitation is very important for macroscopic objects and over macroscopic distances for the following reasons. Gravitation:

- Is the only interaction that acts on all particles having mass, energy and/or momentum
- Has an infinite range, like electromagnetism but unlike strong and weak interaction
- Cannot be absorbed, transformed, or shielded against

- Always attracts and never repels

Even though electromagnetism is far stronger than gravitation, electrostatic attraction is not relevant for large celestial bodies, such as planets, stars, and galaxies, simply because such bodies contain equal numbers of protons and electrons and so have a net electric charge of zero. Nothing "cancels" gravity, since it is only attractive, unlike electric forces which can be attractive or repulsive. On the other hand, all objects having mass are subject to the gravitational force, which only attracts. Therefore, only gravitation matters on the large-scale structure of the universe.

The long range of gravitation makes it responsible for such large-scale phenomena as the structure of galaxies and black holes and it retards the expansion of the universe. Gravitation also explains astronomical phenomena on more modest scales, such as planetary orbits, as well as everyday experience: objects fall; heavy objects act as if they were glued to the ground, and animals can only jump so high.

Gravitation was the first interaction to be described mathematically. In ancient times, Aristotle hypothesized that objects of different masses fall at different rates. During the Scientific Revolution, Galileo Galilei experimentally determined that this was not the case – neglecting the friction due to air resistance, and buoyancy forces if an atmosphere is present (e.g. the case of a dropped air-filled balloon vs a water-filled balloon) all objects accelerate toward the Earth at the same rate. Isaac Newton's law of Universal Gravitation (1687) was a good approximation of the behaviour of gravitation. Our present-day understanding of gravitation stems from Albert Einstein's General Theory of Relativity of 1915, a more accurate (especially for cosmological masses and distances) description of gravitation in terms of the geometry of spacetime.

Merging general relativity and quantum mechanics (or quantum field theory) into a more general theory of quantum gravity is an area of active research. It is hypothesized that gravitation is mediated by a massless spin-2 particle called the graviton.

Although general relativity has been experimentally confirmed (at least for weak fields) on all but the smallest scales, there are rival theories of gravitation. Those taken seriously by the physics community all reduce to general relativity in some limit, and the focus of observational work is to establish limitations on what deviations from general relativity are possible.

Proposed extra dimensions could explain why the gravity force is so weak.

Electroweak Interaction

Electromagnetism and weak interaction appear to be very different at everyday low energies. They can be modeled using two different theories. However, above unification energy, on the order of 100 GeV, they would merge into a single electroweak force.

Electroweak theory is very important for modern cosmology, particularly on how the universe evolved. This is because shortly after the Big Bang, the temperature was approximately above 10^{15} K. Electromagnetic force and weak force were merged into a combined electroweak force.

For contributions to the unification of the weak and electromagnetic interaction between elementary particles, Abdus Salam, Sheldon Glashow and Steven Weinberg were awarded the Nobel Prize in Physics in 1979.

Electromagnetism

Electromagnetism is the force that acts between electrically charged particles. This phenomenon includes the electrostatic force acting between charged particles at rest, and the combined effect of electric and magnetic forces acting between charged particles moving relative to each other.

Electromagnetism is infinite-ranged like gravity, but vastly stronger, and therefore describes a number of macroscopic phenomena of everyday experience such as friction, rainbows, lightning, and all human-made devices using electric current, such as television, lasers, and computers. Electromagnetism fundamentally determines all macroscopic, and many atomic levels, properties of the chemical elements, including all chemical bonding.

In a four kilogram (~1 gallon) jug of water there are

$$4000\ \mathrm{g}H_2O \cdot \frac{1\ \mathrm{mol}H_2O}{18\ \mathrm{g}H_2O} \cdot \frac{10\ \mathrm{mole}^-}{1\ \mathrm{mol}H_2O} \cdot \frac{96{,}000\ \mathrm{C}}{1\ \mathrm{mole}^-} = 2.1\times 10^8 C$$

of total electron charge. Thus, if we place two such jugs a meter apart, the electrons in one of the jugs repel those in the other jug with a force of

$$\frac{1}{4\pi\varepsilon_0}\frac{(2.1\times 10^8 C)^2}{(1m)^2} = 4.1\times 10^{26} N.$$

This is larger than the planet Earth would weigh if weighed on another Earth. The atomic nuclei in one jug also repel those in the other with the same force. However, these repulsive forces are canceled by the attraction of the electrons in jug A with the nuclei in jug B and the attraction of the nuclei in jug A with the electrons in jug B, resulting in no net force. Electromagnetic forces are tremendously stronger than gravity but cancel out so that for large bodies gravity dominates.

Electrical and magnetic phenomena have been observed since ancient times, but it was only in the 19th century that it was discovered that electricity and magnetism are two aspects of the same fundamental interaction. By 1864, Maxwell's equations had rigorously quantified this unified interaction. Maxwell's theory, restated using vector calculus, is the classical theory of electromagnetism, suitable for most technological purposes.

The constant speed of light in a vacuum (customarily described with the letter "c") can be derived from Maxwell's equations, which are consistent with the theory of special relativity. Einstein's 1905 theory of special relativity, however, which flows from the observation that the speed of light is constant no matter how fast the observer is moving, showed that the theoretical result implied by Maxwell's equations has profound implications far beyond electromagnetism on the very nature of time and space.

In another work that departed from classical electro-magnetism, Einstein also explained the photoelectric effect by hypothesizing that light was transmitted in quanta, which we now call photons. Starting around 1927, Paul Dirac combined quantum mechanics with the relativistic theory of electromagnetism. Further work in the 1940s, by Richard Feynman, Freeman Dyson, Julian Schwinger, and Sin-Itiro Tomonaga, completed this theory, which is now called quantum electrodynamics, the revised theory of electromagnetism. Quantum electrodynamics and quantum mechanics provide a theoretical basis for electromagnetic behavior such as quantum tunneling, in which a certain percentage of electrically charged particles move in ways that would be impossible under the classical electromagnetic theory, that is necessary for everyday electronic devices such as transistors to function.

Weak Interaction

The *weak interaction* or *weak nuclear force* is responsible for some nuclear phenomena such as beta decay. Electromagnetism and the weak force are now understood to be two aspects of a unified electroweak interaction — this discovery was the first step toward the unified theory known as the Standard Model. In the theory of the electroweak interaction, the carriers of the weak force are the massive gauge bosons called the W and Z bosons. The weak interaction is the only known interaction which does not conserve parity; it is left-right asymmetric. The weak interaction even violates CP symmetry but does conserve CPT.

Strong Interaction

The *strong interaction*, or *strong nuclear force*, is the most complicated interaction, mainly because of the way it varies with distance. At distances greater than 10 femtometers, the strong force is practically unobservable. Moreover, it holds only inside the atomic nucleus.

After the nucleus was discovered in 1908, it was clear that a new force, today known as the nuclear force, was needed to overcome the electrostatic repulsion, a manifestation of electromagnetism, of the positively charged protons. Otherwise, the nucleus could not exist. Moreover, the force had to be strong enough to squeeze the protons into a volume that is about 10^{-15} m, much smaller than that of the entire atom. From the short range of this force, Hideki Yukawa predicted that it was associated with a massive particle, whose mass is approximately 100 MeV.

The 1947 discovery of the pion ushered in the modern era of particle physics. Hundreds of hadrons were discovered from the 1940s to 1960s, and an extremely complicated theory of hadrons as strongly interacting particles was developed. Most notably:

- The pions were understood to be oscillations of vacuum condensates;
- Jun John Sakurai proposed the rho and omega vector bosons to be force carrying particles for approximate symmetries of isospin and hypercharge;
- Geoffrey Chew, Edward K. Burdett and Steven Frautschi grouped the heavier hadrons into families that could be understood as vibrational and rotational excitations of strings.

While each of these approaches offered deep insights, no approach led directly to a fundamental theory.

Murray Gell-Mann along with George Zweig first proposed fractionally charged quarks in 1961. Throughout the 1960s, different authors considered theories similar to the modern fundamental theory of quantum chromodynamics (QCD) as simple models for the interactions of quarks. The first to hypothesize the gluons of QCD were Moo-Young Han and Yoichiro Nambu, who introduced the quark color charge and hypothesized that it might be associated with a force-carrying field. At that time, however, it was difficult to see how such a model could permanently confine quarks. Han and Nambu also assigned each quark color an integer electrical charge, so that the quarks were fractionally charged only on average, and they did not expect the quarks in their model to be permanently confined.

In 1971, Murray Gell-Mann and Harald Fritzsch proposed that the Han/Nambu color gauge field was the correct theory of the short-distance interactions of fractionally charged quarks. A little later, David Gross, Frank Wilczek, and David Politzer discovered that this theory had the property of asymptotic freedom, allowing them to make contact with experimental evidence. They concluded that QCD was the complete theory of the strong interactions, correct at all distance scales. The discovery of asymptotic freedom led most physicists to accept QCD since it became clear that even the long-distance properties of the strong interactions could be consistent with experiment if the quarks are permanently confined.

Assuming that quarks are confined, Mikhail Shifman, Arkady Vainshtein and Valentine Zakharov were able to compute the properties of many low-lying hadrons directly from QCD, with only a few extra parameters to describe the vacuum. In 1980, Kenneth G. Wilson published computer calculations based on the first principles of QCD, establishing, to a level of confidence tantamount to certainty, that QCD will confine quarks. Since then, QCD has been the established theory of the strong interactions.

QCD is a theory of fractionally charged quarks interacting by means of 8 bosonic particles called gluons. The gluons interact with each other, not just with the quarks, and at long distances the lines of force collimate into strings. In this way, the mathematical theory of QCD not only explains how quarks interact over short distances but also the string-like behavior, discovered by Chew and Frautschi, which they manifest over longer distances.

Beyond The Standard Model

Numerous theoretical efforts have been made to systematize the existing four fundamental interactions on the model of electroweak unification.

Grand Unified Theories (GUTs) are proposals to show that all of the fundamental interactions, other than gravity, arise from a single interaction with symmetries that break down at low energy levels. GUTs predict relationships among constants of nature that are unrelated in the SM. GUTs also predict gauge coupling unification for the relative strengths of the electromagnetic, weak, and strong forces, a prediction verified at the Large Electron–Positron Collider in 1991 for supersymmetric theories.

Theories of everything, which integrate GUTs with a quantum gravity theory face a greater barrier, because no quantum gravity theories, which include string theory, loop quantum gravity, and twistor theory, have secured wide acceptance. Some theories look for a graviton to complete the Standard Model list of force-carrying particles, while others, like loop quantum gravity, emphasize the possibility that time-space itself may have a quantum aspect to it.

Some theories beyond the Standard Model include a hypothetical fifth force, and the search for such a force is an ongoing line of experimental research in physics. In supersymmetric theories, there are particles that acquire their masses only through supersymmetry breaking effects and these particles, known as moduli can mediate new forces. Another reason to look for new forces is the recent discovery that the expansion of the universe is accelerating (also known as dark energy), giving rise to a need to explain a nonzero cosmological constant, and possibly to other modifications of general relativity. Fifth forces have also been suggested to explain phenomena such as CP violations, dark matter, and dark flow.

In December 2015, two observations in the ATLAS and CMS detectors at the Large Hadron Collider hinted at the existence of a new particle six times heavier than the Higgs Boson. However, after obtaining more experimental data, the anomaly appeared to not be significant.

References

- Corder, Gregory, "Using an Unconventional History of the Battery to engage students and explore the importance of evidence", Virginia Journal of Science Education 1
- Elizabeth Gibney (August 5, 2016). "Hopes for revolutionary new LHC particle dashed". Nature. doi:10.1038/nature.2016.20376. Retrieved August 18, 2016
- Morris, Simon C. (2003), Life's Solution: Inevitable Humans in a Lonely Universe, Cambridge University Press, pp. 182–185, ISBN 0-521-82704-3
- Tsverava, G. K. 1981. "FARADEI, GENRI, I OTKRYTIE INDUKTIROVANNYKH TOKOV." Voprosy Istorii Estestvoznaniia i Tekhniki no. 3: 99-106. Historical Abstracts, EBSCOhost . Retrieved October 17, 2009
- Ronalds, B.F. (2016). "Sir Francis Ronalds and the Electric Telegraph". Int. J. for the History of Engineering & Technology. doi:10.1080/17581206.2015.1119481
- Krebs, Robert E. (2003), Groundbreaking Scientific Experiments, Inventions, and Discoveries of the 18th Century, Greenwood Publishing Group, p. 82, ISBN 0-313-32015-2
- 1998. "Joseph Henry." Issues in Science & Technology 14, no. 3: 96. Associates Programs Source, EBSCOhost. Retrieved October 17, 2009
- Guarnieri, M. (2015). "How the Genie of Electronics Sprung Out". IEEE Industrial Electronics Magazine. 9 (1): 77–79. doi:10.1109/MIE.2014.2387945
- Keithley, Joseph F. (1999), The Story of Electrical and Magnetic Measurements: From 500 B.C. to the 1940s, Wiley, ISBN 0-7803-1193-0
- A Wind Energy Pioneer: Charles F. Brush Archived 2008-09-08 at the Wayback Machine., Danish Wind Industry Association. Retrieved 2007-05-02
- Lorentz, Hendrik Antoon (1921), "Deux Mémoires de Henri Poincaré sur la Physique Mathématique" [Two Papers of Henri Poincaré on Mathematical Physics], Acta Mathematica, 38 (1): 293–308, doi:10.1007/BF02392073
- Ronalds, B.F. (2016). Sir Francis Ronalds: Father of the Electric Telegraph. London: Imperial College Press. ISBN 978-1-78326-917-4
- Lorentz, H. A.; Lorentz, H. A. (1928), "Conference on the Michelson-Morley Experiment", The Astrophysical Journal, 68: 345–351, Bibcode:1928ApJ....68..341M, doi:10.1086/143148
- "NIOSH Fact Sheet: EMFs in the Workplace". United States National Institute for Occupational Safety and Health. 1996. Retrieved 31 August 2015
- F. Bloch; A. Nordsieck (1937). "Note on the Radiation Field of the Electron". Physical Review. 52: 54–59. Bibcode:1937PhRv...52...54B. doi:10.1103/PhysRev.52.54

- Pais, Abraham (1982), Subtle is the Lord. The Science and the Life of Albert Einstein, Oxford University Press, pp. 382–386, ISBN 0-19-520438-7
- F. J. Hasert; et al. (1973). "Search for elastic muon-neutrino electron scattering". Physics Letters B. 46: 121. Bibcode:1973PhLB...46..121H. doi:10.1016/0370-2693(73)90494-2

2

Understanding Classical Electromagnetism

The interaction that takes place between electric charges and currents is studied under the subject of classical electromagnetism. Electric charge, charge conservation and Liénard–Wiechert potential are some topics discussed in regard to classical electromagnetism. This chapter will provide an integrated understanding of classical electromagnetism.

Classical Electromagnetism

Classical electromagnetism or classical electrodynamics is a branch of theoretical physics that studies the interactions between electric charges and currents using an extension of the classical Newtonian model. The theory provides an excellent description of electromagnetic phenomena whenever the relevant length scales and field strengths are large enough that quantum mechanical effects are negligible. For small distances and low field strengths, such interactions are better described by quantum electrodynamics.

Fundamental physical aspects of classical electrodynamics are presented in many texts, such as those by Feynman, Leighton and Sands, Griffiths, Panofsky and Phillips, and Jackson.

History

The physical phenomena that electromagnetism describes have been studied as separate fields since antiquity. For example, there were many advances in the field of optics centuries before light was understood to be an electromagnetic wave. However, the theory of electromagnetism, as it is currently understood, grew out of Michael Faraday's experiments suggesting an electromagnetic field and James Clerk Maxwell's use of differential equations to describe it in his *A Treatise on Electricity and Magnetism* (1873). For a detailed historical account, consult Pauli, Whittaker, Pais, and Hunt.

Lorentz Force

The electromagnetic field exerts the following force (often called the Lorentz force) on charged particles:

$$\boldsymbol{F} = q\boldsymbol{E} + q\boldsymbol{v} \times \boldsymbol{B}$$

where all boldfaced quantities are vectors: F is the force that a particle with charge q experiences, E is the electric field at the location of the particle, v is the velocity of the particle, B is the magnetic field at the location of the particle.

The above equation illustrates that the Lorentz force is the sum of two vectors. One is the cross product of the velocity and magnetic field vectors. Based on the properties of the cross product, this produces a vector that is perpendicular to both the velocity and magnetic field vectors. The other vector is in the same direction as the electric field. The sum of these two vectors is the Lorentz force.

Therefore, in the absence of a magnetic field, the force is in the direction of the electric field, and the magnitude of the force is dependent on the value of the charge and the intensity of the electric field. In the absence of an electric field, the force is perpendicular to the velocity of the particle and the direction of the magnetic field. If both electric and magnetic fields are present, the Lorentz force is the sum of both of these vectors.

The Electric Field E

The electric field E is defined such that, on a stationary charge:

$$\mathbf{F} = q_0 \mathbf{E}$$

where q_0 is what is known as a test charge. The size of the charge doesn't really matter, as long as it is small enough not to influence the electric field by its mere presence. What is plain from this definition, though, is that the unit of E is N/C (newtons per coulomb). This unit is equal to V/m (volts per meter).

In electrostatics, where charges are not moving, around a distribution of point charges, the forces determined from Coulomb's law may be summed. The result after dividing by q_0 is:

$$\boldsymbol{E}(\boldsymbol{r}) = \frac{1}{4\pi\varepsilon_0} \sum_{i=1}^{n} \frac{q_i (\boldsymbol{r} - \boldsymbol{r}_i)}{|\boldsymbol{r} - \boldsymbol{r}_i|^3}$$

where n is the number of charges, q_i is the amount of charge associated with the ith charge, r_i is the position of the ith charge, r is the position where the electric field is being determined, and ε_0 is the electric constant.

If the field is instead produced by a continuous distribution of charge, the summation becomes an integral:

$$\boldsymbol{E}(\boldsymbol{r}) = \frac{1}{4\pi\varepsilon_0} \int \frac{\rho(\boldsymbol{r}')(\boldsymbol{r} - \boldsymbol{r}')}{|\boldsymbol{r} - \boldsymbol{r}'|^3} \mathrm{d}^3\boldsymbol{r}'$$

where $\rho(\boldsymbol{r}')$ is the charge density and $\boldsymbol{r} - \boldsymbol{r}'$ is the vector that points from the volume element $\mathrm{d}^3\boldsymbol{r}'$ to the point in space where E is being determined.

Both of the above equations are cumbersome, especially if one wants to determine E as a function of position. A scalar function called the electric potential can help. Electric potential, also called voltage (the units for which are the volt), is defined by the line integral

$$\varphi(\boldsymbol{r}) = -\int_C \boldsymbol{E} \cdot \mathrm{d}\boldsymbol{l}$$

where $\varphi(r)$ is the electric potential, and C is the path over which the integral is being taken.

Unfortunately, this definition has a caveat. From Maxwell's equations, it is clear that $\nabla \times E$ is not always zero, and hence the scalar potential alone is insufficient to define the electric field exactly. As a result, one must add a correction factor, which is generally done by subtracting the time derivative of the A vector potential described below. Whenever the charges are quasistatic, however, this condition will be essentially met.

From the definition of charge, one can easily show that the electric potential of a point charge as a function of position is:

$$\varphi(\boldsymbol{r}) = \frac{1}{4\pi\varepsilon_0}\sum_{i=1}^{n}\frac{q_i}{|\boldsymbol{r}-\boldsymbol{r}_i|}$$

where q is the point charge's charge, r is the position at which the potential is being determined, and r_i is the position of each point charge. The potential for a continuous distribution of charge is:

$$\varphi(\mathbf{r}) = \frac{1}{4\pi\varepsilon_0}\int\frac{\rho(\mathbf{r}')}{|\mathbf{r}-\mathbf{r}'|}\mathrm{d}^3\mathbf{r}'$$

where $\rho(\mathbf{r}')$ is the charge density, and $\boldsymbol{r}-\boldsymbol{r}'$ is the distance from the volume element $\mathrm{d}^3\boldsymbol{r}'$ to point in space where φ is being determined.

The scalar φ will add to other potentials as a scalar. This makes it relatively easy to break complex problems down in to simple parts and add their potentials. Taking the definition of φ backwards, we see that the electric field is just the negative gradient (the del operator) of the potential. Or:

$$\boldsymbol{E}(\boldsymbol{r}) = -\nabla\varphi(\boldsymbol{r}).$$

From this formula it is clear that E can be expressed in V/m (volts per meter).

Electromagnetic Waves

A changing electromagnetic field propagates away from its origin in the form of a wave. These waves travel in vacuum at the speed of light and exist in a wide spectrum of wavelengths. Examples of the dynamic fields of electromagnetic radiation (in order of increasing frequency): radio waves, microwaves, light (infrared, visible light and ultraviolet), x-rays and gamma rays. In the field of particle physics this electromagnetic radiation is the manifestation of the electromagnetic interaction between charged particles.

General Field Equations

As simple and satisfying as Coulomb's equation may be, it is not entirely correct in the context of classical electromagnetism. Problems arise because changes in charge distributions require a non-zero amount of time to be "felt" elsewhere (required by special relativity).

For the fields of general charge distributions, the retarded potentials can be computed and differentiated accordingly to yield Jefimenko's Equations.

Retarded potentials can also be derived for point charges, and the equations are known as the Liénard–Wiechert potentials. The scalar potential is:

$$\varphi = \frac{1}{4\pi\varepsilon_0} \frac{q}{\left|\boldsymbol{r}-\boldsymbol{r}_q(t_{ret})\right| - \frac{\boldsymbol{v}_q(t_{ret})}{c}\cdot(\boldsymbol{r}-\boldsymbol{r}_q(t_{ret}))}$$

where q is the point charge's charge and r is the position. r_q and v_q are the position and velocity of the charge, respectively, as a function of retarded time. The vector potential is similar:

$$\boldsymbol{A} = \frac{\mu_0}{4\pi} \frac{q\boldsymbol{v}_q(t_{ret})}{\left|\boldsymbol{r}-\boldsymbol{r}_q(t_{ret})\right| - \frac{\boldsymbol{v}_q(t_{ret})}{c}\cdot(\boldsymbol{r}-\boldsymbol{r}_q(t_{ret}))}.$$

These can then be differentiated accordingly to obtain the complete field equations for a moving point particle.

Models

Branches of classical electromagnetism such as optics, electrical and electronic engineering consist of a collection of relevant mathematical models of different degrees of simplification and idealization to enhance the understanding of specific electrodynamics phenomena, cf. An electrodynamics phenomenon is determined by the particular fields, specific densities of electric charges and currents, and the particular transmission medium. Since there are infinitely many of them, in modeling there is a need for some typical, representative

(a) electrical charges and currents, e.g. moving pointlike charges and electric and magnetic dipoles, electric currents in a conductor etc.;

(b) electromagnetic fields, e.g. voltages, the Liénard–Wiechert potentials, the monochromatic plane waves, optical rays; radio waves, microwaves, infrared radiation, visible light, ultraviolet radiation, X-rays, gamma rays etc.;

(c) transmission media, e.g. electronic components, antennas, electromagnetic waveguides, flat mirrors, mirrors with curved surfaces convex lenses, concave lenses; resistors, inductors, capacitors, switches; wires, electric and optical cables, transmission lines, integrated circuits etc.;

all of which have only few variable characteristics.

Electric Charge

Electric charge is the physical property of matter that causes it to experience a force when placed in an electromagnetic field. There are two types of electric charges: *positive* and *negative* (commonly carried by protons and electrons respectively). Like charges repel and unlike attract. An absence of net charge is referred to as *neutral*. An object is negatively charged if it has an excess of electrons, and is otherwise positively charged or uncharged. The SI derived unit of electric charge is the coulomb (C). In electrical engineering, it is also common to use the ampere-hour (Ah), and, in chemistry, it is common to use the elementary charge (*e*) as a unit. The symbol *Q* often denotes charge. Early knowledge of how charged substances interact is now called classical electrodynamics, and is still accurate for problems that don't require consideration of quantum effects.

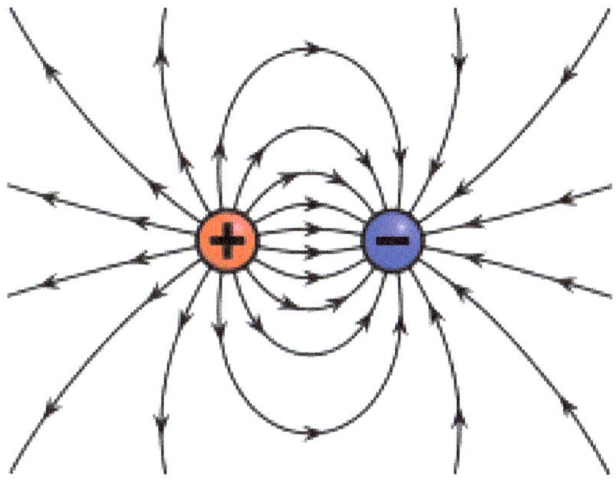

Electric field of a positive and a negative point charge.

The *electric charge* is a fundamental conserved property of some subatomic particles, which determines their electromagnetic interaction. Electrically charged matter is influenced by, and produces, electromagnetic fields. The interaction between a moving charge and an electromagnetic field is the source of the electromagnetic force, which is one of the four fundamental forces.

Twentieth-century experiments demonstrated that electric charge is *quantized*; that is, it comes in integer multiples of individual small units called the elementary charge, *e*, approximately equal to 1.602×10^{-19} coulombs (except for particles called quarks, which have charges that are integer multiples of $1/3e$). The proton has a charge of $+e$, and the electron has a charge of $-e$. The study of charged particles, and how their interactions are mediated by photons, is called quantum electrodynamics.

Overview

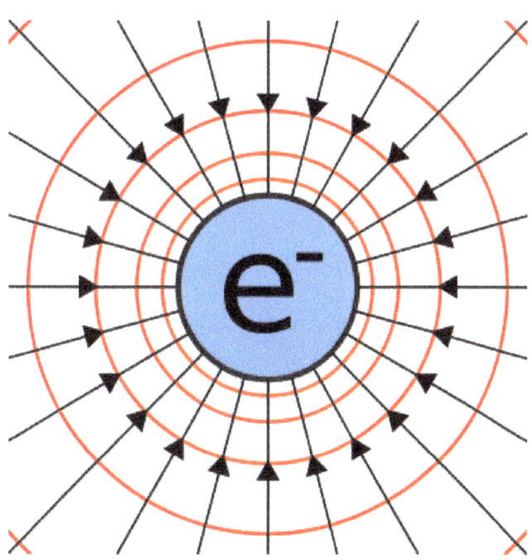

Diagram showing field lines and equipotentials around an electron, a negatively charged particle. In an electrically neutral atom, the number of electrons is equal to the number of protons (which are positively charged), resulting in a net zero overall charge.

Charge is the fundamental property of forms of matter that exhibit electrostatic attraction or repulsion in the presence of other matter. Electric charge is a characteristic property of many subatomic particles. The charges of free-standing particles are integer multiples of the elementary charge *e*; we say that electric charge is *quantized*. Michael Faraday, in his electrolysis experiments, was the first to note the discrete nature of electric charge. Robert Millikan's oil drop experiment demonstrated this fact directly, and measured the elementary charge.

By convention, the charge of an electron is −1, while that of a proton is +1. Charged particles whose charges have the same sign repel one another, and particles whose charges have different signs attract. Coulomb's law quantifies the electrostatic force between two particles by asserting that the force is proportional to the product of their charges, and inversely proportional to the square of the distance between them.

The charge of an antiparticle equals that of the corresponding particle, but with opposite sign. Quarks have fractional charges of either −1/3 or +2/3, but free-standing quarks have never been observed (the theoretical reason for this fact is asymptotic freedom).

The electric charge of a macroscopic object is the sum of the electric charges of the particles that make it up. This charge is often small, because matter is made of atoms, and atoms typically have equal numbers of protons and electrons, in which case their charges cancel out, yielding a net charge of zero, thus making the atom neutral.

An *ion* is an atom (or group of atoms) that has lost one or more electrons, giving it a net positive charge (cation), or that has gained one or more electrons, giving it a net negative charge (anion). *Monatomic ions* are formed from single atoms, while *polyatomic ions* are formed from two or more atoms that have been bonded together, in each case yielding an ion with a positive or negative net charge.

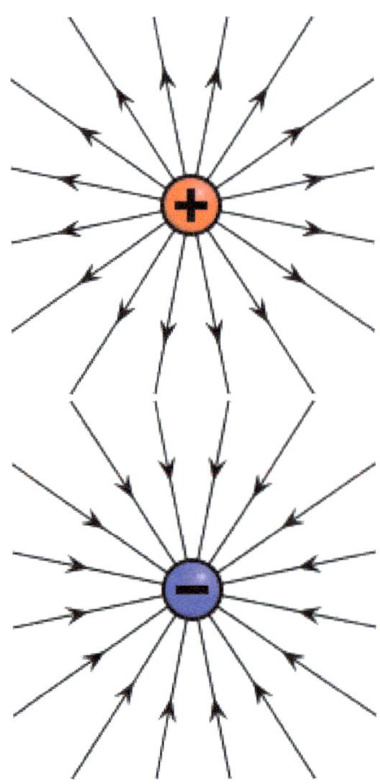

Electric field induced by a positive electric charge (left)
and a field induced by a negative electric charge (right).

During formation of macroscopic objects, constituent atoms and ions usually combine to form structures composed of neutral *ionic compounds* electrically bound to neutral atoms. Thus macroscopic objects tend toward being neutral overall, but macroscopic objects are rarely perfectly net neutral.

Sometimes macroscopic objects contain ions distributed throughout the material, rigidly bound in place, giving an overall net positive or negative charge to the object. Also, macroscopic objects made of conductive elements, can more or less easily (depending on the element) take on or give off electrons, and then maintain a net negative or positive charge indefinitely. When the net electric charge of an object is non-zero and motionless, the phenomenon is known as static electricity. This can easily be produced by rubbing two dissimilar materials together, such as rubbing amber with fur or glass with silk. In this way non-conductive materials can be charged to a significant degree, either positively or negatively. Charge taken from one material is moved to the other material, leaving an opposite charge of the same magnitude behind. The law of *conservation of charge* always applies, giving the object from which a negative charge is taken a positive charge of the same magnitude, and vice versa.

Even when an object's net charge is zero, charge can be distributed non-uniformly in the object (e.g., due to an external electromagnetic field, or bound polar molecules). In such cases the object is said to be polarized. The charge due to polarization is known as bound charge, while charge on an object produced by electrons gained or lost from outside the object is called *free charge*. The motion of electrons in conductive metals in a specific direction is known as electric current.

Units

The SI unit of quantity of electric charge is the coulomb, which is equivalent to about 6.242×10^{18} e (e is the charge of a proton). Hence, the charge of an electron is approximately -1.602×10^{-19} C. The coulomb is defined as the quantity of charge that has passed through the cross section of an electrical conductor carrying one ampere within one second. The symbol Q is often used to denote a quantity of electricity or charge. The quantity of electric charge can be directly measured with an electrometer, or indirectly measured with a ballistic galvanometer.

After finding the quantized character of charge, in 1891 George Stoney proposed the unit 'electron' for this fundamental unit of electrical charge. This was before the discovery of the particle by J.J. Thomson in 1897. The unit is today treated as nameless, referred to as "elementary charge", "fundamental unit of charge", or simply as "e". A measure of charge should be a multiple of the elementary charge e, even if at large scales charge seems to behave as a real quantity. In some contexts it is meaningful to speak of fractions of a charge; for example in the charging of a capacitor, or in the fractional quantum Hall effect.

In systems of units other than SI such as cgs, electric charge is expressed as combination of only three fundamental quantities (length, mass, and time), and not four, as in SI, where electric charge is a combination of length, mass, time, and electric current.

History

As reported by the ancient Greek mathematician Thales of Miletus around 600 BC, charge (or *electricity*) could be accumulated by rubbing fur on various substances, such as amber. The Greeks noted that the charged amber buttons could attract light objects such as hair. They also noted that if they rubbed the amber for long enough, they could even get an electric spark to jump. This property derives from the triboelectric effect.

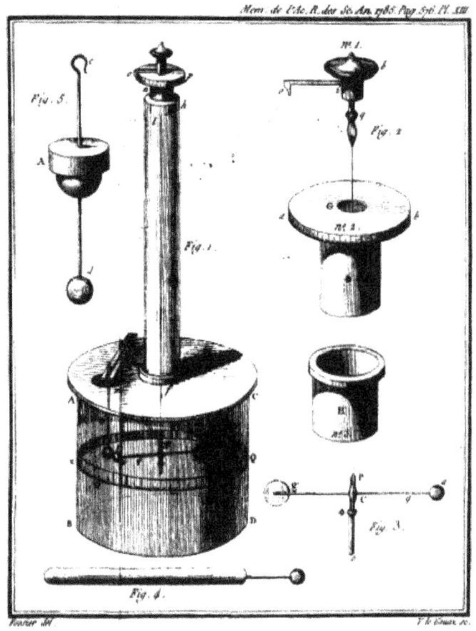
Coulomb's torsion balance

In 1600, the English scientist William Gilbert returned to the subject in *De Magnete*, and coined the New Latin word *electricus* from ἤλεκτρον (ēlektron), the Greek word for *amber*, which soon gave rise to the English words "electric" and "electricity." He was followed in 1660 by Otto von Guericke, who invented what was probably the first electrostatic generator. Other European pioneers were Robert Boyle, who in 1675 stated that electric attraction and repulsion can act across a vacuum; Stephen Gray, who in 1729 classified materials as conductors and insulators; and C. F. du Fay, who proposed in 1733 that electricity comes in two varieties that cancel each other, and expressed this in terms of a two-fluid theory. When glass was rubbed with silk, du Fay said that the glass was charged with *vitreous electricity*, and, when amber was rubbed with fur, the amber was charged with *resinous electricity*. In 1839, Michael Faraday showed that the apparent division between static electricity, current electricity, and bioelectricity was incorrect, and all were a consequence of the behavior of a single kind of electricity appearing in opposite polarities. It is arbitrary which polarity is called positive and which is called negative. Positive charge can be defined as the charge left on a glass rod after being rubbed with silk.

One of the foremost experts on electricity in the 18th century was Benjamin Franklin, who argued in favour of a one-fluid theory of electricity. Franklin imagined electricity as being a type of invisible fluid present in all matter; for example, he believed that it was the glass in a Leyden jar that held the accumulated charge. He posited that rubbing insulating surfaces together caused this fluid to change location, and that a flow of this fluid constitutes an electric current. He also posited that when matter contained too little of the fluid it was "negatively" charged, and when it had an excess it was "positively" charged. For a reason that was not recorded, he identified the term "positive" with vitreous electricity and "negative" with resinous electricity. William Watson arrived at the same explanation at about the same time.

Static Electricity and Electric Current

Static electricity and electric current are two separate phenomena. They both involve electric charge, and may occur simultaneously in the same object. Static electricity refers to the electric charge of an object and the related electrostatic discharge when two objects are brought together that are not at equilibrium. An electrostatic discharge creates a change in the charge of each of the two objects. In contrast, electric current is the flow of electric charge through an object, which produces no net loss or gain of electric charge.

Electrification by Friction

When a piece of glass and a piece of resin—neither of which exhibit any electrical properties—are rubbed together and left with the rubbed surfaces in contact, they still exhibit no electrical properties. When separated, they attract each other.

A second piece of glass rubbed with a second piece of resin, then separated and suspended near the former pieces of glass and resin causes these phenomena:

- The two pieces of glass repel each other.
- Each piece of glass attracts each piece of resin.
- The two pieces of resin repel each other.

This attraction and repulsion is an *electrical phenomena*, and the bodies that exhibit them are said to be *electrified*, or *electrically charged*. Bodies may be electrified in many other ways, as well as by friction. The electrical properties of the two pieces of glass are similar to each other but opposite to those of the two pieces of resin: The glass attracts what the resin repels and repels what the resin attracts.

If a body electrified in any manner whatsoever behaves as the glass does, that is, if it repels the glass and attracts the resin, the body is said to be *vitreously* electrified, and if it attracts the glass and repels the resin it is said to be *resinously* electrified. All electrified bodies are either vitreously or resinously electrified.

An established convention in the scientific community defines vitreous electrification as positive, and resinous electrification as negative. The exactly opposite properties of the two kinds of electrification justify our indicating them by opposite signs, but the application of the positive sign to one rather than to the other kind must be considered as a matter of arbitrary convention—just as it is a matter of convention in mathematical diagram to reckon positive distances towards the right hand.

No force, either of attraction or of repulsion, can be observed between an electrified body and a body not electrified.

Actually, all bodies are electrified, but may appear not electrified because of the relatively similar charge of neighboring objects in the environment. An object further electrified + or − creates an equivalent or opposite charge by default in neighboring objects, until those charges can equalize. The effects of attraction can be observed in high-voltage experiments, while lower voltage effects are merely weaker and therefore less obvious. The attraction and repulsion forces are codified by Coulomb's law (attraction falls off at the square of the distance, which has a corollary for acceleration in a gravitational field, suggesting that gravitation may be merely electrostatic phenomenon between relatively weak charges in terms of scale).

It is now known that the Franklin-Watson model was fundamentally correct. There is only one kind of electrical charge, and only one variable is required to keep track of the amount of charge. On the other hand, just knowing the charge is not a complete description of the situation. Matter is composed of several kinds of electrically charged particles, and these particles have many properties, not just charge.

The most common charge carriers are the positively charged proton and the negatively charged electron. The movement of any of these charged particles constitutes an electric current. In many situations, it suffices to speak of the *conventional current* without regard to whether it is carried by positive charges moving in the direction of the conventional current or by negative charges moving in the opposite direction. This macroscopic viewpoint is an approximation that simplifies electromagnetic concepts and calculations.

At the opposite extreme, if one looks at the microscopic situation, one sees there are many ways of carrying an electric current, including: a flow of electrons; a flow of electron "holes" that act like positive particles; and both negative and positive particles (ions or other charged particles) flowing in opposite directions in an electrolytic solution or a plasma.

Beware that, in the common and important case of metallic wires, the direction of the conventional current is opposite to the drift velocity of the actual charge carriers; i.e., the electrons. This is a source of confusion for beginners.

Conservation of Electric Charge

The total electric charge of an isolated system remains constant regardless of changes within the system itself. This law is inherent to all processes known to physics and can be derived in a local form from gauge invariance of the wave function. The conservation of charge results in the charge-current continuity equation. More generally, the net change in charge density ρ within a volume of integration V is equal to the area integral over the current density J through the closed surface $S = \partial V$, which is in turn equal to the net current I:

$$-\frac{d}{dt}\int_V \rho \mathrm{d}V = \oint\!\!\oint_{\partial V} \boldsymbol{J} \cdot \mathrm{d}\boldsymbol{S} = \int J \mathrm{d}S \cos\theta = I.$$

Thus, the conservation of electric charge, as expressed by the continuity equation, gives the result:

$$I = -\frac{\mathrm{d}Q}{\mathrm{d}t}.$$

The charge transferred between times t_i and t_f is obtained by integrating both sides:

$$Q = \int_{t_i}^{t_f} I \mathrm{d}t$$

where I is the net outward current through a closed surface and Q is the electric charge contained within the volume defined by the surface.

Relativistic Invariance

Aside from the properties described about electromagnetism, charge is a relativistic invariant. This means that any particle that has charge Q, no matter how fast it goes, always has charge Q. This property has been experimentally verified by showing that the charge of *one* helium nucleus (two protons and two neutrons bound together in a nucleus and moving around at high speeds) is the same as *two* deuterium nuclei (one proton and one neutron bound together, but moving much more slowly than they would if they were in a helium nucleus).

Electricity

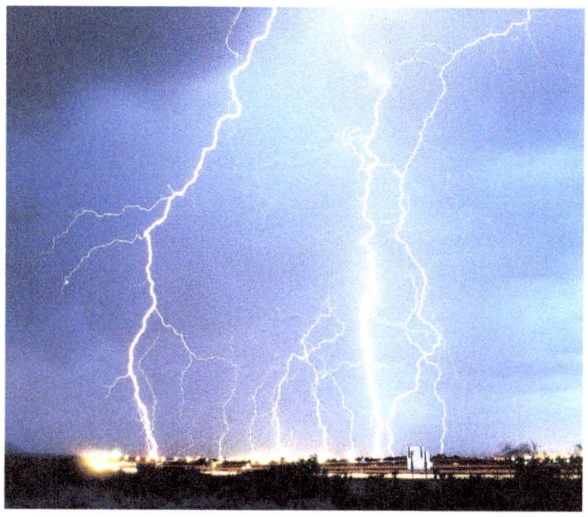

Lightning is one of the most dramatic effects of electricity.

Electricity is the set of physical phenomena associated with the presence of electric charge. Although initially considered a phenomenon separate to magnetism, since the development of Maxwell's Equations both are recognized as part of a single phenomenon: electromagnetism. Various common phenomena are related to electricity, including lightning, static electricity, electric heating, electric discharges and many others. In addition, electricity is at the heart of many modern technologies.

The presence of an electric charge, which can be either positive or negative, produces an electric field. On the other hand, the movement of electric charges, which is known as electric current, produces a magnetic field.

When a charge is placed in a location with non-zero electric field, a force will act on it. The magnitude of this force is given by Coulomb's Law. Thus, if that charge were to move, the electric field would be doing work on the electric charge. Thus we can speak of electric potential at a certain point in space, which is equal to the work done by an external agent in carrying a unit of positive charge from an arbitrarily chosen reference point to that point without any acceleration and is typically measured in volts.

In electrical engineering, electricity is used for:

- electric power where electric current is used to energise equipment;

- electronics which deals with electrical circuits that involve active electrical components such as vacuum tubes, transistors, diodes and integrated circuits, and associated passive interconnection technologies.

Electrical phenomena have been studied since antiquity, though progress in theoretical understanding remained slow until the seventeenth and eighteenth centuries. Even then, practical applications for electricity were few, and it would not be until the late nineteenth century that engineers were able to put it to industrial and residential use. The rapid expansion in electrical technology at this time transformed industry and society. Electricity's extraordinary versatility means it can be put to an almost limitless set of applications which include transport, heating, lighting, communications, and computation. Electrical power is now the backbone of modern industrial society.

History

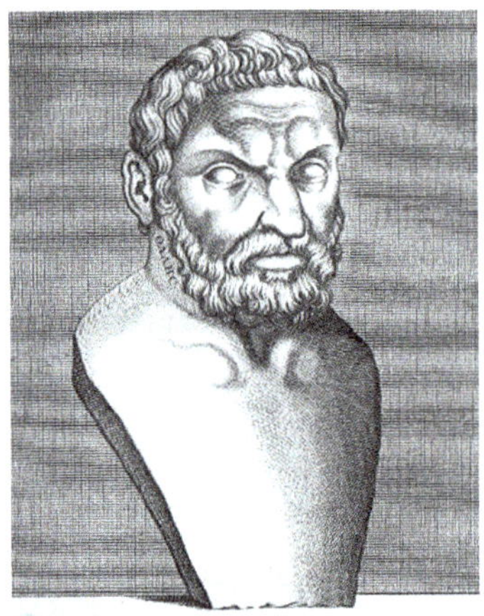

Thales, the earliest known researcher into electricity

Long before any knowledge of electricity existed, people were aware of shocks from electric fish. Ancient Egyptian texts dating from 2750 BCE referred to these fish as the "Thunderer of the Nile", and described them as the "protectors" of all other fish. Electric fish were again reported millennia later by ancient Greek, Roman and Arabic naturalists and physicians. Several ancient writers, such as Pliny the Elder and Scribonius Largus, attested to the numbing effect of electric shocks delivered by catfish and electric rays, and knew that such shocks could travel along conducting objects. Patients suffering from ailments such as gout or headache were directed to touch electric fish in the hope that the powerful jolt might cure them. Possibly the earliest and nearest approach to the discovery of the identity of lightning, and electricity from any other source, is to be attributed to the Arabs, who before the 15th century had the Arabic word for lightning (*raad*) applied to the electric ray.

Ancient cultures around the Mediterranean knew that certain objects, such as rods of amber, could be rubbed with cat's fur to attract light objects like feathers. Thales of Miletus made a series of observations on static electricity around 600 BCE, from which he believed that friction rendered amber magnetic, in contrast to minerals such as magnetite, which needed no rubbing. Thales was incorrect in believing the attraction was due to a magnetic effect, but later science would prove a link between magnetism and electricity. According to a controversial theory, the Parthians may have had knowledge of electroplating, based on the 1936 discovery of the Baghdad Battery, which resembles a galvanic cell, though it is uncertain whether the artifact was electrical in nature.

Electricity would remain little more than an intellectual curiosity for millennia until 1600, when the English scientist William Gilbert made a careful study of electricity and magnetism, distinguishing the lodestone effect from static electricity produced by rubbing amber. He coined the New Latin word *electricus* ("of amber" or "like amber", from ἤλεκτρον, *elektron*, the Greek word for "amber") to refer to the property of attracting small objects after being rubbed. This association gave rise to the English words "electric" and "electricity", which made their first appearance in print in Thomas Browne's *Pseudodoxia Epidemica* of 1646.

Further work was conducted by Otto von Guericke, Robert Boyle, Stephen Gray and C. F. du Fay. In the 18th century, Benjamin Franklin conducted extensive research in electricity, selling his possessions to fund his work. In June 1752 he is reputed to have attached a metal key to the bottom of a dampened kite string and flown the kite in a storm-threatened sky. A succession of sparks jumping from the key to the back of his hand showed that lightning was indeed electrical in nature. He also explained the apparently paradoxical behavior of the Leyden jar as a device for storing large amounts of electrical charge in terms of electricity consisting of both positive and negative charges.

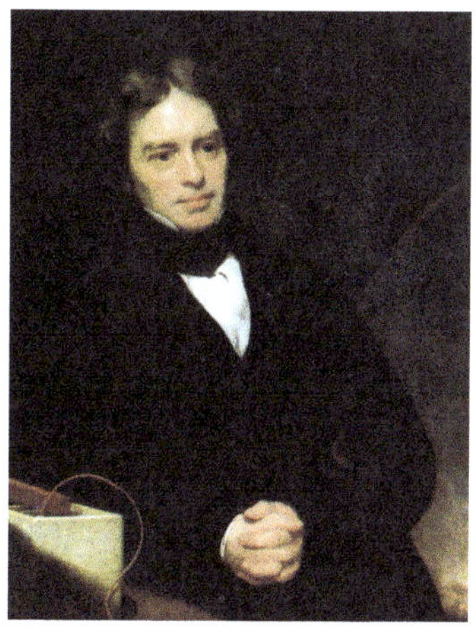

Michael Faraday's discoveries formed the foundation of electric motor technology

In 1791, Luigi Galvani published his discovery of bioelectromagnetics, demonstrating that electricity was the medium by which neurons passed signals to the muscles. Alessandro Volta's battery, or voltaic pile, of 1800, made from alternating layers of zinc and copper, provided scientists with a more reliable source of electrical energy than the electrostatic machines previously used. The recognition of electromagnetism, the unity of electric and magnetic phenomena, is due to Hans Christian Ørsted and André-Marie Ampère in 1819-1820; Michael Faraday invented the electric motor in 1821, and Georg Ohm mathematically analysed the electrical circuit in 1827. Electricity and magnetism (and light) were definitively linked by James Clerk Maxwell, in particular in his "On Physical Lines of Force" in 1861 and 1862.

While the early 19th century had seen rapid progress in electrical science, the late 19th century would see the greatest progress in electrical engineering. Through such people as Alexander Graham Bell, Ottó Bláthy, Thomas Edison, Galileo Ferraris, Oliver Heaviside, Ányos Jedlik, William Thomson, 1st Baron Kelvin, Charles Algernon Parsons, Werner von Siemens, Joseph Swan, Reginald Fessenden, Nikola Tesla and George Westinghouse, electricity turned from a scientific curiosity into an essential tool for modern life, becoming a driving force of the Second Industrial Revolution.

In 1887, Heinrich Hertz discovered that electrodes illuminated with ultraviolet light create electric sparks more easily. In 1905 Albert Einstein published a paper that explained experimental data from the photoelectric effect as being the result of light energy being carried in discrete quantized packets, energising electrons. This discovery led to the quantum revolution. Einstein was awarded the Nobel Prize in Physics in 1921 for "his discovery of the law of the photoelectric effect". The photoelectric effect is also employed in photocells such as can be found in solar panels and this is frequently used to make electricity commercially.

The first solid-state device was the "cat's-whisker detector" first used in the 1900s in radio receivers. A whisker-like wire is placed lightly in contact with a solid crystal (such as a germanium crystal) in order to detect a radio signal by the contact junction effect. In a solid-state component, the current is confined to solid elements and compounds engineered specifically to switch and amplify it. Current flow can be understood in two forms: as negatively charged electrons, and as positively charged electron deficiencies called holes. These charges and holes are understood in terms of quantum physics. The building material is most often a crystalline semiconductor.

The solid-state device came into its own with the invention of the transistor in 1947. Common solid-state devices include transistors, microprocessor chips, and RAM. A specialized type of RAM called flash RAM is used in USB flash drives and more recently, solid-state drives to replace mechanically rotating magnetic disc hard disk drives. Solid state devices became prevalent in the 1950s and the 1960s, during the transition from vacuum tubes to semiconductor diodes, transistors, integrated circuit (IC) and the light-emitting diode (LED).

Concepts

Electric Charge

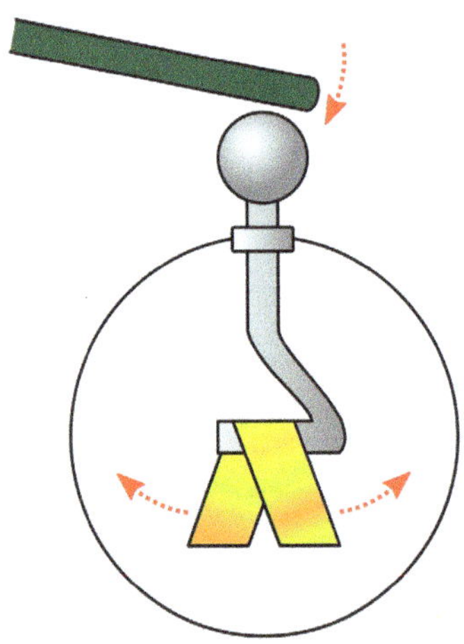

Charge on a gold-leaf electroscope causes the leaves to visibly repel each other

The presence of charge gives rise to an electrostatic force: charges exert a force on each other, an effect that was known, though not understood, in antiquity. A lightweight ball suspended from a string can be charged by touching it with a glass rod that has itself been charged by rubbing with a cloth. If a similar ball is charged by the same glass rod, it is found to repel the first: the charge acts to force the two balls apart. Two balls that are charged with a rubbed amber rod also repel each other. However, if one ball is charged by the glass rod, and the other by an amber rod, the two balls are found to attract each other. These phenomena were investigated in the late eighteenth century by Charles-Augustin de Coulomb, who deduced that charge manifests itself in two opposing forms. This discovery led to the well-known axiom: *like-charged objects repel and opposite-charged objects attract.*

The force acts on the charged particles themselves, hence charge has a tendency to spread itself as evenly as possible over a conducting surface. The magnitude of the electromagnetic force, whether attractive or repulsive, is given by Coulomb's law, which relates the force to the product of the charges and has an inverse-square relation to the distance between them. The electromagnetic force is very strong, second only in strength to the strong interaction, but unlike that force it operates over all distances. In comparison with the much weaker gravitational force, the electromagnetic force pushing two electrons apart is 10^{42} times that of the gravitational attraction pulling them together.

Study has shown that the origin of charge is from certain types of subatomic particles which have the property of electric charge. Electric charge gives rise to and interacts with the electromagnetic force, one of the four fundamental forces of nature. The most familiar carriers of electrical charge are the electron and proton. Experiment has shown charge to be a conserved quantity, that is, the net charge within an isolated system will always remain constant regardless of any changes taking place within that system. Within the system, charge may be transferred between bodies, either by direct contact, or by passing along a conducting material, such as a wire. The informal term static electricity refers to the net presence (or 'imbalance') of charge on a body, usually caused when dissimilar materials are rubbed together, transferring charge from one to the other.

The charge on electrons and protons is opposite in sign, hence an amount of charge may be expressed as being either negative or positive. By convention, the charge carried by electrons is deemed negative, and that by protons positive, a custom that originated with the work of Benjamin Franklin. The amount of charge is usually given the symbol Q and expressed in coulombs; each electron carries the same charge of approximately -1.6022×10^{-19} coulomb. The proton has a charge that is equal and opposite, and thus $+1.6022\times10^{-19}$ coulomb. Charge is possessed not just by matter, but also by antimatter, each antiparticle bearing an equal and opposite charge to its corresponding particle.

Charge can be measured by a number of means, an early instrument being the gold-leaf electroscope, which although still in use for classroom demonstrations, has been superseded by the electronic electrometer.

Electric Current

The movement of electric charge is known as an electric current, the intensity of which is usually measured in amperes. Current can consist of any moving charged particles; most commonly these are electrons, but any charge in motion constitutes a current. Electric current can flow through some things, electrical conductors, but will not flow through an electrical insulator.

By historical convention, a positive current is defined as having the same direction of flow as any positive charge it contains, or to flow from the most positive part of a circuit to the most negative part. Current defined in this manner is called conventional current. The motion of negatively charged electrons around an electric circuit, one of the most familiar forms of current, is thus deemed positive in the *opposite* direction to that of the electrons. However, depending on the conditions, an electric current can consist of a flow of charged particles in either direction, or even in both directions at once. The positive-to-negative convention is widely used to simplify this situation.

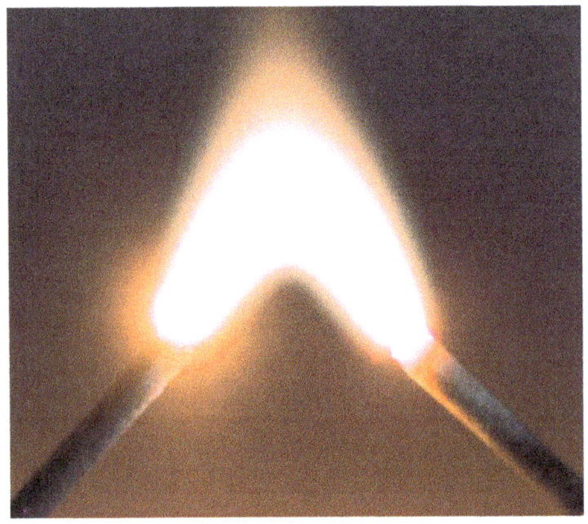

An electric arc provides an energetic demonstration of electric current

The process by which electric current passes through a material is termed electrical conduction, and its nature varies with that of the charged particles and the material through which they are travelling. Examples of electric currents include metallic conduction, where electrons flow through a conductor such as metal, and electrolysis, where ions (charged atoms) flow through liquids, or through plasmas such as electrical sparks. While the particles themselves can move quite slowly, sometimes with an average drift velocity only fractions of a millimetre per second, the electric field that drives them itself propagates at close to the speed of light, enabling electrical signals to pass rapidly along wires.

Current causes several observable effects, which historically were the means of recognising its presence. That water could be decomposed by the current from a voltaic pile was discovered by Nicholson and Carlisle in 1800, a process now known as electrolysis. Their work was greatly expanded upon by Michael Faraday in 1833. Current through a resistance causes localised heating, an effect James Prescott Joule studied mathematically in 1840. One of the most important discoveries relating to current was made accidentally by Hans Christian Ørsted in 1820, when, while preparing a lecture, he witnessed the current in a wire disturbing the needle of a magnetic compass. He had discovered electromagnetism, a fundamental interaction between electricity and magnetics. The level of electromagnetic emissions generated by electric arcing is high enough to produce electromagnetic interference, which can be detrimental to the workings of adjacent equipment.

In engineering or household applications, current is often described as being either direct current (DC) or alternating current (AC). These terms refer to how the current varies in time. Direct current, as produced by example from a battery and required by most electronic devices, is a unidirectional flow from the positive part of a circuit to the negative. If, as is most common, this flow is carried by electrons, they will be travelling in the opposite direction. Alternating current is any current that reverses direction repeatedly; almost always this takes the form of a sine wave. Alternating current thus pulses back and forth within a conductor without the charge moving any net distance over time. The time-averaged value of an alternating current is zero, but it delivers energy in first one direction, and then the reverse. Alternating current is affected by electrical properties that are not observed under steady state direct current, such as inductance and capacitance. These properties however can become important when circuitry is subjected to transients, such as when first energised.

Electric Field

The concept of the electric field was introduced by Michael Faraday. An electric field is created by a charged body in the space that surrounds it, and results in a force exerted on any other charges placed within the field. The electric field acts between two charges in a similar manner to the way that the gravitational field acts between two masses, and like it, extends towards infinity and shows an inverse square relationship with distance. However, there is an important difference. Gravity always acts in attraction, drawing two masses together, while the electric field can result in either attraction or repulsion. Since large bodies such as planets generally carry no net charge, the electric field at a distance is usually zero. Thus gravity is the dominant force at distance in the universe, despite being much weaker.

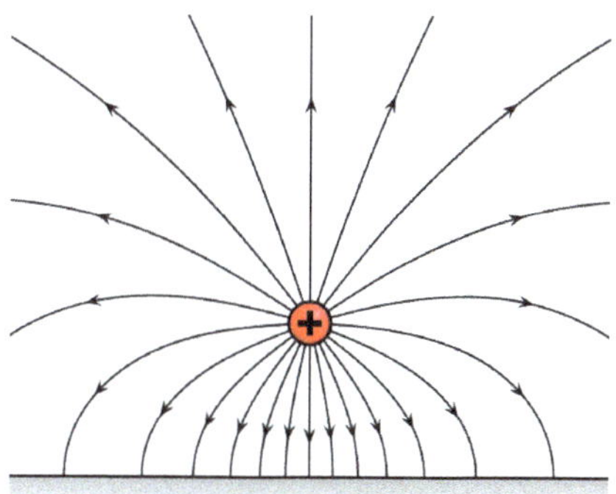

Field lines emanating from a positive charge above a plane conductor

An electric field generally varies in space, and its strength at any one point is defined as the force (per unit charge) that would be felt by a stationary, negligible charge if placed at that point. The conceptual charge, termed a 'test charge', must be vanishingly small to prevent its own electric field disturbing the main field and must also be stationary to prevent the effect of magnetic fields. As the electric field is defined in terms of force, and force is a vector, so it follows that an electric field is also a vector, having both magnitude and direction. Specifically, it is a vector field.

The study of electric fields created by stationary charges is called electrostatics. The field may be visualised by a set of imaginary lines whose direction at any point is the same as that of the field. This concept was introduced by Faraday, whose term 'lines of force' still sometimes sees use. The field lines are the paths that a point positive charge would seek to make as it was forced to move within the field; they are however an imaginary concept with no physical existence, and the field permeates all the intervening space between the lines. Field lines emanating from stationary charges have several key properties: first, that they originate at positive charges and terminate at negative charges; second, that they must enter any good conductor at right angles, and third, that they may never cross nor close in on themselves.

A hollow conducting body carries all its charge on its outer surface. The field is therefore zero at all places inside the body. This is the operating principal of the Faraday cage, a conducting metal shell which isolates its interior from outside electrical effects.

The principles of electrostatics are important when designing items of high-voltage equipment. There is a finite limit to the electric field strength that may be withstood by any medium. Beyond this point, electrical breakdown occurs and an electric arc causes flashover between the charged parts. Air, for example, tends to arc across small gaps at electric field strengths which exceed 30 kV per centimetre. Over larger gaps, its breakdown strength is weaker, perhaps 1 kV per centimetre. The most visible natural occurrence of this is lightning, caused when charge becomes separated in the clouds by rising columns of air, and raises the electric field in the air to greater than it can withstand. The voltage of a large lightning cloud may be as high as 100 MV and have discharge energies as great as 250 kWh.

The field strength is greatly affected by nearby conducting objects, and it is particularly intense when it is forced to curve around sharply pointed objects. This principle is exploited in the lightning conductor, the sharp spike of which acts to encourage the lightning stroke to develop there, rather than to the building it serves to protect.

Electric Potential

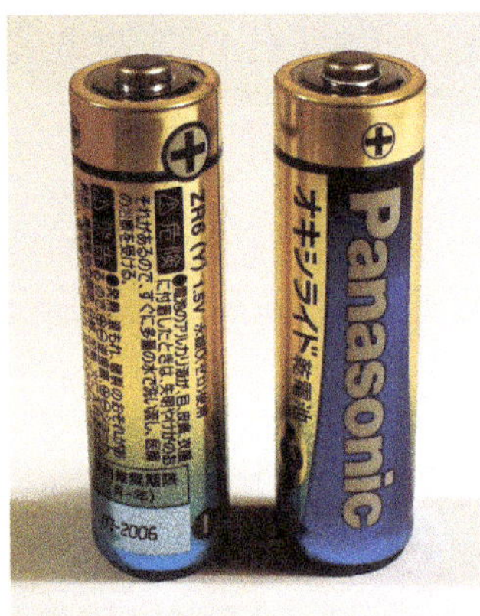

A pair of AA cells. The + sign indicates the polarity of the potential difference between the battery terminals.

The concept of electric potential is closely linked to that of the electric field. A small charge placed within an electric field experiences a force, and to have brought that charge to that point against the force requires work. The electric potential at any point is defined as the energy required to bring a unit test charge from an infinite distance slowly to that point. It is usually measured in volts, and one volt is the potential for which one joule of work must be expended to bring a charge of one coulomb from infinity. This definition of potential, while formal, has little practical application, and a more useful concept is that of electric potential difference, and is the energy required to move a unit charge between two specified points. An electric field has the special property that it is *conservative*, which means that the path taken by the test charge is irrelevant: all paths between two specified points expend the same energy, and thus a unique value for potential difference may be stated. The volt is so strongly identified as the unit of choice for measurement and description of electric potential difference that the term voltage sees greater everyday usage.

For practical purposes, it is useful to define a common reference point to which potentials may be expressed and compared. While this could be at infinity, a much more useful reference is the Earth itself, which is assumed to be at the same potential everywhere. This reference point naturally takes the name earth or ground. Earth is assumed to be an infinite source of equal amounts of positive and negative charge, and is therefore electrically uncharged—and unchargeable.

Electric potential is a scalar quantity, that is, it has only magnitude and not direction. It may be viewed as analogous to height: just as a released object will fall through a difference in heights caused by a gravitational field, so a charge will 'fall' across the voltage caused by an electric field. As relief maps show contour lines marking points of equal height, a set of lines marking points of equal potential (known as equipotentials) may be drawn around an electrostatically charged object. The equipotentials cross all lines of force at right angles. They must also lie parallel to a conductor's surface, otherwise this would produce a force that will move the charge carriers to even the potential of the surface.

The electric field was formally defined as the force exerted per unit charge, but the concept of potential allows for a more useful and equivalent definition: the electric field is the local gradient of the electric potential. Usually expressed in volts per metre, the vector direction of the field is the line of greatest slope of potential, and where the equipotentials lie closest together.

Electromagnets

Ørsted›s discovery in 1821 that a magnetic field existed around all sides of a wire carrying an electric current indicated that there was a direct relationship between electricity and magnetism. Moreover, the interaction seemed different from gravitational and electrostatic forces, the two forces of nature then known. The force on the compass needle did not direct it to or away from the current-carrying wire, but acted at right angles to it. Ørsted's slightly obscure words were that "the electric conflict acts in a revolving manner." The force also depended on the direction of the current, for if the flow was reversed, then the force did too.

Ørsted did not fully understand his discovery, but he observed the effect was reciprocal: a current exerts a force on a magnet, and a magnetic field exerts a force on a current. The phenomenon was further investigated by Ampère, who discovered that two parallel current-carrying wires exerted a force upon each other: two wires conducting currents in the same direction are attracted to each other, while wires containing currents in opposite directions are forced apart. The interaction is mediated by the magnetic field each current produces and forms the basis for the international definition of the ampere.

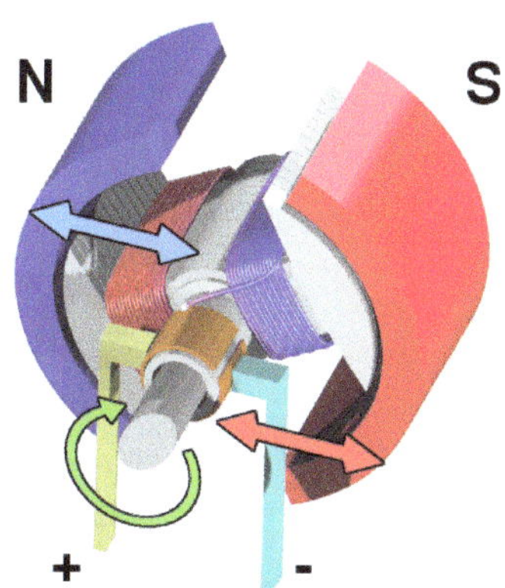

The electric motor exploits an important effect of electromagnetism: a current through a magnetic field experiences a force at right angles to both the field and current.

This relationship between magnetic fields and currents is extremely important, for it led to Michael Faraday's invention of the electric motor in 1821. Faraday's homopolar motor consisted of a permanent magnet sitting in a pool of mercury. A current was allowed through a wire suspended from a pivot above the magnet and dipped into the mercury. The magnet exerted a tangential force on the wire, making it circle around the magnet for as long as the current was maintained.

Experimentation by Faraday in 1831 revealed that a wire moving perpendicular to a magnetic field developed a potential difference between its ends. Further analysis of this process, known as electromagnetic induction, enabled him to state the principle, now known as Faraday's law of induction, that the potential difference induced in a closed circuit is proportional to the rate of change of magnetic flux through the loop. Exploitation of this discovery enabled him to invent the first electrical generator in 1831, in which he converted the mechanical energy of a rotating copper disc to electrical energy. Faraday's disc was inefficient and of no use as a practical generator, but it showed the possibility of generating electric power using magnetism, a possibility that would be taken up by those that followed on from his work.

Electrochemistry

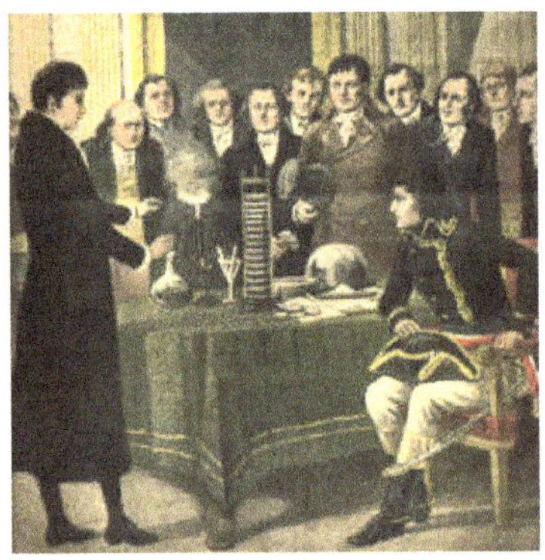

Italian physicist Alessandro Volta showing his *"battery"* to French emperor Napoleon Bonaparte in the early 19th century.

The ability of chemical reactions to produce electricity, and conversely the ability of electricity to drive chemical reactions has a wide array of uses.

Electrochemistry has always been an important part of electricity. From the initial invention of the Voltaic pile, electrochemical cells have evolved into the many different types of batteries, electroplating and electrolysis cells. Aluminium is produced in vast quantities this way, and many portable devices are electrically powered using rechargeable cells.

Electric Circuits

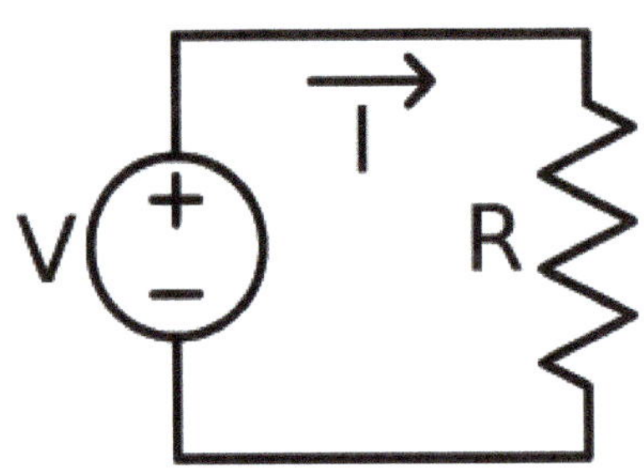

A basic electric circuit. The voltage source *V* on the left drives a current *I* around the circuit, delivering electrical energy into the resistor *R*. From the resistor, the current returns to the source, completing the circuit.

An electric circuit is an interconnection of electric components such that electric charge is made to flow along a closed path (a circuit), usually to perform some useful task.

The components in an electric circuit can take many forms, which can include elements such as resistors, capacitors, switches, transformers and electronics. Electronic circuits contain active components, usually semiconductors, and typically exhibit non-linear behaviour, requiring complex analysis. The simplest electric components are those that are termed passive and linear: while they may temporarily store energy, they contain no sources of it, and exhibit linear responses to stimuli.

The resistor is perhaps the simplest of passive circuit elements: as its name suggests, it resists the current through it, dissipating its energy as heat. The resistance is a consequence of the motion of charge through a conductor: in metals, for example, resistance is primarily due to collisions between electrons and ions. Ohm's law is a basic law of circuit theory, stating that the current passing through a resistance is directly proportional to the potential difference across it. The resistance of most materials is relatively constant over a range of temperatures and currents; materials under these conditions are known as 'ohmic'. The ohm, the unit of resistance, was named in honour of Georg Ohm, and is symbolised by the Greek letter Ω. 1 Ω is the resistance that will produce a potential difference of one volt in response to a current of one amp.

The capacitor is a development of the Leyden jar and is a device that can store charge, and thereby storing electrical energy in the resulting field. It consists of two conducting plates separated by a thin insulating dielectric layer; in practice, thin metal foils are coiled together, increasing the surface area per unit volume and therefore the capacitance. The unit of capacitance is the farad, named after Michael Faraday, and given the symbol F: one farad is the capacitance that develops a potential difference of one volt when it stores a charge of one coulomb. A capacitor connected to a voltage supply initially causes a current as it accumulates charge; this current will however decay in time as the capacitor fills, eventually falling to zero. A capacitor will therefore not permit a steady state current, but instead blocks it.

The inductor is a conductor, usually a coil of wire, that stores energy in a magnetic field in response to the current through it. When the current changes, the magnetic field does too, inducing a voltage between the ends of the conductor. The induced voltage is proportional to the time rate of change of the current. The constant of proportionality is termed the inductance. The unit of inductance is the henry, named after Joseph Henry, a contemporary of Faraday. One henry is the inductance that will induce a potential difference of one volt if the current through it changes at a rate of one ampere per second. The inductor's behaviour is in some regards converse to that of the capacitor: it will freely allow an unchanging current, but opposes a rapidly changing one.

Electric Power

Electric power is the rate at which electric energy is transferred by an electric circuit. The SI unit of power is the watt, one joule per second.

Electric power, like mechanical power, is the rate of doing work, measured in watts, and represented by the letter P. The term *wattage* is used colloquially to mean "electric power in watts." The electric power in watts produced by an electric current I consisting of a charge of Q coulombs every t seconds passing through an electric potential (voltage) difference of V is

$$P = \text{work done per unit time} = \frac{QV}{t} = IV$$

where

Q is electric charge in coulombs

t is time in seconds

I is electric current in amperes

V is electric potential or voltage in volts

Electricity generation is often done with electric generators, but can also be supplied by chemical sources such as electric batteries or by other means from a wide variety of sources of energy. Electric power is generally supplied to businesses and homes by the electric power industry. Electricity is usually sold by the kilowatt hour (3.6 MJ) which is the product of power in kilowatts multiplied by running time in hours. Electric utilities measure power using electricity meters, which keep a running total of the electric energy delivered to a customer. Unlike fossil fuels, electricity is a low entropy form of energy and can be converted into motion or many other forms of energy with high efficiency.

Electronics

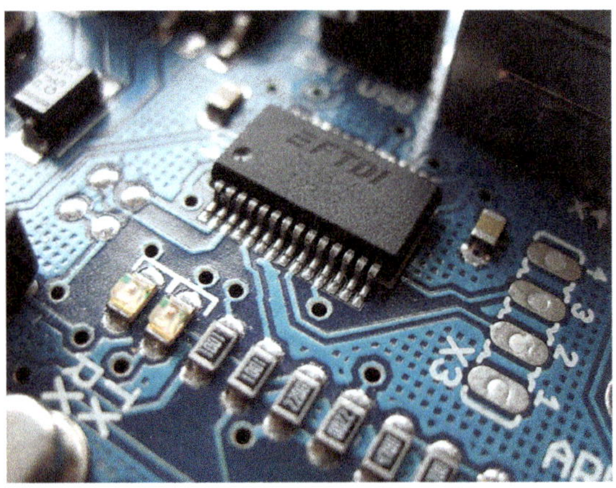

Surface mount electronic components

Electronics deals with electrical circuits that involve active electrical components such as vacuum tubes, transistors, diodes, optoelectronics, sensors and integrated circuits, and associated passive interconnection technologies. The nonlinear behaviour of active components and their ability to control electron flows makes amplification of weak signals possible and electronics is widely used in information processing, telecommunications, and signal processing. The ability of electronic devices to act as switches makes digital information processing possible. Interconnection technologies such as circuit boards, electronics packaging technology, and other varied forms of communication infrastructure complete circuit functionality and transform the mixed components into a regular working system.

Today, most electronic devices use semiconductor components to perform electron control. The study of semiconductor devices and related technology is considered a branch of solid state physics, whereas the design and construction of electronic circuits to solve practical problems come under electronics engineering.

Electromagnetic Wave

Faraday's and Ampère's work showed that a time-varying magnetic field acted as a source of an electric field, and a time-varying electric field was a source of a magnetic field. Thus, when either field is changing in time, then a field of the other is necessarily induced. Such a phenomenon has the properties of a wave, and is naturally referred to as an electromagnetic wave. Electromagnetic waves were analysed theoretically by James Clerk Maxwell in 1864. Maxwell developed a set of equations that could unambiguously describe the interrelationship between electric field, magnetic field, electric charge, and electric current. He could moreover prove that such a wave would necessarily travel at the speed of light, and thus light itself was a form of electromagnetic radiation. Maxwell's Laws, which unify light, fields, and charge are one of the great milestones of theoretical physics.

Thus, the work of many researchers enabled the use of electronics to convert signals into high frequency oscillating currents, and via suitably shaped conductors, electricity permits the transmission and reception of these signals via radio waves over very long distances.

Production and uses

Generation and Transmission

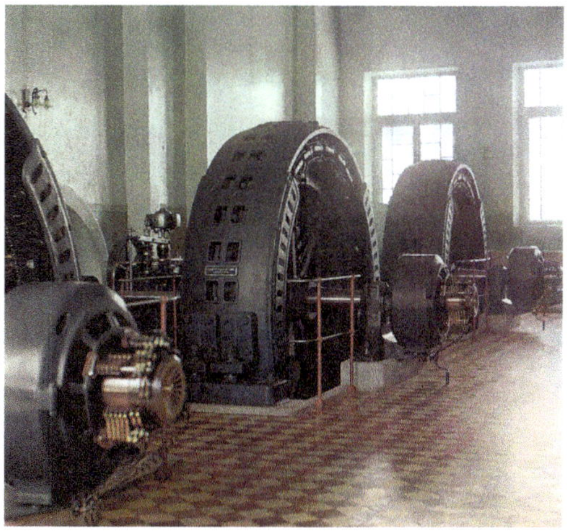

Early 20th-century alternator made in Budapest, Hungary, in the power generating hall of a hydroelectric station (photograph by Prokudin-Gorsky, 1905–1915).

In the 6th century BC, the Greek philosopher Thales of Miletus experimented with amber rods and these experiments were the first studies into the production of electrical energy. While this method, now known as the triboelectric effect, can lift light objects and generate sparks, it is extremely inefficient. It was not until the invention of the voltaic pile in the eighteenth century that a viable source of electricity became available. The voltaic pile, and its modern descendant, the electrical battery, store energy chemically and make it available on demand in the form of electrical energy. The battery is a versatile and very common power source which is ideally suited to many applications, but its energy storage is finite, and once discharged it must be disposed of or recharged. For large electrical demands electrical energy must be generated and transmitted continuously over conductive transmission lines.

Electrical power is usually generated by electro-mechanical generators driven by steam produced from fossil fuel combustion, or the heat released from nuclear reactions; or from other sources such as kinetic energy extracted from wind or flowing water. The modern steam turbine invented by Sir Charles Parsons in 1884 today generates about 80 percent of the electric power in the world using a variety of heat sources. Such generators bear no resemblance to Faraday's homopolar disc generator of 1831, but they still rely on his electromagnetic principle that a conductor linking a changing magnetic field induces a potential difference across its ends. The invention in the late nineteenth century of the transformer meant that electrical power could be transmitted more efficiently at a higher voltage but lower current. Efficient electrical transmission meant in turn that electricity could be generated at centralised power stations, where it benefited from economies of scale, and then be despatched relatively long distances to where it was needed.

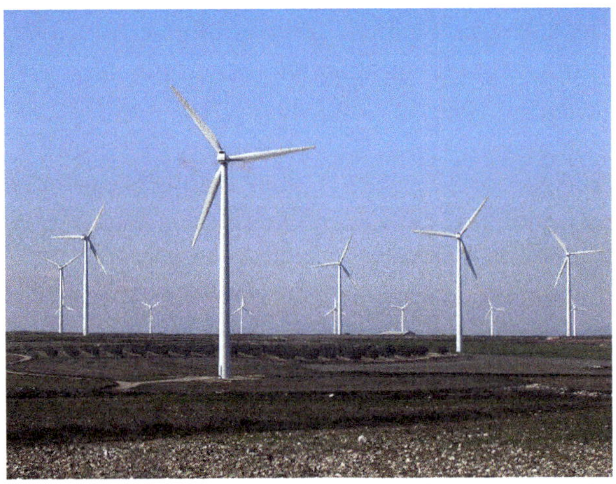

Wind power is of increasing importance in many countries

Since electrical energy cannot easily be stored in quantities large enough to meet demands on a national scale, at all times exactly as much must be produced as is required. This requires electricity utilities to make careful predictions of their electrical loads, and maintain constant co-ordination with their power stations. A certain amount of generation must always be held in reserve to cushion an electrical grid against inevitable disturbances and losses.

Demand for electricity grows with great rapidity as a nation modernises and its economy develops. The United States showed a 12% increase in demand during each year of the first three decades of the twentieth century, a rate of growth that is now being experienced by emerging economies such as those of India or China. Historically, the growth rate for electricity demand has outstripped that for other forms of energy.

Environmental concerns with electricity generation have led to an increased focus on generation from renewable sources, in particular from wind and hydropower. While debate can be expected to continue over the environmental impact of different means of electricity production, its final form is relatively clean.

Applications

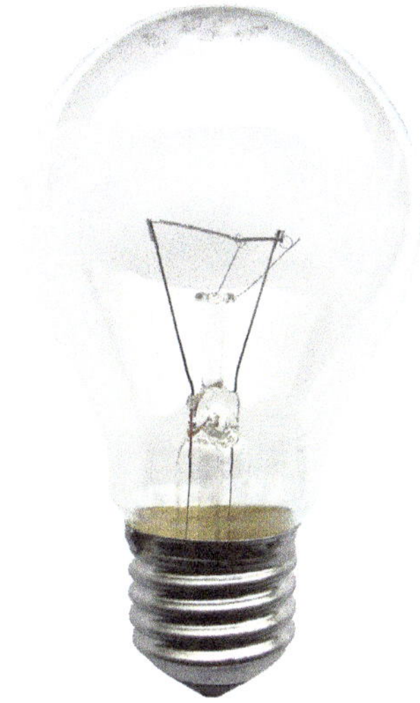

The light bulb, an early application of electricity, operates by Joule heating: the passage of current through resistance generating heat

Electricity is a very convenient way to transfer energy, and it has been adapted to a huge, and growing, number of uses. The invention of a practical incandescent light bulb in the 1870s led to lighting becoming one of the first publicly available applications of electrical power. Although electrification brought with it its own dangers, replacing the naked flames of gas lighting greatly reduced fire hazards within homes and factories. Public utilities were set up in many cities targeting the burgeoning market for electrical lighting. In the late 20th century and in modern times, the trend has started to flow in the direction of deregulation in the electrical power sector.

The resistive Joule heating effect employed in filament light bulbs also sees more direct use in electric heating. While this is versatile and controllable, it can be seen as wasteful, since most electrical generation has already required the production of heat at a power station. A number of countries, such as Denmark, have issued legislation restricting or banning the use of resistive electric heating in new buildings. Electricity is however still a highly practical energy source for heating and refrigeration, with air conditioning/heat pumps representing a growing sector for electricity demand for heating and cooling, the effects of which electricity utilities are increasingly obliged to accommodate.

Electricity is used within telecommunications, and indeed the electrical telegraph, demonstrated commercially in 1837 by Cooke and Wheatstone, was one of its earliest applications. With the construction of first intercontinental, and then transatlantic, telegraph systems in the 1860s, electricity had enabled communications in minutes across the globe. Optical fibre and satellite communication have taken a share of the market for communications systems, but electricity can be expected to remain an essential part of the process.

The effects of electromagnetism are most visibly employed in the electric motor, which provides a clean and efficient means of motive power. A stationary motor such as a winch is easily provided with a supply of power, but a motor that moves with its application, such as an electric vehicle, is obliged to either carry along a power source such as a battery, or to collect current from a sliding contact such as a pantograph.

Electronic devices make use of the transistor, perhaps one of the most important inventions of the twentieth century, and a fundamental building block of all modern circuitry. A modern integrated circuit may contain several billion miniaturised transistors in a region only a few centimetres square.

Electricity is also used to fuel public transportation, including electric buses and trains.

Electricity and the Natural World

Physiological Effects

A voltage applied to a human body causes an electric current through the tissues, and although the relationship is non-linear, the greater the voltage, the greater the current. The threshold for perception varies with the supply frequency and with the path of the current, but is about 0.1 mA to 1 mA for mains-frequency electricity, though a current as low as a microamp can be detected as an electrovibration effect under certain conditions. If the current is sufficiently high, it will cause muscle contraction, fibrillation of the heart, and tissue burns. The lack of any visible sign that a conductor is electrified makes electricity a particular hazard. The pain caused by an electric shock can be intense, leading electricity at times to be employed as a method of torture. Death caused by an electric shock is referred to as electrocution. Electrocution is still the means of judicial execution in some jurisdictions, though its use has become rarer in recent times.

Electrical Phenomena in Nature

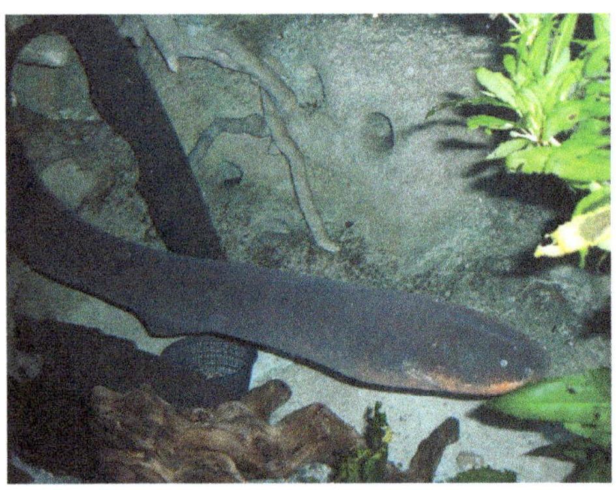

The electric eel, *Electrophorus electricus*

Electricity is not a human invention, and may be observed in several forms in nature, a prominent manifestation of which is lightning. Many interactions familiar at the macroscopic level, such as touch, friction or chemical bonding, are due to interactions between electric fields on the atomic scale. The Earth's magnetic field is thought to arise from a natural dynamo of circulating currents in the planet's core. Certain crystals, such as quartz, or even sugar, generate a potential difference across their faces when subjected to external pressure. This phenomenon is known as piezoelectricity, from the Greek *piezein*, meaning to press, and was discovered in 1880 by Pierre and Jacques Curie. The effect is reciprocal, and when a piezoelectric material is subjected to an electric field, a small change in physical dimensions takes place.

Some organisms, such as sharks, are able to detect and respond to changes in electric fields, an ability known as electroreception, while others, termed electrogenic, are able to generate voltages themselves to serve as a predatory or defensive weapon. The order Gymnotiformes, of which the best known example is the electric eel, detect or stun their prey via high voltages generated from modified muscle cells called electrocytes. All animals transmit information along their cell membranes with voltage pulses called action potentials, whose functions include communication by the nervous system between neurons and muscles. An electric shock stimulates this system, and causes muscles to contract. Action potentials are also responsible for coordinating activities in certain plants.

Cultural Perception

In 1850, William Gladstone asked the scientist Michael Faraday why electricity was valuable. Faraday answered, "One day sir, you may tax it."

In the 19th and early 20th century, electricity was not part of the everyday life of many people, even in the industrialised Western world. The popular culture of the time accordingly often depicts it as a mysterious, quasi-magical force that can slay the living, revive the dead or otherwise bend the laws of nature. This attitude began with the 1771 experiments of Luigi Galvani in which the legs of dead frogs were shown to twitch on application of animal electricity. "Revitalization" or resuscitation of apparently dead or drowned persons was reported in the medical literature shortly after Galvani's work. These results were known to Mary Shelley when she authored *Frankenstein* (1819), although she does not name the method of revitalization of the monster. The revitalization of monsters with electricity later became a stock theme in horror films.

As the public familiarity with electricity as the lifeblood of the Second Industrial Revolution grew, its wielders were more often cast in a positive light, such as the workers who "finger death at their gloves' end as they piece and repiece the living wires" in Rudyard Kipling's 1907 poem *Sons of Martha*. Electrically powered vehicles of every sort featured large in adventure stories such as those of Jules Verne and the *Tom Swift* books. The masters of electricity, whether fictional or real—including scientists such as Thomas Edison, Charles Steinmetz or Nikola Tesla—were popularly conceived of as having wizard-like powers.

With electricity ceasing to be a novelty and becoming a necessity of everyday life in the later half of the 20th century, it required particular attention by popular culture only when it *stops* flowing, an event that usually signals disaster. The people who *keep* it flowing, such as the nameless hero of Jimmy Webb's song "Wichita Lineman" (1968), are still often cast as heroic, wizard-like figures.

Triboelectric Effect

The triboelectric effect (also known as triboelectric charging) is a type of contact electrification in which certain materials become electrically charged after they come into frictional contact with a different material. Rubbing glass with fur, or a plastic comb through the hair, can build up triboelectricity. Most everyday static electricity is triboelectric. The polarity and strength of the charges produced differ according to the materials, surface roughness, temperature, strain, and other properties.

The triboelectric effect is not very predictable, and only broad generalizations can be made. Amber, for example, can acquire an electric charge by contact and separation (or friction) with a material like wool. This property was first recorded by Thales of Miletus. The word "electricity" is derived from William Gilbert's initial coinage, "electra", which originates in the Greek word for amber, *ēlektron*. The prefix *tribo-* (Greek for 'rub') refers to 'friction', as in tribology. Other examples of materials that can acquire a significant charge when rubbed together include glass rubbed with silk, and hard rubber rubbed with fur.

The triboelectric effect is now considered to be related to the phenomenon of adhesion, where two materials composed of different molecules tend to stick together because of attraction between the different molecules. While adhesion is not a chemical bond between atoms, there is an exchange of electrons between the different types of molecules, resulting in an electrostatic attraction between the molecules that holds them together. Physical separation of materials that are adhered together results in friction between the materials. Because the electron transfer between molecules in the different materials is not immediately reversible, the excess electrons in one type of molecule remain left behind, while a deficit of electrons occurs in the other. Thus, a material can develop a positive or negative charge that dissipates after the materials separate.

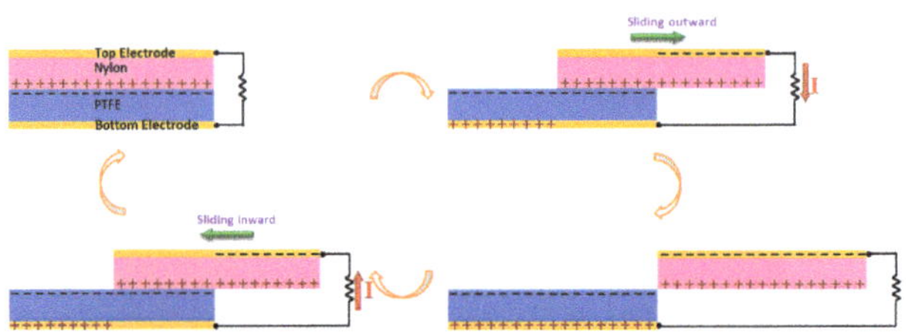

A nanogenerator employing the triboelectric effect to generate electricity

Triboelectric Series

Johan Carl Wilcke published the first triboelectric series in a 1757 paper on static charges. Materials are often listed in order of the polarity of charge separation when they are touched with another object. A material towards the bottom of the series, when touched to a material near the top of the series, will acquire a more negative charge. The farther away two materials are from each other on the series, the greater the charge transferred. Materials near to each other on the series may not exchange any charge, or may even exchange the opposite of what is implied by the list. This can be caused by rubbing, by contaminants or oxides, or other variables. Lists vary somewhat as to the exact order of some materials, since the relative charge varies for nearby materials. From actual tests, there is little or no measurable difference in charge affinity between metals, probably because the rapid motion of conduction electrons cancels such differences.

Cause

Although the part 'tribo-' comes from the Greek for "rubbing", (friction), the two materials only need to come into contact for electrons to be exchanged. After coming into contact, a chemical bond is formed between parts of the two surfaces, called adhesion, and charges move from one material to the other to equalize their electrochemical potential. This is what creates the net charge imbalance between the objects. When separated, some of the bonded atoms have a tendency to keep extra electrons, and some a tendency to give them away, though the imbalance will be partially destroyed by tunneling or electrical breakdown (usually corona discharge). In addition, some materials may exchange ions of differing mobility, or exchange charged fragments of larger molecules.

The triboelectric effect is related to friction only because they both involve adhesion. However, the effect is greatly enhanced by rubbing the materials together, as they touch and separate many times. For surfaces with differing geometry, rubbing may also lead to heating of protrusions, causing pyroelectric charge separation which may add to the existing contact electrification, or which may oppose the existing polarity. Surface nano-effects are not well understood, and the atomic force microscope has enabled rapid progress in this field of physics.

Sparks

Because the surface of the material is now electrically charged, either negatively or positively, any contact with an uncharged conductive object or with an object having substantially different charge may cause an electrical discharge of the built-up static electricity: a spark. A person simply walking across a carpet may build up a potential of many thousands of volts, enough to cause a spark one centimeter long or more. Low humidity in the ambient air increases the voltage at which electrical discharge occurs by increasing the ability of the insulating material to hold charge by decreasing the conductivity of the air, making it difficult for the charge build-up to dissipate gradually. Simply removing a nylon shirt or corset can also create sparks. Car travel can lead to a build-up of charge on the driver and passengers due to friction between the driver's clothes and the leather or plastic furnishings inside the vehicle. This charge can then be relaxed as a spark to the metal car body, fuel dispensers, or nearby door handles, etc. When the vehicle's body itself builds up a static charge (acting as a Faraday cage) it can relax through the carbon in the tires. If it remains charged when parked, sparks may jump from the door frame to occupants as they make contact with the ground.

This type of discharge is often harmless because the energy ($1/2V^2C$) of the spark is very small, being typically several tens of micro joules in cold dry weather, and much less than that in humid conditions. However, such sparks can ignite flammable vapours.

In Aircraft and Spacecraft

Aircraft flying in weather will develop a static charge from air friction on the airframe. The static can be discharged with static dischargers or static wicks.

NASA follows what they call the "Triboelectrification Rule" whereby they will cancel a launch if the launch vehicle is predicted to pass through certain types of clouds. Flying through high-level clouds can generate "P-static" (P for precipitation), which can create static around the launch vehicle that will interfere with radio signals sent by or to the vehicle. This may prevent transmitting of telemetry to the ground or, if the need arises, sending a signal to the vehicle, particularly critical signals for the flight termination system. When a hold is put in place due to the triboelectrification rule, it remains until Space Wing and observer personnel, such as those in reconnaissance aircraft, indicate that the skies are clear.

Risks and Counter-measures

Ignition

The effect is of considerable industrial importance in terms of both safety and potential damage to manufactured goods. Static discharge is a particular hazard in grain elevators owing to the danger of a dust explosion. The spark produced is fully able to ignite flammable vapours, for example, petrol, ether fumes as well as methane gas. For bulk fuel deliveries and aircraft fueling a grounding connection is made between the vehicle and the receiving tank prior to opening the tanks. When fueling vehicles at a retail station touching metal on the car before opening the gas tank or touching the nozzle may decrease one's risk of static ignition of fuel vapors.

In the Workplace

Means have to be provided to discharge static from carts which may carry volatile liquids, flammable gasses, or oxygen in hospitals. Even where only a small charge is produced, it can result in dust particles being attracted to the rubbed surface. In the case of textile manufacture this can lead to a permanent grimy mark where the cloth comes in contact with dust accumulations held by a static charge. Dust attraction may be reduced by treating insulating surfaces with an antistatic cleaning agent.

Damage to Electronics

Some electronic devices, most notably CMOS integrated circuits and MOSFET transistors, can be accidentally destroyed by high-voltage static discharge. Such components are usually stored in a conductive foam for protection. Grounding oneself by touching the workbench, or using a special bracelet or anklet is standard practice while handling unconnected integrated circuits. Another way of dissipating charge is by using conducting materials such as carbon black loaded rubber mats in operating theatres, for example.

Devices containing sensitive components must be protected during normal use, installation, and disconnection, accomplished by designed-in protection at external connections where needed. Protection may be through the use of more robust devices or protective countermeasures at the device's external interfaces. These may be opto-isolators, less sensitive types of transistors, and static bypass devices such as metal oxide varistors.

Charge Conservation

In physics, charge conservation is the principle that electric charge can neither be created nor destroyed. The net quantity of electric charge, the amount of positive charge minus the amount of negative charge in the universe, is always *conserved*. Charge conservation was first proposed by British scientist William Watson in 1746 and American statesman and scientist Benjamin Franklin in 1747, although the first convincing proof was given by Michael Faraday in 1843.

It is now discovered and demonstrated, both here and in Europe, that the Electrical Fire is a real Element, or Species of Matter, not *created* by the Friction, but *collected* only.

—Benjamin Franklin, Letter to Cadwallader Colden

Charge conservation is a physical law that states that the change in the amount of electric charge in any volume of space is exactly equal to the amount of charge flowing into the volume minus the amount of charge flowing out of the volume. In essence, charge conservation is an accounting relationship between the amount of charge in a region and the flow of charge into and out of that region.

Mathematically, we can state the law as a continuity equation:

$$Q(t_2) = Q(t_1) + Q_{IN} - Q_{OUT}.$$

$Q(t)$ is the quantity of electric charge in a specific volume at time t, Q_{IN} is the amount of charge flowing into the volume between time t_1 and t_2, and Q_{OUT} is the amount of charge flowing out of the volume during the same time period.

This does not mean that individual positive and negative charges cannot be created or destroyed. Electric charge is carried by subatomic particles such as electrons and protons, which can be created and destroyed. In particle physics, charge conservation means that in elementary particle reactions that create charged particles, equal numbers of positive and negative particles are always created, keeping the net amount of charge unchanged. Similarly, when particles are destroyed, equal numbers of positive and negative charges are destroyed.

Although conservation of charge requires that the total quantity of charge in the universe is constant, it leaves open the question of what that quantity is. Most evidence indicates that the net charge in the universe is zero; that is, there are equal quantities of positive and negative charge.

Formal Statement of the Law

In electromagnetic field theory, vector calculus can be used to express the law in terms of charge density ρ (in coulombs per cubic meter) and electric current density J (in amperes per square meter). This is called the charge continuity equation

$$\frac{\partial \rho}{\partial t} + \nabla \cdot \boldsymbol{J} = 0.$$

The term on the left is the rate of change of the charge density ρ at a point. The term on the right is the divergence of the current density J at the same point. The equation equates these two factors, which says that the only way for the charge density at a point to change is for a current of charge to flow into or out of the point. This statement is equivalent to a conservation of four-current.

Mathematical Derivation

The net current into a volume is

$$I = -\iint_S \boldsymbol{J} \cdot d\boldsymbol{S}$$

where $S = \partial V$ is the boundary of V oriented by outward-pointing normals, and dS is shorthand for NdS, the outward pointing normal of the boundary ∂V. Here J *is the current density (charge per unit area per unit time) at the surface of the volume. The vector points in the direction of the current.*

From the Divergence theorem this can be written

$$I = -\iiint_V (\nabla \cdot \boldsymbol{J}) dV$$

Charge conservation requires that the net current into a volume must necessarily equal the net change in charge within the volume.

$$\frac{dq}{dt} = -\iiint_V (\nabla \cdot \boldsymbol{J}) dV \qquad (1)$$

The total charge q in volume V is the integral (sum) of the charge density in V

$$q = \iiint_V \rho dV$$

So

$$\frac{dq}{dt} = \iiint_V \frac{d\rho}{dt} dV \qquad (2)$$

Equating (1) and (2) gives

$$0 = \iiint_V \left(\frac{\partial \rho}{\partial t} + \nabla \cdot \mathbf{J} \right) dV.$$

Since this is true for every volume, we have in general

$$\frac{\partial \rho}{\partial t} + \nabla \cdot \boldsymbol{J} = 0.$$

Connection to Gauge Invariance

Charge conservation can also be understood as a consequence of symmetry through Noether's theorem, a central result in theoretical physics that asserts that each conservation law is associated with a symmetry of the underlying physics. The symmetry that is associated with charge conservation is the global gauge invariance of the electromagnetic field. This is related to the fact that the electric and magnetic fields are not changed by different choices of the value representing the zero point of electrostatic potential ϕ. However the full symmetry is more complicated, and also involves the vector potential $\boldsymbol{A}$. The full statement of gauge invariance is that the physics of an electromagnetic field are unchanged when the scalar and vector potential are shifted by the gradient of an arbitrary scalar field χ:

$$\phi' = \phi - \frac{\partial \chi}{\partial t} \qquad \boldsymbol{A}' = \boldsymbol{A} + \nabla \chi.$$

In quantum mechanics the scalar field is equivalent to a phase shift in the wavefunction of the charged particle:

$$\psi' = e^{i\chi}\psi$$

so gauge invariance is equivalent to the well known fact that changes in the phase of a wavefunction are unobservable, and only changes in the magnitude of the wavefunction result in changes to the probability function $|\psi|^2$. This is the ultimate theoretical origin of charge conservation.

Gauge invariance is a very important, well established property of the electromagnetic field and has many testable consequences. The theoretical justification for charge conservation is greatly strengthened by being linked to this symmetry. For example, local gauge invariance also requires that the photon be massless, so the good experimental evidence that the photon has zero mass is also strong evidence that charge is conserved.

Even if gauge symmetry is exact, however, there might be apparent electric charge non-conservation if charge could leak from our normal 3-dimensional space into hidden extra dimensions.

Experimental Evidence

Simple arguments rule out some types of charge nonconservation. For example, the magnitude of the elementary charge on positive and negative particles must be extremely close to equal, differing by no more than a factor of 10^{-21} for the case of protons and electrons. Ordinary matter contains equal numbers of positive and negative particles, protons and electrons, in enormous quantities. If the elementary charge on the electron and proton were even slightly different, all matter would have a large electric charge and would be mutually repulsive.

The best experimental tests of electric charge conservation are searches for particle decays that would be allowed if electric charge is not always conserved. No such decays have ever been seen. The best experimental test comes from searches for the energetic photon from an electron decaying into a neutrino and a single photon:

$e \rightarrow \nu + \gamma$ mean lifetime is greater than 6.6×10^{28} years (90% Confidence Level),

but there are theoretical arguments that such single-photon decays will never occur even if charge is not conserved. Charge disappearance tests are sensitive to decays without energetic photons, other unusual charge violating processes such as an electron spontaneously changing into a positron, and to electric charge moving into other dimensions. The best experimental bounds on charge disappearance are:

$e \rightarrow$ *anything* mean lifetime is greater than 6.4×10^{24} years (68% CL)

$n \rightarrow p + \nu + \nu$ charge non-conserving decays are less than 8×10^{-27} (68% CL) of all neutron decays

Liénard–Wiechert Potential

Liénard–Wiechert potentials describe the classical electromagnetic effect of a moving electric point charge in terms of a vector potential and a scalar potential in the Lorenz gauge. Built directly from Maxwell's equations, these potentials describe the complete, relativistically correct, time-varying electromagnetic field for a point charge in arbitrary motion, but are not corrected for quantum-mechanical effects. Electromagnetic radiation in the form of waves can be obtained from these potentials. These expressions were developed in part by Alfred-Marie Liénard in 1898 and independently by Emil Wiechert in 1900.

Equations

Definition of Liénard–Wiechert Potentials

The Liénard–Wiechert potentials φ (scalar potential field) and $\boldsymbol{A}$ (vector potential field) are for a source point charge q at position $\boldsymbol{r}_s$ traveling with velocity $\boldsymbol{v}_s$:

$$\varphi(r,t) = \frac{1}{4\pi\epsilon_0}\left(\frac{q}{(1-n\cdot\beta_s)|r-r_s|}\right)_{t_r}$$

and

$$A(\mathrm{r},t) = \frac{\mu_0 c}{4\pi}\left(\frac{q\beta_s}{(1-n\cdot\beta_s)|r-r_s|}\right)_{t_r} = \frac{\beta_s(t_r)}{c}\varphi(r,t)$$

where $\beta_s(t) = \frac{v_s(t)}{c}$ and $\boldsymbol{n} = \frac{\boldsymbol{r}-\boldsymbol{r}_s}{|\boldsymbol{r}-\boldsymbol{r}_s|}$.

Corresponding Values of Electric and Magnetic Fields

We can calculate the electric and magnetic fields directly from the potentials using the definitions:

$$\boldsymbol{E} = -\nabla\varphi - \frac{\partial \boldsymbol{A}}{\partial t} \text{ and } \boldsymbol{B} = \nabla\times\boldsymbol{A}$$

The calculation is nontrivial and requires a number of steps. The electric and magnetic fields are (in non-covariant form):

$$E(\mathrm{r},t) = \frac{1}{4\pi\epsilon_0}\left(\frac{q(\mathrm{n}-\beta)}{\gamma^2(1-n\cdot\beta)^3|r-r_s|^2} + \frac{qn\times\big((n-\beta)\times\dot{\beta}\big)}{c(1-n\cdot\beta)^3|r-r_s|}\right)_{t_r}$$

and

$$\mathrm{B}(\mathrm{r},t) = \frac{\mu_0}{4\pi}\left(\frac{qc(\beta\times n)}{\gamma^2(1-n\cdot\beta)^3|r-r_s|^2} + \frac{qn\times\big(n\times\big((n-\beta)\times\dot{\beta}\big)\big)}{(1-n\cdot\beta)^3|r-r_s|}\right)_{t_r} = \frac{\mathrm{n}(t_r)}{c}\times E(\mathrm{r},t)$$

where $\beta(t) = \frac{v_s(t)}{c}$, $\boldsymbol{n}(t) = \frac{\boldsymbol{r}-\boldsymbol{r}_s(t)}{|\boldsymbol{r}-\boldsymbol{r}_s(t)|}$ and $\gamma(t) = \frac{1}{\sqrt{1-|\beta(t)|^2}}$ (the Lorentz factor).

Note that the $n-\beta$ part of the first term updates the direction of the field toward the instantaneous position of the charge, if it continues to move with constant velocity $c\beta$. This term is connected with the "static" part of the electromagnetic field of the charge.

The second term, which is connected with electromagnetic radiation by the moving charge, requires charge acceleration $\dot{\beta}$ and if this is zero, the value of this term is zero, and the charge does not radiate (emit electromagnetic radiation). This term requires additionally that a component of the charge acceleration be in a direction transverse to the line which connects the charge q and the observer of the field $\boldsymbol{E}(\boldsymbol{r},t)$. The direction of the field associated with this radiative term is toward the fully time-retarded position of the charge (i.e. where the charge was when it was accelerated).

Derivation

In the case that there are no boundaries surrounding the sources, the retarded solutions for the scalar and vector potentials (SI units) of the nonhomogeneous wave equations with sources given by the charge and current densities $\rho(\boldsymbol{r},t)$ and $\boldsymbol{J}(\boldsymbol{r},t)$ are in the Lorenz gauge.

$$\varphi(\boldsymbol{r},t)=\frac{1}{4\pi\epsilon_0}\int\frac{\rho(\boldsymbol{r}',t_{r'})}{|\boldsymbol{r}-\boldsymbol{r}'|}d^3\boldsymbol{r}'$$

and

$$\boldsymbol{A}(\boldsymbol{r},t)=\frac{\mu_0}{4\pi}\int\frac{\boldsymbol{J}(\boldsymbol{r}',t_{r'})}{|\boldsymbol{r}-\boldsymbol{r}'|}d^3\boldsymbol{r}'$$

where $t_{r'}=t-\frac{1}{c}|\boldsymbol{r}-\boldsymbol{r}'|$ is the retarded time.

For a moving point charge whose trajectory is given as a function of time by $\boldsymbol{r}_s(t')$, the charge and current densities are as follows:

$$\rho(\boldsymbol{r}',t')=q\delta^3(\boldsymbol{r}'-\boldsymbol{r}_s(t'))$$

$$\boldsymbol{J}(\boldsymbol{r}',t')=q\boldsymbol{v}_s(t')\delta^3(\boldsymbol{r}'-\boldsymbol{r}_s(t'))$$

where δ^3 is the three-dimensional Dirac delta function and $\mathbf{v}_s(t')$ is the velocity of the point charge.

Substituting into the expressions for the potential gives

$$\varphi(\boldsymbol{r},t)=\frac{1}{4\pi\epsilon_0}\int\frac{q\delta^3(\boldsymbol{r}'-\boldsymbol{r}_s(t_{r'}))}{|\boldsymbol{r}-\boldsymbol{r}'|}d^3\boldsymbol{r}'$$

$$\boldsymbol{A}(\boldsymbol{r},t)=\frac{\mu_0}{4\pi}\int\frac{q\boldsymbol{v}_s(t_{r'})\delta^3(\boldsymbol{r}'-\boldsymbol{r}_s(t_{r'}))}{|\boldsymbol{r}-\boldsymbol{r}'|}d^3\boldsymbol{r}'$$

These integrals are difficult to evaluate in their present form, so we will rewrite them by replacing $t_{r'}$ with t' and integrating over the delta distribution $\delta(t'-t_{r'})$:

$$\varphi(\boldsymbol{r},t)=\frac{1}{4\pi\epsilon_0}\iint\frac{q\delta^3(\boldsymbol{r}'-\boldsymbol{r}_s(t'))}{|\boldsymbol{r}-\boldsymbol{r}'|}\delta(t'-t_{r'})dt'd^3\boldsymbol{r}'$$

$$\boldsymbol{A}(\boldsymbol{r},t)=\frac{\mu_0}{4\pi}\iint\frac{q\boldsymbol{v}_s(t')\delta^3(\boldsymbol{r}'-\boldsymbol{r}_s(t'))}{|\boldsymbol{r}-\boldsymbol{r}'|}\delta(t'-t_{r'})dt'd^3\boldsymbol{r}'$$

We exchange the order of integration:

$$\varphi(\boldsymbol{r},t)=\frac{1}{4\pi\epsilon_0}\iint\frac{\delta(t'-t_{r'})}{|\boldsymbol{r}-\boldsymbol{r}'|}q\delta^3(\boldsymbol{r}'-\boldsymbol{r}_s(t'))d^3\boldsymbol{r}'dt'$$

$$\boldsymbol{A}(\boldsymbol{r},t)=\frac{\mu_0}{4\pi}\iint\frac{\delta(t'-t_{r'})}{|\boldsymbol{r}-\boldsymbol{r}'|}q\boldsymbol{v}_s(t')\delta^3(\boldsymbol{r}'-\boldsymbol{r}_s(t'))d^3\boldsymbol{r}'dt'$$

The delta function picks out $\boldsymbol{r}'=\boldsymbol{r}_s(t')$ which allows us to perform the inner integration with ease. Note that $t_{r'}$ is a function of $\mathbf{r}'$, so this integration also fixes $t_r=t_r(\mathbf{r}_s(t'),t')$.

$$\varphi(\boldsymbol{r},t)=\frac{1}{4\pi\epsilon_0}\int q\frac{\delta(t'-t_{r'})}{|\boldsymbol{r}-\boldsymbol{r}_s(t')|}dt'$$

$$\boldsymbol{A}(\boldsymbol{r},t)=\frac{\mu_0}{4\pi}\int q\boldsymbol{v}_s(t')\frac{\delta(t'-t_{r'})}{|\boldsymbol{r}-\boldsymbol{r}_s(t')|}dt'$$

The retarded time $t_{r'}$ is a function of the field point $(\boldsymbol{r},t)$ and the source trajectory $\boldsymbol{r}_s(t')$, and hence depends on t'. To evaluate this integral, therefore, we need the identity

$$\delta(f(t'))=\sum_i\frac{\delta(t'-t_i)}{|f'(t_i)|}$$

where each t_i is a zero of f. Because there is only one retarded time t_r for any given space-time coordinates $(\mathbf{r},t)$ and source trajectory $\boldsymbol{r}_s(t')$, this reduces to:

$$\delta(t'-t_{r'})=\frac{\delta(t'-t_r)}{\frac{\partial}{\partial t'}(t'-t_{r'})|_{t'=t_r}}=\frac{\delta(t'-t_r)}{\frac{\partial}{\partial t'}(t'-(t-\frac{1}{c}|r-r_s(t')|))|_{t'=t_r}}=\frac{\delta(t'-t_r)}{1+\frac{1}{c}(r-r_s(t'))/|r-r_s(t')|\cdot(-v_s(t'))|_{t'=t_r}}=$$
$$=\frac{\delta(t'-t_r)}{1-\beta_s\cdot(r-r_s)/|r-r_s|}$$

where $\beta_s=v_s/c$ and $\boldsymbol{r}_s$ are evaluated at the retarded time, and we have used the identity $|\boldsymbol{x}|'=\hat{\boldsymbol{x}}\cdot\boldsymbol{v}$. Finally, the delta function picks out $t'=t_r$, and

$$\varphi(r,t)=\frac{1}{4\pi\epsilon_0}\left(\frac{q}{|r-r_s|(1-\beta_s\cdot(r-r_s)/|r-r_s|)}\right)_{t_r}=\frac{1}{4\pi\epsilon_0}\left(\frac{q}{(1-n\cdot\beta_s)|r-r_s|}\right)_{t_r}$$

$$A(\mathrm{r},t)=\frac{\mu_0}{4\pi}\left(\frac{qv}{|\mathrm{r}-r_s|(1-\beta_s\cdot(r-r_s)/|r-r_s|)}\right)_{t_r}=\frac{\mu_0 c}{4\pi}\left(\frac{q\beta_s}{(1-n\cdot\beta_s)|r-r_s|}\right)_{t_r}$$

which are the Liénard–Wiechert potentials.

Lorenz Gauge, Electric and Magnetic Fields

In order to calculate the derivatives of φ and A it is convenient to first compute the derivatives of the retarded time. Taking the derivatives of both sides of its defining equation (remembering that $\boldsymbol{r}_s=\boldsymbol{r}_s(t_r)$):

$$t_r+\frac{1}{c}|\mathbf{r}-\mathbf{r_s}|=t$$

Differentiating with respect to t,

$$\frac{t_r}{dt}+\frac{1}{c}\frac{dt_r}{dt}\frac{d|\mathbf{r}-\mathbf{r_s}|}{dt_r}=1$$

$$\frac{dt_r}{dt}(1-n\cdot\beta_s)=1$$

$$\frac{dt_r}{dt}=\frac{1}{(1-\mathrm{n}\cdot\beta_s)}$$

Similarly, Taking the gradient with respect to $\mathbf{r}$ gives

$$\nabla t_r+\frac{1}{c}\nabla|\boldsymbol{r}-\boldsymbol{r}_s|=0$$

$$\nabla t_r+\frac{1}{c}\left(\nabla t_r\frac{d|\boldsymbol{r}-\boldsymbol{r}_s|}{dt_r}+\boldsymbol{n}\right)=0$$

$$\nabla t_r(1-n\cdot\beta_s)=-n/c$$

$$\nabla t_r=-\frac{\mathrm{n}/c}{(1-\mathrm{n}\cdot\beta_s)}$$

It follows that

$$\frac{d|\mathrm{r}-r_s|}{dt}=\frac{dt_r}{dt}\frac{d|r-r_s|}{dt_r}=\frac{-n\cdot\beta_s c}{(1-n\cdot\beta_s)}$$

$$\nabla|r-r_s|=\nabla t_r\frac{d|r-r_s|}{dt_r}+n=\frac{n}{(1-n\cdot\beta_s)}$$

These can be used in calculating the derivatives of the vector potential and the resulting expressions are

$$\frac{d\varphi}{dt} = -\frac{q}{4\pi\epsilon_0}\frac{1}{|\boldsymbol{r}-\boldsymbol{r}_s|^2\left(1-\boldsymbol{n}\cdot\boldsymbol{\beta}_s\right)^2}\frac{d}{dt}\left[(|\boldsymbol{r}-\boldsymbol{r}_s|(1-\boldsymbol{n}\cdot\boldsymbol{\beta}_s)\right]$$

$$= -\frac{q}{4\pi\epsilon_0}\frac{1}{|\boldsymbol{r}-\boldsymbol{r}_s|^2\left(1-\boldsymbol{n}\cdot\boldsymbol{\beta}_s\right)^2}\frac{d}{dt}\left[|\boldsymbol{r}-\boldsymbol{r}_s|-(\boldsymbol{r}-\boldsymbol{r}_s)\cdot\boldsymbol{\beta}_s\right]$$

$$= -\frac{qc}{4\pi\epsilon_0}\frac{1}{|\boldsymbol{r}-\boldsymbol{r}_s|^2\left(1-\boldsymbol{n}\cdot\boldsymbol{\beta}_s\right)^3}\left[-\boldsymbol{n}\cdot\boldsymbol{\beta}_s+\beta_s^2-(\boldsymbol{r}-\boldsymbol{r}_s)\cdot\dot{\boldsymbol{\beta}}_s/c\right]$$

$$\nabla\cdot\boldsymbol{A} = -\frac{q}{4\pi\epsilon_0 c}\frac{1}{|\boldsymbol{r}-\boldsymbol{r}_s|^2\left(1-\boldsymbol{n}\cdot\boldsymbol{\beta}_s\right)^2}\left(\nabla\left[(|\boldsymbol{r}-\boldsymbol{r}_s|-(\boldsymbol{r}-\boldsymbol{r}_s)\cdot\boldsymbol{\beta}_s)\right]\cdot\boldsymbol{\beta}_s-\left[(|\boldsymbol{r}-\boldsymbol{r}_s|-(\boldsymbol{r}-\boldsymbol{r}_s)\cdot\boldsymbol{\beta}_s)\right]\nabla\cdot\boldsymbol{\beta}_s\right)$$

$$= -\frac{q}{4\pi\epsilon_0 c}\frac{1}{|\boldsymbol{r}-\boldsymbol{r}_s|^2\left(1-\boldsymbol{n}\cdot\boldsymbol{\beta}_s\right)^3}\cdot$$

$$\left[(\boldsymbol{n}\cdot\boldsymbol{\beta}_s)-\beta_s^2(1-\boldsymbol{n}\cdot\boldsymbol{\beta}_s)-\beta_s^2\boldsymbol{n}\cdot\boldsymbol{\beta}_s+\left((\boldsymbol{r}-\boldsymbol{r}_s)\cdot\dot{\boldsymbol{\beta}}_s/c\right)(\boldsymbol{n}\cdot\boldsymbol{\beta}_s)+\left(|\boldsymbol{r}-\boldsymbol{r}_s|-(\boldsymbol{r}-\boldsymbol{r}_s)\cdot\boldsymbol{\beta}_s\right)(\boldsymbol{n}\cdot\dot{\boldsymbol{\beta}}_s/c)\right]$$

$$= \frac{q}{4\pi\epsilon_0 c}\frac{1}{|\boldsymbol{r}-\boldsymbol{r}_s|^2\left(1-\boldsymbol{n}\cdot\boldsymbol{\beta}_s\right)^3}\left[\beta_s^2-\boldsymbol{n}\cdot\boldsymbol{\beta}_s-(\boldsymbol{r}-\boldsymbol{r}_s)\cdot\dot{\boldsymbol{\beta}}_s/c\right]$$

These show that the Lorenz gauge is satisfied, namely that $\frac{d\varphi}{dt}+c^2\nabla\cdot\boldsymbol{A}=0$.

Similarly one calculates:

$$\nabla\varphi = -\frac{q}{4\pi\epsilon_0}\frac{1}{|\boldsymbol{r}-\boldsymbol{r}_s|^2\left(1-\boldsymbol{n}\cdot\boldsymbol{\beta}_s\right)^3}\left[\boldsymbol{n}\left(1-\beta_s^2+(\boldsymbol{r}-\boldsymbol{r}_s)\cdot\dot{\boldsymbol{\beta}}_s/c\right)-\boldsymbol{\beta}_s(1-\boldsymbol{n}\cdot\boldsymbol{\beta}_s)\right]$$

$$\frac{dA}{dt} = \frac{q}{4\pi\epsilon_0}\frac{1}{|\boldsymbol{r}-\boldsymbol{r}_s|^2\left(1-\boldsymbol{n}\cdot\boldsymbol{\beta}_s\right)^3}\left[\boldsymbol{\beta}_s\left(\boldsymbol{n}\cdot\boldsymbol{\beta}_s-\beta_s^2+(\boldsymbol{r}-\boldsymbol{r}_s)\cdot\dot{\boldsymbol{\beta}}_s/c\right)+|\boldsymbol{r}-\boldsymbol{r}_s|\dot{\boldsymbol{\beta}}_s(1-\boldsymbol{n}\cdot\boldsymbol{\beta}_s)/c\right]$$

By noting that for any vectors $\boldsymbol{u}$, $\mathbf{v}$, $\boldsymbol{w}$:

$$\boldsymbol{u}\times(\boldsymbol{v}\times\boldsymbol{w}) = (\boldsymbol{u}\cdot\boldsymbol{w})\boldsymbol{v}-(\boldsymbol{u}\cdot\boldsymbol{v})\boldsymbol{w}$$

The expression for the electric field mentioned above becomes

$$\boldsymbol{E}(\boldsymbol{r},t) = \frac{q}{4\pi\epsilon_0}\frac{1}{|\boldsymbol{r}-\boldsymbol{r}_s|^2(1-\boldsymbol{n}\cdot\boldsymbol{\beta}_s)^3}\cdot$$

$$\left[(\boldsymbol{n}-\boldsymbol{\beta}_s)(1-\beta_s^2)+|\boldsymbol{r}-\boldsymbol{r}_s|(\boldsymbol{n}\cdot\dot{\boldsymbol{\beta}}_s/c)(\boldsymbol{n}-\boldsymbol{\beta}_s)-|\boldsymbol{r}-\boldsymbol{r}_s|\left(\boldsymbol{n}\cdot(\boldsymbol{n}-\boldsymbol{\beta}_s)\right)\dot{\boldsymbol{\beta}}_s/c\right]$$

which is easily seen to be equal to $-\nabla\varphi-\dfrac{d\boldsymbol{A}}{dt}$

Similarly $\nabla\times\boldsymbol{A}$ gives the expression of the magnetic field mentioned above:

$$\boldsymbol{B}=\nabla\times\boldsymbol{A}=-\frac{q}{4\pi\epsilon_0 c}\frac{1}{|\boldsymbol{r}-\boldsymbol{r}_s|^2\left(1-\boldsymbol{n}\cdot\boldsymbol{\beta}_s\right)^2}\left(\nabla\left[\left(|\boldsymbol{r}-\boldsymbol{r}_s|-(\boldsymbol{r}-\boldsymbol{r}_s)\cdot\boldsymbol{\beta}_s\right)\right]\times\boldsymbol{\beta}_s-\left[\left(|\boldsymbol{r}-\boldsymbol{r}_s|-(\boldsymbol{r}-\boldsymbol{r}_s)\cdot\boldsymbol{\beta}_s\right)\right]\nabla\times\boldsymbol{\beta}_s\right)$$

$$=-\frac{q}{4\pi\epsilon_0 c}\frac{1}{|\boldsymbol{r}-\boldsymbol{r}_s|^2\left(1-\boldsymbol{n}\cdot\boldsymbol{\beta}_s\right)^3}\cdot$$

$$\left[(\boldsymbol{n}\times\boldsymbol{\beta}_s)-(\boldsymbol{\beta}_s\times\boldsymbol{\beta}_s)(1-\boldsymbol{n}\cdot\boldsymbol{\beta}_s)-\beta_s^2\boldsymbol{n}\times\boldsymbol{\beta}_s+\left((\boldsymbol{r}-\boldsymbol{r}_s)\cdot\dot{\boldsymbol{\beta}}_s/c\right)(\boldsymbol{n}\times\boldsymbol{\beta}_s)+\left(|\boldsymbol{r}-\boldsymbol{r}_s|-(\boldsymbol{r}-\boldsymbol{r}_s)\cdot\boldsymbol{\beta}_s\right)(\boldsymbol{n}\times\dot{\boldsymbol{\beta}}_s/c)\right]$$

$$=-\frac{q}{4\pi\epsilon_0 c}\frac{1}{|\boldsymbol{r}-\boldsymbol{r}_s|^2(1-\boldsymbol{n}\cdot\boldsymbol{\beta}_s)^3}\cdot$$

$$\left[(\boldsymbol{n}\times\boldsymbol{\beta}_s)(1-\beta_s^2)+|\boldsymbol{r}-\boldsymbol{r}_s|(\boldsymbol{n}\cdot\dot{\boldsymbol{\beta}}_s/c)(\boldsymbol{n}\times\boldsymbol{\beta}_s)+|\boldsymbol{r}-\boldsymbol{r}_s|\left(\boldsymbol{n}\cdot(\boldsymbol{n}-\boldsymbol{\beta}_s)\right)\boldsymbol{n}\times\dot{\boldsymbol{\beta}}_s/c\right]=\frac{\boldsymbol{n}}{c}\times\boldsymbol{E}$$

Implications

The study of classical electrodynamics was instrumental in Einstein's development of the theory of relativity. Analysis of the motion and propagation of electromagnetic waves led to the special relativity description of space and time. The Liénard–Wiechert formulation is an important launchpad into more complex analysis of relativistic moving particles.

The Liénard–Wiechert description is accurate for a large (i.e., not quantum mechanical). independent (i.e., free of external influence) moving particle.The Liénard–Wiechert formulation always provides two sets of solutions: Advanced fields are absorbed by the charges and retarded fields are emitted. Schwarzschild and Fokker considered the advanced field of a system of moving charges, and the retarded field of a system of charges having the same geometry and opposite charges. Linearity of Maxwell's equations in vacuum allows one to add both systems, so that the charges disappear: This trick allows Maxwell's equations to become linear in matter. Multiplying electric parameters of both problems by arbitrary real constants produces a coherent interaction of light with matter which generalizes Einstein's theory (A. Einstein, "Zur Quantentheorie der Strahlung." Phys. Z. 18 121-128, 1917) which is now considered as founding theory of lasers: it is not necessary to study a large set of identical molecules to get coherent amplification in the mode obtained by arbitrary multiplications of advanced and retarded fields. To compute energy, it is necessary to use the absolute fields which includes the zero point field; otherwise, an error appears, for instance in photon counting.

It is important to take into account the zero point field discovered by Planck (M. Planck, Deutsche Physikalische Gesellschaft, 1911). It replaces Einstein's "A" coefficient and explains that the classical electron is stable on Rydberg's classical orbits. Moreover, introducing the fluctuations of the zero point field produces Willis E. Lamb's correction of levels of H atom.

Quantum electrodynamics helped bring together the radiative behavior with the quantum constraints. It introduces quantization of normal modes of the electromagnetic field in assumed perfect optical resonators.

Universal Speed Limit

The force on a particle at a given location $\boldsymbol{r}$ and time t depends in a complicated way on the position of the source particles at an earlier time t_r due to the finite speed, c, at which electromagnetic information travels. A particle on Earth 'sees' a charged particle accelerate on the Moon as this acceleration happened 1.5 seconds ago, and a charged particle's acceleration on the Sun as happened 500 seconds ago. This earlier time in which an event happens such that a particle at location $\boldsymbol{r}$ 'sees' this event at a later time t is called the retarded time, t_r. The retarded time varies with position; for example the retarded time at the Moon is 1.5 seconds before the current time and the retarded time on the Sun is 500 s before the current time on the Earth. The retarded time $t_r=t_r(\boldsymbol{r},t)$ is defined implicitly by

$$t_r = t - \frac{R(t_r)}{c}$$

where $R(t_r)$ is the distance of the particle from the source at the retarded time. Only electromagnetic wave effects depend fully on the retarded time.

A novel feature in the Liénard–Wiechert potential is seen in the breakup of its terms into two types of field terms, only one of which depends fully on the retarded time. The first of these is the static electric (or magnetic) field term that depends only on the distance to the moving charge, and does not depend on the retarded time at all, if the velocity of the source is constant. The other term is dynamic, in that it requires that the moving charge be *accelerating* with a component perpendicular to the line connecting the charge and the observer and does not appear unless the source changes velocity. This second term is connected with electromagnetic radiation.

The first term describes near field effects from the charge, and its direction in space is updated with a term that corrects for any constant-velocity motion of the charge on its distant static field, so that the distant static field appears at distance from the charge, with no aberration of light or light-time correction. This term, which corrects for time-retardation delays in the direction of the static field, is required by Lorentz invariance. A charge moving with a constant velocity must appear to a distant observer in exactly the same way as a static charge appears to a moving observer, and in the latter case, the direction of the static field must change instantaneously, with no time-delay. Thus, static fields (the first term) point exactly at the true instantaneous (non-retarded) position of the charged object if its velocity has not changed over the retarded time delay. This is true over any distance separating objects.

The second term, however, which contains information about the acceleration and other unique behavior of the charge that cannot be removed by changing the Lorentz frame (inertial reference frame of the observer), is fully dependent for direction on the time-retarded position of the source. Thus, electromagnetic radiation (described by the second term) always appears to come from the direction of the position of the emitting charge at the retarded time. Only this second term describes information transfer about the behavior of the charge, which transfer occurs (radiates from the charge) at the speed of light. At "far" distances (longer than several wavelengths of radiation), the 1/R dependence of this term makes electromagnetic field effects (the value of this field term) more powerful than "static" field effects, which are described by the $1/R^2$ field of the first (static) term and thus decay more rapidly with distance from the charge.

Existence and Uniqueness of the Retarded Time

Existence

The retarded time is not guaranteed to exist in general. For example, if, in a given frame of reference, an electron has just been created, then at this very moment another electron does not yet feel its electromagnetic force at all. However, under certain conditions, there always exists a retarded time. For example, if the source charge has existed for an unlimited amount of time, during which it has always travelled at a speed not exceeding $v_M < c$, then there exists a valid retarded time t_r. This can be seen by considering the function $f(t') = |\boldsymbol{r} - \boldsymbol{r}_s(t')| - c(t - t')$. At the present time $t' = t$; $f(t') = |\boldsymbol{r} - \boldsymbol{r}_s(t')| - c(t - t') = |\boldsymbol{r} - \boldsymbol{r}_s(t')| \geq 0$. The derivative $f'(t')$ is given by

$$f'(t') = \frac{\boldsymbol{r} - \boldsymbol{r}_s(t_r)}{|\boldsymbol{r} - \boldsymbol{r}_s(t_r)|} \cdot (-\boldsymbol{v}_s(t')) + c \geq c - \left| \frac{\boldsymbol{r} - \boldsymbol{r}_s(t_r)}{|\boldsymbol{r} - \boldsymbol{r}_s(t_r)|} \right| |\boldsymbol{v}_s(t')| = c - |\boldsymbol{v}_s(t')| \geq c - v_M > 0$$

By the mean value theorem, $f(t - \Delta t) \leq f(t) - f'(t)\Delta t \leq f(t) - (c - v_M)\Delta t$. By making Δt sufficiently large, this can become negative, *i.e.*, at some point in the past, $f(t') < 0$. By the intermediate value theorem, there exists an intermediate t_r with $f(t_r) = 0$, the defining equation of the retarded time. Intuitively, as the source charge moves back in time, the cross section of its light cone at present time expands faster than it can recede, so eventually it must reach the point $\boldsymbol{r}$. This is not necessarily true if the source charge's speed is allowed to be arbitrarily close to c, *i.e.*, if for any given speed $v < c$ there was some time in the past when the charge was moving at this speed. In this case the cross section of the light cone at present time approaches the point $\boldsymbol{r}$ as the observer travels back in time but does not necessarily ever reach it.

Uniqueness

For a given point $(\boldsymbol{r}, t)$ and trajectory of the point source $\boldsymbol{r}_s(t')$, there is at most one value of the retarded time t_r, *i.e.*, one value t_r such that $|\boldsymbol{r} - \boldsymbol{r}_s(t_r)| = c(t - t_r)$. This can be realized by assuming that there are two retarded times t_1 and t_2, with $t_1 \leq t_2$. Then, $|\boldsymbol{r} - \boldsymbol{r}_s(t_1)| = c(t - t_1)$ and $|\boldsymbol{r} - \boldsymbol{r}_s(t_2)| = c(t - t_2)$. Subtracting gives $c(t_2 - t_1) = |\boldsymbol{r} - \boldsymbol{r}_s(t_1)| - |\boldsymbol{r} - \boldsymbol{r}_s(t_2)| \leq |\boldsymbol{r}_s(t_2) - \boldsymbol{r}_s(t_1)|$ by the triangle inequality. Unless $t_2 = t_1$, this then implies that the average velocity of the charge between t_1 and t_2 is $|\boldsymbol{r}_s(t_2) - \boldsymbol{r}_s(t_1)| / (t_2 - t_1) \geq c$, which is impossible. The intuitive interpretation is that one can only ever "see" the point source at one location/time at once unless it travels at least at the speed of light to another location. As the source moves forward in time, the cross section of its light cone at present time contracts faster than the source can approach, so it can never intersect the point $\boldsymbol{r}$ again.

The conclusion is that, under certain conditions, the retarded time exists and is unique.

3

Measurement Units in Electromagnetism

Ampere, coulomb, charge number, tesla, Siemens, farad, ohm, watt, volt and weber are some measurement units in electromagnetism. The base unit of electric current is known as ampere whereas the unit used for electric charge is known as coulomb. The measurement units in electromagnetism are discussed in this chapter.

Ampere

The ampere (SI unit symbol: A, dimension symbol: I), often shortened to "amp", is a unit of electric current. In the International System of Units (SI) the ampere is one of the seven SI base units. It is named after André-Marie Ampère (1775–1836), French mathematician and physicist, considered the father of electrodynamics.

SI defines the ampere in terms of other base units by measuring the electromagnetic force between electrical conductors carrying electric current. The earlier CGS measurement system had two different definitions of current, one essentially the same as the SI's and the other using electric charge as the base unit, with the unit of charge defined by measuring the force between two charged metal plates. The ampere was then defined as one coulomb of charge per second. In SI, the unit of charge, the coulomb, is defined as the charge carried by one ampere during one second.

In the future, the SI definition may shift back to charge as the base unit, with the coulomb defined in terms of the elementary charge on electrons and protons (one coulomb equals the charge of roughly 6.242×10^{18} protons).

Definition

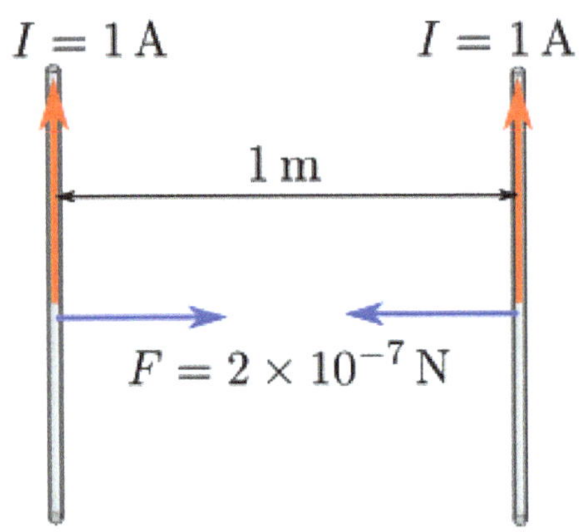

Illustration of the definition of the ampere unit

SI defines ampere as follows:

The ampere is that constant current which, if maintained in two straight parallel conductors of infinite length, of negligible circular cross-section, and placed one metre apart in vacuum, would produce between these conductors a force equal to 2×10^{-7} newtons per metre of length.

Ampère's force law states that there is an attractive or repulsive force between two parallel wires carrying an electric current. This force is used in the formal definition of the ampere.

The SI unit of charge, the coulomb, "is the quantity of electricity carried in 1 second by a current of 1 ampere". Conversely, a current of one ampere is one coulomb of charge going past a given point per second:

$$1A = 1\frac{C}{S}$$

In general, charge Q is determined by steady current I flowing for a time t as $Q = It$.

Constant, instantaneous and average current are expressed in amperes (as in "the charging current is 1.2 A") and the charge accumulated, or passed through a circuit over a period of time is expressed in coulombs (as in "the battery charge is 30000 C"). The relation of the ampere (C/s) to the coulomb is the same as that of the watt (J/s) to the joule.

History

The ampere was originally defined as one tenth of the unit of electric current in the centimetre–gram–second system of units. That unit, now known as the abampere, was defined as the amount of current that generates a force of two dynes per centimetre of length between two wires one centimetre apart. The size of the unit was chosen so that the units derived from it in the MKSA system would be conveniently sized.

The "international ampere" was an early realization of the ampere, defined as the current that would deposit 0.001118 grams of silver per second from a silver nitrate solution. Later, more accurate measurements revealed that this current is 0.99985 A.

Realization

The standard ampere is most accurately realized using a watt balance, but is in practice maintained via Ohm's law from the units of electromotive force and resistance, the volt and the ohm, since the latter two can be tied to physical phenomena that are relatively easy to reproduce, the Josephson junction and the quantum Hall effect, respectively.

At present, techniques to establish the realization of an ampere have a relative uncertainty of approximately a few parts in 10^7, and involve realizations of the watt, the ohm and the volt.

Proposed Future Definition

Rather than a definition in terms of the force between two current-carrying wires, it has been proposed that the ampere should be defined in terms of the rate of flow of elementary charges. Since a coulomb is approximately equal to 6.2415093×10^{18} elementary charges (such as those carried by protons, or the negative of those carried by electrons), one ampere is approximately equivalent to 6.2415093×10^{18} elementary charges moving past a boundary in one second. (6.2415093×10^{18} is the reciprocal of the value of the elementary charge in coulombs.) The proposed change would define 1 A as being the current in the direction of flow of a particular number of elementary charges per second. In 2005, the International Committee for Weights and Measures (CIPM) agreed to study the proposed change. The new definition was discussed at the 25th General Conference on Weights and Measures (CGPM) in 2014 but for the time being was not adopted.

Everyday Examples

The current drawn by typical constant-voltage energy distribution systems is usually dictated by the power (watt) consumed by the system and the operating voltage. For this reason the examples given below are grouped by voltage level.

Portable Devices

- Hearing aid (typically 1 mW at 1.4 V): 700 μA
- USB charging cable (typically 10.5 W at 5.0 V): 2.1 A

Internal Combustion Engine Vehicles – 12 V DC

A typical motor vehicle has a 12 V battery. The various accessories that are powered by the battery might include:

- Instrument panel light (typically 2 W): 166 mA
- Headlight (each, typically 60 W): 5 A
- Starter motor (typically 1–2 kW): 80–160 A

North American Domestic Supply – 120 V AC

Most Canada, Mexico and United States domestic power suppliers run at 120 V.

Household circuit breakers typically provide a maximum of 15 A or 20 A of current to a given set of outlets.

- 22-inch/56-centimeter portable television (35 W): 290 mA
- Tungsten light bulb (60–100 W): 500–830 mA
- Toaster, kettle (1.5 kW): 12.5 A
- Hair dryer (1.8 kW): 15 A
- USB cell phone charger (typically 10 W): 83 mA

European & Commonwealth Domestic Supply – 230–240 V AC

Most European domestic power supplies run at 230 V, and most Commonwealth domestic power supplies run at 240 V. For the same amount of power (in watts), the current drawn by a particular European or Commonwealth appliance (in Europe or a Commonwealth country) will be less than for an equivalent North American appliance. Typical circuit breakers will provide 16 A.

The current drawn by a number of typical appliances are:

- 22-inch/56-centimeter portable television (35 W): 145–150 mA
- Tungsten light bulb (60–100 W): 240–450 mA
- Compact fluorescent lamp (11–30 W): 56–112 mA
- Toaster, kettle (2 kW): 9 A
- Immersion heater (4.6 kW): 19–20 A

Coulomb

The coulomb (unit symbol: C) is the International System of Units (SI) unit of electric charge. It is the charge (symbol: Q or q) transported by a constant current of one ampere in one second:

$$1\,\mathrm{C} = 1\,\mathrm{A} \cdot 1\,\mathrm{s}$$

Thus, it is also the amount of excess charge on a capacitor of one farad charged to a potential difference of one volt:

$$1\,\mathrm{C} = 1\,\mathrm{F} \cdot 1\,\mathrm{V}$$

It is equivalent to the charge of approximately 6.242×10^{18} (1.036×10^{-5} mol) protons, and −1 C is equivalent to the charge of approximately 6.242×10^{18} electrons.

Name and Notation

This SI unit is named after Charles-Augustin de Coulomb. As with every International System of Units (SI) unit named for a person, the first letter of its symbol is upper case (C). However, when an SI unit is spelled out in English, it should always begin with a lower case letter (*coulomb*)—except in a situation where *any* word in that position would be capitalized, such as at the beginning of a sentence or in material using title case. Note that "degree Celsius" conforms to this rule because the "d" is lowercase.— based on *The International System of Units*.

Definition

The SI system defines the coulomb in terms of the ampere and second: 1 C = 1 A × 1 s. The second is defined in terms of a frequency naturally emitted by caesium atoms. The ampere is defined using Ampère's force law; the definition relies in part on the mass of the international prototype kilogram, a metal cylinder housed in France. In practice, the watt balance is used to measure amperes with the highest possible accuracy.

Since the charge of one electron is known to be about 1.6021766208(98)×10^{-19} C, 1 C can also be considered the charge of roughly 6.241509×10^{18} electrons (or +1 C the charge of that many positrons or protons), where the number is the reciprocal of 1.602177×10^{-19}.

The proposed redefinition of the ampere and other SI base units would have the effect of fixing the numerical value of the elementary charge to an explicit constant expressed in coulombs, and therefore it would implicitly fix the value of the coulomb when expressed as a multiple of the fundamental charge (the numerical values of those quantities are the multiplicative inverses of each other).

SI Prefixes

SI multiples for coulomb (C)						
Submultiples				**Multiples**		
Value	**SI symbol**	**Name**		**Value**	**SI symbol**	**Name**
10^{-1} C	dC	decicoulomb		10^{1} C	daC	decacoulomb
10^{-2} C	cC	centicoulomb		10^{2} C	hC	hectocoulomb
10^{-3} C	mC	millicoulomb		10^{3} C	kC	kilocoulomb
10^{-6} C	μC	microcoulomb		10^{6} C	MC	megacoulomb
10^{-9} C	nC	nanocoulomb		10^{9} C	GC	gigacoulomb
10^{-12} C	pC	picocoulomb		10^{12} C	TC	teracoulomb
10^{-15} C	fC	femtocoulomb		10^{15} C	PC	petacoulomb
10^{-18} C	aC	attocoulomb		10^{18} C	EC	exacoulomb
10^{-21} C	zC	zeptocoulomb		10^{21} C	ZC	zettacoulomb
10^{-24} C	yC	yoctocoulomb		10^{24} C	YC	yottacoulomb
Common multiples are in bold face.						

Conversions

- One coulomb is the magnitude (absolute value) of electrical charge in 6.24150934(14)×10^{18} protons or electrons.
- The inverse of this number gives the elementary charge of 1.6021766208(98)×10^{-19} C.
- The magnitude of the electrical charge of one mole of elementary charges (approximately 6.022×10^{23}, or Avogadro's number) is known as a faraday unit of charge (closely related to the Faraday constant). One faraday equals 96485.3399 coulombs. In terms of Avogadro's number (N_A), one coulomb is equal to approximately 1.036 × N_A×10^{-5} elementary charges.
- One ampere-hour = 3600 C, 1 mA·h = 3.6 C.
- One statcoulomb (statC), the obsolete CGS electrostatic unit of charge (esu), is approximately 3.3356×10^{-10} C or about one-third of a nanocoulomb.

Relation to Elementary Charge

The elementary charge, the charge of a proton (equivalently, the negative of the charge of an electron), is approximately 1.6021766208(98)×10^{-19} C. In SI, the elementary charge in coulombs is an approximate value: no experiment can be infinitely accurate. However, in other unit systems, the elementary charge has an *exact* value by definition, and other charges are ultimately measured relative to the elementary charge. For example, in conventional electrical units, the values of the Josephson constant K_J and von Klitzing constant R_K are exact defined values (written $K_{J\text{-}90}$ and $R_{K\text{-}90}$), and it follows that the elementary charge $e = 2/(K_J R_K)$ is also an exact defined value in this unit system. Specifically, $e_{90} = (2\times10^{-9})/(25812.807 \times 483597.9)$ C exactly. SI itself may someday change its definitions in a similar way. For example, one possible proposed redefinition is "the ampere...is [defined] such that the value of the elementary charge *e* (charge on a proton) is exactly $1.602176487\times10^{-19}$ coulombs», (in which the numeric value is the 2006 CODATA recommended value, since superseded). This proposal is not yet accepted as part of the SI.

In Everyday Terms

- The charges in static electricity from rubbing materials together are typically a few microcoulombs.
- The amount of charge that travels through a lightning bolt is typically around 15 C, although large bolts can be up to 350 C.
- The amount of charge that travels through a typical alkaline AA battery from being fully charged to discharged is about 5 kC = 5000 C ≈ 1400 mA·h.
- The hydraulic analogy uses everyday terms to illustrate movement of charge and the transfer of energy. The analogy equates charge to a volume of water, and voltage to pressure. One coulomb equals (the negative of) the charge of 6.24×10^{18} electrons. The amount of energy transferred by the flow of 1 coulomb can vary; for example, 300 times fewer electrons flow through a lightning bolt than in the discharge of an AA battery, but the total energy transferred by the flow of the lightning›s electrons is 300 million times greater.

Charge Number

Charge number (z) refers to a quantized value of electric charge, with the quantum of electric charge being the elementary charge, so that the charge number equals the electric charge (q) in coulombs divided by the elementary-charge constant (e), or $z = q/e$. The charge numbers for ions (and also subatomic particles) are written in superscript, e.g. Na^+ is a sodium ion with charge number positive one (an electric charge of one elementary charge). Atomic numbers (Z) are a special case of charge numbers, referring to the charge number of an atomic nucleus, as opposed to the net charge of an atom or ion. All particles of ordinary matter have integer-value charge numbers, with the exception of quarks, which cannot exist in isolation under ordinary circumstances (the strong force keeps them bound into hadrons of integer charge numbers).

Charge Numbers in Chemistry

Charge number or valence of an ion is the coefficient that, when multiplied by the elementary charge, gives the ion's charge.

For example, the charge on a chloride ion, Cl^-, is $-1 \cdot e$, where e is the elementary charge. This means that the charge number for the ion is -1.

z is used as the symbol for the charge number. In that case, the charge of an ion could be written as $Q = ze$.

The charge number in chemistry normally relates to an electric charge. This is a property of specific subatomic atoms. Theses elements define the electromagnetic contact between the two elements.

A chemical charge can be found by using the periodic table. An element's placement on the periodic table indicates whether its chemical charge is negative or positive. Looking at the equation, one can see that the positive charges are on the left side of the table and the negative charges are on the right side of the table. Charges that are positive are called cations. Charges that are negative are called anions. Elements in the same group have the same charge. A group in the periodic table is a term used to represent the vertical columns.

The noble gases of the periodic table do not have a charge because they are nonreactive. Noble gases are considered stable since they contain the desired eight electrons. The other atoms or ions have charges because they are very reactive and want to react with another atom or ion to become stable. When elements are bonded, they can either be bonded by ionic bonding or covalent bonding. When elements bond between positive and negative charged atoms, their charges will be switched and carried down on the other element to combine them equally. This is shown below. Using the chart provided, if ammonium with a plus 1 charge is combined with an acetate ion with a negative 1 charge, the charges will be cancelled out, shown in the equation.

$$[NH]_4^+ + C_2\,H_3\,O_2^- \rightarrow [NH]_4\,C_2\,H_3\,O_2$$

When two ions are combined with different charges, the charges do not get canceled out. They get carried over and placed at the end of the other ion. This is shown below between ammonium and carbonate.

$$2[NH]_4^+ + [C\,O]_3^{(2-)} \rightarrow [(NH)_4]_2\,[C\,O]_3$$

The ammonium part on the product side has to have parenthesis in order to distinguish between the ammonium subscript 4 compared to the 2 charge that has been dropped down, connected to it.

$$[NH]_4^+ + C_2\,H_3\,O_2^- \rightarrow [NH]_4\,C_2\,H_3\,O_2$$

When two ions are combined with different charges, the charges do not get canceled out. They get carried over and placed at the end of the other ion. This is shown below between ammonium and carbonate.

$$[NH]_4^+ + [CO]_3^{(2-)} \rightarrow [(NH)_4]_2\,[CO]_3$$

The ammonium part on the product side has to have parenthesis in order to distinguish between the ammonium subscript 4 compared to the 2 charge that has been dropped down, connected to it.

Charge numbers also help to determine other aspects of chemistry. One example is that someone can use the charge of an ion to find the oxidation number of a monatomic ion. For example, the oxidation number of $[Li]^+$ is +1. This helps when trying to solve oxidation questions.

A charge number also can help when drawing Lewis dot structures. For example, if the structure is an ion, the charge will be included outside of the Lewis dot structure.

Since there is a negative charge on the outside of the Lewis dot structure, one electron needs to be added to the structure. If the charge was positive, an electron would be lost and taken away.

Charge Numbers in Nuclear and Hadron Physics

For an atomic nucleus, which can be regarded as an ion having stripped off all electrons, the charge number is identical with the atomic number Z, which corresponds to the number of protons in ordinary atomic nuclei.

Unlike in chemistry, subatomic particles with electric charges of two elementary charges (e.g. some delta baryons) are indicated with a superscript "++" or "−−". In chemistry, the same charge numbers are usually indicated as superscript "+2" or "−2".

Charge Numbers in Elementary-particle Physics

In particle physics, the charge number is a (derived) flavor quantum number. For color-charged particles like quarks and hypothetical leptoquarks, the charge number is a multiple of 1/3.

Tesla (Unit)

The tesla (symbol T) is a unit of measurement of the strength of a magnetic field. It is a derived unit of the International System of Units, the modern form of the metric system.

One tesla is equal to one weber per square metre. The unit was announced during the General Conference on Weights and Measures in 1960 and is named in honour of Nikola Tesla, upon the proposal of the Slovenian electrical engineer France Avčin.

The strongest fields encountered from permanent magnets are from Halbach spheres and can be over 4.5 T. The strongest field trapped in a laboratory superconductor as of June 2014 is 21 T. The record magnetic field has been produced by scientists at the Los Alamos National Laboratory campus of the National High Magnetic Field Laboratory, the world's first 100-tesla non-destructive magnetic field.

Definition

A particle, carrying a charge of one coulomb, and passing through a magnetic field of one tesla, at a speed of one metre per second, perpendicular to said field, experiences a force with magnitude one newton, according to the Lorentz force law. As an SI derived unit, the tesla can also be expressed as:

$$\mathrm{T} = \frac{\mathrm{V \cdot s}}{\mathrm{m^2}} = \frac{\mathrm{N}}{\mathrm{A \cdot m}} = \frac{\mathrm{J}}{\mathrm{A \cdot m^2}} = \frac{\mathrm{H \cdot A}}{\mathrm{m^2}} = \frac{\mathrm{Wb}}{\mathrm{m^2}} = \frac{\mathrm{kg}}{\mathrm{C \cdot s}} = \frac{\mathrm{N \cdot s}}{\mathrm{C \cdot m}} = \frac{\mathrm{kg}}{\mathrm{A \cdot s^2}}$$

(The last equivalent is in SI base units).

Units used:

A = ampere

C = coulomb

kg = kilogram

m = metre

N = newton

s = second

H = henry

V = volt

J = joule

Wb = weber

Electric vs. Magnetic Field

In the production of the Lorentz force, the difference between these fields is that a force from a magnetic field on a charged particle is generally due to the charged particle's movement, while the force imparted by an electric field on a charged particle is not due to the charged particle's movement. This may be appreciated by looking at the units for each. The unit of electric field in the MKS system of units is newtons per coulomb, N/C, while the magnetic field (in teslas) can be written as N/(C·m/s). The dividing factor between the two types of field is metres per second (m/s), which is velocity. This relationship immediately highlights the fact that whether a static electromagnetic field is seen as purely magnetic, or purely electric, or some combination of these, is dependent upon one's reference frame (that is, one's velocity relative to the field).

In ferromagnets, the movement creating the magnetic field is the electron spin (and to a lesser extent electron orbital angular momentum). In a current-carrying wire (electromagnets) the movement is due to electrons moving through the wire (whether the wire is straight or circular).

Conversions

One tesla is equivalent to:

10,000 (or 10^4) G (gauss), used in the CGS system. Thus, 10 kG = 1 T (tesla), and 1 G = 10^{-4} T.

1,000,000,000 (or 10^9) γ (gamma), used in geophysics. Thus, 1 γ = 1 nT (nanotesla).

42.6 MHz of the ^{1}H nucleus frequency, in NMR. Thus, the magnetic field associated with NMR at 1 GHz is 23.5 T.

One tesla is equal to 1 V·s/m^2. This can be shown by starting with the speed of light in vacuum, *c*

= $(\varepsilon_0\mu_0)^{-1/2}$, and inserting the SI values and units for *c* (2.998×10^8 m/s), the vacuum permittivity ε_0 (8.85×10^{-12} A·s/(V·m)), and the vacuum permeability μ_0 (12.566×10^{-7} T·m/A). Cancellation of numbers and units then produces this relation.

For those concerned with low-frequency electromagnetic radiation in the home, the following conversions are needed most:

1000 nT (nanotesla) = 1 µT (microtesla) = 10 mG (milligauss),

1,000,000 µT = 1 T.

Siemens (Unit)

The siemens (SI unit symbol: S) is the unit of electric conductance, electric susceptance and electric admittance in the International System of Units (SI). Conductance, susceptance, and admittance are the reciprocals of resistance, reactance, and impedance respectively; hence one siemens is equal to the reciprocal of one ohm, and is also referred to as the *mho*. The 14th General Conference on Weights and Measures approved the addition of the siemens as a derived unit in 1971.

The unit is named after Ernst Werner von Siemens. In English, the same form *siemens* is used both for the singular and plural.

Definition

For a conducting or semiconducting element, electrical resistance *R* and electrical conductance *G* are defined as

$$G = \frac{1}{R} = \frac{I}{V}$$

where *I* is the electric current through the object and *V* is the voltage (electrical potential difference) across the object.

The unit siemens for the conductance *G* is defined by

$$\mathrm{S} = \Omega^{-1} = \frac{\mathrm{A}}{\mathrm{V}}$$

where Ω is the ohm, A is the ampere, and V is the volt.

For a device with a conductance of one siemens, the electric current through the device will increase by one ampere for every increase of one volt of electric potential difference across the device.

The conductance of a resistor with a resistance of five ohms, for example, is $(5\ \Omega)^{-1}$, which is equal to 200 mS.

Mho

Mho /moʊ/ is an alternative name of the same unit, the reciprocal of one ohm. Mho is derived from spelling *ohm* backwards (a semordnilap) and is written with an upside-down capital Greek letter Omega: ℧, Unicode symbol U+2127 (℧). According to Maver the term *mho* was suggested by Sir William Thomson (Lord Kelvin). The *mho* was officially renamed to the *siemens*, replacing the old meaning of the "*siemens* unit", at a conference in 1881.

The term *siemens*, as it is an SI term, is used universally in science and often in electrical applications, while *mho* is still used primarily in electronic applications. The inverted Omega, while not an official SI abbreviation, has the advantage of being less likely to be confused with a variable than the letter S when doing algebraic calculations by hand, where the usual typographical distinctions (such as italic for variables and Roman for unit names) are difficult to maintain. Likewise, it is difficult to distinguish the symbol *S* from the lower-case *s* where *second* is meant, potentially causing confusion. So, for example, a pentode's transconductance of 2.2 mS might alternatively be written as 2.2 m℧ or 2200 micromhos (most common in the 1930's) or 2.2 mA/V.

Farad

The farad (symbol: F) is the SI derived unit of electrical capacitance, the ability of a body to store an electrical charge. It is named after the English physicist Michael Faraday.

Definition

One farad is defined as the capacitance across which, when charged with one coulomb, there is a potential difference of one volt. Equally, one farad can be described as the capacitance which stores a one-coulomb charge across a potential difference of one volt.

The relationship between capacitance, charge and potential difference is linear. For example, if the potential difference across a capacitor is halved, the quantity of charge stored by that capacitor will also be halved.

For most applications, the farad is an impractically large unit of capacitance. Most electrical and electronic applications are covered by the following SI prefixes:

- 1 mF (millifarad, one thousandth (10^{-3}) of a farad) = 1000 μF = 1000000 nF
- 1 μF (microfarad, one millionth (10^{-6}) of a farad) = 0.000 001 F = 1000 nF = 1000000 pF
- 1 nF (nanofarad, one billionth (10^{-9}) of a farad) = 0.001 μF = 1000 pF
- 1 pF (picofarad, one trillionth (10^{-12}) of a farad)

Equalities

A farad has the base SI representation of: $s^4 \times A^2 \times m^{-2} \times kg^{-1}$

It can further be expressed as:

$$\mathrm{F} = \frac{\mathrm{A}\cdot\mathrm{s}}{V} = \frac{\mathrm{J}}{V^2} = \frac{\mathrm{W}\cdot\mathrm{s}}{V^2} = \frac{\mathrm{C}}{V} = \frac{\mathrm{C}^2}{J} = \frac{\mathrm{C}^2}{N\cdot m} = \frac{\mathrm{s}^2\cdot\mathrm{C}^2}{m^2\cdot kg} = \frac{\mathrm{s}^4\cdot\mathrm{A}^2}{m^2\cdot kg} = \frac{\mathrm{s}}{\Omega} = \frac{\mathrm{s}^2}{\mathrm{H}}$$

where F=farad, A=ampere, V=volt, C=coulomb, J=joule, m=metre, N=newton, s=second, W=watt, kg=kilogram, Ω=ohm, H=henry.

History

The term “farad” was originally coined by Latimer Clark and Charles Bright in 1861, in honor of Michael Faraday, for a unit of quantity of charge but by 1873, the farad had become a unit of capacitance. In 1881 at the International Congress of Electricians in Paris, the name farad was officially used for the unit of electrical capacitance.

Explanation

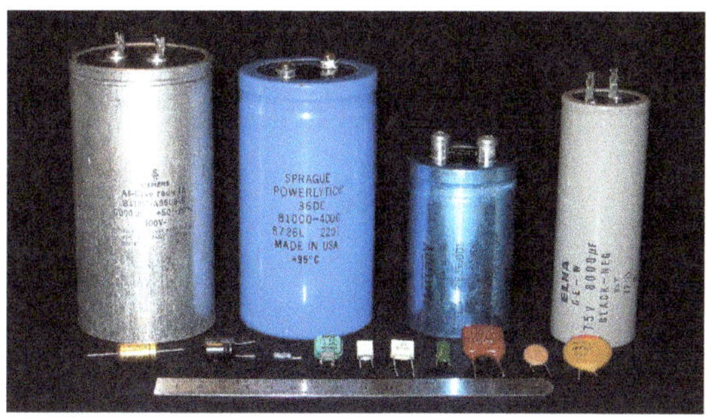

Examples of different types of capacitors

A capacitor generally consists of two conducting surfaces, frequently referred to as plates, separated by an insulating layer usually referred to as a dielectric. The original capacitor was the Leyden jar developed in the 18th century. It is the accumulation of electric charge on the plates that results in capacitance. Modern capacitors are constructed using a range of manufacturing techniques and materials to provide the extraordinarily wide range of capacitance values used in electronics applications from femtofarads to farads, with maximum-voltage ratings ranging from a few volts to several kilovolts.

Values of capacitors are usually specified in farads (F), microfarads (μF), nanofarads (nF) and picofarads (pF). The millifarad is rarely used in practice (a capacitance of 4.7 mF (0.0047 F), for example, is instead written as 4700 μF), while the nanofarad is uncommon in North America. The size of commercially available capacitors ranges from around 0.1 pF to 5000F (5 kF) supercapacitors. Parasitic capacitance in high-performance integrated circuits can be measured in femtofarads (1 fF = 0.001 pF = 10^{-15} F), while high-performance test equipment can detect changes in capacitance on the order of tens of attofarads (1 aF = 10^{-18} F).

A value of 0.1 pF is about the smallest available in capacitors for general use in electronic design, since smaller ones would be dominated by the parasitic capacitances of other components, wiring or printed circuit boards. Capacitance values of 1 pF or lower can be achieved by twisting two short lengths of insulated wire together.

The capacitance of the Earth’s ionosphere with respect to the ground is calculated to be about 1 F.

Informal and Deprecated Terminology

The picofarad is sometimes colloquially pronounced as "puff" or "pic", as in "a ten-puff capacitor". Similarly, "mic" (pronounced "mike") is sometimes used informally to signify microfarads. If the Greek letter μ is not available, the notation "uF" is often used as a substitute for "μF" in electronics literature. A "micro-microfarad" (μμF, and confusingly often mmf or MMF), an obsolete unit sometimes found in older texts, is the equivalent of a picofarad. In texts prior to 1960, and on capacitor packages even much more recently, mf or MFD rather than the modern μF frequently represented microfarads. Similarly, mmf or MMFD represented picofarads.

Related Concepts

The reciprocal of capacitance is called electrical elastance, the (non-standard, non-SI) unit of which is the daraf.

CGS units

The abfarad (abbreviated abF) is an obsolete CGS unit of capacitance equal to 10^9 farads (1 gigafarad, GF).

The statfarad (abbreviated statF) is a rarely used CGS unit equivalent to the capacitance of a capacitor with a charge of 1 statcoulomb across a potential difference of 1 statvolt. It is $1/(10^{-5}c^2)$ farad, approximately 1.1126 picofarads.

Henry (Unit)

The henry (symbol H) is the SI derived unit of electrical inductance. The unit is named after Joseph Henry (1797–1878), the American scientist who discovered electromagnetic induction independently of and at about the same time as Michael Faraday (1791–1867) in England. The magnetic permeability of vacuum is $4\pi \times 10^{-7}$ H·m^{-1} (henry per metre).

Definition

The inductance of an electric circuit is one henry when an electric current that is changing at one ampere per second results in an electromotive force of one volt across the inductor:

$$v(t) = L\frac{di}{dt},$$

where $v(t)$ denotes the resulting voltage across the circuit, $i(t)$ is the current through the circuit, and L is the inductance of the circuit.

The henry is a derived unit based on four of the seven base units of the International System of Units: kilogram (kg), meter (m), second (s), and ampere (A). Expressed in combinations of SI units, the henry is:

$$H = \frac{kg \cdot m^2}{s^2 \cdot A^2} = \frac{kg \cdot m^2}{C^2} = \frac{J}{A^2} = \frac{T \cdot m^2}{A} = \frac{Wb}{A} = \frac{V \cdot s}{A} = \frac{s^2}{F} = \frac{1}{F \cdot Hz^2} = \Omega \cdot s$$

where

Wb = weber,

T = tesla,

J = joule,

m = meter,

s = second,

A = ampere,

V = volt,

C = coulomb,

F = farad,

Hz = hertz,

Ω = ohm.

Use

As with every International System of Units (SI) unit named for a person, the first letter of its symbol is upper case (H). However, when an SI unit is spelled out in English, it should always begin with a lower case letter (henry)—except in a situation where any word in that position would be capitalized, such as at the beginning of a sentence or in material using title case.

The United States National Institute of Standards and Technology recommends English-speaking users of SI to write the plural as *henries*.

Ohm

The ohm (symbol: Ω) is the SI derived unit of electrical resistance, named after German physicist Georg Simon Ohm. Although several empirically derived standard units for expressing electrical resistance were developed in connection with early telegraphy practice, the British Association for the Advancement of Science proposed a unit derived from existing units of mass, length and time and of a convenient size for practical work as early as 1861. The definition of the ohm was revised several times. Today the definition of the ohm is expressed from the quantum Hall effect.

Definition

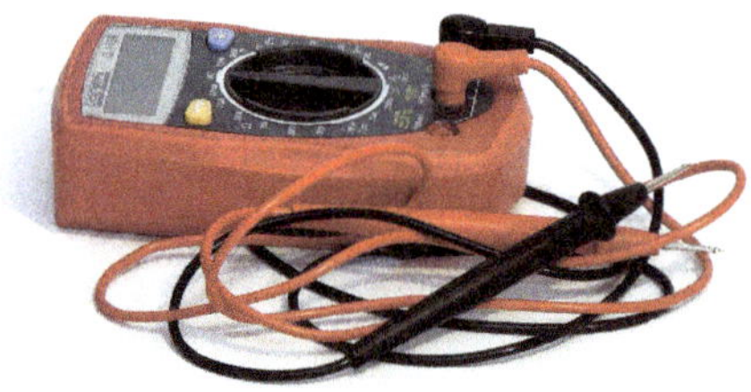

A multimeter can be used to measure resistance in ohms, among other things.

The ohm is defined as an electrical resistance between two points of a conductor when a constant potential difference of 1 volt, applied to these points, produces in the conductor a current of 1 ampere, the conductor not being the seat of any electromotive force.

$$\Omega = \frac{V}{A} = \frac{1}{S} = \frac{W}{A^2} = \frac{V^2}{W} = \frac{s}{F} = \frac{J \cdot s}{C^2} = \frac{kg \cdot m^2}{s \cdot C^2} = \frac{J}{s \cdot A^2} = \frac{kg \cdot m^2}{s^3 \cdot A^2}$$

in which the following units appear: volt (V), ampere (A), siemens (S), watt (W), second (s), farad (F), joule (J), kilogram (kg), metre (m), and coulomb (C).

In many cases the resistance of a conductor in ohms is approximately constant within a certain range of voltages, temperatures, and other parameters. These are called linear resistors. In other cases resistance varies (e.g., thermistors).

Commonly used multiples and submultiples in electrical and electronic usage are the microohm, milliohm, kilohm, megohm, and gigaohm; the term "gigohm", though not official, is in common use for the latter.

In alternating current circuits, electrical impedance is also measured in ohms.

Conversions

The siemens (symbol: S) is the SI derived unit of electric conductance and admittance, also known as the mho (ohm spelled backwards, symbol is ℧); it is the reciprocal of resistance in ohms (Ω).

Power as a Function of Resistance

The power dissipated by a resistor may be calculated from its resistance, and the voltage or current involved. The formula is a combination of Ohm's Law and Joule's law:

$$P = V \cdot I = \frac{V^2}{R} = I^2 \cdot R$$

where:

P = power in watts

R = resistance in ohms

V = voltage across the resistor

I = current through the resistor in amps

A linear resistor has a constant resistance value over all applied voltages or currents; many practical resistors are linear over a useful range of currents. Non-linear resistors have a value that may vary depending on the applied voltage (or current). Where alternating current is applied to the circuit,(or where the resistance value is a function of time), the relation above is true at any instant but calculation of average power over an interval of time will require integration of "instantaneous" power over that interval.

History

The rapid rise of electrotechnology in the last half of the 19th century created a demand for a rational, coherent, consistent, and international system of units for electrical quantities. Telegraphers and other early users of electricity in the 19th century needed a practical standard unit of measurement for resistance. Resistance was often expressed as a multiple of the resistance of a standard length of telegraph wires; different agencies used different bases for a standard, so units were not readily interchangeable. Electrical units so defined were not a coherent system with the units for energy, mass, length, and time, requiring conversion factors to be used in calculations relating energy or power to resistance.

Two different methods of establishing a system of electrical units can be chosen. Various artifacts, such as a length of wire or a standard electrochemical cell, could be specified as producing defined quantities for resistance, voltage, and so on. Alternatively, the electrical units can be related to the mechanical units by defining, for example, a unit of current that gives a specified force between two wires, or a unit of charge that gives a unit of force between two unit charges. This latter method ensures coherence with the units of energy. Defining a unit for resistance that is coherent with units of energy and time in effect also requires defining units for potential and current. It is desirable that one unit of electrical potential will force one unit of electric current through one unit of electrical resistance, doing one unit of work in one unit of time, otherwise all electrical calculations will require conversion factors.

Since so-called "absolute" units of charge and current are expressed as combinations of units of mass, length, and time, dimensional analysis of the relations between potential, current, and resistance show that resistance is expressed in units of length per time — a velocity. Some early definitions of a unit of resistance, for example, defined a unit resistance as one quadrant of the Earth per second.

The absolute-units system related magnetic and electrostatic quantities to metric base units of mass, time, and length. These units had the great advantage of simplifying the equations used in the solution of electromagnetic problems, and eliminated conversion factors in calculations about electrical quantities. However, the centimeter-gram-second, CGS, units turned out to have impractical sizes for practical measurements.

Various artifact standards were proposed as the definition of the unit of resistance. In 1860 Werner Siemens (1816–1892) published a suggestion for a reproducible resistance standard in Poggendorffs Annalen der Physik und Chemie. He proposed a column of pure mercury, of one square millimetre cross section, one metre long: Siemens mercury unit. However, this unit was not coherent with other units. One proposal was to devise a unit based on a mercury column that would be coherent – in effect, adjusting the length to make the resistance one ohm. Not all users of units had the resources to carry out metrology experiments to the required precision, so working standards notionally based on the physical definition were required.

In 1861, Latimer Clark (1822–1898) and Sir Charles Bright (1832–1888) presented a paper at the British Association for the Advancement of Science meeting suggesting that standards for electrical units be established and suggesting names for these units derived from eminent philosophers, 'Ohma', 'Farad' and 'Volt'. The BAAS in 1861 appointed a committee including Maxwell and Thomson to report upon Standards of Electrical Resistance. Their objectives were to devise a unit that was of convenient size, part of a complete system for electrical measurements, coherent with the units for energy, stable, reproducible and based on the French metrical system. In the third report of the committee, 1864, the resistance unit is referred to as "B.A. unit, or Ohmad". By 1867 the unit is referred to as simply Ohm.

The B.A. ohm was intended to be 10^9 CGS units but owing to an error in calculations the definition was 1.3% too small. The error was significant for preparation of working standards.

On September 21, 1881 the *Congrès internationale d'électriciens* (international conference of electricians) defined a *practical* unit of Ohm for the resistance, based on CGS units, using a mercury column at zero deg. Celsius, similar to the apparatus suggested by Siemens.

A *legal* ohm, a reproducible standard, was defined by the international conference of electricians at Paris in 1884 as the resistance of a mercury column of specified weight and 106 cm long; this was a compromise value between the B. A. unit (equivalent to 104.7 cm), the Siemens unit (100 cm by definition), and the CGS unit. Although called "legal", this standard was not adopted by any national legislation. The "international" ohm was defined as a mercury column 106.3 cm long of mass 14.4521 grams and 0 °C at the International Electrical Conference 1893 in Chicago. This definition became the basis for the legal definition of the ohm in several countries. In 1908, the next Electrical Conference confirmed this definition. The mercury column standard was maintained until the 1948 General Conference on Weights and Measures, at which the ohm was redefined in absolute terms instead of as an artifact standard.

By the end of the 19th century, units were well-understood and consistent. Definitions would change with little effect on commercial uses of the units. Advances in metrology allowed definitions to be formulated with a high degree of precision and repeatability.

Historical Units of Resistance

Unit	Definition	Value in B.A. ohms	Remarks
Absolute foot/second x 10^7	using Imperial units	.3048	considered obsolete even in 1884
Thomson's unit	using Imperial units	.3202	100 million feet/second, considered obsolete even in 1884
Jacobi copper unit	A specified copper wire 25 feet long weighing 345 grains	.6367	Used in 1850s

Weber's absolute unit × 10^7	Based on the metre and the second	0.9191	
Siemens mercury unit	1860. A column of pure mercury	.9537	100 cm and 1 mm^2 cross section at 0 °C
British Association (B.A.) "ohm"	1863	1.000	Standard coils deposited at Kew Observatory in 1863
Digney, Breguet, Swiss		9.266–10.420	Iron wire 1 km long and 4 square mm cross section
Matthiessen		13.59	One mile of 1/16 inch diameter pure annealed copper wire at 15.5 °C
Varley		25.61	One mile of special 1/16 inch diameter copper wire
German mile		57.44	A German mile (8,238 yard) of iron wire 1/6th inch diameter
Abohm		10^{-9}	Electromagnetic absolute unit in cm-gram-second units
Statohm		$8.987551787 \times 10^{11}$	Electrostatic absolute unit in cm-gram-second units

Realization of Standards

The mercury column method of realizing a physical standard ohm turned out to be difficult to reproduce, owing to the effects of non-constant cross section of the glass tubing. Various resistance coils were constructed by the British Association and others, to serve as physical artifact standards for the unit of resistance. The long-term stability and reproducibility of these artifacts was an ongoing field of research, as the effects of temperature, air pressure, humidity, and time on the standards were detected and analyzed.

Artifact standards are still used, but metrology experiments relating accurately-dimensioned inductors and capacitors provided a more fundamental basis for the definition of the ohm. Since 1990 the quantum Hall effect has been used to define the ohm with high precision and repeatability. The quantum Hall experiments are used to check the stability of working standards that have convenient values for comparison.

Symbol

The symbol Ω was suggested, because of the similar sound of ohm and omega, by William Henry Preece in 1867. In documents printed before WWII the unit symbol often consisted of the raised lowercase omega (ω), such that 56 Ω was written as 56^{ω}.

When preparing electronic documents, some document editing software applications have used the Symbol typeface to render the character Ω. Where the font is not supported, a W is displayed instead ("10 W" instead of "10 Ω", for instance). As W represents the watt, the SI unit of power, this can lead to confusion.

In the electronics industry it is common to use the character R instead of the Ω symbol, thus, a 10 Ω resistor may be represented as 10R. This is the British standard BS 1852 code. It is used in many instances where the value has a decimal place. For example, 5.6 Ω is listed as 5R6. This method avoids overlooking the decimal period, which may not be rendered reliably on components or when duplicating documents.

Unicode encodes the symbol as U+2126 Ω OHM SIGN, distinct from Greek omega among letterlike symbols, but it is only included for backwards compatibility and the Greek uppercase omega character U+03A9 Ω GREEK CAPITAL LETTER OMEGA (HTML Ω · Ω) is preferred. In DOS and Windows, the alt code ALT 234 may produce the Ω symbol. In Mac OS, ⌥ Opt+Z does the same.

Volt

The volt (symbol: V) is the derived unit for electric potential, electric potential difference (voltage), and electromotive force.

Definition

One volt is defined as the difference in electric potential between two points of a conducting wire when an electric current of one ampere dissipates one watt of power between those points. It is also equal to the potential difference between two parallel, infinite planes spaced 1 meter apart that create an electric field of 1 newton per coulomb. Additionally, it is the potential difference between two points that will impart one joule of energy per coulomb of charge that passes through it. It can be expressed in terms of SI base units (m, kg, s, and A) as

$$\mathrm{V} = \frac{\text{potential energy}}{\text{charge}} = \frac{\mathrm{N \cdot m}}{\text{coulomb}} = \frac{\mathrm{m \cdot kg \cdot m}}{\mathrm{A \cdot s \cdot s^2}} = \frac{\mathrm{kg \cdot m^2}}{\mathrm{A \cdot s^3}}.$$

It can also be expressed as amperes times ohms (current times resistance, Ohm's law), watts per ampere (power per unit current, Joule's law), or joules per coulomb (energy per unit charge), which is also equivalent to electronvolts per elementary charge:

$$\mathrm{V} = \mathrm{A} \cdot \Omega = \frac{\mathrm{W}}{\mathrm{A}} = \frac{\mathrm{J}}{\mathrm{C}} = \frac{\mathrm{eV}}{e}.$$

Josephson Junction Definition

The "conventional" volt, V_{90}, defined in 1988 by the 18th General Conference on Weights and Measures and in use from 1990, is implemented using the Josephson effect for exact frequency-to-voltage conversion, combined with the caesium frequency standard. For the Josephson constant, $K_J = 2e/h$ (where e is the elementary charge and h is the Planck constant), the "conventional" value $K_{J\text{-}90}$ is used:

$$K_{J\text{-}90} = 0.4835979 \frac{\mathrm{GHz}}{\mu\mathrm{V}}.$$

This standard is typically realized using a series-connected array of several thousand or tens of thousands of junctions, excited by microwave signals between 10 and 80 GHz (depending on the array design). Empirically, several experiments have shown that the method is independent of device design, material, measurement setup, etc., and no correction terms are required in a practical implementation.

Water-flow Analogy

In the *water-flow analogy* sometimes used to explain electric circuits by comparing them with water-filled pipes, voltage (difference in electric potential) is likened to difference in water pressure. Current is proportional to the diameter of the pipe or the amount of water flowing at that pressure. A resistor would be a reduced diameter somewhere in the piping and a capacitor/inductor could be likened to a "U" shaped pipe where a higher water level on one side could store energy temporarily.

The relationship between voltage and current is defined (in ohmic devices like resistors) by Ohm's Law. Ohm's Law is analogous to the Hagen–Poiseuille equation, as both are linear models relating flux and potential in their respective systems.

Common Voltages

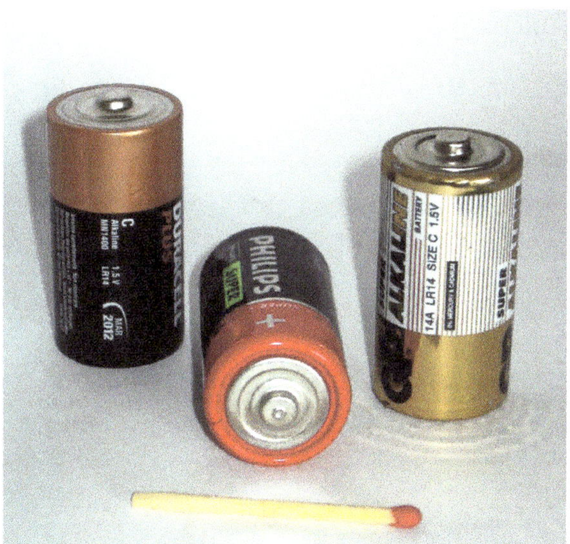

1.5 V C-cell batteries

The voltage produced by each electrochemical cell in a battery is determined by the chemistry of that cell. Cells can be combined in series for multiples of that voltage, or additional circuitry added to adjust the voltage to a different level. Mechanical generators can usually be constructed to any voltage in a range of feasibility.

Nominal voltages of familiar sources:

- Nerve cell resting potential: around −75 mV
- Single-cell, rechargeable NiMH or NiCd battery: 1.2 V

- Single-cell, non-rechargeable (e.g., AAA, AA, C and D cells): alkaline battery: 1.5 V; zinc-carbon battery: 1.56 V if fresh and unused
- $LiFePO_4$ rechargeable battery: 3.3 V
- Lithium polymer rechargeable battery: 3.75 V
- Transistor-transistor logic/CMOS (TTL) power supply: 5 V
- USB: 5 V DC
- PP3 battery: 9 V
- Internal Combustion Automobile electrical system: nominal 12 V, about 11.8 V discharged, 12.8 V charged, and 13.8–14.4 V while charging (vehicle running).
- Electric Car Battery: 400 V when fully charged
- Trucks/lorries: 24 V DC (Europe), 12 V DC (North America)
- Household mains electricity AC:
  - 100 V in Japan
  - 120 V in North America,
  - 230 V in Europe, Asia, Africa and Australia
- Rapid transit third rail: 600–750 V
- High-speed train overhead power lines: 25 kV at 50 Hz, but refer to the directory of current systems for electric rail traction and 25 kV at 60 Hz for exceptions.
- High-voltage electric power transmission lines: 110 kV and up (1.15 MV was the record as of 2005)
- Lightning: Varies greatly, often around 100 MV.

History

In 1800, as the result of a professional disagreement over the galvanic response advocated by Luigi Galvani, Alessandro Volta developed the so-called voltaic pile, a forerunner of the battery, which produced a steady electric current. Volta had determined that the most effective pair of dissimilar metals to produce electricity was zinc and silver. In 1861, Latimer Clark and Sir Charles Bright coined the name “volt” for the unit of resistance. By 1873, the British Association for the Advancement of Science had defined the volt, ohm, and farad. In 1881, the International Electrical Congress, now the International Electrotechnical Commission (IEC), approved the volt as the unit for electromotive force. They made the volt equal to 10^8 cgs units of voltage, the cgs system at the time being the customary system of units in science. They chose such a ratio because the cgs unit of voltage is inconveniently small and one volt in this definition is approximately the emf of a Daniell cell, the standard source of voltage in the telegraph systems of the day. At that time, the volt was defined as the potential difference [i.e., what is nowadays called the "voltage (difference)"] across a conductor when a current of one ampere dissipates one watt of power.

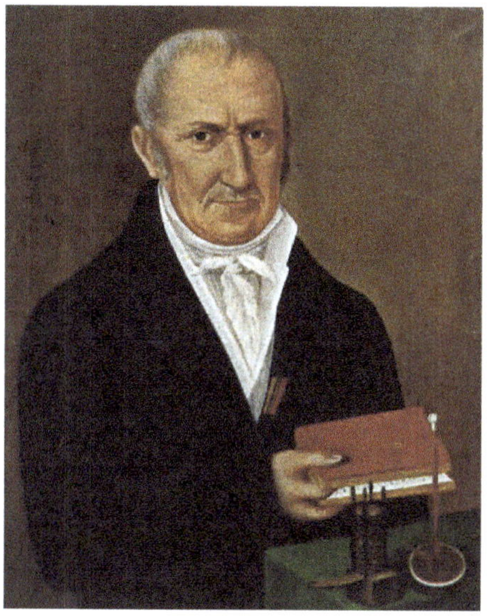

Alessandro Volta

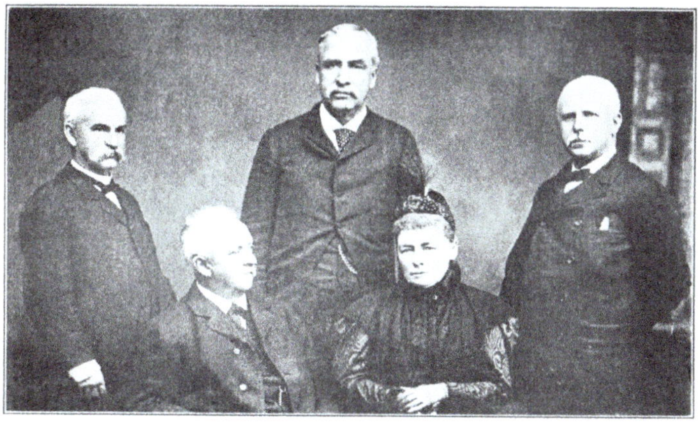

Group photograph of Herman Helmholtz, his wife (seated) and academic friends Hugo Kronecker (left), Thomas Corwin Mendenhall (right), Henry Villard (center) during the International Electrical Congress

The international volt was defined in 1893 as 1/1.434 of the emf of a Clark cell. This definition was abandoned in 1908 in favor of a definition based on the international ohm and international ampere until the entire set of "reproducible units" was abandoned in 1948.

Prior to the development of the Josephson junction voltage standard, the volt was maintained in national laboratories using specially constructed batteries called standard cells. The United States used a design called the Weston cell from 1905 to 1972.

This SI unit is named after Alessandro Volta. As with every International System of Units (SI) unit named for a person, the first letter of its symbol is upper case (V). However, when an SI unit is spelled out in English, it should always begin with a lower case letter (*volt*)—except in a situation where *any* word in that position would be capitalized, such as at the beginning of a sentence or in material using title case. Note that "degree Celsius" conforms to this rule because the "d" is lowercase— based on *The International System of Units.*

Watt

The watt (symbol: W) is a derived unit of power in the International System of Units (SI) defined as 1 joule per second and can be used to quantify the rate of energy transfer. Power has dimensions of ML^2T^{-3}.

Examples

When an object's velocity is held constant at one meter per second against constant opposing force of one newton the rate at which work is done is 1 watt.

$$W = 1\frac{J}{s} = 1\frac{N \cdot m}{s} = 1\frac{kg \cdot m^2}{s^3}$$

In terms of electromagnetism, one watt is the rate at which work is done when one ampere (A) of current flows through an electrical potential difference of one volt (V).

$$1\,W = 1\,V \cdot A$$

Two additional unit conversions for watt can be found using the above equation and Ohm's Law.

$$1\,W = 1\frac{V^2}{\Omega} = 1\,A^2 \cdot \Omega$$

Where ohm (Ω) is the SI derived unit of electrical resistance.

- A person having a mass of 100 kilograms who climbs a 3-meter-high ladder in 5 seconds is doing work at a rate of about 600 watts. Mass times acceleration due to gravity times height divided by the time it takes to lift the object to the given height gives the *rate of doing work* or *power*.
- A laborer over the course of an 8-hour day can sustain an average output of about 75 watts; higher power levels can be achieved for short intervals and by athletes.

Origin and Adoption as an SI unit

The watt is named after the Scottish inventor James Watt for his contributions to the development of the steam engine. The measurement unit was recognized by the Second Congress of the British Association for the Advancement of Science in 1882, concurrent with the start of commercial power production from both water and steam. In 1960 the 11th General Conference on Weights and Measures adopted it for the measurement of power into the International System of Units (SI).

Multiples

SI multiples for watt (W)						
Submultiples				**Multiples**		
Value	**SI symbol**	**Name**		**Value**	**SI symbol**	**Name**
10^{-1} W	dW	deciwatt		10^{1} W	daW	decawatt
10^{-2} W	cW	centiwatt		10^{2} W	hW	hectowatt
10^{-3} W	**mW**	**milliwatt**		10^{3} W	**kW**	**kilowatt**
10^{-6} W	µW	**microwatt**		10^{6} W	**MW**	**megawatt**
10^{-9} W	**nW**	**nanowatt**		10^{9} W	**GW**	**gigawatt**
10^{-12} W	**pW**	**picowatt**		10^{12} W	**TW**	**terawatt**
10^{-15} W	fW	femtowatt		10^{15} W	PW	petawatt
10^{-18} W	aW	attowatt		10^{18} W	EW	exawatt
10^{-21} W	zW	zeptowatt		10^{21} W	ZW	zettawatt
10^{-24} W	yW	yoctowatt		10^{24} W	YW	yottawatt
Common multiples are in **bold** face						

Femtowatt

The femtowatt is equal to one quadrillionth (10^{-15}) of a watt. Technologically important powers that are measured in femtowatts are typically found in reference(s) to radio and radar receivers. For example, meaningful FM tuner performance figures for sensitivity, quieting and signal-to-noise require that the RF energy applied to the antenna input be specified. These input levels are often stated in dBf (decibels referenced to 1 femtowatt). This is 0.2739 microvolt across a 75-ohm load or 0.5477 microvolt across a 300-ohm load; the specification takes into account the RF input impedance of the tuner.

Picowatt

The picowatt is equal to one trillionth (10^{-12}) of a watt. Technologically important powers that are measured in picowatts are typically used in reference to radio and radar receivers, acoustics and in the science of radio astronomy.

Nanowatt

The nanowatt is equal to one billionth (10^{-9}) of a watt. Important powers that are measured in nanowatts are also typically used in reference to radio and radar receivers.

Microwatt

The microwatt is equal to one millionth (10^{-6}) of a watt. Important powers that are measured in microwatts are typically stated in medical instrumentation systems such as the EEG and the ECG, in a wide variety of scientific and engineering instruments and also in reference to radio and radar receivers. Compact solar cells for devices such as calculators and watches are typically measured in microwatts.

Milliwatt

The milliwatt is equal to one thousandth (10^{-3}) of a watt. A typical laser pointer outputs about five milliwatts of light power, whereas a typical hearing aid for people uses less than one milliwatt. Audio signals and other electronic signal levels are often measured in dBm, referenced to one milliwatt.

Kilowatt

The kilowatt is equal to one thousand (10^3) watts. This unit is typically used to express the output power of engines and the power of electric motors, tools, machines, and heaters. It is also a common unit used to express the electromagnetic power output of broadcast radio and television transmitters.

One kilowatt is approximately equal to 1.34 horsepower. A small electric heater with one heating element can use 1.0 kilowatt. The average electric power consumption of a household in the United States is about one kilowatt.

Also, kilowatts of light power can be measured in the output pulses of some lasers.

A surface area of one square meter on Earth receives typically about one kilowatt of sunlight from the sun (the solar irradiance) (on a clear day at mid day, close to the equator).

Megawatt

The megawatt is equal to one million (10^6) watts. Many events or machines produce or sustain the conversion of energy on this scale, including large electric motors; large warships such as aircraft carriers, cruisers, and submarines; large server farms or data centers; and some scientific research equipment, such as supercolliders, and the output pulses of very large lasers. A large residential or commercial building may use several megawatts in electric power and heat. On railways, modern high-powered electric locomotives typically have a peak power output of 5 or 6 MW, although some produce much more. The Eurostar, for example, uses more than 12 MW, while heavy diesel-electric locomotives typically produce/use 3 to 5 MW. U.S. nuclear power plants have net summer capacities between about 500 and 1300 MW.

The earliest citing of the megawatt in the *Oxford English Dictionary* (OED) is a reference in the 1900 *Webster's International Dictionary of English Language*. The OED also states that megawatt appeared in a 28 November 1947 article in the journal *Science*.

Gigawatt

The gigawatt is equal to one billion (10^9) watts or 1 gigawatt = 1000 megawatts. This unit is often used for large power plants or power grids. For example, by the end of 2010 power shortages in China's Shanxi province were expected to increase to 5–6 GW and the installed capacity of wind power in Germany was 25.8 GW. The largest unit (out of four) of the Belgian Doel Nuclear Power Station has a peak output of 1.04 GW. HVDC converters have been built with power ratings of up to 2 GW.

Terawatt

The terawatt is equal to one trillion (10^{12}) watts. The total power used by humans worldwide is commonly measured in terawatts. The most powerful lasers from the mid-1960s to the mid-1990s produced power in terawatts, but only for nanosecond time frames. The average lightning strike peaks at 1 terawatt, but these strikes only last for 30 microseconds.

Petawatt

The petawatt is equal to one quadrillion (10^{15}) watts and can be produced by the current generation of lasers for time-scales on the order of picoseconds (10^{-12} s). One such laser is the Lawrence Livermore's Nova laser, which achieved a power output of 1.25 PW (1.25×10^{15} W) by a process called chirped pulse amplification. The duration of the pulse was roughly 0.5 ps (5×10^{-13} s), giving a total energy of 600 J, or enough energy to power a 100 W light bulb for six seconds. Another example is the Laser for Fast Ignition Experiments (LFEX) at the Institute of Laser Engineering (ILE), Osaka University, which achieved a power output of 2 PW (2×10^{15} W) for a duration of approximately 1 ps.

Based on the average total solar irradiance of 1.366 kW/m², the total power of sunlight striking Earth's atmosphere is estimated at 174 PW.

Conventions in the Electric Power Industry

In the electric power industry, *megawatt electrical* (MWe or MW_e) refers by convention to the electric power produced by a generator, while *megawatt thermal* or *thermal megawatt* (MWt, MW_t, or MWth, MW_{th}) refers to thermal power produced by the plant. For example, the Embalse nuclear power plant in Argentina uses a fission reactor to generate 2109 MW_t (i.e. heat), which creates steam to drive a turbine, which generates 648 MW_e (i.e. electricity). Other SI prefixes are sometimes used, for example *gigawatt electrical* (GW_e). The International Bureau of Weights and Measures, which maintains the SI-standard, states that further information about a quantity should not be attached to the unit symbol but instead to the quantity symbol (i.e., $P_{\text{thermal}} = 270$ W rather than $P = 270\ W_{th}$) and so these units are non-SI. In compliance with SI the energy company DONG Energy uses the unit megawatt for produced electrical power and the equivalent unit megajoule/s for delivered heating power in a combined heat and power station such as Avedøre Power Station.

When describing alternating current (AC) electricity, another distinction is made between the watt and the volt-ampere. While these units are equivalent for simple resistive circuits, they differ when loads exhibit electrical reactance.

Radio Transmission

Radio stations usually report the power of their transmitters in units of watts, referring to the effective radiated power. It refers to the relative power of the transmission when it is directed towards the horizon for maximum geographic coverage, rather than uniformly broadcast in all directions.

Confusion of Watts, Watt-hours and Watts Per Hour

The terms power and energy are frequently confused. Power is the rate at which energy is generated or consumed and hence is measured in units (e.g. watts) that represent energy *per unit time*.

For example, when a light bulb with a power rating of 100W is turned on for one hour, the energy used is 100 watt hours (W·h), 0.1 kilowatt hour, or 360 kJ. This same amount of energy would light a 40-watt bulb for 2.5 hours, or a 50-watt bulb for 2 hours. A power station would be *rated* in multiples of watts (for example, the Three Gorges Dam is rated at approximately 22 gigawatts), but its annual energy *sales* or *output* would be in multiples of watt *hours*. Major energy production or consumption is often expressed as terawatt hours for a given period that is often a calendar year or financial year. One terawatt hour is equal to a sustained power of approximately 114 megawatts for a period of one year.

The watt second is a unit of energy, equal to the joule. One kilowatt hour is 3 600 000 watt seconds. The watt second is used, for example, to rate the energy storage of flash lamps used in photography, although the term *joule* is generally employed.

Terms such as *watts per hour* (W/h) are often misused when *watts* would be correct. Watts per hour properly refers to a *change* of power per hour. Watts per hour might be useful to characterize the ramp-up behavior of power plants. For example, a power plant that changes its power output from 0 MW to 1 MW in 15 minutes has a ramp-up rate of 4 MW/h. Hydroelectric power plants have a very high ramp-up rate, which makes them particularly useful in peak load and emergency situations. The misnomer watts per hour is essentially the derivative of power and should be called rate of watt change per hour.

Weber (Unit)

In physics, the weber is the SI unit of magnetic flux. A *flux density* of one Wb/m^2 (one weber per square metre) is one tesla.

The weber is named after the German physicist Wilhelm Eduard Weber (1804–1891).

Definition

SI multiples for weber (Wb)						
Submultiples				Multiples		
Value	SI symbol	Name		Value	SI symbol	Name
10^{-1} Wb	dWb	deciweber		10^{1} Wb	daWb	decaweber
10^{-2} Wb	cWb	centiweber		10^{2} Wb	hWb	hectoweber
10^{-3} Wb	**mWb**	**milliweber**		10^{3} Wb	kWb	kiloweber
10^{-6} Wb	µWb	**microweber**		10^{6} Wb	MWb	megaweber
10^{-9} Wb	**nWb**	**nanoweber**		10^{9} Wb	GWb	gigaweber
10^{-12} Wb	pWb	picoweber		10^{12} Wb	TWb	teraweber
10^{-15} Wb	fWb	femtoweber		10^{15} Wb	PWb	petaweber
10^{-18} Wb	aWb	attoweber		10^{18} Wb	EWb	exaweber
10^{-21} Wb	zWb	zeptoweber		10^{21} Wb	ZWb	zettaweber
10^{-24} Wb	yWb	yoctoweber		10^{24} Wb	YWb	yottaweber
Common multiples are in bold face.						

The weber may be defined in terms of Faraday's law, which relates a changing magnetic flux through a loop to the electric field around the loop. A change in flux of one weber per second will induce an electromotive force of one volt (produce an electric potential difference of one volt across two open-circuited terminals).

Officially,

Weber (unit of magnetic flux) — The weber is the magnetic flux that, linking a circuit of one turn, would produce in it an electromotive force of 1 volt if it were reduced to zero at a uniform rate in 1 second.

The weber is commonly expressed in a multitude of other units:

$$\mathrm{Wb} = \frac{\mathrm{kg} \cdot \mathrm{m}^2}{\mathrm{s}^2 \cdot \mathrm{A}} = \mathrm{V} \cdot \mathrm{s} = \mathrm{H} \cdot \mathrm{A} = \mathrm{T} \cdot \mathrm{m}^2 = \frac{\mathrm{J}}{\mathrm{A}} = 10^8 \,\mathrm{Mx}$$

where Wb = weber,

V = volt,

T = tesla,

J = joule,

m = meter,

s = second,

A = ampere,

H = henry,

Mx = maxwell.

This SI unit is named after Wilhelm Eduard Weber. As with every International System of Units (SI) unit named for a person, the first letter of its symbol is upper case (Wb). However, when an SI unit is spelled out in English, it should always begin with a lower case letter (*weber*)—except in a situation where *any* word in that position would be capitalized, such as at the beginning of a sentence or in material using title case. Note that "degree Celsius" conforms to this rule because the "d" is lowercase — Based on *The International System of Units.*

History

In 1861, the British Association for the Advancement of Science (known as "The BA") established a committee under William Thomson (later Lord Kelvin) to study electrical units. In a February 1902 manuscript, with handwritten notes of Oliver Heaviside, Giovanni Giorgi proposed a set of rational units of electromagnetism including the weber, noting that "the product of the volt into the second has been called the *weber* by the B. A."

The International Electrotechnical Commission began work on terminology in 1909 and established Technical Committee 1 in 1911, its oldest established committee, "to sanction the terms and definitions used in the different electrotechnical fields and to determine the equivalence of the terms used in the different languages."

It was not until 1927 that TC1 dealt with the study of various outstanding problems concerning electrical and magnetic quantities and units. Discussions of a theoretical nature were opened at which eminent electrical engineers and physicists considered whether magnetic field strength and magnetic flux density were in fact quantities of the same nature. As disagreement continued, the IEC decided on an effort to remedy the situation. It instructed a task force to study the question in readiness for the next meeting.

In 1930, TC1 decided that the magnetic field strength (H) is of a different nature from the magnetic flux density (B), and took up the question of naming the units for these fields and related quantities, among them the integral of magnetic flux density.

In 1935, TC 1 recommended names for several electrical units, including the weber for the practical unit of magnetic flux (and the maxwell for the CGS unit).

It was decided to extend the existing series of practical units into a complete comprehensive system of physical units, the recommendation being adopted in 1935 "that the system with four fundamental units proposed by Professor Giorgi be adopted subject to the fourth fundamental unit being eventually selected". This system was given the designation of "Giorgi system".

Also in 1936 , TC1 passed responsibility for "electric and magnetic magnitudes and units" to the new TC24. This "led eventually to the universal adoption of the Giorgi system, which unified electromagnetic units with the MKS dimensional system of units, the whole now known simply as the SI system (Système International d'unités)."

In 1938, TC24 "recommended as a connecting link [from mechanical to electrical units] the permeability of free space with the value of $\mu_0 = 4\pi\times10^{-7}$ H/m. This group also recognized that any one of the practical units already in use (ohm, ampere, volt, henry, farad, coulomb, and weber), could equally serve as the fourth fundamental unit. "After consultation, the ampere was adopted as the fourth unit of the Giorgi system in Paris in 1950."

References

- Serway, Raymond A; Jewett, JW (2006). Serway's principles of physics: a calculus based text (Fourth ed.). Belmont, CA: Thompson Brooks/Cole. p. 746. ISBN 0-53449143-X
- Preece, William Henry (1867), "The B.A. unit for electrical measurements", Philosophical Magazine, 33, p. 397, retrieved 26 February 2017
- Werner Siemens (1860), "Vorschlag eines reproducirbaren Widerstandsmaaßes", Annalen der Physik und Chemie (in German), 186 (5), pp. 1–20, doi:10.1002/andp.18601860502
- Tunbridge, Paul (1992). Lord Kelvin : his influence on electrical measurements and units. London: Peregrinus. pp. 26, 39–40. ISBN 9780863412370. Retrieved 5 May 2015
- Rowlett, Russ. "How Many? A Dictionary of Units of Measurement. M". University of North Carolina at Chapel Hill. Retrieved 2017-03-04
- Hill, Paul Horowitz; Winfield; Winfield, Hill (2015). The Art of Electronics (3. ed.). Cambridge [u.a.]: Cambridge Univ. Press. p. 689. ISBN 978-0-521-809269

- Williams, L. L. (January 1999). "Electrical Properties of the Fair-Weather Atmosphere and the Possibility of Observable Discharge on Moving Objects" (PDF). Retrieved 2012-08-13
- Keller, Mark W (2008-01-18), "Current status of the quantum metrology triangle" (PDF), Metrologia, 45 (1): 102–109, Bibcode:2008Metro..45..102K, ISSN 0026-1394, doi:10.1088/0026-1394/45/1/014
- Avallone, Eugene A; et. al, eds. (2007), Marks' Standard Handbook for Mechanical Engineers (11th ed.), New York: Mc-Graw Hill, pp. 9–4, ISBN 0-07-142867-4
- Ambler Thompson & Barry N. Taylor (2008). "NIST Special Publication 811: Guide for the Use of the International System of Units (SI)" (PDF). National Institute of Standards and Technology. Retrieved 2013-03-21
- International Bureau of Weights and Measures (2006), The International System of Units (SI) (PDF) (8th ed.), p. 132, ISBN 92-822-2213-6
- Clark, Latimer; Bright, Sir Charles (1861-11-09). "Measurement of Electrical Quantities and Resistance". The Electrician. 1 (1): 3–4. Retrieved 27 February 2014
- "Construction of a Composite Total Solar Irradiance (TSI) Time Series from 1978 to present". CH: PMODWRC. Retrieved 2005-10-05

4

An Overview of Superconductivity

The ability of some materials to conduct electricity with no resistance is known as superconductivity. There are a number of criteria used in classifying superconductors. Some of these are response to a magnetic field, by critical temperature, by material and by theory of operation. The chapter on superconductivity offers an insightful focus, keeping in mind the complex subject matter.

Superconductivity

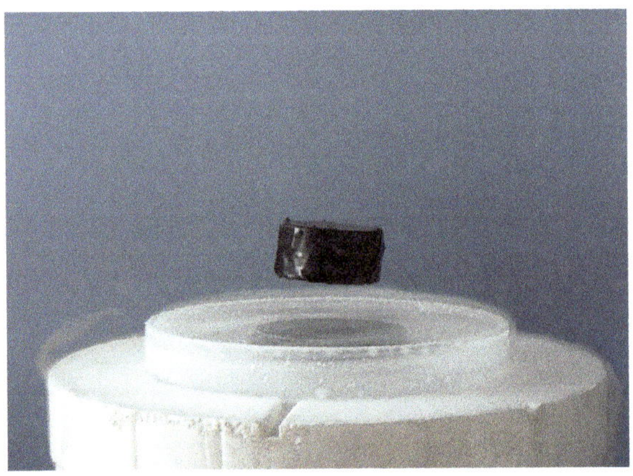

A magnet levitating above a high-temperature superconductor, cooled with liquid nitrogen. Persistent electric current flows on the surface of the superconductor, acting to exclude the magnetic field of the magnet (Faraday's law of induction). This current effectively forms an electromagnet that repels the magnet.

Superconductivity is a phenomenon of exactly zero electrical resistance and expulsion of magnetic flux fields occurring in certain materials, called superconductors, when cooled below a characteristic critical temperature. It was discovered by Dutch physicist Heike Kamerlingh Onnes on April 8, 1911, in Leiden. Like ferromagnetism and atomic spectral lines, superconductivity is a quantum mechanical phenomenon. It is characterized by the Meissner effect, the complete ejection of magnetic field lines from the interior of the superconductor as it transitions into the superconducting state. The occurrence of the Meissner effect indicates that superconductivity cannot be understood simply as the idealization of *perfect conductivity* in classical physics.

The electrical resistance of a metallic conductor decreases gradually as temperature is lowered. In ordinary conductors, such as copper or silver, this decrease is limited by impurities and other defects. Even near absolute zero, a real sample of a normal conductor shows some resistance. In a superconductor; the resistance drops abruptly to zero when the material is cooled below its critical temperature. An electric current flowing through a loop of superconducting wire can persist indefinitely with no power source.

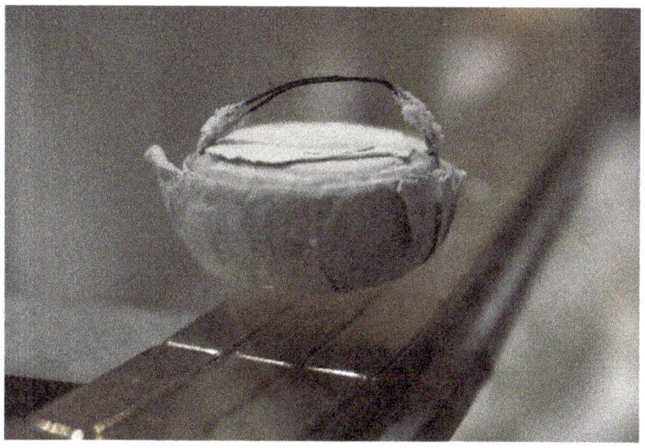

A high-temperature superconductor levitating above a magnet

In 1986, it was discovered that some cuprate-perovskite ceramic materials have a critical temperature above 90 K (−183 °C). Such a high transition temperature is theoretically impossible for a conventional superconductor, leading the materials to be termed high-temperature superconductors. The cheaply-available coolant liquid nitrogen boils at 77 K, and thus superconduction at higher temperatures than this facilitates many experiments and applications that are less practical at lower temperatures.

Classification

There are many criteria by which superconductors are classified. The most common are:

Response to a Magnetic Field

A superconductor can be *Type I*, meaning it has a single critical field, above which all superconductivity is lost; or *Type II*, meaning it has two critical fields, between which it allows partial penetration of the magnetic field.

By Theory of Operation

It is *conventional* if it can be explained by the BCS theory or its derivatives, or *unconventional*, otherwise.

By Critical Temperature

A superconductor is generally considered *high-temperature* if it reaches a superconducting state when cooled using liquid nitrogen – that is, at only T_c > 77 K) – or *low-temperature* if more aggressive cooling techniques are required to reach its critical temperature.

By Material

Superconductor material classes include chemical elements (e.g. mercury or lead), alloys (such as niobium-titanium, germanium-niobium, and niobium nitride), ceramics (YBCO and magnesium diboride), superconducting pnictides (like fluorine-doped LaOFeAs) or organic superconductors (fullerenes and carbon nanotubes; though perhaps these examples should be included among the chemical elements, as they are composed entirely of carbon).

Elementary Properties of Superconductors

Most of the physical properties of superconductors vary from material to material, such as the heat capacity and the critical temperature, critical field, and critical current density at which superconductivity is destroyed.

On the other hand, there is a class of properties that are independent of the underlying material. For instance, all superconductors have *exactly* zero resistivity to low applied currents when there is no magnetic field present or if the applied field does not exceed a critical value. The existence of these "universal" properties implies that superconductivity is a thermodynamic phase, and thus possesses certain distinguishing properties which are largely independent of microscopic details.

Zero Electrical DC Resistance

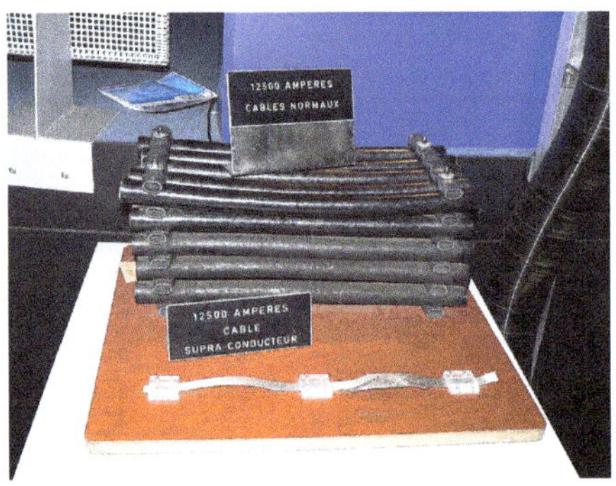

Electric cables for accelerators at CERN. Both the massive and slim cables are rated for 12,500 A. *Top:* conventional cables for LEP; *bottom:* superconductor-based cables for the LHC

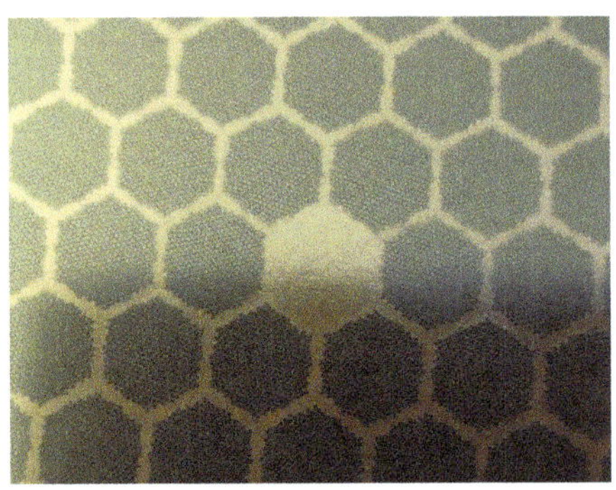

Cross section of a preform superconductor rod from abandoned Texas Superconducting Super Collider (SSC).

The simplest method to measure the electrical resistance of a sample of some material is to place it in an electrical circuit in series with a current source I and measure the resulting voltage V across the sample. The resistance of the sample is given by Ohm's law as $R = V / I$. If the voltage is zero, this means that the resistance is zero.

Superconductors are also able to maintain a current with no applied voltage whatsoever, a property exploited in superconducting electromagnets such as those found in MRI machines. Experiments have demonstrated that currents in superconducting coils can persist for years without any measurable degradation. Experimental evidence points to a current lifetime of at least 100,000 years. Theoretical estimates for the lifetime of a persistent current can exceed the estimated lifetime of the universe, depending on the wire geometry and the temperature.

In a normal conductor, an electric current may be visualized as a fluid of electrons moving across a heavy ionic lattice. The electrons are constantly colliding with the ions in the lattice, and during each collision some of the energy carried by the current is absorbed by the lattice and converted into heat, which is essentially the vibrational kinetic energy of the lattice ions. As a result, the energy carried by the current is constantly being dissipated. This is the phenomenon of electrical resistance and Joule heating.

The situation is different in a superconductor. In a conventional superconductor, the electronic fluid cannot be resolved into individual electrons. Instead, it consists of bound *pairs* of electrons known as Cooper pairs. This pairing is caused by an attractive force between electrons from the exchange of phonons. Due to quantum mechanics, the energy spectrum of this Cooper pair fluid possesses an *energy gap*, meaning there is a minimum amount of energy ΔE that must be supplied in order to excite the fluid. Therefore, if ΔE is larger than the thermal energy of the lattice, given by kT, where k is Boltzmann's constant and T is the temperature, the fluid will not be scattered by the lattice. The Cooper pair fluid is thus a superfluid, meaning it can flow without energy dissipation.

In a class of superconductors known as type II superconductors, including all known high-temperature superconductors, an extremely small amount of resistivity appears at temperatures not too far below the nominal superconducting transition when an electric current is applied in conjunction with a strong magnetic field, which may be caused by the electric current. This is due to the motion of magnetic vortices in the electronic superfluid, which dissipates some of the energy carried by the current. If the current is sufficiently small, the vortices are stationary, and the resistivity vanishes. The resistance due to this effect is tiny compared with that of non-superconducting materials, but must be taken into account in sensitive experiments. However, as the temperature decreases far enough below the nominal superconducting transition, these vortices can become frozen into a disordered but stationary phase known as a "vortex glass". Below this vortex glass transition temperature, the resistance of the material becomes truly zero.

Superconducting Phase Transition

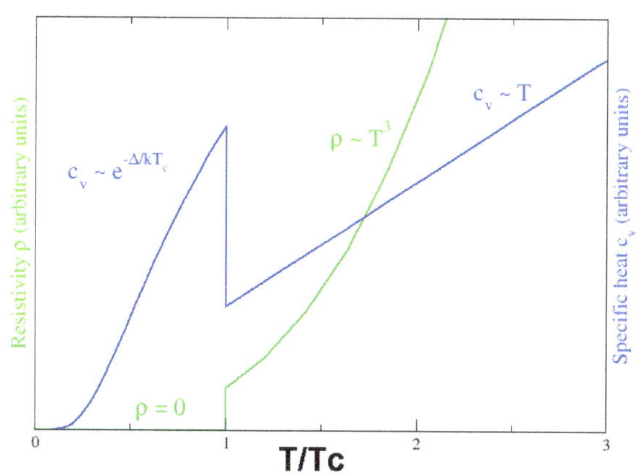

Behavior of heat capacity (c_v, blue) and resistivity (ρ, green) at the superconducting phase transition

In superconducting materials, the characteristics of superconductivity appear when the temperature T is lowered below a critical temperature T_c. The value of this critical temperature varies from material to material. Conventional superconductors usually have critical temperatures ranging from around 20 K to less than 1 K. Solid mercury, for example, has a critical temperature of 4.2 K.

As of 2009, the highest critical temperature found for a conventional superconductor is 39 K for magnesium diboride (MgB_2), although this material displays enough exotic properties that there is some doubt about classifying it as a "conventional" superconductor. Cuprate superconductors can have much higher critical temperatures: $YBa_2Cu_3O_7$, one of the first cuprate superconductors to be discovered, has a critical temperature of 92 K, and mercury-based cuprates have been found with critical temperatures in excess of 130 K. The explanation for these high critical temperatures remains unknown. Electron pairing due to phonon exchanges explains superconductivity in conventional superconductors, but it does not explain superconductivity in the newer superconductors that have a very high critical temperature.

Similarly, at a fixed temperature below the critical temperature, superconducting materials cease to superconduct when an external magnetic field is applied which is greater than the *critical magnetic field*. This is because the Gibbs free energy of the superconducting phase increases quadratically with the magnetic field while the free energy of the normal phase is roughly independent of the magnetic field. If the material superconducts in the absence of a field, then the superconducting phase free energy is lower than that of the normal phase and so for some finite value of the magnetic field (proportional to the square root of the difference of the free energies at zero magnetic field) the two free energies will be equal and a phase transition to the normal phase will occur. More generally, a higher temperature and a stronger magnetic field lead to a smaller fraction of the electrons in the superconducting band and consequently a longer London penetration depth of external magnetic fields and currents. The penetration depth becomes infinite at the phase transition.

The onset of superconductivity is accompanied by abrupt changes in various physical properties, which is the hallmark of a phase transition. For example, the electronic heat capacity is proportional to the temperature in the normal (non-superconducting) regime. At the superconducting transition, it suffers a discontinuous jump and thereafter ceases to be linear. At low temperatures, it varies instead as $e^{-\alpha/T}$ for some constant, α. This exponential behavior is one of the pieces of evidence for the existence of the energy gap.

The order of the superconducting phase transition was long a matter of debate. Experiments indicate that the transition is second-order, meaning there is no latent heat. However, in the presence of an external magnetic field there is latent heat, because the superconducting phase has a lower entropy below the critical temperature than the normal phase. It has been experimentally demonstrated that, as a consequence, when the magnetic field is increased beyond the critical field, the resulting phase transition leads to a decrease in the temperature of the superconducting material.

Calculations in the 1970s suggested that it may actually be weakly first-order due to the effect of long-range fluctuations in the electromagnetic field. In the 1980s it was shown theoretically with the help of a disorder field theory, in which the vortex lines of the superconductor play a major role, that the transition is of second order within the type II regime and of first order (i.e., latent heat) within the type I regime, and that the two regions are separated by a tricritical point. The results were strongly supported by Monte Carlo computer simulations.

Meissner Effect

When a superconductor is placed in a weak external magnetic field H, and cooled below its transition temperature, the magnetic field is ejected. The Meissner effect does not cause the field to be completely ejected but instead the field penetrates the superconductor but only to a very small distance, characterized by a parameter λ, called the London penetration depth, decaying exponentially to zero within the bulk of the material. The Meissner effect is a defining characteristic of superconductivity. For most superconductors, the London penetration depth is on the order of 100 nm.

The Meissner effect is sometimes confused with the kind of diamagnetism one would expect in a perfect electrical conductor: according to Lenz's law, when a *changing* magnetic field is applied to a conductor, it will induce an electric current in the conductor that creates an opposing magnetic field. In a perfect conductor, an arbitrarily large current can be induced, and the resulting magnetic field exactly cancels the applied field.

The Meissner effect is distinct from this—it is the spontaneous expulsion which occurs during transition to superconductivity. Suppose we have a material in its normal state, containing a constant internal magnetic field. When the material is cooled below the critical temperature, we would observe the abrupt expulsion of the internal magnetic field, which we would not expect based on Lenz's law.

The Meissner effect was given a phenomenological explanation by the brothers Fritz and Heinz London, who showed that the electromagnetic free energy in a superconductor is minimized provided

$$\nabla^2\mathbf{H} = \lambda^{-2}\mathbf{H}$$

where H is the magnetic field and λ is the London penetration depth.

This equation, which is known as the London equation, predicts that the magnetic field in a superconductor decays exponentially from whatever value it possesses at the surface.

A superconductor with little or no magnetic field within it is said to be in the Meissner state. The Meissner state breaks down when the applied magnetic field is too large. Superconductors can be divided into two classes according to how this breakdown occurs. In Type I superconductors, superconductivity is abruptly destroyed when the strength of the applied field rises above a critical value H_c. Depending on the geometry of the sample, one may obtain an intermediate state consisting of a baroque pattern of regions of normal material carrying a magnetic field mixed with regions of superconducting material containing no field. In Type II superconductors, raising the applied field past a critical value H_{c1} leads to a mixed state (also known as the vortex state) in which an increasing amount of magnetic flux penetrates the material, but there remains no resistance to the flow of electric current as long as the current is not too large. At a second critical field strength H_{c2}, superconductivity is destroyed. The mixed state is actually caused by vortices in the electronic superfluid, sometimes called fluxons because the flux carried by these vortices is quantized. Most pure elemental superconductors, except niobium and carbon nanotubes, are Type I, while almost all impure and compound superconductors are Type II.

London Moment

Conversely, a spinning superconductor generates a magnetic field, precisely aligned with the spin axis. The effect, the London moment, was put to good use in Gravity Probe B. This experiment measured the magnetic fields of four superconducting gyroscopes to determine their spin axes. This was critical to the experiment since it is one of the few ways to accurately determine the spin axis of an otherwise featureless sphere.

History of Superconductivity

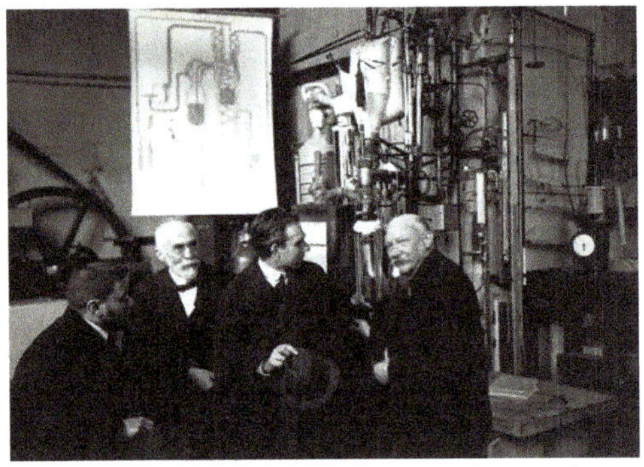

Heike Kamerlingh Onnes (right), the discoverer of superconductivity. Paul Ehrenfest, Hendrik Lorentz, Niels Bohr stand to his left.

Superconductivity was discovered on April 8, 1911 by Heike Kamerlingh Onnes, who was studying the resistance of solid mercury at cryogenic temperatures using the recently produced liquid helium as a refrigerant. At the temperature of 4.2 K, he observed that the resistance abruptly disappeared. In the same experiment, he also observed the superfluid transition of helium at 2.2 K, without recognizing its significance. The precise date and circumstances of the discovery were only reconstructed a century later, when Onnes's notebook was found. In subsequent decades, superconductivity was observed in several other materials. In 1913, lead was found to superconduct at 7 K, and in 1941 niobium nitride was found to superconduct at 16 K.

Great efforts have been devoted to finding out how and why superconductivity works; the important step occurred in 1933, when Meissner and Ochsenfeld discovered that superconductors expelled applied magnetic fields, a phenomenon which has come to be known as the Meissner effect. In 1935, Fritz and Heinz London showed that the Meissner effect was a consequence of the minimization of the electromagnetic free energy carried by superconducting current.

London Theory

The first phenomenological theory of superconductivity was London theory. It was put forward by the brothers Fritz and Heinz London in 1935, shortly after the discovery that magnetic fields are expelled from superconductors. A major triumph of the equations of this theory is their ability to explain the Meissner effect, wherein a material exponentially expels all internal magnetic fields as it crosses the superconducting threshold. By using the London equation, one can obtain the dependence of the magnetic field inside the superconductor on the distance to the surface.

There are two London equations:

$$\frac{\partial \boldsymbol{j}_s}{\partial t} = \frac{n_s e^2}{m} \boldsymbol{E}, \qquad \nabla \times \boldsymbol{j}_s = -\frac{n_s e^2}{m} \boldsymbol{B}.$$

The first equation follows from Newton's second law for superconducting electrons.

Conventional Theories (1950s)

During the 1950s, theoretical condensed matter physicists arrived at an understanding of "conventional" superconductivity, through a pair of remarkable and important theories: the phenomenological Ginzburg-Landau theory (1950) and the microscopic BCS theory (1957).

In 1950, the phenomenological Ginzburg-Landau theory of superconductivity was devised by Landau and Ginzburg. This theory, which combined Landau's theory of second-order phase transitions with a Schrödinger-like wave equation, had great success in explaining the macroscopic properties of superconductors. In particular, Abrikosov showed that Ginzburg-Landau theory predicts the division of superconductors into the two categories now referred to as Type I and Type II. Abrikosov and Ginzburg were awarded the 2003 Nobel Prize for their work (Landau had received the 1962 Nobel Prize for other work, and died in 1968). The four-dimensional extension of the Ginzburg-Landau theory, the Coleman-Weinberg model, is important in quantum field theory and cosmology.

Also in 1950, Maxwell and Reynolds *et al.* found that the critical temperature of a superconductor depends on the isotopic mass of the constituent element. This important discovery pointed to the electron-phonon interaction as the microscopic mechanism responsible for superconductivity.

The complete microscopic theory of superconductivity was finally proposed in 1957 by Bardeen, Cooper and Schrieffer. This BCS theory explained the superconducting current as a superfluid of Cooper pairs, pairs of electrons interacting through the exchange of phonons. For this work, the authors were awarded the Nobel Prize in 1972.

The BCS theory was set on a firmer footing in 1958, when N. N. Bogolyubov showed that the BCS wavefunction, which had originally been derived from a variational argument, could be obtained using a canonical transformation of the electronic Hamiltonian. In 1959, Lev Gor'kov showed that the BCS theory reduced to the Ginzburg-Landau theory close to the critical temperature.

Generalizations of BCS theory for conventional superconductors form the basis for understanding of the phenomenon of superfluidity, because they fall into the lambda transition universality class. The extent to which such generalizations can be applied to unconventional superconductors is still controversial.

Further History

The first practical application of superconductivity was developed in 1954 with Dudley Allen Buck's invention of the cryotron. Two superconductors with greatly different values of critical magnetic field are combined to produce a fast, simple switch for computer elements.

Soon after discovering superconductivity in 1911, Kamerlingh Onnes attempted to make an electromagnet with superconducting windings but found that relatively low magnetic fields destroyed superconductivity in the materials he investigated. Much later, in 1955, G.B. Yntema succeeded in constructing a small 0.7-tesla iron-core electromagnet with superconducting niobium wire windings. Then, in 1961, J.E. Kunzler, E. Buehler, F.S.L. Hsu, and J.H. Wernick made the startling discovery that, at 4.2 kelvin, a compound consisting of three parts niobium and one part tin, was capable of supporting a current density of more than 100,000 amperes per square centimeter in a magnetic field of 8.8 tesla. Despite being brittle and difficult to fabricate, niobium-tin has since proved extremely useful in supermagnets generating magnetic fields as high as 20 tesla. In 1962 T.G. Berlincourt and R.R. Hake discovered that alloys of niobium and titanium are suitable for applications up to 10 tesla. Promptly thereafter, commercial production of niobium-titanium supermagnet wire commenced at Westinghouse Electric Corporation and at Wah Chang Corporation. Although niobium-titanium boasts less-impressive superconducting properties than those of niobium-tin, niobium-titanium has, nevertheless, become the most widely used "workhorse" supermagnet material, in large measure a consequence of its very-high ductility and ease of fabrication. However, both niobium-tin and niobium-titanium find wide application in MRI medical imagers, bending and focusing magnets for enormous high-energy-particle accelerators, and a host of other applications. Conectus, a European superconductivity consortium, estimated that in 2014, global economic activity for which superconductivity was indispensable amounted to about five billion euros, with MRI systems accounting for about 80% of that total.

In 1962, Josephson made the important theoretical prediction that a supercurrent can flow between two pieces of superconductor separated by a thin layer of insulator. This phenomenon, now called the Josephson effect, is exploited by superconducting devices such as SQUIDs. It is used in the most accurate available measurements of the magnetic flux quantum $\Phi_0 = h/(2e)$, where h is the Planck constant. Coupled with the quantum Hall resistivity, this leads to a precise measurement of the Planck constant. Josephson was awarded the Nobel Prize for this work in 1973.

In 2008, it was proposed that the same mechanism that produces superconductivity could produce a superinsulator state in some materials, with almost infinite electrical resistance.

High-temperature Superconductivity

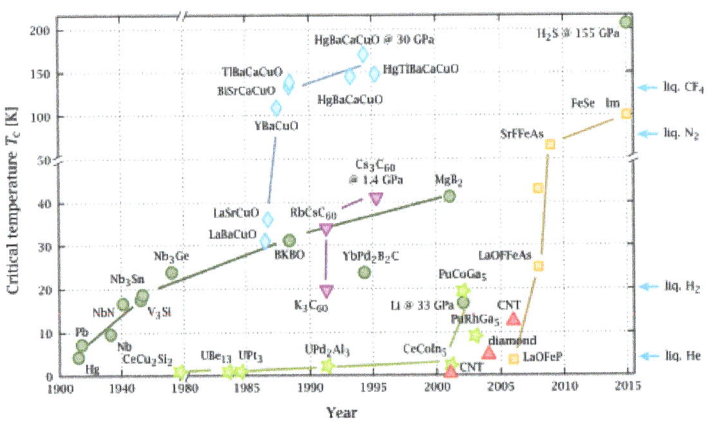

Timeline of superconducting materials

Until 1986, physicists had believed that BCS theory forbade superconductivity at temperatures above about 30 K. In that year, Bednorz and Müller discovered superconductivity in a lanthanum-based cuprate perovskite material, which had a transition temperature of 35 K (Nobel Prize in Physics, 1987). It was soon found that replacing the lanthanum with yttrium (i.e., making YBCO) raised the critical temperature to 92 K.

This temperature jump is particularly significant, since it allows liquid nitrogen as a refrigerant, replacing liquid helium. This can be important commercially because liquid nitrogen can be produced relatively cheaply, even on-site. Also, the higher temperatures help avoid some of the problems that arise at liquid helium temperatures, such as the formation of plugs of frozen air that can block cryogenic lines and cause unanticipated and potentially hazardous pressure buildup.

Many other cuprate superconductors have since been discovered, and the theory of superconductivity in these materials is one of the major outstanding challenges of theoretical condensed matter physics. There are currently two main hypotheses – the resonating-valence-bond theory, and spin fluctuation which has the most support in the research community. The second hypothesis proposed that electron pairing in high-temperature superconductors is mediated by short-range spin waves known as paramagnons.

Since about 1993, the highest-temperature superconductor has been a ceramic material consisting of mercury, barium, calcium, copper and oxygen ($HgBa_2Ca_2Cu_3O_{8+\delta}$) with T_c = 133–138 K. The latter experiment (138 K) still awaits experimental confirmation, however.

In February 2008, an iron-based family of high-temperature superconductors was discovered. Hideo Hosono, of the Tokyo Institute of Technology, and colleagues found lanthanum oxygen fluorine iron arsenide ($LaO_{1-x}F_xFeAs$), an oxypnictide that superconducts below 26 K. Replacing the lanthanum in $LaO_{1-x}F_xFeAs$ with samarium leads to superconductors that work at 55 K.

In May 2014, hydrogen sulfide (H_2S) was predicted to be a high-temperature superconductor with a transition temperature of 80 K at 160 gigapascals of pressure. In 2015, H_2S has been observed to exhibit superconductivity at below 203 K but at extremely high pressures — around 150 gigapascals.

Applications

Superconducting magnets are some of the most powerful electromagnets known. They are used in MRI/NMR machines, mass spectrometers, the beam-steering magnets used in particle accelerators and plasma confining magnets in some tokamaks. They can also be used for magnetic separation, where weakly magnetic particles are extracted from a background of less or non-magnetic particles, as in the pigment industries.

In the 1950s and 1960s, superconductors were used to build experimental digital computers using cryotron switches. More recently, superconductors have been used to make digital circuits based on rapid single flux quantum technology and RF and microwave filters for mobile phone base stations.

Superconductors are used to build Josephson junctions which are the building blocks of SQUIDs (superconducting quantum interference devices), the most sensitive magnetometers known. SQUIDs are used in scanning SQUID microscopes and magnetoencephalography. Series of Josephson devices are used to realize the SI volt. Depending on the particular mode of operation, a superconductor-insulator-superconductor Josephson junction can be used as a photon detector or as a mixer. The large resistance change at the transition from the normal- to the superconducting state is used to build thermometers in cryogenic micro-calorimeter photon detectors. The same effect is used in ultrasensitive bolometers made from superconducting materials.

Other early markets are arising where the relative efficiency, size and weight advantages of devices based on high-temperature superconductivity outweigh the additional costs involved. For example, in wind turbines the lower weight and volume of superconducting generators could lead to savings in construction and tower costs, offsetting the higher costs for the generator and lowering the total LCOE.

Promising future applications include high-performance smart grid, electric power transmission, transformers, power storage devices, electric motors (e.g. for vehicle propulsion, as in vactrains or maglev trains), magnetic levitation devices, fault current limiters, enhancing spintronic devices with superconducting materials, and superconducting magnetic refrigeration. However, superconductivity is sensitive to moving magnetic fields so applications that use alternating current (e.g. transformers) will be more difficult to develop than those that rely upon direct current. Compared to traditional power lines superconducting transmission lines are more efficient and require only a fraction of the space, which would not only lead to a better environmental performance but could also improve public acceptance for expansion of the electric grid.

History of Superconductivity

Superconductivity is the phenomenon of certain materials exhibiting zero electrical resistance and the expulsion of magnetic fields below a characteristic temperature. The history of superconductivity began with Dutch physicist Heike Kamerlingh Onnes's discovery of superconductivity in mercury in 1911. Since then, many other superconducting materials have been discovered and the theory of superconductivity has been developed. These subjects remain active areas of study in the field of condensed matter physics.

Exploring Ultra-cold Phenomena (to 1908)

James Dewar initiated research into electrical resistance at low temperatures. Dewar and John Ambrose Fleming predicted that at absolute zero, pure metals would become perfect electromagnetic conductors (though, later, Dewar altered his opinion on the disappearance of resistance, believing that there would always be some resistance). Walther Hermann Nernst developed the third law of thermodynamics and stated that absolute zero was unattainable. Carl von Linde and William Hampson, both commercial researchers, nearly at the same time filed for patents on the Joule–Thomson effect for the liquefaction of gases. Linde's patent was the climax of 20 years of systematic investigation of established facts, using a regenerative counterflow method. Hampson's designs was also of a regenerative method. The combined process became known as the Hampson–Linde liquefaction process.

Onnes purchased a Linde machine for his research. On March 21, 1900, Nikola Tesla was granted a US patent for the means for increasing the intensity of electrical oscillations by lowering the temperature, which was caused by lowered resistance. Within this patent it describes the increased intensity and duration of electric oscillations of a low temperature resonating circuit. It is believed that Tesla had intended that Linde's machine would be used to attain the cooling agents.

A milestone was achieved on July 10, 1908 when Heike Kamerlingh Onnes at Leiden University in the Netherlands produced, for the first time, liquified helium, which has a boiling point of 4.2 kelvin at atmospheric pressure.

Sudden and Fundamental Disappearance

Heike Kamerlingh Onnes and Jacob Clay reinvestigated Dewar's earlier experiments on the reduction of resistance at low temperatures. Onnes began the investigations with platinum and gold, replacing these later with mercury (a more readily refinable material). Onnes's research into the resistivity of solid mercury at cryogenic temperatures was accomplished by using liquid helium as a refrigerant. On April 8, 1911, 16:00 hours Onnes noted "Kwik nagenoeg nul", which translates as "[Resistance of] mercury almost zero." At the temperature of 4.19 K, he observed that the resistivity abruptly disappeared (the measuring device Onnes was using did not indicate any resistance). Onnes disclosed his research in 1911, in a paper titled "*On the Sudden Rate at Which the Resistance of Mercury Disappears.*" Onnes stated in that paper that the "specific resistance" became thousands of times less in amount relative to the best conductor at ordinary temperature. Onnes later reversed the process and found that at 4.2 K, the resistance returned to the material. The next year, Onnes published more articles about the phenomenon. Initially, Onnes called the phenomenon "*supraconductivity*" (1913) and, only later, adopted the term "*superconductivity.*" For his research, he was awarded the Nobel Prize in Physics in 1913.

Onnes conducted an experiment, in 1912, on the usability of superconductivity. Onnes introduced an electric current into a superconductive ring and removed the battery that generated it. Upon measuring the electric current, Onnes found that its intensity did not diminish with the time. The current persisted due to the superconductive state of the conductive medium. In subsequent decades, superconductivity was found in several other materials. In 1913, lead was found to superconduct at 7 K, and in 1941 niobium nitride was found to superconduct at 16 K.

Enigmas and Solutions

The next important step in understanding superconductivity occurred in 1933, when Walther Meissner and Robert Ochsenfeld discovered that superconductors expelled applied magnetic fields, a phenomenon that has come to be known as the Meissner effect. In 1935, brothers Fritz London and Heinz London showed that the Meissner effect was a consequence of the minimization of the electromagnetic free energy carried by superconducting current. In 1950, the phenomenological Ginzburg-Landau theory of superconductivity was devised by Lev Landau and Vitaly Ginzburg.

The Ginzburg-Landau theory, which combined Landau's theory of second-order phase transitions with a Schrödinger-like wave equation, had great success in explaining the macroscopic properties of superconductors. In particular, Alexei Abrikosov showed that Ginzburg-Landau theory predicts the division of superconductors into the two categories now referred to as Type I and Type II. Abrikosov and Ginzburg were awarded the 2003 Nobel Prize in Physics for their work (Landau having died in 1968). Also in 1950, Emanuel Maxwell and, almost simultaneously, C.A. Reynolds *et al.* found that the critical temperature of a superconductor depends on the isotopic mass of the constituent element. This important discovery pointed to the electron-phonon interaction as the microscopic mechanism responsible for superconductivity.

BCS Theory

The complete microscopic theory of superconductivity was finally proposed in 1957 by John Bardeen, Leon N. Cooper, and Robert Schrieffer. This BCS theory explained the superconducting current as a superfluid of Cooper pairs, pairs of electrons interacting through the exchange of phonons. For this work, the authors were awarded the Nobel Prize in Physics in 1972. The BCS theory was set on a firmer footing in 1958, when Nikolai Nikolaevich Bogolyubov showed that the BCS wavefunction, which had originally been derived from a variational argument, could be obtained using a canonical transformation of the electronic Hamiltonian. In 1959, Lev Gor'kov showed that the BCS theory reduced to the Ginzburg-Landau theory close to the critical temperature.

Gor'kov was the first to derive the superconducting phase evolution equation $2eV = \hbar \frac{\partial \phi}{\partial t}$.

Little-Parks Effect

The Little-Parks effect was discovered in 1962 in experiments with empty and thin-walled superconducting cylinders subjected to a parallel magnetic field. The electrical resistance of such cylinders shows a periodic oscillation with the magnetic flux through the cylinder, the period being $h/2e = 2.07 \times 10^{-15}$ V·s. The explanation provided by William Little and Ronald Parks is that the resistance oscillation reflects a more fundamental phenomenon, i.e. periodic oscillation of the superconducting critical temperature (T_c). This is the temperature at which the sample becomes superconducting. The Little-Parks effect is a result of collective quantum behavior of superconducting electrons. It reflects the general fact that it is the fluxoid rather than the flux which is quantized in superconductors. The Little-Parks effect demonstrates that the vector potential couples to an observable physical quantity, namely the superconducting critical temperature.

Commercial Activity

Soon after discovering superconductivity in 1911, Kamerlingh Onnes attempted to make an electromagnet with superconducting windings but found that relatively low magnetic fields destroyed superconductivity in the materials he investigated. Much later, in 1955, George Yntema succeeded in constructing a small 0.7-tesla iron-core electromagnet with superconducting niobium wire windings. Then, in 1961, J. E. Kunzler, E. Buehler, F. S. L. Hsu, and J. H. Wernick made the startling discovery that at 4.2 kelvins, a compound consisting of three parts niobium and one part tin was capable of supporting a current density of more than 100,000 amperes per square centimeter in a magnetic field of 8.8 tesla. Despite being brittle and difficult to fabricate, niobium-tin has since proved extremely useful in supermagnets generating magnetic fields as high as 20 teslas. In 1962, Ted Berlincourt and Richard Hake discovered that alloys of niobium and titanium are suitable for applications up to 10 teslas. Promptly thereafter, commercial production of niobium-titanium supermagnet wire commenced at Westinghouse Electric Corporation and at Wah Chang Corporation. Although niobium-titanium boasts less-impressive superconductng properties than those of niobium-tin, niobium-titanium has, nevertheless, become the most widely used "workhorse" supermagnet material, in large measure a consequence of its very high ductility and ease of fabrication. However, both niobium-tin and niobium-titanium find wide application in MRI medical imagers, bending and focusing magnets for enormous high-energy particle accelerators, and a host of other applications. Conectus, a European consortium for superconductivity, estimated that in 2014, global economic activity, for which superconductivity was indispensable, amounted to about five billion euros, with MRI systems accounting for about 80% of that total.

In 1962, Brian Josephson made the important theoretical prediction that a supercurrent can flow between two pieces of superconductor separated by a thin layer of insulator. This phenomenon, now called the Josephson effect, is exploited by superconducting devices such as SQUIDs. It is used in the most accurate available measurements of the magnetic flux quantum $h/2e$, and thus (coupled with the quantum Hall resistivity) for Planck's constant h. Josephson was awarded the Nobel Prize in Physics for this work in 1973.

In 1973 Nb_3Ge found to have T_c of 23 K, which remained the highest ambient-pressure T_c until the discovery of the cuprate high-temperature superconductors in 1986.

High-temperature Superconductors

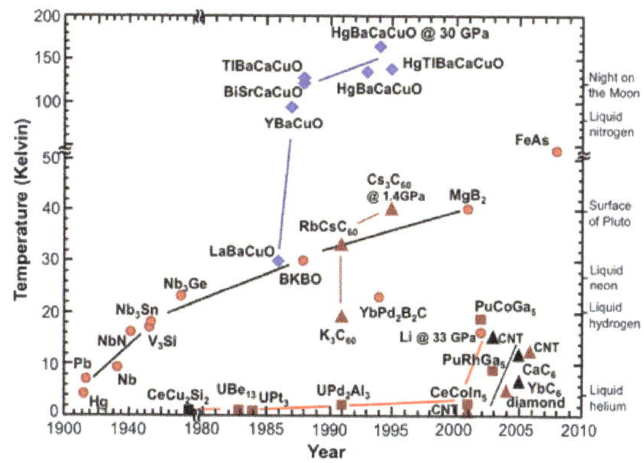

Superconductor timeline

In 1986, J. Georg Bednorz and K. Alex Mueller discovered superconductivity in a lanthanum-based cuprate perovskite material, which had a transition temperature of 35 K (Nobel Prize in Physics, 1987) and was the first of the high-temperature superconductors. It was shortly found (by Ching-Wu Chu) that replacing the lanthanum with yttrium, i.e. making YBCO, raised the critical temperature to 92 K, which was important because liquid nitrogen could then be used as a refrigerant (at atmospheric pressure, the boiling point of nitrogen is 77 K). This is important commercially because liquid nitrogen can be produced cheaply on-site with no raw materials, and is not prone to some of the problems (solid air plugs, etc.) of helium in piping. Many other cuprate superconductors have since been discovered, and the theory of superconductivity in these materials is one of the major outstanding challenges of theoretical condensed-matter physics.

In March 2001, superconductivity of magnesium diboride (MgB_2) was found with $T_c = 39$ K.

In 2008, the oxypnictide or iron-based superconductors were discovered, which led to a flurry of work in the hope that studying them would provide a theory of the cuprate superconductors.

In 2013, room-temperature superconductivity was attained in YBCO for picoseconds, using short pulses of infrared laser light to deform the material's crystal structure.

Electrical Resistance and Conductance

The electrical resistance of an electrical conductor is a measure of the difficulty to pass an electric current through that conductor. The inverse quantity is electrical conductance, and is the ease with which an electric current passes. Electrical resistance shares some conceptual parallels with the notion of mechanical friction. The SI unit of electrical resistance is the ohm (Ω), while electrical conductance is measured in siemens (S).

An object of uniform cross section has a resistance proportional to its resistivity and length and inversely proportional to its cross-sectional area. All materials show some resistance, except for superconductors, which have a resistance of zero.

The resistance (R) of an object is defined as the ratio of voltage across it (*V*) to current through it (*I*), while the conductance (G) is the inverse:

$$R = \frac{V}{I}, \qquad G = \frac{I}{V} = \frac{1}{R}$$

For a wide variety of materials and conditions, *V* and *I* are directly proportional to each other, and therefore *R* and *G* are constant (although they can depend on other factors like temperature or strain). This proportionality is called Ohm's law, and materials that satisfy it are called *ohmic* materials.

In other cases, such as a diode or battery, *V* and *I* are *not* directly proportional. The ratio V/I is sometimes still useful, and is referred to as a "chordal resistance" or "static resistance", since it corresponds to the inverse slope of a chord between the origin and an *I–V* curve. In other situations, the derivative $\frac{dV}{dI}$ may be most useful; this is called the "differential resistance".

Introduction

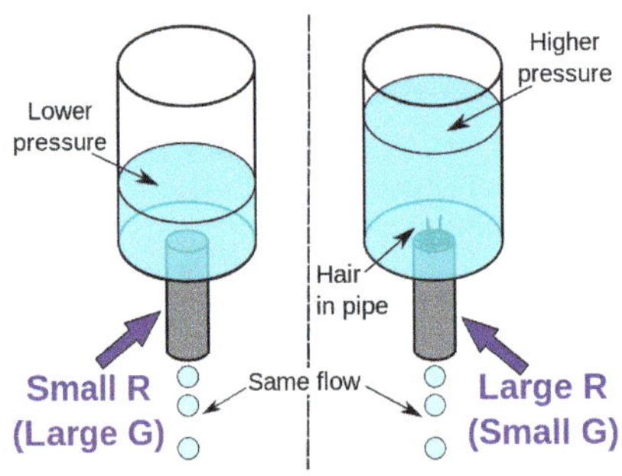

The hydraulic analogy compares electric current flowing through circuits to water flowing through pipes. When a pipe (left) is filled with hair (right), it takes a larger pressure to achieve the same flow of water. Pushing electric current through a large resistance is like pushing water through a pipe clogged with hair: It requires a larger push (electromotive force) to drive the same flow (electric current).

In the hydraulic analogy, current flowing through a wire (or resistor) is like water flowing through a pipe, and the voltage drop across the wire is like the pressure drop that pushes water through the pipe. Conductance is proportional to how much flow occurs for a given pressure, and resistance is proportional to how much pressure is required to achieve a given flow. (Conductance and resistance are reciprocals.)

The voltage *drop* (i.e., difference between voltages on one side of the resistor and the other), not the voltage itself, provides the driving force pushing current through a resistor. In hydraulics, it is similar: The pressure *difference* between two sides of a pipe, not the pressure itself, determines the flow through it. For example, there may be a large water pressure above the pipe, which tries to push water down through the pipe. But there may be an equally large water pressure below the pipe, which tries to push water back up through the pipe. If these pressures are equal, no water flows. (In the image at right, the water pressure below the pipe is zero.)

The resistance and conductance of a wire, resistor, or other element is mostly determined by two properties:

- geometry (shape), and
- material

Geometry is important because it is more difficult to push water through a long, narrow pipe than a wide, short pipe. In the same way, a long, thin copper wire has higher resistance (lower conductance) than a short, thick copper wire.

Materials are important as well. A pipe filled with hair restricts the flow of water more than a clean pipe of the same shape and size. Similarly, electrons can flow freely and easily through a copper wire, but cannot flow as easily through a steel wire of the same shape and size, and they essentially cannot flow at all through an insulator like rubber, regardless of its shape. The difference between copper, steel, and rubber is related to their microscopic structure and electron configuration, and is quantified by a property called resistivity.

In addition to geometry and material, there are various other factors that influence resistance and conductance, such as temperature.

Conductors and Resistors

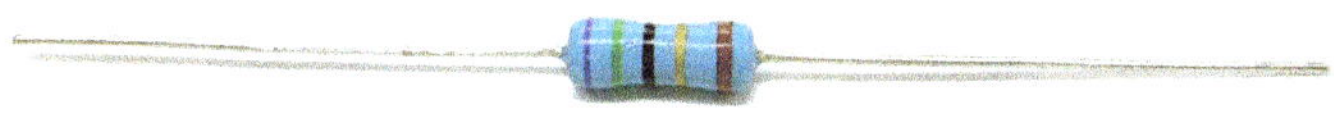

A 6.5 MΩ resistor, as identified by its electronic color code (blue–green–black-yellow-red). An ohmmeter could be used to verify this value.

Substances in which electricity can flow are called conductors. A piece of conducting material of a particular resistance meant for use in a circuit is called a resistor. Conductors are made of high-conductivity materials such as metals, in particular copper and aluminium. Resistors, on the other hand, are made of a wide variety of materials depending on factors such as the desired resistance, amount of energy that it needs to dissipate, precision, and costs.

Ohm's Law

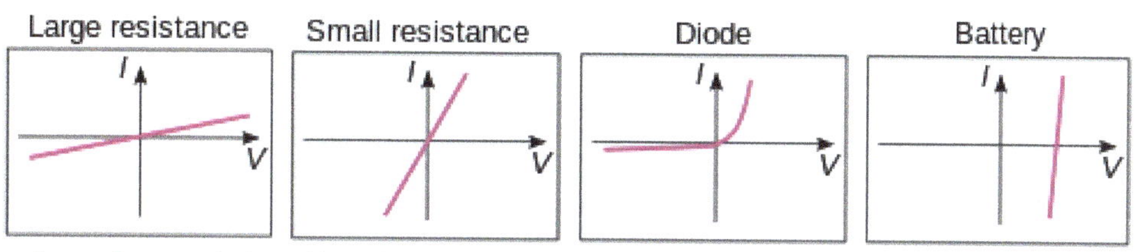

The current-voltage characteristics of four devices: Two resistors, a diode, and a battery. The horizontal axis is voltage drop, the vertical axis is current. Ohm's law is satisfied when the graph is a straight line through the origin. Therefore, the two resistors are *ohmic*, but the diode and battery are not.

Ohm's law is an empirical law relating the voltage V across an element to the current I through it:

$$I \propto V$$

(I is directly proportional to V). This law is not always true: For example, it is false for diodes, batteries, and other devices whose conductance is not constant. However, it is true to a very good approximation for wires and resistors (assuming that other conditions, including temperature, are held constant). Materials or objects where Ohm's law is true are called *ohmic*, whereas objects that do not obey Ohm's law are *non-ohmic.*

Relation to Resistivity and Conductivity

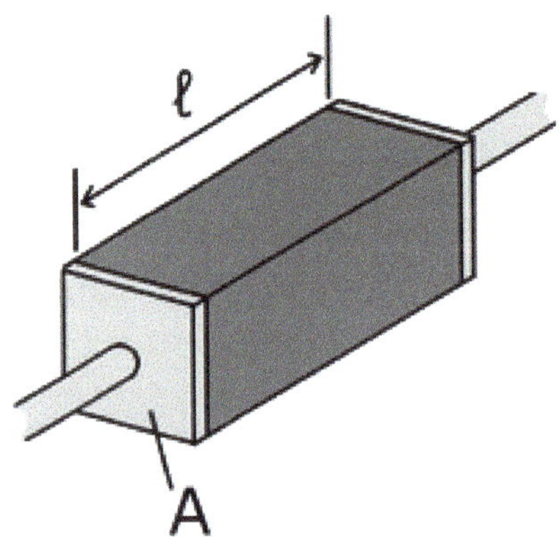

A piece of resistive material with electrical contacts on both ends.

The resistance of a given object depends primarily on two factors: What material it is made of, and its shape. For a given material, the resistance is inversely proportional to the cross-sectional area; for example, a thick copper wire has lower resistance than an otherwise-identical thin copper wire. Also, for a given material, the resistance is proportional to the length; for example, a long copper wire has higher resistance than an otherwise-identical short copper wire. The resistance R and conductance G of a conductor of uniform cross section, therefore, can be computed as

$$R = \rho \frac{\ell}{A},$$

$$G = \sigma \frac{A}{\ell}.$$

where ℓ is the length of the conductor, measured in metres [m], A is the cross-sectional area of the conductor measured in square metres [m^2], σ (sigma) is the electrical conductivity measured in siemens per meter (S·m^{-1}), and ρ (rho) is the electrical resistivity (also called *specific electrical resistance*) of the material, measured in ohm-metres (Ω·m). The resistivity and conductivity are proportionality constants, and therefore depend only on the material the wire is made of, not the geometry of the wire. Resistivity and conductivity are reciprocals: $\rho = 1/\sigma$. Resistivity is a measure of the material's ability to oppose electric current.

This formula is not exact, as it assumes the current density is totally uniform in the conductor, which is not always true in practical situations. However, this formula still provides a good approximation for long thin conductors such as wires.

Another situation for which this formula is not exact is with alternating current (AC), because the skin effect inhibits current flow near the center of the conductor. For this reason, the *geometrical* cross-section is different from the *effective* cross-section in which current actually flows, so resistance is higher than expected. Similarly, if two conductors near each other carry AC current, their resistances increase due to the proximity effect. At commercial power frequency, these effects are significant for large conductors carrying large currents, such as busbars in an electrical substation, or large power cables carrying more than a few hundred amperes.

What Determines Resistivity?

The resistivity of different materials varies by an enormous amount: For example, the conductivity of teflon is about 10^{30} times lower than the conductivity of copper. Why is there such a difference? Loosely speaking, a metal has large numbers of "delocalized" electrons that are not stuck in any one place, but free to move across large distances, whereas in an insulator (like teflon), each electron is tightly bound to a single molecule, and a great force is required to pull it away. Semiconductors lie between these two extremes.

Resistivity varies with temperature. In semiconductors, resistivity also changes when exposed to light.

Measuring Resistance

An instrument for measuring resistance is called an ohmmeter. Simple ohmmeters cannot measure low resistances accurately because the resistance of their measuring leads causes a voltage drop that interferes with the measurement, so more accurate devices use four-terminal sensing.

Typical Resistances

Component	Resistance (Ω)
1 meter of copper wire with 1 mm diameter	0.02
1 km overhead power line (*typical*)	0.03
AA battery (*typical internal resistance*)	0.1
Incandescent light bulb filament (*typical*)	200–1000
Human body	1000 to 100,000

Static and Differential Resistance

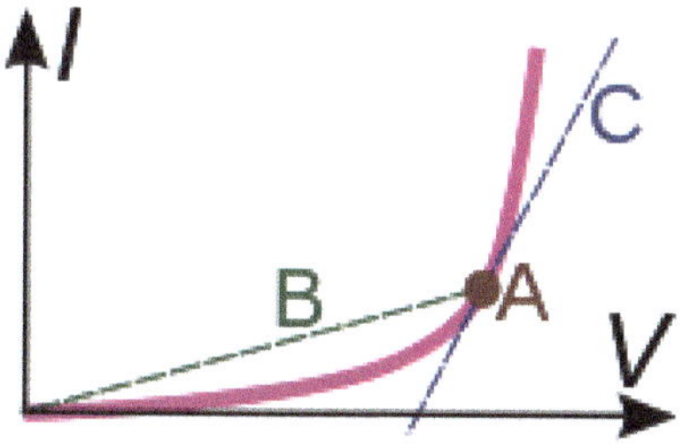

The IV curve of a non-ohmic device (purple). The static resistance at point *A* is the inverse slope of line *B* through the origin. The differential resistance at *A* is the inverse slope of tangent line *C*.

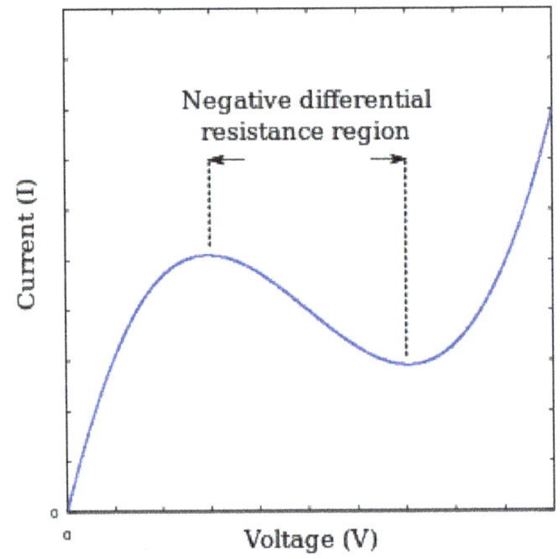

The IV curve of a component with negative differential resistance, an unusual phenomenon where the IV curve is non-monotonic.

Many electrical elements, such as diodes and batteries do *not* satisfy Ohm's law. These are called *non-ohmic* or *non-linear*, and their *I–V* curves are *not* straight lines through the origin.

Resistance and conductance can still be defined for non-ohmic elements. However, unlike ohmic resistance, non-linear resistance is not constant but varies with the voltage or current through the device; i.e., its operating point. There are two types of resistance:

- Static resistance (also called *chordal* or *DC resistance*) - This corresponds to the usual definition of resistance; the voltage divided by the current

  $$R_{\text{static}} = \frac{V}{I}$$

  It is the slope of the line (chord) from the origin through the point on the curve. Static resistance determines the power dissipation in an electrical component. Points on the *IV* curve located in the 2nd or 4th quadrants, for which the slope of the chordal line is negative, have *negative static resistance*. Passive devices, which have no source of energy, cannot have negative static resistance. However active devices such as transistors or op-amps can synthesize negative static resistance with feedback, and it is used in some circuits such as gyrators.

- Differential resistance (also called *dynamic, incremental* or *small signal resistance*) - Differential resistance is the derivative of the voltage with respect to the current; the slope of the *IV* curve at a point

  $$R_{\text{diff}} = \frac{dV}{dI}$$

  If the *IV* curve is nonmonotonic (with peaks and troughs), the curve has a negative slope in some regions—so in these regions the device has *negative differential resistance*. Devices with negative differential resistance can amplify a signal applied to them, and are used to make amplifiers and oscillators. These include tunnel diodes, Gunn diodes, IMPATT diodes, magnetron tubes, and unijunction transistors.

AC Circuits

Impedance and Admittance

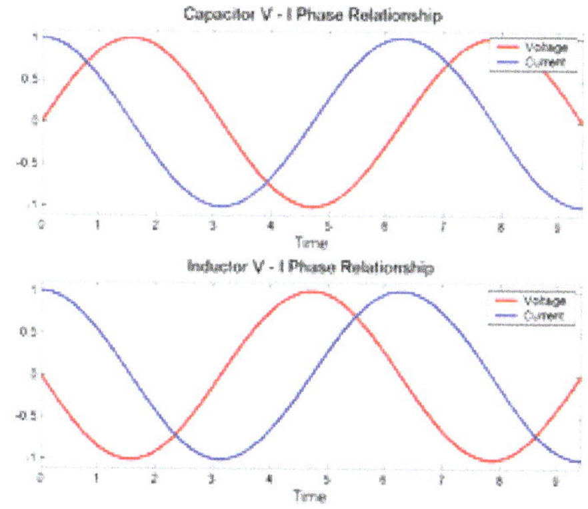

The voltage (red) and current (blue) versus time (horizontal axis) for a capacitor (top) and inductor (bottom). Since the amplitude of the current and voltage sinusoids are the same, the absolute value of impedance is 1 for both the capacitor and the inductor (in whatever units the graph is using). On the other hand, the phase difference between current and voltage is -90° for the capacitor; therefore, the complex phase of the impedance of the capacitor is -90°. Similarly, the phase difference between current and voltage is +90° for the inductor; therefore, the complex phase of the impedance of the inductor is +90°.

When an alternating current flows through a circuit, the relation between current and voltage across a circuit element is characterized not only by the ratio of their magnitudes, but also the difference in their phases. For example, in an ideal resistor, the moment when the voltage reaches its maximum, the current also reaches its maximum (current and voltage are oscillating in phase). But for a capacitor or inductor, the maximum current flow occurs as the voltage passes through zero and vice versa (current and voltage are oscillating 90° out of phase). Complex numbers are used to keep track of both the phase and magnitude of current and voltage:

$$V(t) = \mathrm{Re}(V_0 e^{j\omega t}), \quad I(t) = \mathrm{Re}(I_0 e^{j\omega t}), \quad Z = \frac{V_0}{I_0}, \quad Y = \frac{I_0}{V_0}$$

where:

- t is time,
- $V(t)$ and $I(t)$ are, respectively, voltage and current as a function of time,
- V_o, I_o, Z, and Y are complex numbers,
- Z is called impedance,
- Y is called admittance,
- Re indicates real part,
- ω is the angular frequency of the AC current,
- $j = \sqrt{-1}$ is the imaginary unit.

The impedance and admittance may be expressed as complex numbers that can be broken into real and imaginary parts:

$$Z = R + jX, \quad Y = G + jB$$

where R and G are resistance and conductance respectively, X is reactance, and B is susceptance. For ideal resistors, Z and Y reduce to R and G respectively, but for AC networks containing capacitors and inductors, X and B are nonzero.

$Z = 1/Y$ for AC circuits, just as $R = 1/G$ for DC circuits.

Frequency Dependence of Resistance

Another complication of AC circuits is that the resistance and conductance can be frequency-dependent. One reason, mentioned above is the skin effect (and the related proximity effect). Another reason is that the resistivity itself may depend on frequency.

Energy Dissipation and Joule Heating

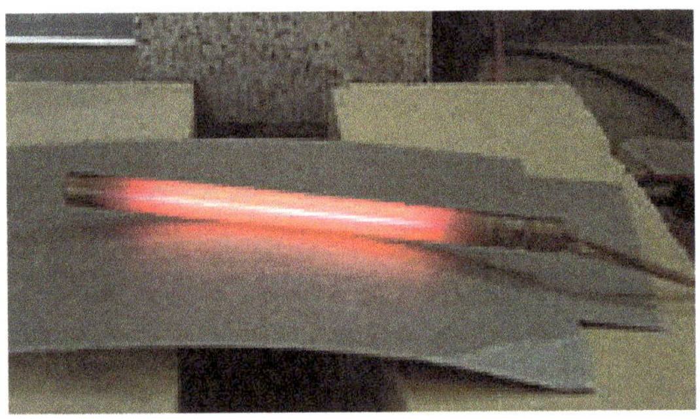

Running current through a material with high resistance creates heat, in a phenomenon called Joule heating. In this picture, a cartridge heater, warmed by Joule heating, is glowing red hot.

Resistors (and other elements with resistance) oppose the flow of electric current; therefore, electrical energy is required to push current through the resistance. This electrical energy is dissipated, heating the resistor in the process. This is called *Joule heating* (after James Prescott Joule), also called *ohmic heating* or *resistive heating*.

The dissipation of electrical energy is often undesired, particularly in the case of transmission losses in power lines. High voltage transmission helps reduce the losses by reducing the current for a given power.

On the other hand, Joule heating is sometimes useful, for example in electric stoves and other electric heaters (also called *resistive heaters*). As another example, incandescent lamps rely on Joule heating: the filament is heated to such a high temperature that it glows "white hot" with thermal radiation (also called incandescence).

The formula for Joule heating is:

$$P = I^2 R$$

where P is the power (energy per unit time) converted from electrical energy to thermal energy, R is the resistance, and I is the current through the resistor.

Dependence of Resistance on Other Conditions

Temperature Dependence

Near room temperature, the resistivity of metals typically increases as temperature is increased, while the resistivity of semiconductors typically decreases as temperature is increased. The resistivity of insulators and electrolytes may increase or decrease depending on the system. For the detailed behavior and explanation.

As a consequence, the resistance of wires, resistors, and other components often change with temperature. This effect may be undesired, causing an electronic circuit to malfunction at extreme temperatures. In some cases, however, the effect is put to good use. When temperature-dependent resistance of a component is used purposefully, the component is called a resistance thermometer or thermistor. (A resistance thermometer is made of metal, usually platinum, while a thermistor is made of ceramic or polymer.)

Resistance thermometers and thermistors are generally used in two ways. First, they can be used as thermometers: By measuring the resistance, the temperature of the environment can be inferred. Second, they can be used in conjunction with Joule heating (also called self-heating): If a large current is running through the resistor, the resistor's temperature rises and therefore its resistance changes. Therefore, these components can be used in a circuit-protection role similar to fuses, or for feedback in circuits, or for many other purposes. In general, self-heating can turn a resistor into a nonlinear and hysteretic circuit element.

If the temperature T does not vary too much, a linear approximation is typically used:

$$R(T) = R_0[1+\alpha(T-T_0)]$$

where α is called the *temperature coefficient of resistance*, T_0 is a fixed reference temperature (usually room temperature), and R_0 is the resistance at temperature T_0. The parameter α is an empirical parameter fitted from measurement data. Because the linear approximation is only an approximation, α is different for different reference temperatures. For this reason it is usual to specify the temperature that α was measured at with a suffix, such as α_{15}, and the relationship only holds in a range of temperatures around the reference.

The temperature coefficient α is typically $+3\times10^{-3}$ K^{-1} to $+6\times10^{-3}$ K^{-1} for metals near room temperature. It is usually negative for semiconductors and insulators, with highly variable magnitude.

Strain Dependence

Just as the resistance of a conductor depends upon temperature, the resistance of a conductor depends upon strain. By placing a conductor under tension (a form of stress that leads to strain in the form of stretching of the conductor), the length of the section of conductor under tension increases and its cross-sectional area decreases. Both these effects contribute to increasing the resistance of the strained section of conductor. Under compression (strain in the opposite direction), the resistance of the strained section of conductor decreases.

Light Illumination Dependence

Some resistors, particularly those made from semiconductors, exhibit *photoconductivity*, meaning that their resistance changes when light is shining on them. Therefore, they are called *photoresistors* (or *light dependent resistors*). These are a common type of light detector.

Superconductivity

Superconductors are materials that have exactly zero resistance and infinite conductance, because they can have V=0 and I≠0. This also means there is no joule heating, or in other words no dissipation of electrical energy. Therefore, if superconductive wire is made into a closed loop, current flows around the loop forever. Superconductors require cooling to temperatures near 4 K with liquid helium for most metallic superconductors like NbSn alloys, or cooling to temperatures near 77K with liquid nitrogen for the expensive, brittle and delicate ceramic high temperature superconductors. Nevertheless, there are many technological applications of superconductivity, including superconducting magnets.

Magnetic Field

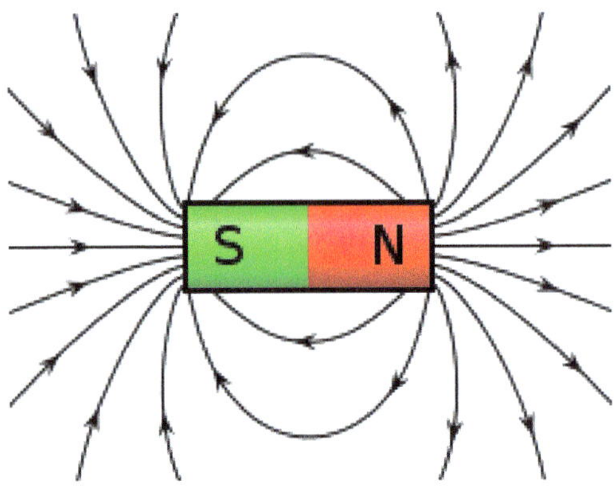

Magnetic field of an ideal cylindrical magnet with its axis of symmetry inside the image plane. The magnetic field is represented by magnetic field lines, which show the direction of the field at different points.

A magnetic field is the magnetic effect of electric currents and magnetic materials. The magnetic field at any given point is specified by both a *direction* and a *magnitude* (or strength); as such it is represented by a vector field. The term is used for two distinct but closely related fields denoted by the symbols B and H, where H is measured in units of amperes per meter (symbol: $A{\cdot}m^{-1}$ or A/m) in the SI. B is measured in teslas (symbol: T) and newtons per meter per ampere (symbol: $N{\cdot}m^{-1}{\cdot}A^{-1}$ or N/(m·A)) in the SI. B is most commonly defined in terms of the Lorentz force it exerts on moving electric charges.

Magnetic fields can be produced by moving electric charges and the intrinsic magnetic moments of elementary particles associated with a fundamental quantum property, their spin. In special relativity, electric and magnetic fields are two interrelated aspects of a single object, called the electromagnetic tensor; the split of this tensor into electric and magnetic fields depends on the relative velocity of the observer and charge. In quantum physics, the electromagnetic field is quantized and electromagnetic interactions result from the exchange of photons.

In everyday life, magnetic fields are most often encountered as a force created by permanent magnets, which pull on ferromagnetic materials such as iron, cobalt, or nickel, and attract or repel other magnets. Magnetic fields are widely used throughout modern technology, particularly in electrical engineering and electromechanics. The Earth produces its own magnetic field, which is important in navigation, and it shields the Earth's atmosphere from solar wind. Rotating magnetic fields are used in both electric motors and generators. Magnetic forces give information about the charge carriers in a material through the Hall effect. The interaction of magnetic fields in electric devices such as transformers is studied in the discipline of magnetic circuits.

History

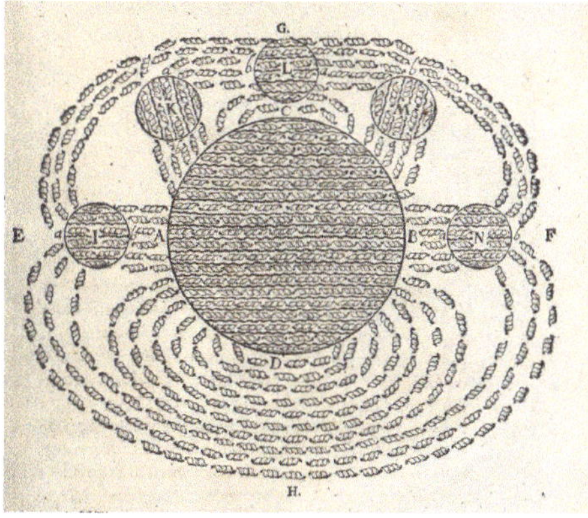

One of the first drawings of a magnetic field, by René Descartes, 1644, showing the Earth attracting lodestones. It illustrated his theory that magnetism was caused by the circulation of tiny helical particles, "threaded parts", through threaded pores in magnets.

Although magnets and magnetism were known much earlier, the study of magnetic fields began in 1269 when French scholar Petrus Peregrinus de Maricourt mapped out the magnetic field on the surface of a spherical magnet using iron needles. Noting that the resulting field lines crossed at two points he named those points 'poles' in analogy to Earth's poles. He also clearly articulated the principle that magnets always have both a north and south pole, no matter how finely one slices them.

Almost three centuries later, William Gilbert of Colchester replicated Petrus Peregrinus' work and was the first to state explicitly that Earth is a magnet. Published in 1600, Gilbert's work, *De Magnete*, helped to establish magnetism as a science.

In 1750, John Michell stated that magnetic poles attract and repel in accordance with an inverse square law. Charles-Augustin de Coulomb experimentally verified this in 1785 and stated explicitly that the north and south poles cannot be separated. Building on this force between poles, Siméon Denis Poisson (1781–1840) created the first successful model of the magnetic field, which he presented in 1824. In this model, a magnetic H-field is produced by 'magnetic poles' and magnetism is due to small pairs of north/south magnetic poles.

Three discoveries challenged this foundation of magnetism, though. First, in 1819, Hans Christian Ørsted discovered that an electric current generates a magnetic field encircling it. Then in 1820, André-Marie Ampère showed that parallel wires having currents in the same direction attract one another. Finally, Jean-Baptiste Biot and Félix Savart discovered the Biot–Savart law in 1820, which correctly predicts the magnetic field around any current-carrying wire.

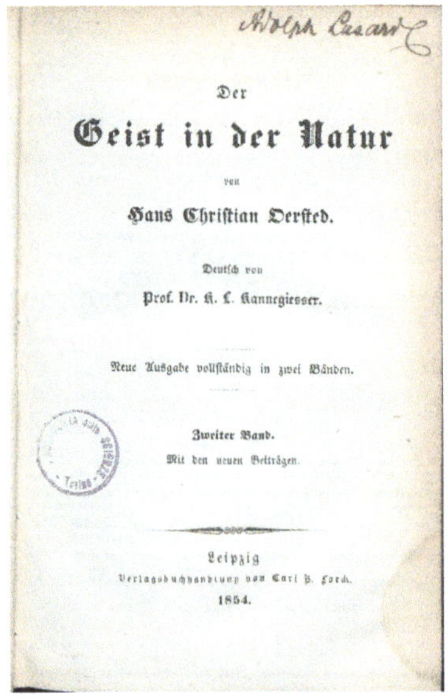

Der
Geist in der Natur
von
Hans Christian Oersted.
Deutsch von
Prof. Dr. K. L. Kannegiesser.
Neue Ausgabe vollständig in zwei Bänden.
Zweiter Band.
Mit den neuen Beiträgen.
Leipzig
Verlagsbuchhandlung von Carl B. Lorck.
1854.

Hans Christian Ørsted, *Der Geist in der Natur*, 1854.

Extending these experiments, Ampère published his own successful model of magnetism in 1825. In it, he showed the equivalence of electrical currents to magnets and proposed that magnetism is due to perpetually flowing loops of current instead of the dipoles of magnetic charge in Poisson's model. This has the additional benefit of explaining why magnetic charge can not be isolated. Further, Ampère derived both Ampère's force law describing the force between two currents and Ampère's law, which, like the Biot–Savart law, correctly described the magnetic field generated by a steady current. Also in this work, Ampère introduced the term electrodynamics to describe the relationship between electricity and magnetism.

In 1831, Michael Faraday discovered electromagnetic induction when he found that a changing magnetic field generates an encircling electric field. He described this phenomenon in what is known as Faraday's law of induction. Later, Franz Ernst Neumann proved that, for a moving conductor in a magnetic field, induction is a consequence of Ampère's force law. In the process he introduced the magnetic vector potential, which was later shown to be equivalent to the underlying mechanism proposed by Faraday.

In 1850, Lord Kelvin, then known as William Thomson, distinguished between two magnetic fields now denoted H and B. The former applied to Poisson's model and the latter to Ampère's model and induction. Further, he derived how H and B relate to each other.

The reason H and B are used for the two magnetic fields has been a source of some debate among science historians. Most agree that Kelvin avoided M to prevent confusion with the SI fundamental unit of length, the Metre, abbreviated "m". Others believe the choices were purely random.

Between 1861 and 1865, James Clerk Maxwell developed and published Maxwell's equations, which explained and united all of classical electricity and magnetism. The first set of these equations was published in a paper entitled *On Physical Lines of Force* in 1861. These equations were valid although incomplete. Maxwell completed his set of equations in his later 1865 paper *A Dynamical Theory of the Electromagnetic Field* and demonstrated the fact that light is an electromagnetic wave. Heinrich Hertz experimentally confirmed this fact in 1887.

The twentieth century extended electrodynamics to include relativity and quantum mechanics. Albert Einstein, in his paper of 1905 that established relativity, showed that both the electric and magnetic fields are part of the same phenomena viewed from different reference frames. Finally, the emergent field of quantum mechanics was merged with electrodynamics to form quantum electrodynamics (QED).

Definitions, Units, and Measurement

The B-field

Alternative names for B

- Magnetic flux density
- Magnetic field

Alternative names for H

- Magnetic field intensity
- Magnetic field strength
- Magnetic field
- Magnetizing field

The magnetic field can be defined in several equivalent ways based on the effects it has on its environment.

Often the magnetic field is defined by the force it exerts on a moving charged particle. It is known from experiments in electrostatics that a particle of charge q in an electric field E experiences a force F = qE. However, in other situations, such as when a charged particle moves in the vicinity of a current-carrying wire, the force also depends on the velocity of that particle. Fortunately, the velocity dependent portion can be separated out such that the force on the particle satisfies the *Lorentz force law*,

$$\boldsymbol{F} = q(\boldsymbol{E} + \boldsymbol{v} \times \boldsymbol{B}).$$

Here v is the particle's velocity and × denotes the cross product. The vector B is termed the magnetic field, and it is *defined* as the vector field necessary to make the Lorentz force law correctly describe the motion of a charged particle. This definition allows the determination of B in the following way.

The command, "Measure the direction and magnitude of the vector B at such and such a place," calls for the following operations: Take a particle of known charge q. Measure the force on q at rest, to determine E. Then measure the force on the particle when its velocity is v; repeat with v in some other direction. Now find a B that makes the Lorentz force law fit all these results—that is the magnetic field at the place in question.

Alternatively, the magnetic field can be defined in terms of the torque it produces on a magnetic dipole.

The H-field

In addition to B, there is a quantity H, which is also sometimes called the *magnetic field.* In a vacuum, B and H are proportional to each other, with the multiplicative constant depending on the physical units. Inside a material they are different (H and B inside and outside of magnetic materials). The term "magnetic field" is historically reserved for H while using other terms for B. Informally, though, and formally for some recent textbooks mostly in physics, the term 'magnetic field' is used to describe B as well as or in place of H. There are many alternative names for both.

Units

In SI units, B is measured in teslas (symbol: T) and correspondingly Φ_B (magnetic flux) is measured in webers (symbol: Wb) so that a flux density of 1 Wb/m^2 is 1 tesla. The SI unit of tesla is equivalent to (newton·second)/(coulomb·metre). In Gaussian-cgs units, B is measured in gauss (symbol: G). (The conversion is 1 T = 10,000 G.) One nanotesla is also called a gamma (symbol: γ). The H-field is measured in amperes per metre (A/m) in SI units, and in oersteds (Oe) in cgs units.

Measurement

The precision attained for a magnetic field measurement for Gravity Probe B experiment is 5 attoteslas (5×10^{-18} T); the largest magnetic field produced in a laboratory is 2.8 kT (VNIIEF in Sarov, Russia, 1998). The magnetic field of some astronomical objects such as magnetars are much higher; magnetars range from 0.1 to 100 GT (10^8 to 10^{11} T).

Devices used to measure the local magnetic field are called magnetometers. Important classes of magnetometers include using induction magnetometer (or search-coil magnetometer) which measure only varying magnetic field, rotating coil magnetometer, Hall effect magnetometers, NMR magnetometers, SQUID magnetometers, and fluxgate magnetometers. The magnetic fields of distant astronomical objects are measured through their effects on local charged particles. For instance, electrons spiraling around a field line produce synchrotron radiation that is detectable in radio waves.

Magnetic Field Lines

Mapping the magnetic field of an object is simple in principle. First, measure the strength and direction of the magnetic field at a large number of locations (or at every point in space). Then, mark each location with an arrow (called a vector) pointing in the direction of the local magnetic field with its magnitude proportional to the strength of the magnetic field.

An alternative method to map the magnetic field is to 'connect' the arrows to form magnetic *field lines.* The direction of the magnetic field at any point is parallel to the direction of nearby field lines, and the local density of field lines can be made proportional to its strength.

Magnetic field lines are like streamlines in fluid flow, in that they represent something continuous, and a different resolution would show more or fewer lines. An advantage of using magnetic field lines as a representation is that many laws of magnetism (and electromagnetism) can be stated completely and concisely using simple concepts such as the 'number' of field lines through a surface. These concepts can be quickly 'translated' to their mathematical form. For example, the number of field lines through a given surface is the surface integral of the magnetic field.

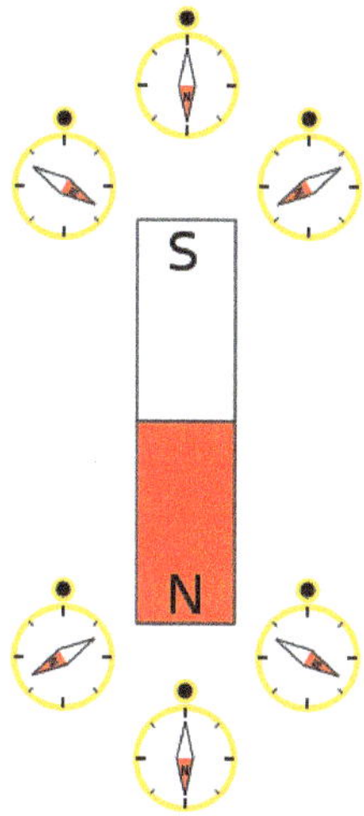

Compasses reveal the direction of the local magnetic field. As seen here, the magnetic field points towards a magnet's south pole and away from its north pole.

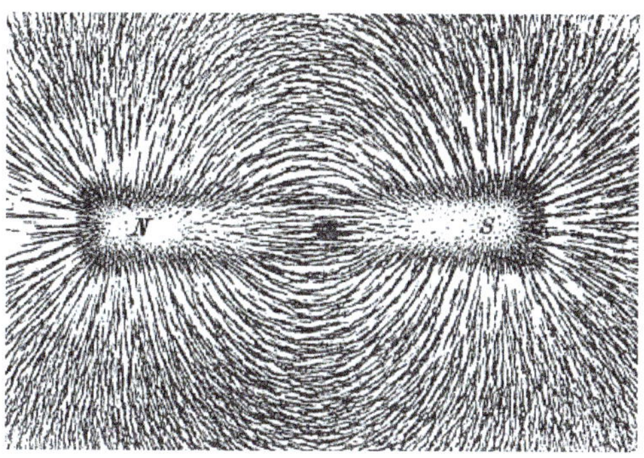

The direction of magnetic field lines represented by the alignment of iron filings sprinkled on paper placed above a bar magnet.

Various phenomena have the effect of "displaying" magnetic field lines as though the field lines were physical phenomena. For example, iron filings placed in a magnetic field, form lines that correspond to 'field lines'. Magnetic field "lines" are also visually displayed in polar auroras, in which plasma particle dipole interactions create visible streaks of light that line up with the local direction of Earth's magnetic field.

Field lines can be used as a qualitative tool to visualize magnetic forces. In ferromagnetic substances like iron and in plasmas, magnetic forces can be understood by imagining that the field lines exert a tension, (like a rubber band) along their length, and a pressure perpendicular to their length on neighboring field lines. 'Unlike' poles of magnets attract because they are linked by many field lines; 'like' poles repel because their field lines do not meet, but run parallel, pushing on each other. The rigorous form of this concept is the electromagnetic stress–energy tensor.

Magnetic Field and Permanent Magnets

Permanent magnets are objects that produce their own persistent magnetic fields. They are made of ferromagnetic materials, such as iron and nickel, that have been magnetized, and they have both a north and a south pole.

Magnetic Field of Permanent Magnets

The magnetic field of permanent magnets can be quite complicated, especially near the magnet. The magnetic field of a small straight magnet is proportional to the magnet's *strength* (called its magnetic dipole moment m). The equations are non-trivial and also depend on the distance from the magnet and the orientation of the magnet. For simple magnets, m points in the direction of a line drawn from the south to the north pole of the magnet. Flipping a bar magnet is equivalent to rotating its m by 180 degrees.

The magnetic field of larger magnets can be obtained by modelling them as a collection of a large number of small magnets called dipoles each having their own m. The magnetic field produced by the magnet then is the net magnetic field of these dipoles. And, any net force on the magnet is a result of adding up the forces on the individual dipoles.

There are two competing models for the nature of these dipoles. These two models produce two different magnetic fields, H and B. Outside a material, though, the two are identical (to a multiplicative constant) so that in many cases the distinction can be ignored. This is particularly true for magnetic fields, such as those due to electric currents, that are not generated by magnetic materials.

Magnetic Pole Model and the H-field

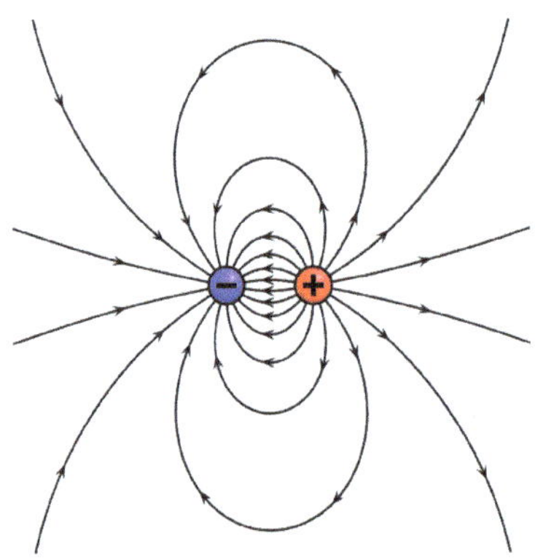

The magnetic pole model: two opposing poles, North (+) and South (−), separated by a distance d produce an H-field (lines).

It is sometimes useful to model the force and torques between two magnets as due to magnetic poles repelling or attracting each other in the same manner as the Coulomb force between electric charges. This is called the Gilbert model of magnetism, after William Gilbert. In this model, a magnetic H-field is produced by *magnetic charges* that are 'smeared' around each pole. These *magnetic charges* are in fact related to the magnetization field M.

The H-field, therefore, is analogous to the electric field E, which starts at a positive electric charge and ends at a negative electric charge. Near the north pole, therefore, all H-field lines point away from the north pole (whether inside the magnet or out) while near the south pole (whether inside the magnet or out) all H-field lines point toward the south pole. A north pole, then, feels a force in the direction of the H-field while the force on the south pole is opposite to the H-field.

In the magnetic pole model, the elementary magnetic dipole m is formed by two opposite magnetic poles of pole strength q_m separated by a small distance vector d, such that m = q_m d. The magnetic pole model predicts correctly the field H both inside and outside magnetic materials, in particular the fact that H is opposite to the magnetization field M inside a permanent magnet.

Since it is based on the fictitious idea of a *magnetic charge density*, the Gilbert model has limitations. Magnetic poles cannot exist apart from each other as electric charges can, but always come in north/south pairs. If a magnetized object is divided in half, a new pole appears on the surface of each piece, so each has a pair of complementary poles. The magnetic pole model does not account for magnetism that is produced by electric currents.

Amperian Loop Model and the B-field

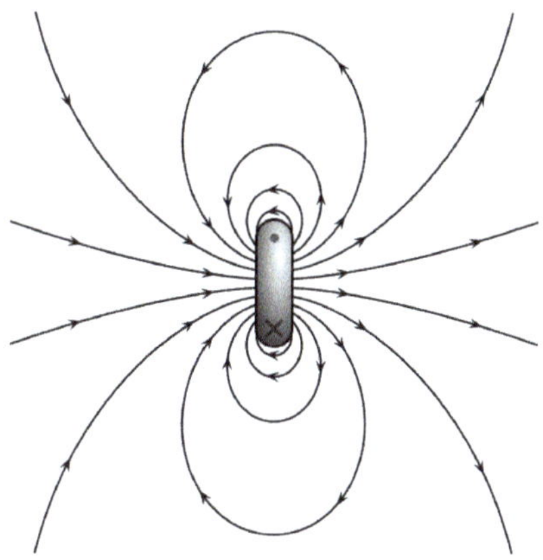

The Amperian loop model: A current loop (ring) that goes into the page at the x and comes out at the dot produces a B-field (lines). The north pole is to the right and the south to the left.

After Ørsted discovered that electric currents produce a magnetic field and Ampere discovered that electric currents attracted and repelled each other similar to magnets, it was natural to hypothesize that all magnetic fields are due to electric current loops. In this model developed by Ampere, the elementary magnetic dipole that makes up all magnets is a sufficiently small Amperian loop of current I. The dipole moment of this loop is $m = IA$ where A is the area of the loop.

These magnetic dipoles produce a magnetic B-field. One important property of the B-field produced this way is that magnetic B-field lines neither start nor end (mathematically, B is a solenoidal vector field); a field line either extends to infinity or wraps around to form a closed curve. To date no exception to this rule has been found. Magnetic field lines exit a magnet near its north pole and enter near its south pole, but inside the magnet B-field lines continue through the magnet from the south pole back to the north. If a B-field line enters a magnet somewhere it has to leave somewhere else; it is not allowed to have an end point. Magnetic poles, therefore, always come in N and S pairs.

More formally, since all the magnetic field lines that enter any given region must also leave that region, subtracting the 'number' of field lines that enter the region from the number that exit gives identically zero. Mathematically this is equivalent to:

$$\oint_S \boldsymbol{B} \cdot \mathrm{d}\boldsymbol{A} = 0,$$

where the integral is a surface integral over the closed surface S (a closed surface is one that completely surrounds a region with no holes to let any field lines escape). Since dA points outward, the dot product in the integral is positive for B-field pointing out and negative for B-field pointing in.

There is also a corresponding differential form of this equation covered in Maxwell's equations below.

Force Between Magnets

The force between two small magnets is quite complicated and depends on the strength and orientation of both magnets and the distance and direction of the magnets relative to each other. The force is particularly sensitive to rotations of the magnets due to magnetic torque. The force on each magnet depends on its magnetic moment and the magnetic field of the other.

To understand the force between magnets, it is useful to examine the *magnetic pole model* given above. In this model, the *H-field* of one magnet pushes and pulls on *both* poles of a second magnet. If this H-field is the same at both poles of the second magnet then there is no net force on that magnet since the force is opposite for opposite poles. If, however, the magnetic field of the first magnet is *nonuniform* (such as the H near one of its poles), each pole of the second magnet sees a different field and is subject to a different force. This difference in the two forces moves the magnet in the direction of increasing magnetic field and may also cause a net torque.

This is a specific example of a general rule that magnets are attracted (or repulsed depending on the orientation of the magnet) into regions of higher magnetic field. Any non-uniform magnetic field, whether caused by permanent magnets or electric currents, exerts a force on a small magnet in this way.

The details of the Amperian loop model are different and more complicated but yield the same result: that magnetic dipoles are attracted/repelled into regions of higher magnetic field. Mathematically, the force on a small magnet having a magnetic moment m due to a magnetic field B is:

$$\boldsymbol{F} = \nabla(\boldsymbol{m} \cdot \boldsymbol{B}),$$

where the gradient ∇ is the change of the quantity m · B per unit distance and the direction is that of maximum increase of m · B. To understand this equation, note that the dot product m · B = $mB\cos(\theta)$, where m and B represent the magnitude of the m and B vectors and θ is the angle between them. If m is in the same direction as B then the dot product is positive and the gradient points 'uphill' pulling the magnet into regions of higher B-field (more strictly larger m · B). This equation is strictly only valid for magnets of zero size, but is often a good approximation for not too large magnets. The magnetic force on larger magnets is determined by dividing them into smaller regions each having their own m then summing up the forces on each of these very small regions.

Magnetic Torque on Permanent Magnets

If two like poles of two separate magnets are brought near each other, and one of the magnets is allowed to turn, it promptly rotates to align itself with the first. In this example, the magnetic field of the stationary magnet creates a *magnetic torque* on the magnet that is free to rotate. This magnetic torque τ tends to align a magnet's poles with the magnetic field lines. A compass, therefore, turns to align itself with Earth's magnetic field.

Magnetic torque is used to drive electric motors. In one simple motor design, a magnet is fixed to a freely rotating shaft and subjected to a magnetic field from an array of electromagnets. By continuously switching the electric current through each of the electromagnets, thereby flipping the polarity of their magnetic fields, like poles are kept next to the rotor; the resultant torque is transferred to the shaft.

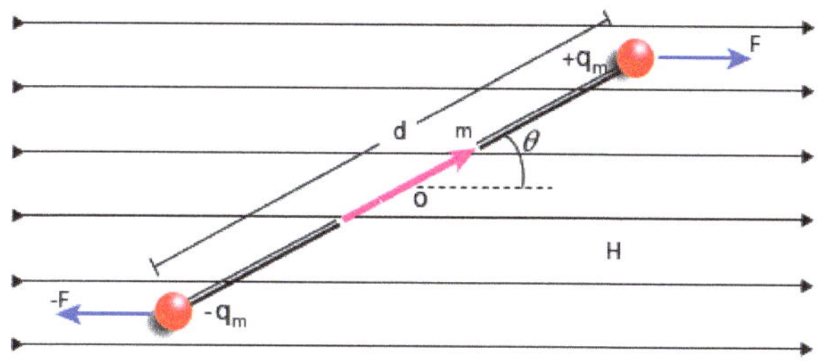

torque on a dipole: An H field (to right) causes equal but opposite forces on a N pole ($+q$) and a S pole ($-q$) creating a torque.

As is the case for the force between magnets, the magnetic pole model leads more readily to the correct equation. Here, two equal and opposite magnetic charges experiencing the same H also experience equal and opposite forces. Since these equal and opposite forces are in different locations, this produces a torque proportional to the distance (perpendicular to the force) between them. With the definition of m as the pole strength times the distance between the poles, this leads to $\tau = \mu_0 mH\sin\theta$, where μ_0 is a constant called the vacuum permeability, measuring $4\pi\times10^{-7}$ V·s/(A·m) and θ is the angle between H and m.

The Amperian loop model also predicts the same magnetic torque. Here, it is the B field interacting with the Amperian current loop through a Lorentz force described below. Again, the results are the same although the models are completely different.

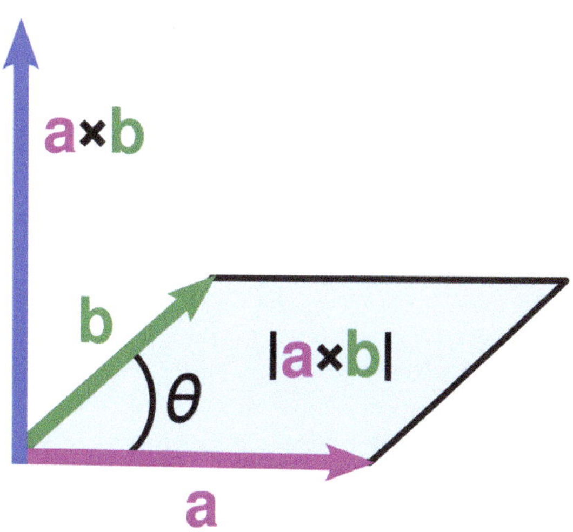

Cross product: $|a \times b| = a\, b \sin\theta$.

Mathematically, the torque τ on a small magnet is proportional both to the applied magnetic field and to the magnetic moment m of the magnet:

$$\tau = m \times B = \mu_0 m \times H,$$

where × represents the vector cross product. Note that this equation includes all of the qualitative information included above. There is no torque on a magnet if m is in the same direction as the magnetic field. (The cross product is zero for two vectors that are in the same direction.) Further, all other orientations feel a torque that twists them toward the direction of magnetic field.

Magnetic Field and Electric Currents

Currents of electric charges both generate a magnetic field and feel a force due to magnetic B-fields.

Magnetic Field Due to Moving Charges and Electric Currents

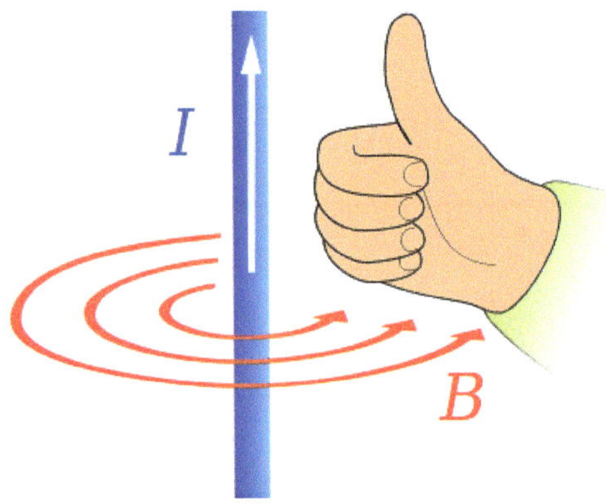

Right hand grip rule: a current flowing in the direction of the white arrow produces a magnetic field shown by the red arrows.

All moving charged particles produce magnetic fields. Moving point charges, such as electrons, produce complicated but well known magnetic fields that depend on the charge, velocity, and acceleration of the particles.

Magnetic field lines form in concentric circles around a cylindrical current-carrying conductor, such as a length of wire. The direction of such a magnetic field can be determined by using the "right hand grip rule" . The strength of the magnetic field decreases with distance from the wire. (For an infinite length wire the strength is inversely proportional to the distance.)

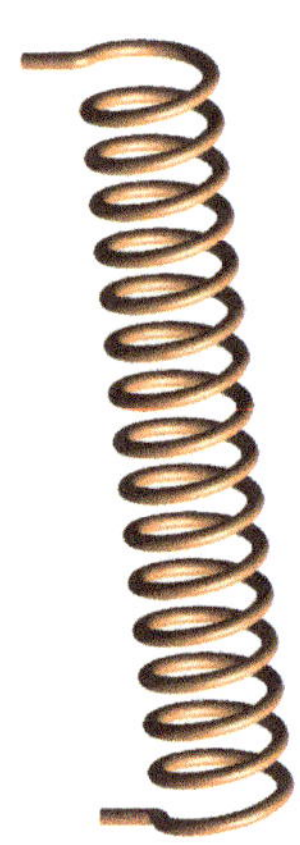

Solenoid

Bending a current-carrying wire into a loop concentrates the magnetic field inside the loop while weakening it outside. Bending a wire into multiple closely spaced loops to form a coil or "solenoid" enhances this effect. A device so formed around an iron core may act as an *electromagnet*, generating a strong, well-controlled magnetic field. An infinitely long cylindrical electromagnet has a uniform magnetic field inside, and no magnetic field outside. A finite length electromagnet produces a magnetic field that looks similar to that produced by a uniform permanent magnet, with its strength and polarity determined by the current flowing through the coil.

The magnetic field generated by a steady current I (a constant flow of electric charges, in which charge neither accumulates nor is depleted at any point) is described by the *Biot–Savart law*:

$$\boldsymbol{B} = \frac{\mu_0 I}{4\pi}\int_{\text{wire}} \frac{\mathrm{d}\ell \times \hat{\boldsymbol{r}}}{r^2},$$

where the integral sums over the wire length where vector $\mathrm{d}\ell$ is the vector line element with direction in the same sense as the current *I*, μ_0 is the magnetic constant, *r* is the distance between the location of $\mathrm{d}\ell$ and the location where the magnetic field is calculated, and $\hat{\mathrm{r}}$ is a unit vector in the direction of r. In the case of a sufficiently long wire, this becomes:

$$\boldsymbol{B} = \frac{\mu_0 I}{2\pi r}$$

where *r* is the distance from the wire.

A slightly more general way of relating the current I to the B-field is through Ampère's law:

$$\oint \mathbf{B} \cdot \mathrm{d}\ell = \mu_0 I_{\text{enc}},$$

where the line integral is over any arbitrary loop and I_{enc} is the current enclosed by that loop. Ampère's law is always valid for steady currents and can be used to calculate the B-field for certain highly symmetric situations such as an infinite wire or an infinite solenoid.

In a modified form that accounts for time varying electric fields, Ampère's law is one of four Maxwell's equations that describe electricity and magnetism.

Force on a Charged Particle

A charged particle moving in a B-field experiences a *sideways* force that is proportional to the strength of the magnetic field, the component of the velocity that is perpendicular to the magnetic field and the charge of the particle. This force is known as the *Lorentz force*, and is given by

$$\boldsymbol{F} = q\boldsymbol{E} + q\boldsymbol{v} \times \boldsymbol{B},$$

where F is the force, q is the electric charge of the particle, v is the instantaneous velocity of the particle, and B is the magnetic field (in teslas).

The Lorentz force is always perpendicular to both the velocity of the particle and the magnetic field that created it. When a charged particle moves in a static magnetic field, it traces a helical path in which the helix axis is parallel to the magnetic field, and in which the speed of the particle remains constant. Because the magnetic force is always perpendicular to the motion, the magnetic field can do no work on an isolated charge. It can only do work indirectly, via the electric field generated by a changing magnetic field. It is often claimed that the magnetic force can do work to a non-elementary magnetic dipole, or to charged particles whose motion is constrained by other forces, but this is incorrect because the work in those cases is performed by the electric forces of the charges deflected by the magnetic field.

Force on Current-carrying Wire

The force on a current carrying wire is similar to that of a moving charge as expected since a charge carrying wire is a collection of moving charges. A current-carrying wire feels a force in the presence of a magnetic field. The Lorentz force on a macroscopic current is often referred to as the *Laplace force*. Consider a conductor of length ℓ, cross section A, and charge q due to electric current i. If this conductor is placed in a magnetic field of magnitude B that makes an angle θ with the velocity of charges in the conductor, the force exerted on a single charge q is

$$F = qvB\sin\theta,$$

so, for N charges where

$$N = n\ell A,$$

the force exerted on the conductor is

$$f = FN = qvBn\ell A\sin\theta = Bi\ell\sin\theta,$$

where $i = nqvA$.

Direction of Force

The direction of force on a charge or a current can be determined by a mnemonic known as the *right-hand rule*. Using the right hand and pointing the thumb in the direction of the moving positive charge or positive current and the fingers in the direction of the magnetic field the resulting force on the charge points outwards from the palm. The force on a negatively charged particle is in the opposite direction. If both the speed and the charge are reversed then the direction of the force remains the same. For that reason a magnetic field measurement (by itself) cannot distinguish whether there is a positive charge moving to the right or a negative charge moving to the left. (Both of these cases produce the same current.) On the other hand, a magnetic field combined with an electric field *can* distinguish between these.

An alternative mnemonic to the right hand rule Flemings's left hand rule.

Relation Between H and B

The formulas derived for the magnetic field above are correct when dealing with the entire current. A magnetic material placed inside a magnetic field, though, generates its own bound current, which can be a challenge to calculate. (This bound current is due to the sum of atomic sized current loops and the spin of the subatomic particles such as electrons that make up the material.) The H-field as defined above helps factor out this bound current; but to see how, it helps to introduce the concept of *magnetization* first.

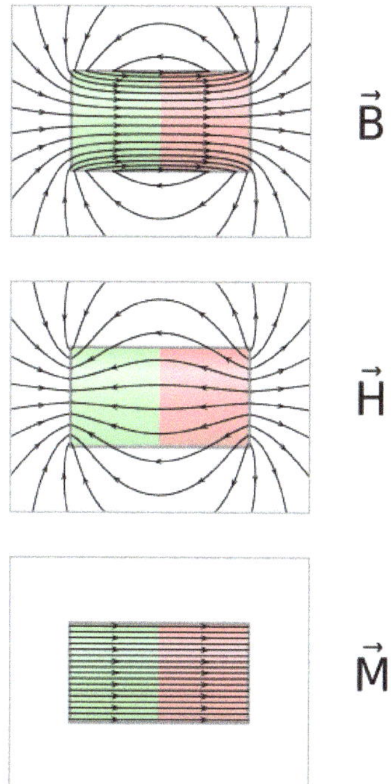

B-field, H-field and magnetization of a cylindrical bar magnet.

Magnetization

The *magnetization* vector field M represents how strongly a region of material is magnetized. It is defined as the net magnetic dipole moment per unit volume of that region. The magnetization of a uniform magnet is therefore a material constant, equal to the magnetic moment m of the magnet divided by its volume. Since the SI unit of magnetic moment is A·m^2, the SI unit of magnetization M is ampere per meter, identical to that of the H-field.

The magnetization M field of a region points in the direction of the average magnetic dipole moment in that region. Magnetization field lines, therefore, begin near the magnetic south pole and ends near the magnetic north pole. (Magnetization does not exist outside of the magnet.)

In the Amperian loop model, the magnetization is due to combining many tiny Amperian loops to form a resultant current called *bound current*. This bound current, then, is the source of the magnetic B field due to the magnet. Given the definition of the magnetic dipole, the magnetization field follows a similar law to that of Ampere's law:

$$\oint \boldsymbol{M} \cdot \mathrm{d}\ell = I_\mathrm{b},$$

where the integral is a line integral over any closed loop and I_b is the 'bound current' enclosed by that closed loop.

In the magnetic pole model, magnetization begins at and ends at magnetic poles. If a given region, therefore, has a net positive 'magnetic pole strength' (corresponding to a north pole) then it has more magnetization field lines entering it than leaving it. Mathematically this is equivalent to:

$$\oint_S \mu_0 \mathbf{M} \cdot d\mathbf{A} = -q_M$$

where the integral is a closed surface integral over the closed surface S and q_M is the 'magnetic charge' (in units of magnetic flux) enclosed by S. (A closed surface completely surrounds a region with no holes to let any field lines escape.) The negative sign occurs because the magnetization field moves from south to north.

H-field and Magnetic Materials

In SI units, the H-field is related to the B-field by

$$\boldsymbol{H} \equiv \frac{\boldsymbol{B}}{\mu_0} - \boldsymbol{M}.$$

In terms of the H-field, Ampere's law is

$$\oint \boldsymbol{H} \cdot d\ell = \oint \left(\frac{\boldsymbol{B}}{\mu_0} - \boldsymbol{M} \right) \cdot d\ell = I_{tot} - I_b = I_f,$$

where I_f represents the 'free current' enclosed by the loop so that the line integral of H does not depend at all on the bound currents.

For the differential equivalent of this equation refer to Maxwell's equations. Ampere's law leads to the boundary condition

$$\left(\mathbf{H}_1^{\parallel} - \mathbf{H}_2^{\parallel} \right) = \mathbf{K}_f \times \hat{\mathbf{n}},$$

where K_f is the surface free current density and the unit normal $\hat{n}$ points in the direction from medium 2 to medium 1.

Similarly, a surface integral of H over any closed surface is independent of the free currents and picks out the "magnetic charges" within that closed surface:

$$\oint_S \mu_0 \boldsymbol{H} \cdot d\boldsymbol{A} = \oint_S (\boldsymbol{B} - \mu_0 \boldsymbol{M}) \cdot d\boldsymbol{A} = 0 - (-q_M) = q_M,$$

which does not depend on the free currents.

The H-field, therefore, can be separated into two independent parts:

$$\boldsymbol{H} = \boldsymbol{H}_0 + \boldsymbol{H}_d,$$

where H_0 is the applied magnetic field due only to the free currents and H_d is the demagnetizing field due only to the bound currents.

The magnetic H-field, therefore, re-factors the bound current in terms of "magnetic charges". The H field lines loop only around 'free current' and, unlike the magnetic B field, begins and ends near magnetic poles as well.

Magnetism

Most materials respond to an applied B-field by producing their own magnetization M and therefore their own B-field. Typically, the response is weak and exists only when the magnetic field is applied. The term *magnetism* describes how materials respond on the microscopic level to an applied magnetic field and is used to categorize the magnetic phase of a material. Materials are divided into groups based upon their magnetic behavior:

- Diamagnetic materials produce a magnetization that opposes the magnetic field.
- Paramagnetic materials produce a magnetization in the same direction as the applied magnetic field.
- Ferromagnetic materials and the closely related ferrimagnetic materials and antiferromagnetic materials can have a magnetization independent of an applied B-field with a complex relationship between the two fields.
- Superconductors (and ferromagnetic superconductors) are materials that are characterized by perfect conductivity below a critical temperature and magnetic field. They also are highly magnetic and can be perfect diamagnets below a lower critical magnetic field. Superconductors often have a broad range of temperatures and magnetic fields (the so-named mixed state) under which they exhibit a complex hysteretic dependence of M on B.

In the case of paramagnetism and diamagnetism, the magnetization M is often proportional to the applied magnetic field such that:

$$\mathbf{B} = \mu \mathbf{H},$$

where μ is a material dependent parameter called the permeability. In some cases the permeability may be a second rank tensor so that H may not point in the same direction as B. These relations between B and H are examples of constitutive equations. However, superconductors and ferromagnets have a more complex B to H relation;

Energy Stored in Magnetic Fields

Energy is needed to generate a magnetic field both to work against the electric field that a changing magnetic field creates and to change the magnetization of any material within the magnetic field. For non-dispersive materials this same energy is released when the magnetic field is destroyed so that this energy can be modeled as being stored in the magnetic field.

For linear, non-dispersive, materials (such that B = μH where μ is frequency-independent), the energy density is:

$$u = \frac{\boldsymbol{B} \cdot \boldsymbol{H}}{2} = \frac{\boldsymbol{B} \cdot \boldsymbol{B}}{2\mu} = \frac{\mu \boldsymbol{H} \cdot \boldsymbol{H}}{2}.$$

If there are no magnetic materials around then μ can be replaced by μ_0. The above equation cannot be used for nonlinear materials, though; a more general expression given below must be used.

In general, the incremental amount of work per unit volume δW needed to cause a small change of magnetic field δB is:

$$\delta W = \boldsymbol{H} \cdot \delta \boldsymbol{B}.$$

Once the relationship between H and B is known this equation is used to determine the work needed to reach a given magnetic state. For hysteretic materials such as ferromagnets and superconductors, the work needed also depends on how the magnetic field is created. For linear non-dispersive materials, though, the general equation leads directly to the simpler energy density equation given above.

Electromagnetism: The Relationship between Magnetic and Electric Fields

Faraday's Law: Electric Force Due to a Changing B-field

A changing magnetic field, such as a magnet moving through a conducting coil, generates an electric field (and therefore tends to drive a current in such a coil). This is known as *Faraday's law* and forms the basis of many electrical generators and electric motors.

Mathematically, Faraday's law is:

$$\mathcal{E} = -\frac{\mathrm{d}\Phi_{\mathrm{m}}}{\mathrm{d}t},$$

where $\mathcal{E}$ is the electromotive force (or *EMF*, the voltage generated around a closed loop) and Φ_{m} is the *magnetic flux*—the product of the area times the magnetic field normal to that area. (This definition of magnetic flux is why B is often referred to as *magnetic flux density*.)

The negative sign represents the fact that any current generated by a changing magnetic field in a coil produces a magnetic field that *opposes* the *change* in the magnetic field that induced it. This phenomenon is known as Lenz's law.

This integral formulation of Faraday's law can be converted into a differential form, which applies under slightly different conditions. This form is covered as one of Maxwell's equations below.

Maxwell's Correction to Ampère's Law: The Magnetic Field due to a Changing Electric Field

Similar to the way that a changing magnetic field generates an electric field, a changing electric field generates a magnetic field. This fact is known as *Maxwell's correction to Ampère's law* and is applied as an additive term to Ampere's law as given above. This additional term is proportional to the time rate of change of the electric flux and is similar to Faraday's law above but with a different and positive constant out front. (The electric flux through an area is proportional to the area times the perpendicular part of the electric field.)

The full law including the correction term is known as the Maxwell–Ampère equation. It is not commonly given in integral form because the effect is so small that it can typically be ignored in most cases where the integral form is used.

The Maxwell term *is* critically important in the creation and propagation of electromagnetic waves. Maxwell's correction to Ampère's Law together with Faraday's law of induction describes how mutually changing electric and magnetic fields interact to sustain each other and thus to form electromagnetic waves, such as light: a changing electric field generates a changing magnetic field, which generates a changing electric field again. These, though, are usually described using the differential form of this equation given below.

Maxwell's Equations

Like all vector fields, a magnetic field has two important mathematical properties that relates it to its *sources*. (For B the *sources* are currents and changing electric fields.) These two properties, along with the two corresponding properties of the electric field, make up *Maxwell's Equations*. Maxwell's Equations together with the Lorentz force law form a complete description of classical electrodynamics including both electricity and magnetism.

The first property is the divergence of a vector field A, $\nabla \cdot A$, which represents how A 'flows' outward from a given point. As discussed above, a B-field line never starts or ends at a point but instead forms a complete loop. This is mathematically equivalent to saying that the divergence of B is zero. (Such vector fields are called solenoidal vector fields.) This property is called Gauss's law for magnetism and is equivalent to the statement that there are no isolated magnetic poles or magnetic monopoles. The electric field on the other hand begins and ends at electric charges so that its divergence is non-zero and proportional to the charge density.

The second mathematical property is called the curl, such that $\nabla \times A$ represents how A curls or 'circulates' around a given point. The result of the curl is called a 'circulation source'. The equations for the curl of B and of E are called the Ampère–Maxwell equation and Faraday's law respectively. They represent the differential forms of the integral equations given above.

The complete set of Maxwell's equations then are:

$$\nabla \cdot \boldsymbol{B} = 0,$$

$$\nabla \cdot \boldsymbol{E} = \frac{\rho}{\varepsilon_0},$$

$$\nabla \times \boldsymbol{B} = \mu_0 \boldsymbol{J} + \mu_0 \varepsilon_0 \frac{\partial \boldsymbol{E}}{\partial t},$$

$$\nabla \times \boldsymbol{E} = -\frac{\partial \boldsymbol{B}}{\partial t},$$

where J = complete microscopic current density and ρ is the charge density.

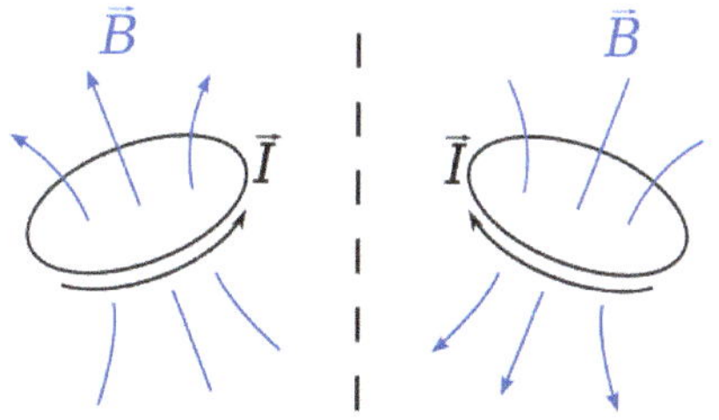

Magnetic field, like all pseudovectors, changes sign when reflected in a mirror: When a current carrying loop (black) is reflected in a mirror (dotted line), its magnetic field (blue) is reflected *and* reversed.

Technically, B is a pseudovector (also called an *axial vector*) due to being defined by a vector cross product.

As discussed above, materials respond to an applied electric E field and an applied magnetic B field by producing their own internal 'bound' charge and current distributions that contribute to E and B but are difficult to calculate. To circumvent this problem, H and D fields are used to re-factor Maxwell's equations in terms of the *free current density* J_f and *free charge density* ρ_f:

$$\nabla \cdot \boldsymbol{B} = 0,$$

$$\nabla \cdot \boldsymbol{D} = \rho_f,$$

$$\nabla \times \boldsymbol{H} = \boldsymbol{J}_f + \frac{\partial \boldsymbol{D}}{\partial t},$$

$$\nabla \times \boldsymbol{E} = -\frac{\partial \boldsymbol{B}}{\partial t}.$$

These equations are not any more general than the original equations (if the 'bound' charges and currents in the material are known). They also must be supplemented by the relationship between B and H as well as that between E and D. On the other hand, for simple relationships between these quantities this form of Maxwell's equations can circumvent the need to calculate the bound charges and currents.

Electric and Magnetic Fields: Different Aspects of the Same Phenomenon

According to the special theory of relativity, the partition of the electromagnetic force into separate electric and magnetic components is not fundamental, but varies with the observational frame of reference: An electric force perceived by one observer may be perceived by another (in a different frame of reference) as a magnetic force, or a mixture of electric and magnetic forces.

Formally, special relativity combines the electric and magnetic fields into a rank-2 tensor, called the *electromagnetic tensor*. Changing reference frames *mixes* these components. This is analogous to the way that special relativity *mixes* space and time into spacetime, and mass, momentum and energy into four-momentum.

Magnetic Vector Potential

In advanced topics such as quantum mechanics and relativity it is often easier to work with a potential formulation of electrodynamics rather than in terms of the electric and magnetic fields. In this representation, the *vector potential* A, and the scalar potential φ, are defined such that:

$$\boldsymbol{B} = \nabla \times \boldsymbol{A},$$

$$\boldsymbol{E} = -\nabla \varphi - \frac{\partial \boldsymbol{A}}{\partial t}.$$

The vector potential A may be interpreted as a *generalized potential momentum per unit charge* just as φ is interpreted as a *generalized potential energy per unit charge.*

Maxwell's equations when expressed in terms of the potentials can be cast into a form that agrees with special relativity with little effort. In relativity A together with φ forms the four-potential, analogous to the four-momentum that combines the momentum and energy of a particle. Using the four potential instead of the electromagnetic tensor has the advantage of being much simpler—and it can be easily modified to work with quantum mechanics.

Quantum Electrodynamics

In modern physics, the electromagnetic field is understood to be not a *classical* field, but rather a quantum field; it is represented not as a vector of three numbers at each point, but as a vector of three quantum operators at each point. The most accurate modern description of the electromagnetic interaction (and much else) is *quantum electrodynamics* (QED), which is incorporated into a more complete theory known as the *Standard Model of particle physics*.

In QED, the magnitude of the electromagnetic interactions between charged particles (and their antiparticles) is computed using perturbation theory. These rather complex formulas produce a remarkable pictorial representation as Feynman diagrams in which virtual photons are exchanged.

Predictions of QED agree with experiments to an extremely high degree of accuracy: currently about 10^{-12} (and limited by experimental errors). This makes QED one of the most accurate physical theories constructed thus far.

All equations are in the classical approximation, which is less accurate than the quantum description mentioned here. However, under most everyday circumstances, the difference between the two theories is negligible.

Important uses and Examples of Magnetic Field

Earth's Magnetic Field

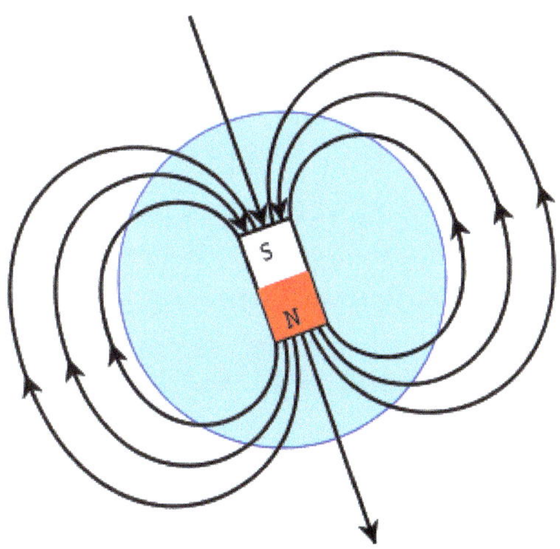

A sketch of Earth's magnetic field representing the source of the field as a magnet. The geographic north pole of Earth is near the top of the diagram, the south pole near the bottom. The south pole of that magnet is deep in Earth's interior below Earth's North Magnetic Pole.

The Earth's magnetic field is thought to be produced by convection currents in the outer liquid of Earth's core. The Dynamo theory proposes that these movements produce electric currents that, in turn, produce the magnetic field.

The presence of this field causes a compass, placed anywhere within it, to rotate so that the "north pole" of the magnet in the compass points roughly north, toward Earth's North Magnetic Pole. This is the traditional definition of the "north pole" of a magnet, although other equivalent definitions are also possible.

One confusion that arises from this definition is that, if Earth itself is considered as a magnet, the *south* pole of that magnet would be the one nearer the north magnetic pole, and vice versa. The north magnetic pole is so-named not because of the polarity of the field there but because of its geographical location. The north and south poles of a permanent magnet are so-called because they are "north-seeking" and "south-seeking", respectively.

The figure is a sketch of Earth's magnetic field represented by field lines. For most locations, the magnetic field has a significant up/down component in addition to the north/south component. (There is also an east/west component, as Earth's magnetic and geographical poles do not coincide.) The magnetic field can be visualised as a bar magnet buried deep in Earth's interior.

Earth's magnetic field is not constant—the strength of the field and the location of its poles vary. Moreover, the poles periodically reverse their orientation in a process called geomagnetic reversal. The most recent reversal occurred 780,000 years ago.

Rotating Magnetic Fields

The *rotating magnetic field* is a key principle in the operation of alternating-current motors. A permanent magnet in such a field rotates so as to maintain its alignment with the external field. This effect was conceptualized by Nikola Tesla, and later utilized in his, and others', early AC (alternating current) electric motors.

A rotating magnetic field can be constructed using two orthogonal coils with 90 degrees phase difference in their AC currents. However, in practice such a system would be supplied through a three-wire arrangement with unequal currents.

This inequality would cause serious problems in standardization of the conductor size and so, to overcome it, three-phase systems are used where the three currents are equal in magnitude and have 120 degrees phase difference. Three similar coils having mutual geometrical angles of 120 degrees create the rotating magnetic field in this case. The ability of the three-phase system to create a rotating field, utilized in electric motors, is one of the main reasons why three-phase systems dominate the world's electrical power supply systems.

Synchronous motors use DC-voltage-fed rotor windings, which lets the excitation of the machine be controlled—and induction motors use short-circuited rotors (instead of a magnet) following the rotating magnetic field of a multicoiled stator. The short-circuited turns of the rotor develop eddy currents in the rotating field of the stator, and these currents in turn move the rotor by the Lorentz force.

In 1882, Nikola Tesla identified the concept of the rotating magnetic field. In 1885, Galileo Ferraris independently researched the concept. In 1888, Tesla gained U.S. Patent 381,968 for his work. Also in 1888, Ferraris published his research in a paper to the *Royal Academy of Sciences* in Turin.

Hall Effect

The charge carriers of a current-carrying conductor placed in a transverse magnetic field experience a sideways Lorentz force; this results in a charge separation in a direction perpendicular to the current and to the magnetic field. The resultant voltage in that direction is proportional to the applied magnetic field. This is known as the *Hall effect*.

The *Hall effect* is often used to measure the magnitude of a magnetic field. It is used as well to find the sign of the dominant charge carriers in materials such as semiconductors (negative electrons or positive holes).

Magnetic Circuits

An important use of H is in *magnetic circuits* where $B = \mu H$ inside a linear material. Here, μ is the magnetic permeability of the material. This result is similar in form to Ohm's law $J = \sigma E$, where J is the current density, σ is the conductance and E is the electric field. Extending this analogy, the counterpart to the macroscopic Ohm's law ($I = V/R$) is:

$$\Phi = \frac{F}{R_m},$$

where $\Phi = \int \boldsymbol{B} \cdot dA$ is the magnetic flux in the circuit, $F = \int \boldsymbol{H} \cdot d\ell$ is the magnetomotive force applied to the circuit, and R_m is the reluctance of the circuit. Here the reluctance R_m is a quantity similar in nature to resistance for the flux.

Using this analogy it is straightforward to calculate the magnetic flux of complicated magnetic field geometries, by using all the available techniques of circuit theory.

Magnetic Field Shape Descriptions

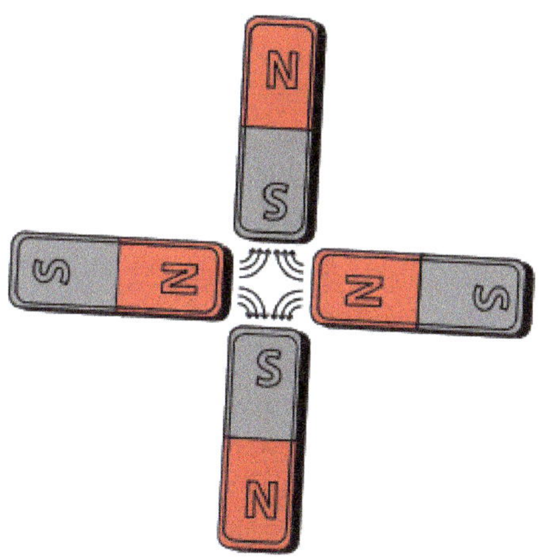

Schematic quadrupole magnet ("*four-pole*") magnetic field. There are four steel pole tips, two opposing magnetic north poles and two opposing magnetic south poles.

- An *azimuthal* magnetic field is one that runs east–west.
- A *meridional* magnetic field is one that runs north–south. In the solar dynamo model of the Sun, differential rotation of the solar plasma causes the meridional magnetic field to

stretch into an azimuthal magnetic field, a process called the *omega-effect*. The reverse process is called the *alpha-effect*.

- A *dipole* magnetic field is one seen around a bar magnet or around a charged elementary particle with nonzero spin.
- A *quadrupole* magnetic field is one seen, for example, between the poles of four bar magnets. The field strength grows linearly with the radial distance from its longitudinal axis.
- A *solenoidal* magnetic field is similar to a dipole magnetic field, except that a solid bar magnet is replaced by a hollow electromagnetic coil magnet.
- A *toroidal* magnetic field occurs in a doughnut-shaped coil, the electric current spiraling around the tube-like surface, and is found, for example, in a tokamak.
- A *poloidal* magnetic field is generated by a current flowing in a ring, and is found, for example, in a tokamak.
- A *radial* magnetic field is one in which field lines are directed from the center outwards, similar to the spokes in a bicycle wheel. An example can be found in a loudspeaker transducers (driver).
- A *helical* magnetic field is corkscrew-shaped, and sometimes seen in space plasmas such as the Orion Molecular Cloud.

Magnetic Dipoles

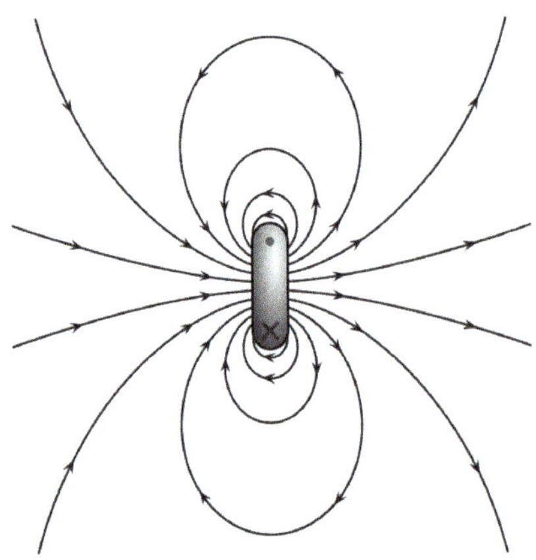

Magnetic field lines around a "magnetostatic dipole" pointing to the right.

The magnetic field of a magnetic dipole is depicted in the figure. From outside, the ideal magnetic dipole is identical to that of an ideal electric dipole of the same strength. Unlike the electric dipole, a magnetic dipole is properly modeled as a current loop having a current I and an area a. Such a current loop has a magnetic moment of:

$$m = Ia,$$

where the direction of m is perpendicular to the area of the loop and depends on the direction of the current using the right-hand rule. An ideal magnetic dipole is modeled as a real magnetic dipole whose area a has been reduced to zero and its current I increased to infinity such that the product $m = Ia$ is finite. This model clarifies the connection between angular momentum and magnetic moment, which is the basis of the Einstein–de Haas effect *rotation by magnetization* and its inverse, the Barnett effect or *magnetization by rotation*. Rotating the loop faster (in the same direction) increases the current and therefore the magnetic moment, for example.

It is sometimes useful to model the magnetic dipole similar to the electric dipole with two equal but opposite magnetic charges (one south the other north) separated by distance d. This model produces an H-field not a B-field. Such a model is deficient, though, both in that there are no magnetic charges and in that it obscures the link between electricity and magnetism. Further, as discussed above it fails to explain the inherent connection between angular momentum and magnetism.

Magnetic Monopole (Hypothetical)

A *magnetic monopole* is a hypothetical particle (or class of particles) that has, as its name suggests, only one magnetic pole (either a north pole or a south pole). In other words, it would possess a "magnetic charge" analogous to an electric charge. Magnetic field lines would start or end on magnetic monopoles, so if they exist, they would give exceptions to the rule that magnetic field lines neither start nor end.

Modern interest in this concept stems from particle theories, notably Grand Unified Theories and superstring theories, that predict either the existence, or the possibility, of magnetic monopoles. These theories and others have inspired extensive efforts to search for monopoles. Despite these efforts, no magnetic monopole has been observed to date.

In recent research, materials known as spin ices can simulate monopoles, but do not contain actual monopoles.

High-temperature Superconductivity

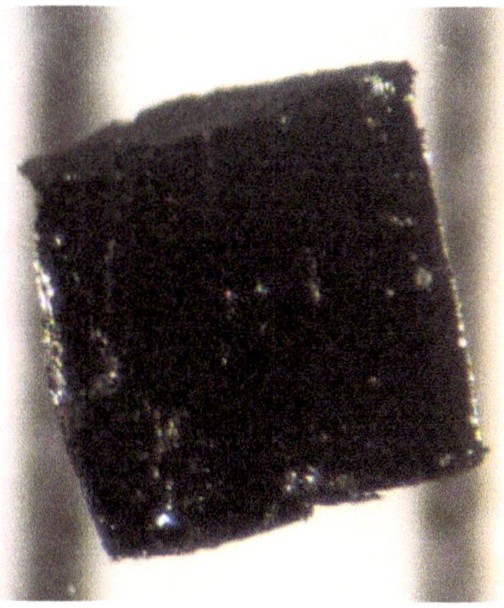

A small sample of the high-temperature superconductor BSCCO-2223.

High-temperature superconductors (abbreviated high-T_c or HTS) are materials that behave as superconductors at unusually high temperatures. The first high-T_c superconductor was discovered in 1986 by IBM researchers Georg Bednorz and K. Alex Müller, who were awarded the 1987 Nobel Prize in Physics "for their important break-through in the discovery of superconductivity in ceramic materials".

Whereas "ordinary" or metallic superconductors usually have transition temperatures (temperatures below which they are superconductive) below 30 K (−243.2 °C), and must be cooled using liquid helium in order to achieve superconductivity, HTS have been observed with transition temperatures as high as 138 K (−135 °C), and can be cooled to superconductivity using liquid nitrogen. Until 2008, only certain compounds of copper and oxygen (so-called "cuprates") were believed to have HTS properties, and the term high-temperature superconductor was used interchangeably with cuprate superconductor for compounds such as bismuth strontium calcium copper oxide (BSCCO) and yttrium barium copper oxide (YBCO). Several iron-based compounds (the iron pnictides) are now known to be superconducting at high temperatures.

In 2015, hydrogen sulfide (H_2S) under extremely high pressure (around 150 gigapascals) was found to undergo superconducting transition near 203 K (-70 °C), the highest temperature superconductor known to date.

For an explanation about T_c (the critical temperature for superconductivity), refer to Superconductivity, Superconducting phase transition and the second bullet item of BCS theory, Successes of the BCS theory.

History

The phenomenon of superconductivity was discovered by Kamerlingh Onnes in 1911, in metallic mercury below 4 K (−269.15 °C). Ever since, researchers have attempted to observe superconductivity at increasing temperatures with the goal of finding a room-temperature superconductor. In the late 1970s, superconductivity was observed in certain metal oxides at temperatures as high as 13 K (−260.1 °C), which were much higher than those for elemental metals. In 1986, J. Georg Bednorz and K. Alex Müller, working at the IBM research lab near Zurich, Switzerland were exploring a new class of ceramics for superconductivity. Bednorz encountered a barium-doped compound of lanthanum and copper oxide whose resistance dropped to zero at a temperature around 35 K (−238.2 °C). Their results were soon confirmed by many groups, notably Paul Chu at the University of Houston and Shoji Tanaka at the University of Tokyo.

Shortly after, P. W. Anderson, at Princeton University came up with the first theoretical description of these materials, using the resonating valence bond theory, but a full understanding of these materials is still developing today. These superconductors are now known to possess a *d*-wave pair symmetry. The first proposal that high-temperature cuprate superconductivity involves *d*-wave pairing was made in 1987 by Bickers, Scalapino and Scalettar, followed by three subsequent theories in 1988 by Inui, Doniach, Hirschfeld and Ruckenstein, using spin-fluctuation theory, and by Gros, Poilblanc, Rice and Zhang, and by Kotliar and Liu identifying *d*-wave pairing as a natural consequence of the RVB theory. The confirmation of the *d*-wave nature of the cuprate superconductors was made by a variety of experiments, including the direct observation of the *d*-wave nodes in the excitation spectrum through Angle Resolved Photoemission Spectroscopy, the observation of a half-integer flux in tunneling experiments, and indirectly from the temperature dependence of the penetration depth, specific heat and thermal conductivity.

Until 2015 the superconductor with the highest transition temperature that had been confirmed by multiple independent research groups (a prerequisite to be called a discovery, verified by peer review) was mercury barium calcium copper oxide ($HgBa_2Ca_2Cu_3O_8$) at around 133 K.

After more than twenty years of intensive research, the origin of high-temperature superconductivity is still not clear, but it seems that instead of *electron-phonon* attraction mechanisms, as in conventional superconductivity, one is dealing with genuine *electronic* mechanisms (e.g. by antiferromagnetic correlations), and instead of conventional, purely *s*-wave pairing, more exotic pairing symmetries are thought to be involved (*d*-wave in the case of the cuprates; primarily extended *s*-wave, but occasionally *d*-wave, in the case of the iron-based superconductors). In 2014, evidence showing that fractional particles can happen in quasi two-dimensional magnetic materials, was found by EPFL scientists lending support for Anderson's theory of high-temperature superconductivity.

Crystal Structures of High-temperature Ceramic Superconductors

The structure of high-T_c copper oxide or cuprate superconductors are often closely related to perovskite structure, and the structure of these compounds has been described as a distorted, oxygen deficient multi-layered perovskite structure. One of the properties of the crystal structure of oxide superconductors is an alternating multi-layer of CuO_2 planes with superconductivity taking place between these layers. The more layers of CuO_2, the higher T_c. This structure causes a large anisotropy in normal conducting and superconducting properties, since electrical currents are carried by holes induced in the oxygen sites of the CuO_2 sheets. The electrical conduction is highly anisotropic, with a much higher conductivity parallel to the CuO_2 plane than in the perpendicular direction. Generally, critical temperatures depend on the chemical compositions, cations substitutions and oxygen content. They can be classified as superstripes; i.e., particular realizations of superlattices at atomic limit made of superconducting atomic layers, wires, dots separated by spacer layers, that gives multiband and multigap superconductivity.

YBaCuO Superconductors

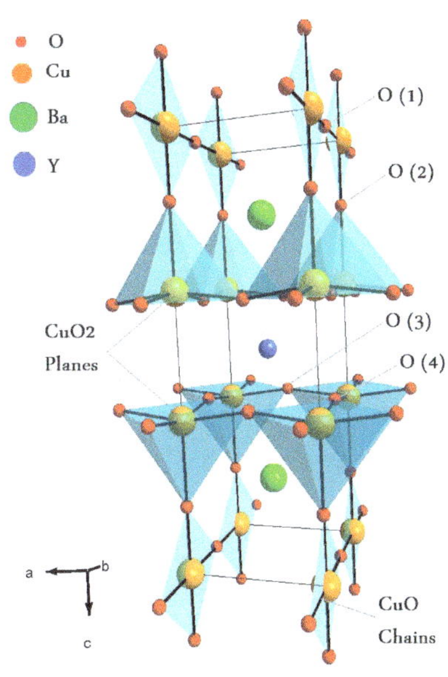

YBCO unit cell

The first superconductor found with T_c > 77 K (liquid nitrogen boiling point) is yttrium barium copper oxide ($YBa_2Cu_3O_{7-x}$); the proportions of the three different metals in the $YBa_2Cu_3O_7$ superconductor are in the mole ratio of 1 to 2 to 3 for yttrium to barium to copper, respectively. Thus, this particular superconductor is often referred to as the 123 superconductor.

The unit cell of $YBa_2Cu_3O_7$ consists of three pseudocubic elementary perovskite unit cells. Each perovskite unit cell contains a Y or Ba atom at the center: Ba in the bottom unit cell, Y in the middle one, and Ba in the top unit cell. Thus, Y and Ba are stacked in the sequence [Ba–Y–Ba] along the c-axis. All corner sites of the unit cell are occupied by Cu, which has two different coordinations, Cu(1) and Cu(2), with respect to oxygen. There are four possible crystallographic sites for oxygen: O(1), O(2), O(3) and O(4). The coordination polyhedra of Y and Ba with respect to oxygen are different. The tripling of the perovskite unit cell leads to nine oxygen atoms, whereas $YBa_2Cu_3O_7$ has seven oxygen atoms and, therefore, is referred to as an oxygen-deficient perovskite structure. The structure has a stacking of different layers: (CuO)(BaO)(CuO_2)(Y)(CuO_2)(BaO)(CuO). One of the key feature of the unit cell of $YBa_2Cu_3O_{7-x}$ (YBCO) is the presence of two layers of CuO_2. The role of the Y plane is to serve as a spacer between two CuO_2 planes. In YBCO, the Cu–O chains are known to play an important role for superconductivity. T_c is maximal near 92 K when $x \approx 0.15$ and the structure is orthorhombic. Superconductivity disappears at $x \approx 0.6$, where the structural transformation of YBCO occurs from orthorhombic to tetragonal.

Bi-, Tl- and Hg-based high-T_c Superconductors

The crystal structure of Bi-, Tl- and Hg-based high-T_c superconductors are very similar. Like YBCO, the perovskite-type feature and the presence of CuO_2 layers also exist in these superconductors. However, unlike YBCO, Cu–O chains are not present in these superconductors. The YBCO superconductor has an orthorhombic structure, whereas the other high-T_c superconductors have a tetragonal structure.

The Bi–Sr–Ca–Cu–O system has three superconducting phases forming a homologous series as $Bi_2Sr_2Ca_{n-1}Cu_nO_{4+2n+x}$ (n=1, 2 and 3). These three phases are Bi-2201, Bi-2212 and Bi-2223, having transition temperatures of 20, 85 and 110 K, respectively, where the numbering system represent number of atoms for Bi, Sr, Ca and Cu respectively. The two phases have a tetragonal structure which consists of two sheared crystallographic unit cells. The unit cell of these phases has double Bi–O planes which are stacked in a way that the Bi atom of one plane sits below the oxygen atom of the next consecutive plane. The Ca atom forms a layer within the interior of the CuO_2 layers in both Bi-2212 and Bi-2223; there is no Ca layer in the Bi-2201 phase. The three phases differ with each other in the number of CuO_2 planes; Bi-2201, Bi-2212 and Bi-2223 phases have one, two and three CuO_2 planes, respectively. The c axis lattice constants of these phases increases with the number of CuO_2 planes. The coordination of the Cu atom is different in the three phases. The Cu atom forms an octahedral coordination with respect to oxygen atoms in the 2201 phase, whereas in 2212, the Cu atom is surrounded by five oxygen atoms in a pyramidal arrangement. In the 2223 structure, Cu has two coordinations with respect to oxygen: one Cu atom is bonded with four oxygen atoms in square planar configuration and another Cu atom is coordinated with five oxygen atoms in a pyramidal arrangement.

Tl–Ba–Ca–Cu–O superconductor: The first series of the Tl-based superconductor containing one Tl–O layer has the general formula $TlBa_2Ca_{n-1}Cu_nO_{2n+3}$, whereas the second series containing two

Tl–O layers has a formula of $Tl_2Ba_2Ca_{n-1}Cu_nO_{2n+4}$ with n =1, 2 and 3. In the structure of $Tl_2Ba_2CuO_6$ (Tl-2201), there is one CuO_2 layer with the stacking sequence (Tl–O) (Tl–O) (Ba–O) (Cu–O) (Ba–O) (Tl–O) (Tl–O). In $Tl_2Ba_2CaCu_2O_8$ (Tl-2212), there are two Cu–O layers with a Ca layer in between. Similar to the $Tl_2Ba_2CuO_6$ structure, Tl–O layers are present outside the Ba–O layers. In $Tl_2Ba_2Ca_2Cu_3O_{10}$ (Tl-2223), there are three CuO2 layers enclosing Ca layers between each of these. In Tl-based superconductors, T_c is found to increase with the increase in CuO_2 layers. However, the value of T_c decreases after four CuO_2 layers in $TlBa_2Ca_{n-1}Cu_nO_{2n+3}$, and in the $Tl_2Ba_2Ca_{n-1}Cu_nO_{2n+4}$ compound, it decreases after three CuO_2 layers.

Hg–Ba–Ca–Cu–O superconductor: The crystal structure of $HgBa_2CuO_4$ (Hg-1201), $HgBa_2CaCu_2O_6$ (Hg-1212) and $HgBa_2Ca_2Cu_3O_8$ (Hg-1223) is similar to that of Tl-1201, Tl-1212 and Tl-1223, with Hg in place of Tl. It is noteworthy that the T_c of the Hg compound (Hg-1201) containing one CuO_2 layer is much larger as compared to the one-CuO_2-layer compound of thallium (Tl-1201). In the Hg-based superconductor, T_c is also found to increase as the CuO_2 layer increases. For Hg-1201, Hg-1212 and Hg-1223, the values of T_c are 94, 128 and the record value at ambient pressure 134 K, respectively, as shown in table below. The observation that the T_c of Hg-1223 increases to 153 K under high pressure indicates that the T_c of this compound is very sensitive to the structure of the compound.

Critical temperature (T_c), crystal structure and lattice constants of some high-T_c superconductors

Formula	Notation	T_c (K)	No. of Cu-O planes in unit cell	Crystal structure
$YBa_2Cu_3O_7$	123	92	2	Orthorhombic
$Bi_2Sr_2CuO_6$	Bi-2201	20	1	Tetragonal
$Bi_2Sr_2CaCu_2O_8$	Bi-2212	85	2	Tetragonal
$Bi_2Sr_2Ca_2Cu_3O_{10}$	Bi-2223	110	3	Tetragonal
$Tl_2Ba_2CuO_6$	Tl-2201	80	1	Tetragonal
$Tl_2Ba_2CaCu_2O_8$	Tl-2212	108	2	Tetragonal
$Tl_2Ba_2Ca_2Cu_3O_{10}$	Tl-2223	125	3	Tetragonal
$TlBa_2Ca_3Cu_4O_{11}$	Tl-1234	122	4	Tetragonal
$HgBa_2CuO_4$	Hg-1201	94	1	Tetragonal
$HgBa_2CaCu_2O_6$	Hg-1212	128	2	Tetragonal
$HgBa_2Ca_2Cu_3O_8$	Hg-1223	134	3	Tetragonal

Preparation of High-T_c Superconductors

The simplest method for preparing high-T_c superconductors is a solid-state thermochemical reaction involving mixing, calcination and sintering. The appropriate amounts of precursor powders, usually oxides and carbonates, are mixed thoroughly using a Ball mill. Solution chemistry processes such as coprecipitation, freeze-drying and sol-gel methods are alternative ways for preparing a homogeneous mixture. These powders are calcined in the temperature range from 800 °C to 950 °C for several hours. The powders are cooled, reground and calcined again. This process is repeated several times to get homogeneous material. The powders are subsequently compacted to pellets and sintered. The sintering environment such as temperature, annealing time, atmosphere and cooling rate play a very important role in getting good high-T_c superconducting materials. The $YBa_2Cu_3O_{7-x}$ compound is prepared by calcination and sintering of a homogeneous mixture of

Y_2O_3, $BaCO_3$ and CuO in the appropriate atomic ratio. Calcination is done at 900–950 °C, whereas sintering is done at 950 °C in an oxygen atmosphere. The oxygen stoichiometry in this material is very crucial for obtaining a superconducting $YBa_2Cu_3O_{7-x}$ compound. At the time of sintering, the semiconducting tetragonal $YBa_2Cu_3O_6$ compound is formed, which, on slow cooling in oxygen atmosphere, turns into superconducting $YBa_2Cu_3O_{7-x}$. The uptake and loss of oxygen are reversible in $YBa_2Cu_3O_{7-x}$. A fully oxygenated orthorhombic $YBa_2Cu_3O_{7-x}$ sample can be transformed into tetragonal $YBa_2Cu_3O_6$ by heating in a vacuum at temperature above 700 °C.

The preparation of Bi-, Tl- and Hg-based high-T_c superconductors is difficult compared to YBCO. Problems in these superconductors arise because of the existence of three or more phases having a similar layered structure. Thus, syntactic intergrowth and defects such as stacking faults occur during synthesis and it becomes difficult to isolate a single superconducting phase. For Bi–Sr–Ca–Cu–O, it is relatively simple to prepare the Bi-2212 ($T_c \approx 85$ K) phase, whereas it is very difficult to prepare a single phase of Bi-2223 ($T_c \approx 110$ K). The Bi-2212 phase appears only after few hours of sintering at 860–870 °C, but the larger fraction of the Bi-2223 phase is formed after a long reaction time of more than a week at 870 °C. Although the substitution of Pb in the Bi–Sr–Ca–Cu–O compound has been found to promote the growth of the high-T_c phase, a long sintering time is still required.

Properties

"High-temperature" has two common definitions in the context of superconductivity:

1. Above the temperature of 30 K that had historically been taken as the upper limit allowed by BCS theory(1957). This is also above the 1973 record of 23 K that had lasted until copper-oxide materials were discovered in 1986.

2. Having a transition temperature that is a larger fraction of the Fermi temperature than for conventional superconductors such as elemental mercury or lead. This definition encompasses a wider variety of unconventional superconductors and is used in the context of theoretical models.

The label high-T_c may be reserved by some authors for materials with critical temperature greater than the boiling point of liquid nitrogen (77 K or −196 °C). However, a number of materials – including the original discovery and recently discovered pnictide superconductors – had critical temperatures below 77 K but are commonly referred to in publication as being in the high-T_c class.

Technological applications could benefit from both the higher critical temperature being above the boiling point of liquid nitrogen and also the higher critical magnetic field (and critical current density) at which superconductivity is destroyed. In magnet applications, the high critical magnetic field may prove more valuable than the high T_c itself. Some cuprates have an upper critical field of about 100 tesla. However, cuprate materials are brittle ceramics which are expensive to manufacture and not easily turned into wires or other useful shapes. Also, high-temperature superconductors do not form large, continuous superconducting domains, but only clusters of microdomains within which superconductivity occurs. They are therefore unsuitable for applications requiring actual superconducted currents, such as magnets for magnetic resonance spectrometers.

After two decades of intense experimental and theoretical research, with over 100,000 published papers on the subject, several common features in the properties of high-temperature superconductors have been identified. As of 2011, no widely accepted theory explains their properties. Relative to conventional superconductors, such as elemental mercury or lead that are adequately explained by the BCS theory, cuprate superconductors (and other unconventional superconductors) remain distinctive. There also has been much debate as to high-temperature superconductivity coexisting with magnetic ordering in YBCO, iron-based superconductors, several ruthenocuprates and other exotic superconductors, and the search continues for other families of materials. HTS are Type-II superconductors, which allow magnetic fields to penetrate their interior in quantized units of flux, meaning that much higher magnetic fields are required to suppress superconductivity. The layered structure also gives a directional dependence to the magnetic field response.

Cuprates

Cuprate superconductors are generally considered to be quasi-two-dimensional materials with their superconducting properties determined by electrons moving within weakly coupled copper-oxide (CuO_2) layers. Neighbouring layers containing ions such as lanthanum, barium, strontium, or other atoms act to stabilize the structure and dope electrons or holes onto the copper-oxide layers. The undoped "parent" or "mother" compounds are Mott insulators with long-range antiferromagnetic order at low enough temperature. Single band models are generally considered to be sufficient to describe the electronic properties.

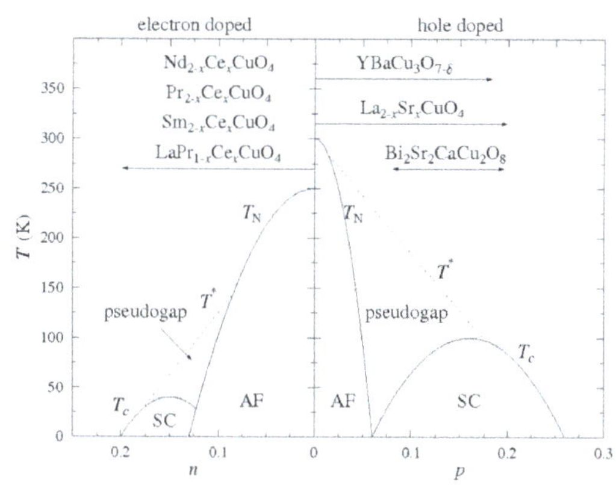

Simplified doping dependent phase diagram of cuprate superconductors for both electron (n) and hole (p) doping. The phases shown are the antiferromagnetic (AF) phase close to zero doping, the superconducting phase around optimal doping, and the pseudogap phase. Doping ranges possible for some common compounds are also shown.

The cuprate superconductors adopt a perovskite structure. The copper-oxide planes are checkerboard lattices with squares of O^{2-} ions with a Cu^{2+} ion at the centre of each square. The unit cell is rotated by 45° from these squares. Chemical formulae of superconducting materials generally contain fractional numbers to describe the doping required for superconductivity. There are several families of cuprate superconductors and they can be categorized by the elements they contain and the number of adjacent copper-oxide layers in each superconducting block. For example, YBCO and BSCCO can alternatively be referred to as Y123 and Bi2201/Bi2212/Bi2223 depending on the number of layers in each superconducting block (n). The superconducting transition temperature has been found to peak at an optimal doping value (p=0.16) and an optimal number of layers in each superconducting block, typically n=3.

Possible mechanisms for superconductivity in the cuprates are still the subject of considerable debate and further research. Certain aspects common to all materials have been identified. Similarities between the antiferromagnetic low-temperature state of the undoped materials and the superconducting state that emerges upon doping, primarily the $d_{x^2-y^2}$ orbital state of the Cu^{2+} ions, suggest that electron-electron interactions are more significant than electron-phonon interactions in cuprates – making the superconductivity unconventional. Recent work on the Fermi surface has shown that nesting occurs at four points in the antiferromagnetic Brillouin zone where spin waves exist and that the superconducting energy gap is larger at these points. The weak isotope effects observed for most cuprates contrast with conventional superconductors that are well described by BCS theory.

Similarities and differences in the properties of hole-doped and electron doped cuprates:

- Presence of a pseudogap phase up to at least optimal doping.
- Different trends in the Uemura plot relating transition temperature to the superfluid density. The inverse square of the London penetration depth appears to be proportional to the critical temperature for a large number of underdoped cuprate superconductors, but the constant of proportionality is different for hole- and electron-doped cuprates. The linear trend implies that the physics of these materials is strongly two-dimensional.
- Universal hourglass-shaped feature in the spin excitations of cuprates measured using inelastic neutron diffraction.
- Nernst effect evident in both the superconducting and pseudogap phases.

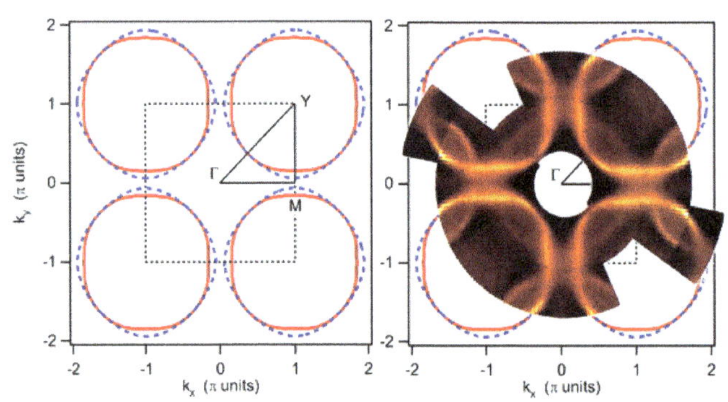

The Fermi surface of bi-layer BSCCO, calculated (left) and measured by ARPES (right). The dashed rectangle represents the first Brillouin zone.

The electronic structure of superconducting cuprates is highly anisotropic. Therefore, the Fermi surface of HTSC is very close to the Fermi surface of the doped CuO_2 plane (or multi-planes, in case of multi-layer cuprates) and can be presented on the 2D reciprocal space (or momentum space) of the CuO_2 lattice. The typical Fermi surface within the first CuO_2 Brillouin zone is sketched in Fig. (left). It can be derived from the band structure calculations or measured by angle resolved photoemission spectroscopy (ARPES). Fig (right) shows the Fermi surface of BSCCO measured by ARPES. In a wide range of charge carrier concentration (doping level), in which the hole-doped HTSC are superconducting, the Fermi surface is hole-like (*i.e.* open, as shown in Fig.). This results in an inherent in-plane anisotropy of the electronic properties of HTSC.

Iron-based Superconductors

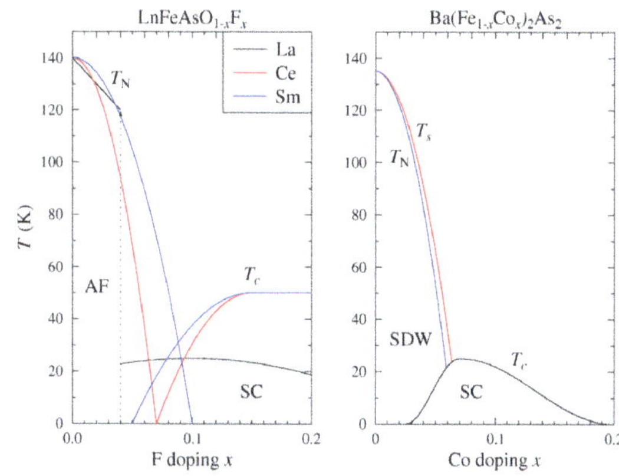

Simplified doping dependent phase diagrams of iron-based superconductors for both Ln-1111 and Ba-122 materials. The phases shown are the antiferromagnetic/spin density wave (AF/SDW) phase close to zero doping and the superconducting phase around optimal doping. The Ln-1111 phase diagrams for La and Sm were determined using muon spin spectroscopy, the phase diagram for Ce was determined using neutron diffraction. The Ba-122 phase diagram is based on.

Iron-based superconductors contain layers of iron and a pnictogen—such as arsenic or phosphorus—or a chalcogen. This is currently the family with the second highest critical temperature, behind the cuprates. Interest in their superconducting properties began in 2006 with the discovery of superconductivity in LaFePO at 4 K and gained much greater attention in 2008 after the analogous material LaFeAs(O,F) was found to superconduct at up to 43 K under pressure. The highest critical temperatures in the iron-based superconductor family exist in thin films of FeSe, where a critical temperature in excess of 100 K has recently been reported.

Since the original discoveries several families of iron-based superconductors have emerged:

- LnFeAs(O,F) or $LnFeAsO_{1-x}$ (Ln=lanthanide) with T_c up to 56 K, referred to as 1111 materials. A fluoride variant of these materials was subsequently found with similar T_c values.
- $(Ba,K)Fe_2As_2$ and related materials with pairs of iron-arsenide layers, referred to as 122 compounds. T_c values range up to 38 K. These materials also superconduct when iron is replaced with cobalt
- LiFeAs and NaFeAs with T_c up to around 20 K. These materials superconduct close to stoichiometric composition and are referred to as 111 compounds.
- FeSe with small off-stoichiometry or tellurium doping.

Most undoped iron-based superconductors show a tetragonal-orthorhombic structural phase transition followed at lower temperature by magnetic ordering, similar to the cuprate superconductors. However, they are poor metals rather than Mott insulators and have five bands at the Fermi surface rather than one. The phase diagram emerging as the iron-arsenide layers are doped is remarkably similar, with the superconducting phase close to or overlapping the magnetic phase. Strong evidence that the T_c value varies with the As-Fe-As bond angles has already emerged and shows that the optimal T_c value is obtained with undistorted $FeAs_4$ tetrahedra. The symmetry of the pairing wavefunction is still widely debated, but an extended *s*-wave scenario is currently favoured.

Hydrogen Sulfide

At pressures above 90 GPa (Gigapascals), hydrogen sulfide becomes a metallic conductor of electricity. When cooled below a critical temperature this high-pressure phase exhibits superconductivity. The critical temperature increases with pressure, ranging from 23 K at 100 GPa to 150 K at 200 GPa. If hydrogen sulfide is pressurized at higher temperatures, then cooled, the critical temperature reaches 203 K (−70 °C), the highest accepted superconducting critical temperature as of 2015. It has been predicted that by substituting a small part of sulfur with phosphorus and using even higher pressures it may be possible to raise the critical temperature to above 0 °C (273 K) and achieve room-temperature superconductivity.

Other Materials Sometimes Referred to as high-temperature Superconductors

Magnesium diboride is occasionally referred to as a high-temperature superconductor because its T_c value of 39 K is above that historically expected for BCS superconductors. However, it is more generally regarded as the highest-T_c conventional superconductor, the increased T_c resulting from two separate bands being present at the Fermi level.

Fulleride superconductors where alkali-metal atoms are intercalated into C_{60} molecules show superconductivity at temperatures of up to 38 K for Cs_3C_{60}.

Some organic superconductors and heavy fermion compounds are considered to be high-temperature superconductors because of their high T_c values relative to their Fermi energy, despite the T_c values being lower than for many conventional superconductors. This description may relate better to common aspects of the superconducting mechanism than the superconducting properties.

Metallic Hydrogen

Theoretical work by Neil Ashcroft in 1968 predicted that solid metallic hydrogen at extremely high pressure should become superconducting at approximately room-temperature because of its extremely high speed of sound and expected strong coupling between the conduction electrons and the lattice vibrations. As of 2016 this prediction is yet to be experimentally verified.

Magnetic Properties

All known high-T_c superconductors are Type-II superconductors. In contrast to Type-I superconductors, which expel all magnetic fields due to the Meissner effect, Type-II superconductors allow magnetic fields to penetrate their interior in quantized units of flux, creating "holes" or "tubes" of normal metallic regions in the superconducting bulk called vortices. Consequently, high-T_c superconductors can sustain much higher magnetic fields.

Ongoing Research

The question of how superconductivity arises in high-temperature superconductors is one of the major unsolved problems of theoretical condensed matter physics. The mechanism that causes the electrons in these crystals to form pairs is not known. Despite intensive research and many promising leads, an explanation has so far eluded scientists. One reason for this is that the materials in question are generally very complex, multi-layered crystals (for example, BSCCO), making theoretical modelling difficult.

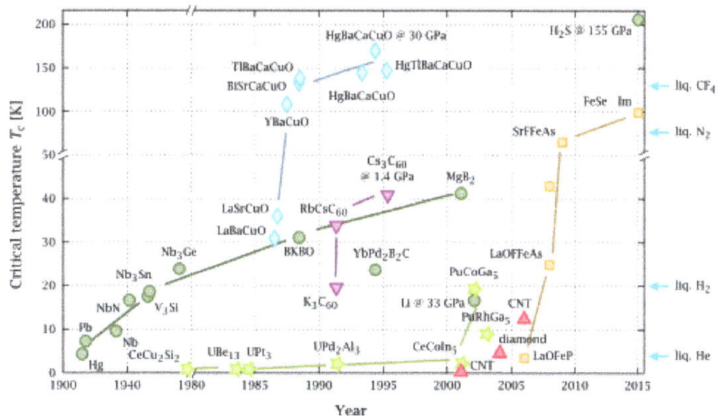

Superconductor timeline

Improving the quality and variety of samples also gives rise to considerable research, both with the aim of improved characterisation of the physical properties of existing compounds, and synthesizing new materials, often with the hope of increasing T_c. Technological research focuses on making HTS materials in sufficient quantities to make their use economically viable and optimizing their properties in relation to applications.

Possible Mechanism

There have been two representative theories for high-temperature or unconventional superconductivity. Firstly, weak coupling theory suggests superconductivity emerges from antiferromagnetic spin fluctuations in a doped system. According to this theory, the pairing wave function of the cuprate HTS should have a $d_{x^2-y^2}$ symmetry. Thus, determining whether the pairing wave function has *d*-wave symmetry is essential to test the spin fluctuation mechanism. That is, if the HTS order parameter (pairing wave function) does not have *d*-wave symmetry, then a pairing mechanism related to spin fluctuations can be ruled out. (Similar arguments can be made for iron-based superconductors but the different material properties allow a different pairing symmetry.) Secondly, there was the interlayer coupling model, according to which a layered structure consisting of BCS-type (*s*-wave symmetry) superconductors can enhance the superconductivity by itself. By introducing an additional tunnelling interaction between each layer, this model successfully explained the anisotropic symmetry of the order parameter as well as the emergence of the HTS. Thus, in order to solve this unsettled problem, there have been numerous experiments such as photoemission spectroscopy, NMR, specific heat measurements, etc. Up to date the results were ambiguous, some reports supported the *d* symmetry for the HTS whereas others supported the *s* symmetry. This muddy situation possibly originated from the indirect nature of the experimental evidence, as well as experimental issues such as sample quality, impurity scattering, twinning, etc.

Junction Experiment Supporting the d Symmetry

An experiment based on flux quantization of a three-grain ring of $YBa_2Cu_3O_7$ (YBCO) was proposed to test the symmetry of the order parameter in the HTS. The symmetry of the order parameter could best be probed at the junction interface as the Cooper pairs tunnel across a Josephson junction or weak link. It was expected that a half-integer flux, that is, a spontaneous magnetization could only occur for a junction of *d* symmetry superconductors. But, even if the junction experiment is the strongest method to determine the symmetry of the HTS order parameter, the results have been ambiguous. J. R. Kirtley and C. C. Tsuei thought that the ambiguous results came from the defects inside the HTS, so that they designed an experiment where both clean limit (no defects) and dirty limit (maximal defects) were considered simultaneously. In the experiment, the spontaneous magnetization was clearly observed in YBCO, which supported the *d* symmetry of the order parameter in YBCO. But, since YBCO is orthorhombic, it might inherently have an admixture of *s* symmetry. So, by tuning their technique further, they found that there was an admixture of *s* symmetry in YBCO within about 3%. Also, they found that there was a pure $d_{x^2-y^2}$ order parameter symmetry in the tetragonal $Tl_2Ba_2CuO_6$.

Qualitative Explanation of The Spin-fluctuation Mechanism

Despite all these years, the mechanism of high-T_c superconductivity is still highly controversial, mostly due to the lack of exact theoretical computations on such strongly interacting electron systems. However, most rigorous theoretical calculations, including phenomenological and diagrammatic approaches, converge on magnetic fluctuations as the pairing mechanism for these systems. The qualitative explanation is as follows:

In a superconductor, the flow of electrons cannot be resolved into individual electrons, but instead consists of many pairs of bound electrons, called Cooper pairs. In conventional superconductors, these pairs are formed when an electron moving through the material distorts the surrounding crystal lattice, which in turn attracts another electron and forms a bound pair. This is sometimes called the "water bed" effect. Each Cooper pair requires a certain minimum energy to be displaced, and if the thermal fluctuations in the crystal lattice are smaller than this energy the pair can flow without dissipating energy. This ability of the electrons to flow without resistance leads to superconductivity.

In a high-T_c superconductor, the mechanism is extremely similar to a conventional superconductor, except, in this case, phonons virtually play no role and their role is replaced by spin-density waves. Just as all known conventional superconductors are strong phonon systems, all known high-T_c superconductors are strong spin-density wave systems, within close vicinity of a magnetic transition to, for example, an antiferromagnet. When an electron moves in a high-T_c superconductor, its spin creates a spin-density wave around it. This spin-density wave in turn causes a nearby electron to fall into the spin depression created by the first electron (water-bed effect again). Hence, again, a Cooper pair is formed. When the system temperature is lowered, more spin density waves and Cooper pairs are created, eventually leading to superconductivity. Note that in high-T_c systems, as these systems are magnetic systems due to the Coulomb interaction, there is a strong Coulomb repulsion between electrons. This Coulomb repulsion prevents pairing of the Cooper pairs on the same lattice site. The pairing of the electrons occur at near-neighbor lattice sites as a result. This is the so-called *d*-wave pairing, where the pairing state has a node (zero) at the origin.

Meissner Effect

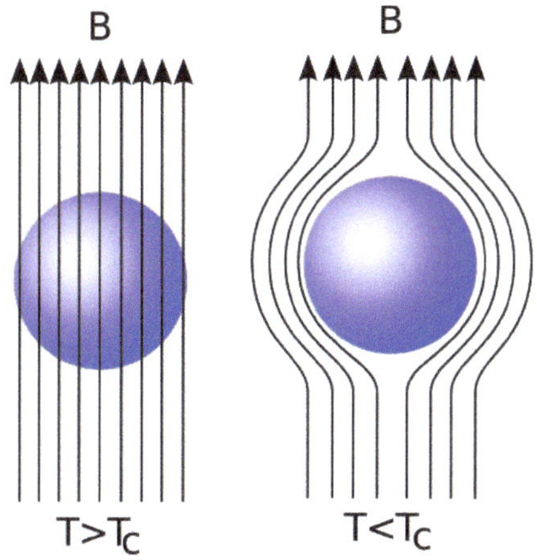

Diagram of the Meissner effect. Magnetic field lines, represented as arrows, are excluded from a superconductor when it is below its critical temperature.

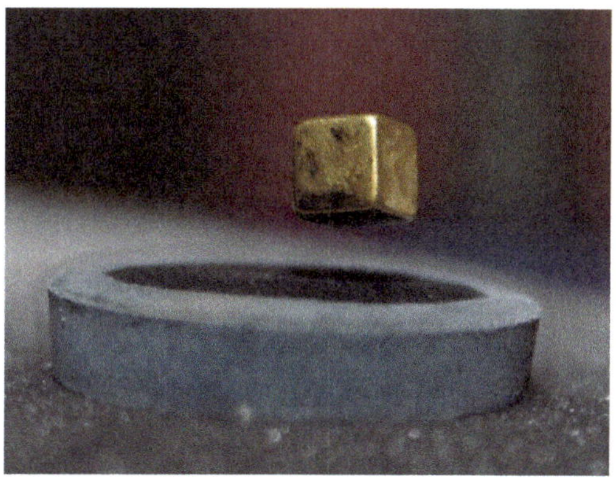

The Meissner effect demonstrated by levitating a magnet above a cuprate superconductor, which is cooled by liquid nitrogen

The Meissner effect is the expulsion of a magnetic field from a superconductor during its transition to the superconducting state. The German physicists Walther Meissner and Robert Ochsenfeld discovered this phenomenon in 1933 by measuring the magnetic field distribution outside superconducting tin and lead samples. The samples, in the presence of an applied magnetic field, were cooled below their superconducting transition temperature. Below the transition temperature the samples cancelled nearly all interior magnetic fields. They detected this effect only indirectly because the magnetic flux is conserved by a superconductor: when the interior field decreases, the exterior field increases. The experiment demonstrated for the first time that superconductors were more than just perfect conductors and provided a uniquely defining property of the superconductor state.

A superconductor with little or no magnetic field within it is said to be in the Meissner state. The Meissner state breaks down when the applied magnetic field is too large. Superconductors can be divided into two classes according to how this breakdown occurs. In Type I superconductors, superconductivity is abruptly destroyed when the strength of the applied field rises above a critical value H_c. Depending on the geometry of the sample, one may obtain an intermediate state consisting of a baroque pattern of regions of normal material carrying a magnetic field mixed with regions of superconducting material containing no field. In Type II superconductors, raising the applied field past a critical value H_{c1} leads to a mixed state (also known as the vortex state) in which an increasing amount of magnetic flux penetrates the material, but there remains no resistance to the flow of electric current as long as the current is not too large. At a second critical field strength H_{c2}, superconductivity is destroyed. The mixed state is actually caused by vortices in the electronic superfluid, sometimes called fluxons because the flux carried by these vortices is quantized. Most pure elemental superconductors, except niobium and carbon nanotubes, are Type I, while almost all impure and compound superconductors are Type II.

Explanation

The Meissner effect was given a phenomenological explanation by the brothers Fritz and Heinz London, who showed that the electromagnetic free energy in a superconductor is minimized provided

$$\nabla^2 \boldsymbol{H} = \lambda^{-2} \boldsymbol{H}$$

where H is the magnetic field and λ is the London penetration depth.

This equation, which is known as the London equation, predicts that the magnetic field in a superconductor decays exponentially from whatever value it possesses at the surface.

In a weak applied field, a superconductor "expels" nearly all magnetic flux. It does this by setting up electric currents near its surface. The magnetic field of these surface currents cancels the applied magnetic field within the bulk of the superconductor. As the field expulsion, or cancellation, does not change with time, the currents producing this effect (called persistent currents) do not decay with time. Therefore, the conductivity can be thought of as infinite: a superconductor.

Near the surface, within the London penetration depth, the magnetic field is not completely cancelled. Each superconducting material has its own characteristic penetration depth.

Any perfect conductor will prevent any change to magnetic flux passing through its surface due to ordinary electromagnetic induction at zero resistance. The Meissner effect is distinct from this: when an ordinary conductor is cooled so that it makes the transition to a superconducting state in the presence of a constant applied magnetic field, the magnetic flux is expelled during the transition. This effect cannot be explained by infinite conductivity alone. Its explanation is more complex and was first given in the London equations by the brothers Fritz and Heinz London. It should thus be noted that the placement and subsequent levitation of a magnet above an already superconducting material does not demonstrate the Meissner effect, while an initially stationary magnet later being repelled by a superconductor as it is cooled through its critical temperature does.

Perfect Diamagnetism

Superconductors in the Meissner state exhibit perfect diamagnetism, or superdiamagnetism, meaning that the total magnetic field is very close to zero deep inside them (many penetration depths from the surface). This means that their magnetic susceptibility, $\chi_v = -1$. Diamagnetics are defined by the generation of a spontaneous magnetization of a material which directly opposes the direction of an applied field. However, the fundamental origins of diamagnetism in superconductors and normal materials are very different. In normal materials diamagnetism arises as a direct result of the orbital spin of electrons about the nuclei of an atom induced electromagnetically by the application of an applied field. In superconductors the illusion of perfect diamagnetism arises from persistent screening currents which flow to oppose the applied field (the Meissner effect); not solely the orbital spin.

Consequences

The discovery of the Meissner effect led to the phenomenological theory of superconductivity by Fritz and Heinz London in 1935. This theory explained resistanceless transport and the Meissner effect, and allowed the first theoretical predictions for superconductivity to be made. However, this theory only explained experimental observations—it did not allow the microscopic origins of the superconducting properties to be identified. This was done successfully by the BCS theory in 1957, from which the penetration depth and the Meissner effect result. However, some physicists argue that BCS theory does not explain the Meissner effect.

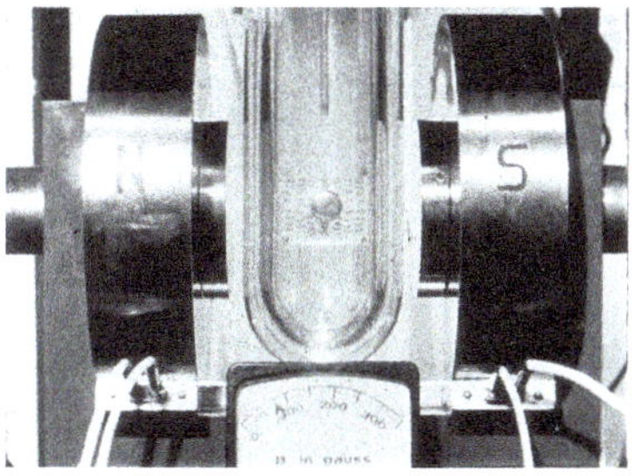

A tin cylinder—in a Dewar flask filled with liquid helium—has been placed between the poles of an electromagnet. The magnetic field is about 8 millitesla (80 G).

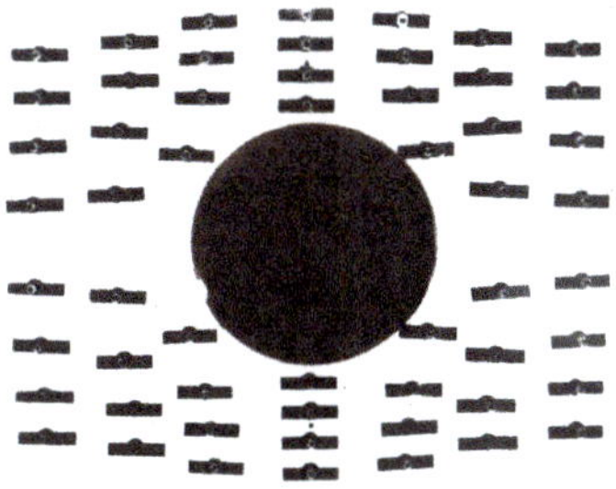

T = 4.2 K, **B** = 8 mT (80 G). Tin is in the normally conducting state. The compass needles indicate that magnetic flux permeates the cylinder.

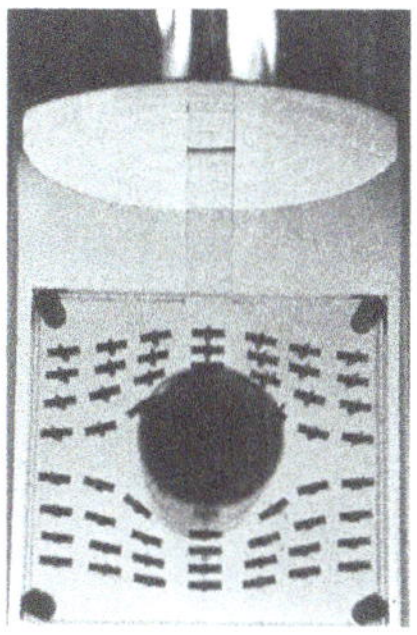

The cylinder has been cooled from 4.2 K to 1.6 K. The current in the electromagnet has been kept constant,but the tin became superconducting at about 3 K. Magnetic flux has been expelled from the cylinder (the Meissner effect).

Paradigm for The Higgs Mechanism

The Meissner superconductivity effect serves as an important paradigm for the generation mechanism of a mass M (i.e. a reciprocal *range*, $\lambda_M := h/(Mc)$ where h is the Planck constant and c is the speed of light) for a gauge field. In fact, this analogy is an abelian example for the Higgs mechanism, which generates the masses of the electroweak W± and Z gauge particles in high-energy physics. The length λ_M is identical with the London penetration depth in the theory of superconductivity.

Type-I Superconductor

The interior of a bulk superconductor cannot be penetrated by a weak magnetic field, a phenomenon known as the Meissner effect. When the applied magnetic field becomes too large, superconductivity breaks down. Superconductors can be divided into two types according to how this breakdown occurs. In type-I superconductors, superconductivity is abruptly destroyed via a first order phase transition when the strength of the applied field rises above a critical value H_c. This type of superconductivity is normally exhibited by pure metals, e.g. aluminium, lead, and mercury. The only alloy known up to now which exhibits type I superconductivity is $TaSi_2$. The covalent superconductor SiC:B, silicon carbide heavily doped with boron, is also type-I.

Depending on the demagnetization factor, one may obtain an intermediate state. This state, first described by Lev Landau, is a phase separation into macroscopic non-superconducting and superconducting domains forming a Husimi Q representation.

This behavior is different from type-II superconductors which exhibit two critical magnetic fields. The first, lower critical field occurs when magnetic flux vortices penetrate the material but the material remains superconducting outside of these microscopic vortices. When the vortex density becomes too large, the entire material becomes non-superconducting; this corresponds to the second, higher critical field.

The ratio of the London penetration depth λ to the superconducting coherence length ξ determines whether a superconductor is type-I or type-II. Type-I superconductors are those with $0 < \lambda/\xi < 1/\sqrt{2}$, and type-II superconductors are those with $\lambda/\xi > 1/\sqrt{2}$.

Type-II Superconductor

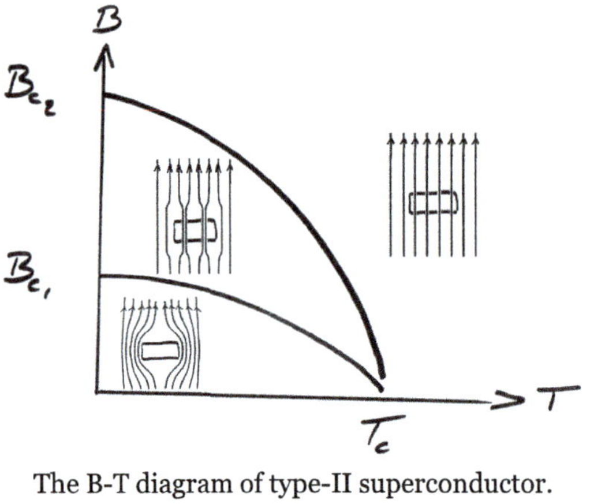

The B-T diagram of type-II superconductor.

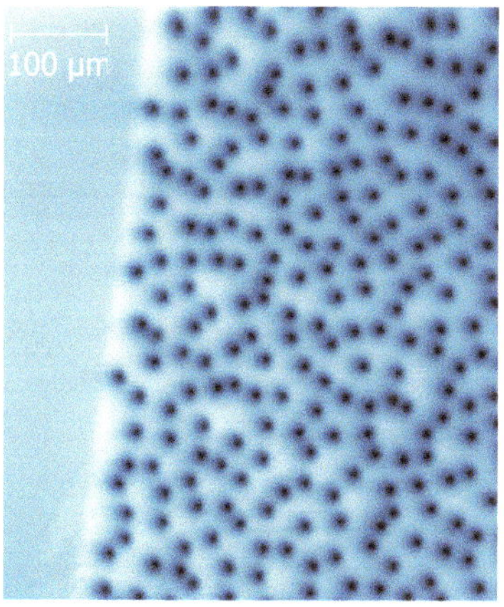

Vortices in a 200-nm-thick YBCO film imaged by scanning SQUID microscopy

In superconductivity, a type-II superconductor is characterized by the formation of magnetic vortices in an applied magnetic field. This occurs above a certain critical field strength H_{c1}. The vortex density increases with increasing field strength. At a higher critical field H_{c2}, superconductivity is destroyed. Type-II superconductors do not exhibit a complete Meissner effect.

History

In 1935, Rjabinin, Lev Shubnikov experimentally discovered the Type-II superconductors. In 1950, the theory of the two types of superconductors was further developed by Lev Landau and Vitaly Ginzburg in their paper on Ginzburg-Landau theory. In their argument, a type-I superconductor had positive free energy of the superconductor-normal metal boundary. Ginzburg and Landau pointed out the possibility of type-II superconductors that should form inhomogeneous state in strong magnetic fields. However, at that time, all known superconductors were type-I, and they commented that there was no experimental motivation to consider precise structure of type-II superconducting state. The theory for the behavior of the Type-II superconducting state in magnetic field was greatly improved by Alexei Alexeyevich Abrikosov, who was elaborating on the ideas by Lars Onsager and Richard Feynman of quantum vortices in superfluids. Quantum vortex solution in a superconductor is also very closely related to Fritz London's work on magnetic flux quantization in superconductors. The Nobel Prize in Physics was awarded for the theory of Type-II superconductivity in 2003.

Vortex State

Ginzburg–Landau theory defines two parameters: The superconducting coherence length and the London magnetic field penetration depth. In a type-II superconductor, the coherence length is smaller than the penetration depth. This leads to negative energy of the interface between superconducting and normal phases. The existence of the negative interface energy was known since the mid-1930s from the early works by the London brothers. A negative interface energy suggests that the system should be unstable against maximizing the number of such interfaces, which was not observed in first experiments on superconductors, before the experiments of Shubnikov in 1936 where two critical fields were found. In 1952 observation of type-II superconductivity was also reported by Zavaritskii. As was later discussed by A. A. Abrikosov, these interfaces manifest as lines of magnetic flux passing through the material, turning a region of the superconductor normal. This normal region is separated from the rest of the superconductor by a circulating supercurrent. In analogy with fluid dynamics, the swirling supercurrent creates what is known as a *vortex*, or an Abrikosov vortex, after Alexei Alexeyevich Abrikosov. In the limit of very short coherence length the vortex solution is identical to London's fluxoid, where vortex core is approximated by sharp cutoff rather than gradually vanishing of superconducting condensate near the vortex center. Abrikosov found that the vortices arrange themselves into a regular array known as a *vortex lattice*.

In the extreme type-II limit, the problem of type-II superconductor in magnetic field is exactly equivalent to that of vortex state in rotating superfluid helium, which was discussed earlier by Richard Feynman in 1955.

Flux Pinning

In the vortex state, a phenomenon known as flux pinning, where a superconductor is pinned in space above a magnet, becomes possible. This is not possible with type-I superconductors, since they cannot be penetrated by magnetic fields. Since the superconductor is pinned above the magnet away from any surfaces, there is the potential for a frictionless joint. The worth of flux pinning is seen through many implementations such as lifts, frictionless joints, and transportation. The thinner the superconducting layer, the stronger the pinning that occurs when exposed to magnetic fields.

Materials

Type-II superconductors are usually made of metal alloys or complex oxide ceramics. All high temperature superconductors are type-II superconductors. While most elemental superconductors are type-I, niobium, vanadium, and technetium are elemental type-II superconductors. Boron-doped diamond and silicon are also type-II superconductors. Metal alloy superconductors also exhibit type-II behavior (*e.g.* niobium-titanium and niobium-tin).

Other type-II examples are the cuprate-perovskite ceramic materials which have achieved the highest superconducting critical temperatures. These include $La_{1.85}Ba_{0.15}CuO_4$, BSCCO, and YBCO (Yttrium-Barium-Copper-Oxide), which is famous as the first material to achieve superconductivity above the boiling point of liquid nitrogen (77 K). Due to strong vortex pinning, the cuprates are close to ideally hard superconductors.

Important uses

Strong superconducting electromagnets (used in MRI scanners, NMR machines, and particle accelerators) often use niobium-titanium or, for higher fields, niobium-tin.

Iron-based Superconductor

Iron-based superconductors (FeSC) are iron-containing chemical compounds whose superconducting properties were discovered in 2006. In 2008, led by recently discovered iron pnictide compounds (originally known as oxypnictides), they were in the first stages of experimentation and implementation. (Previously most high-temperature superconductors were cuprates and being based on layers of copper and oxygen sandwiched between other substances (La, Ba, Hg)).

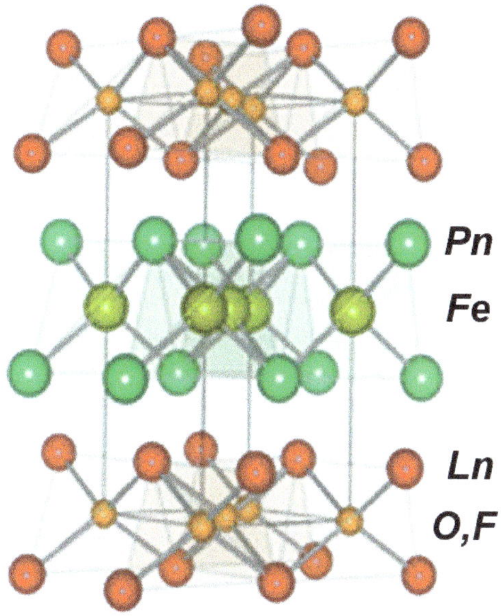

Crystal structure of LnFeAsOF, a 1111-type ferropnictide compound. Ln = lanthanide (La, Ce, etc.), Pn = pnictide (As, P, etc.)

This new type of superconductors is based instead on conducting layers of iron and a pnictide (chemical elements in group 15 of the periodic table, here typically arsenic (As) and phosphorus (P)) and seems to show promise as the next generation of high temperature superconductors.

Much of the interest is because the new compounds are very different from the cuprates and may help lead to a theory of non-BCS-theory superconductivity.

More recently these have been called the ferropnictides. The first ones found belong to the group of oxypnictides. Some of the compounds have been known since 1995, and their semiconductive properties have been known and patented since 2006.

It has also been found that some iron chalcogens superconduct. The undoped β-FeSe is the simplest iron-based superconductor but with the diverse properties. It has a critical temperature (T_c) of 8 K at normal pressure, and 36.7 K under high pressure and by means of intercalation. The combination of both intercalation and pressure results in re-emerging superconductivity at 48.

A subset of iron-based superconductors with properties similar to the oxypnictides, known as the 122 iron arsenides, attracted attention in 2008 due to their relative ease of synthesis.

The oxypnictides such as LaOFeAs are often referred to as the '1111' pnictides.

The crystalline material, known chemically as LaOFeAs, stacks iron and arsenic layers, where the electrons flow, between planes of lanthanum and oxygen. Replacing up to 11 percent of the oxygen with fluorine improved the compound — it became superconductive at 26 kelvin, the team reports in the March 19, 2008 Journal of the American Chemical Society. Subsequent research from other groups suggests that replacing the lanthanum in LaOFeAs with other rare earth elements such as cerium, samarium, neodymium and praseodymium leads to superconductors that work at 52 kelvin.

Oxypnictide	T_c (K)
$LaO_{0.89}F_{0.11}FeAs$	26
$LaO_{0.9}F_{0.2}FeAs$	28.5
$CeFeAsO_{0.84}F_{0.16}$	41
$SmFeAsO_{0.9}F_{0.1}$	43
$La_{0.5}Y_{0.5}FeAsO_{0.6}$	43.1
$NdFeAsO_{0.89}F_{0.11}$	52
$PrFeAsO_{0.89}F_{0.11}$	52
$ErFeAsO_{1-y}$	45
Al-32522 (CaAlOFeAs)	30(As), 16.6 (P)
Al-42622 (CaAlOFeAs)	28.3(As), 17.2 (P)
$GdFeAsO_{0.85}$	53.5
$BaFe_{1.8}Co_{0.2}As_2$	25.3
$SmFeAsO_{\sim 0.85}$	55

Non-oxypnictide	T_c (K)
$Ba_{0.6}K_{0.4}Fe_2As_2$	38
$Ca_{0.6}Na_{0.4}Fe_2As_2$	26
$CaFe_{0.9}Co_{0.1}AsF$	22
$Sr_{0.5}Sm_{0.5}FeAsF$	56
LiFeAs	18
NaFeAs	9–25
FeSe	<27

Iron pnictide superconductors crystallize into the [FeAs] layered structure alternating with spacer or charge reservoir block. The compounds can thus be classified into "1111" system RFeAsO (R: the rare earth element) including LaFeAsO, SmFeAsO, PrFeAsO, etc.; "122" type $BaFe_2As_2$, $SrFe_2As_2$ or $CaFe_2As_2$; "111" type LiFeAs, NaFeAs, and LiFeP. Doping or applied pressure will transform the compounds into superconductors.

Compounds such as $Sr_2ScFePO_3$ discovered in 2009 are referred to as the '42622' family, as $FePSr_2ScO_3$. Noteworthy is the synthesis of $(Ca_4Al_2O_{6-y})(Fe_2Pn_2)$ (or Al-42622(Pn); Pn = As and P) using high-pressure synthesis technique. Al-42622(Pn) exhibit superconductivity for both Pn = As and P with the transition temperatures of 28.3 K and 17.1 K, respectively. The a-lattice parameters of Al-42622(Pn) (a = 3.713 Å and 3.692 Å for Pn = As and P, respectively) are smallest among the iron-pnictide superconductors. Correspondingly, Al-42622(As) has the smallest As-Fe-As bond angle (102.1°) and the largest As distance from the Fe planes (1.5 Å). High-pressure technique also yields $(Ca_3Al_2O_{5-y})(Fe_2Pn_2)$ (Pn = As and P), the first reported iron-based superconductors with the perovskite-based '32522' structure. The transition temperature (T_c) is 30.2 K for Pn = As and 16.6 K for Pn = P. The emergence of superconductivity is ascribed to the small tetragonal a-axis lattice constant of these materials. From these results, an empirical relationship was established between the a-axis lattice constant and T_c in iron-based superconductors.

In 2009, it was shown that undoped iron pnictides had a magnetic quantum critical point deriving from competition between electronic localization and itinerancy.

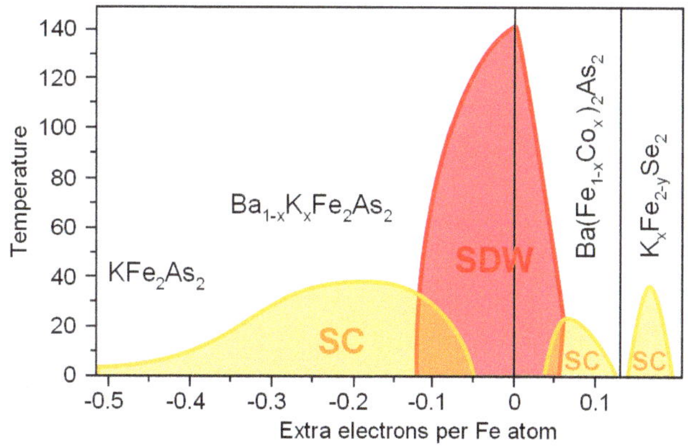

Phase diagram of the 122 family of ferro-pnictides complemented by the 122(Se) family as a generalized phase diagram for the iron based superconductors.

Phase Diagrams

Similarly to superconducting cuprates, the properties of iron based superconductors change dramatically with doping. Parent compounds of FeSC are usually metals (unlike the cuprates) but, similarly to cuprates, are ordered antiferromagnetically that often termed as a spin-density wave (SDW). The superconductivity (SC) emerges upon either hole or electron doping. In general, the phase diagram is similar to the cuprates.

Superconductivity

Superconducting transition temperatures are listed in the tables (some at high pressure). $BaFe_{1.8}Co_{0.2}As_2$ is predicted to have an upper critical field of 43 tesla from the measured coherence length of 2.8 nm.

In 2011, Japanese scientists stumbled across a discovery which increased a metal compound's superconductivity by immersing iron-based compounds in hot alcoholic beverages such as red wine. Earlier reports indicated that excess Fe is the cause of the bicollinear antiferromagnetic order and is not in favor of superconductivity. Further investigation revealed that weak acid has the ability to deintercalate the excess Fe from the interlayer sites. Therefore,weak acid annealing suppresses the antiferromagnetic correlation by deintercalating the excess Fe and, hence superconductivity is achieved

Technological Applications of Superconductivity

Some of the technological applications of superconductivity include:

- the production of sensitive magnetometers based on SQUIDs
- fast digital circuits (including those based on Josephson junctions and rapid single flux quantum technology),

- powerful superconducting electromagnets used in maglev trains, Magnetic Resonance Imaging (MRI) and Nuclear magnetic resonance (NMR) machines, magnetic confinement fusion reactors (e.g. tokamaks), and the beam-steering and focusing magnets used in particle accelerators
- low-loss power cables
- RF and microwave filters (e.g., for mobile phone base stations, as well as military ultra-sensitive/selective receivers)
- fast fault current limiters
- high sensitivity particle detectors, including the transition edge sensor, the superconducting bolometer, the superconducting tunnel junction detector, the kinetic inductance detector, and the superconducting nanowire single-photon detector
- railgun and coilgun magnets
- electric motors and generators

Low-temperature Superconductivity

Magnetic Resonance Imaging (MRI) and Nuclear Magnetic Resonance (NMR)

The biggest application for superconductivity is in producing the large-volume, stable, and high-intensity magnetic fields required for MRI and NMR. This represents a multi-billion-US$ market for companies such as Oxford Instruments and Siemens. The magnets typically use low-temperature superconductors (LTS) because high-temperature superconductors are not yet cheap enough to cost-effectively deliver the high, stable, and large-volume fields required, notwithstanding the need to cool LTS instruments to liquid helium temperatures. Superconductors are also used in high field scientific magnets.

Particle Accelerators and Magnetic Fusion Devices

Particle accelerators such as the Large Hadron Collider can include many high field electromagnets requiring large quantities of LTS. To construct the LHC magnets required more than 28 percent of the world's niobium-titanium wire production for five years, with large quantities of NbTi also used in the magnets for the LHC's huge experiment detectors.

A small number of magnetic fusion devices (mostly tokamaks) have used SC coils. The current construction of ITER has required unprecedented amounts of LTS (e.g. 500 tonnes, causing a 7 fold increase in the world's annual production capacity).

High-temperature Superconductivity (HTS)

The commercial applications so far for high temperature superconductors (HTS) have been limited.

HTS can superconduct at temperatures above the boiling point of liquid nitrogen, which makes them cheaper to cool than low temperature superconductors (LTS). However, the problem with

HTS technology is that the currently known high temperature superconductors are brittle ceramics which are expensive to manufacture and not easily formed into wires or other useful shapes. Therefore, the applications for HTS have been where it has some other intrinsic advantage, e.g. in

- low thermal loss current leads for LTS devices (low thermal conductivity),
- RF and microwave filters (low resistance to RF), and
- increasingly in specialist scientific magnets, particularly where size and electricity consumption are critical (while HTS wire is much more expensive than LTS in these applications, this can be offset by the relative cost and convenience of cooling); the ability to ramp field is desired (the higher and wider range of HTS's operating temperature means faster changes in field can be managed); or cryogen free operation is desired (LTS generally requires liquid helium that is becoming more scarce and expensive).

HTS-based Systems

HTS has application in scientific and industrial magnets, including use in NMR and MRI systems. Commercial systems are now available in each category.

Also one intrinsic attribute of HTS is that it can withstand much higher magnetic fields than LTS, so HTS at liquid helium temperatures are being explored for very high-field inserts inside LTS magnets.

Promising future industrial and commercial HTS applications include Induction heaters, transformers, fault current limiters, power storage, motors and generators, fusion reactors and magnetic levitation devices.

Early applications will be where the benefit of smaller size, lower weight or the ability to rapidly switch current (fault current limiters) outweighs the added cost. Longer-term as conductor price falls HTS systems should be competitive in a much wider range of applications on energy efficiency grounds alone.

Holbrook Superconductor Project

The Holbrook Superconductor Project is a project to design and build the world's first production superconducting transmission power cable. The cable was commissioned in late June 2008. The suburban Long Island electrical substation is fed by about 600-meter-long underground cable system consists of about 99 miles of high-temperature superconductor wire manufactured by American Superconductor, installed underground and chilled with liquid nitrogen greatly reducing the costly right-of-way required to deliver additional power.

Tres Amigas Project

American Superconductor was chosen for The Tres Amigas Project, the United States' first renewable energy market hub. The Tres Amigas renewable energy market hub will be a multi-mile, triangular electricity pathway of superconductor electricity pipelines capable of transferring and balancing many gigawatts of power between three U.S. power grids (the Eastern Interconnection, the Western Interconnection and the Texas Interconnection). Unlike traditional powerlines, it will transfer power as DC instead of AC current. It will be located in Clovis, New Mexico.

Magnesium Diboride

Magnesium diboride is a much cheaper superconductor than either BSCCO or YBCO in terms of cost per current-carrying capacity per length (cost/(kA*m)), in the same ballpark as LTS, and on this basis many manufactured wires are already cheaper than copper. Furthermore, MgB_2 superconducts at temperatures higher than LTS (its critical temperature is 39 K, compared with less than 10 K for NbTi and 18.3 K for Nb_3Sn), introducing the possibility of using it at 10-20 K in cryogen-free magnets or perhaps eventually in liquid hydrogen. However MgB_2 is limited in the magnetic field it can tolerate at these higher temperatures, so further research is required to demonstrate its competitiveness in higher field applications.

Trapped Field Magnets

Exposing superconducting materials to a brief magnetic field can trap the field for use in machines such as generators. In some applications they could replace traditional permanent magnets.

References

- "International system of units (SI)". NIST reference on constants, units, and uncertainty. National Institute of Standards and Technology. Retrieved 9 May 2012
- Lev D. Landau; Evgeny M. Lifschitz (1984). Electrodynamics of Continuous Media. Course of Theoretical Physics. 8. Oxford: Butterworth-Heinemann. ISBN 0-7506-2634-8
- Li, Yinwei; Hao, Jian; Liu, Hanyu; Li, Yanling; Ma, Yanming (2014-05-07). "The metallization and superconductivity of dense hydrogen sulfide". The Journal of Chemical Physics. 140 (17): 174712
- John Bardeen; Leon Cooper; J. R. Schriffer (December 1, 1957). "Theory of Superconductivity". Physical Review. 8 (5): 1178. Bibcode:1957PhRv..108.1175B. ISBN 9780677000800. doi:10.1103/physrev.108.1175. Retrieved June 6
- "Newly discovered fundamental state of matter, a superinsulator, has been created.". Science Daily. April 9, 2008. Retrieved 2008-10-23
- Kamihara, Yoichi; Watanabe, Takumi; Hirano, Masahiro; Hosono, Hideo (2008). "Iron-Based Layered Superconductor $La[O_{1-x}F_x]FeAs$ ($x = 0.05–0.12$) with $T_c = 26$ K". Journal of the American Chemical Society. 130 (11): 3296–3297. PMID 18293989. doi:10.1021/ja800073m
- John Daintith (2009). The Facts on File Dictionary of Physics (4th ed.). Infobase Publishing. p. 238. ISBN 1438109490
- Ishida, Kenji; Nakai, Yusuke; Hosono, Hideo (2009). "To What Extent Iron-Pnictide New Superconductors Have Been Clarified: A Progress Report". Journal of the Physical Society of Japan. 78 (6): 062001. Bibcode:-2009JPSJ...78f2001I. arXiv:0906.2045. doi:10.1143/JPSJ.78.062001
- Buck, Dudley A. "The Cryotron - A Superconductive Computer Component" (PDF). Lincoln Laboratory, Massachusetts Institute of Technology. Retrieved 10 August 2014
- Feynman, Richard Phillips; Leighton, Robert B.; Sands, Matthew (1964). The Feynman Lectures on Physics. 2. California Institute of Technology. pp. 1.7–1.8. ISBN 0465079989
- Hamish Johnston (17 February 2009). "Type-1.5 superconductor shows its stripes". Physics World. Institute of Physics. Retrieved 2009-10-28

- Amikam Aharoni (2000). Introduction to the theory of ferromagnetism (2 ed.). Oxford University Press. p. 27. ISBN 0-19-850808-5
- Mourachkine, A. (2004). Room-Temperature Superconductivity. Cambridge International Science Publishing. ISBN 1-904602-27-4. arXiv:cond-mat/0606187
- Pumplin, Jon; Pratt, Scott. "Magnetic field of a long wire". pa.msu.edu. MSU Department of Physics and Astronomy. Retrieved April 13, 2017

Permissions

All chapters in this book are published with permission under the Creative Commons Attribution Share Alike License or equivalent. Every chapter published in this book has been scrutinized by our experts. Their significance has been extensively debated. The topics covered herein carry significant information for a comprehensive understanding. They may even be implemented as practical applications or may be referred to as a beginning point for further studies.

We would like to thank the editorial team for lending their expertise to make the book truly unique. They have played a crucial role in the development of this book. Without their invaluable contributions this book wouldn't have been possible. They have made vital efforts to compile up to date information on the varied aspects of this subject to make this book a valuable addition to the collection of many professionals and students.

This book was conceptualized with the vision of imparting up-to-date and integrated information in this field. To ensure the same, a matchless editorial board was set up. Every individual on the board went through rigorous rounds of assessment to prove their worth. After which they invested a large part of their time researching and compiling the most relevant data for our readers.

The editorial board has been involved in producing this book since its inception. They have spent rigorous hours researching and exploring the diverse topics which have resulted in the successful publishing of this book. They have passed on their knowledge of decades through this book. To expedite this challenging task, the publisher supported the team at every step. A small team of assistant editors was also appointed to further simplify the editing procedure and attain best results for the readers.

Apart from the editorial board, the designing team has also invested a significant amount of their time in understanding the subject and creating the most relevant covers. They scrutinized every image to scout for the most suitable representation of the subject and create an appropriate cover for the book.

The publishing team has been an ardent support to the editorial, designing and production team. Their endless efforts to recruit the best for this project, has resulted in the accomplishment of this book. They are a veteran in the field of academics and their pool of knowledge is as vast as their experience in printing. Their expertise and guidance has proved useful at every step. Their uncompromising quality standards have made this book an exceptional effort. Their encouragement from time to time has been an inspiration for everyone.

The publisher and the editorial board hope that this book will prove to be a valuable piece of knowledge for students, practitioners and scholars across the globe.

Index